D0912941

The Pediatric Upper Extremity

DIAGNOSIS AND MANAGEMENT

F. William Bora, Jr., M.D.

Professor of Orthopedic Surgery
University of Pennsylvania School of Medicine
Chief of Hand Surgery
Hospital of the University of Pennsylvania
Consultant in Orthopedic Surgery and
Formerly Chief of Hand Surgery (1962–1982)
Children's Hospital of Philadelphia
Philadelphia, Pennsylvania

Released From
Samford University Library
Howard College

1986
W.B. SAUNDERS COMPANY
Philadelphia London Toronto Mexico City
Rio de Janeiro Sydney Tokyo Hong Kong

Samford University Library

W. B. Saunders Company: West Washington Square
                          Philadelphia, PA 19105

Library of Congress Cataloging-in-Publication Data
Main entry under title:

The pediatric upper extremity.

   1. Extremities, Upper—Wounds and injuries.
2. Extremities, Upper—Diseases. 3. Extremities,
Upper—Abnormalities. 4. Children—Surgery.
I. Bora, F. William. [DNLM: 1. Arm Injuries—in
infancy & childhood. 2. Extremities—abnormalities.
3. Hand Injuries—in infancy & childhood. WE 805 P371]
RD557.P43   1986   618.92′09757   85-19615
ISBN 0-7216-1872-3

Editor: Suzanne Boyd
Designer: Bill Donnelly
Production Managers: Laura Tarves and Frank Polizzano
Manuscript Editor: Lorraine Zawodny
Illustration Coordinator: Walter Verbitski

The Pediatric Upper Extremity: Diagnosis and Management   ISBN 0-7216-1872-3

© 1986 by W. B. Saunders Company. Copyright under the Uniform Copyright Convention. Simultaneously published in Canada. All rights reserved. This book is protected by copyright.
No part of it may be reproduced, stored in a retrieval system, or transmitted in any form or by any
means, electronic, mechanical, photocopying, recording, or otherwise, without written permission
from the publisher. Made in the United States of America. Press of W. B. Saunders Company.
Library of Congress catalog card number 85-19615.

Last digit is the print number: 9   8   7   6   5   4   3   2   1

RD
557
.P43
1986

Dedication

To Ann

Contributors

Balu H. Athreya, M.D.
Associate Professor of Pediatrics, University of Pennsylvania School of Medicine; Chief, Pediatric Rheumatology Center, Children's Hospital of Philadelphia, Philadelphia, Pennsylvania
Rheumatoid Diseases

F. William Bora, Jr., M.D.
Professor of Orthopaedic Surgery, University of Pennsylvania School of Medicine; Chief, Hand Surgery, Hospital of the University of Pennsylvania; Consultant, Orthopaedic Surgery, Children's Hospital of Philadelphia; Attending Physician, Veterans Administration Hospital, Attending Physician, Fitzgerald Mercy Hospital, Attending Physician, Graduate Hospital; Philadelphia, Pennsylvania
Embryology of the Upper Extremities; Congenital Anomalies of the Upper Limb; Injuries to Nerves; Injuries to and Developmental Deformities of the Elbow; Rheumatic Diseases

William H. Bowers, M.D.
Attending Hand Surgeon, Memorial Mission Hospital; St. Joseph's Hospital, Asheville, North Carolina
Fractures, Ligamentous Injuries to the Hand

Carl T. Brighton, M.D., Ph.D.
Professor and Chairman, Department of Orthopaedic Surgery, University of Pennsylvania School of Medicine and Hospital of the University of Pennsylvania; Chairman of the Department of Orthopaedic Surgery, Hospital of the University of Pennsylvania, Philadelphia, Pennsylvania
Biology of the Growth Plate

Paul J. Carniol, M.D.
Clinical Assistant, College of Physicians and Surgeons, Columbia University, New York, New York; Attending Physician in Plastic and Reconstructive Surgery, Overlook Hospital, Summit, New Jersey
Embryology of the Upper Extremity; Congenital Anomalies of the Upper Limb

William P. Cooney, M.D.
Associate Professor, Orthopedic Surgery, Mayo Graduate School, Mayo Clinic; Consultant Surgeon, St. Mary's Hospital, Rochester, Minnesota
Arthrogryposis Multiplex Congenita

Richard P. DuShuttle, M.D.
Kent General Hospital, Milford Memorial Hospital, Dover, Delaware
Rheumatic Diseases

Richard S. Fox, M.D.
Attending Physician, Division of Plastic and Reconstructive Surgery, St. Lukes
Hospital; Parkwood Hospital; New Bedford, Massachusetts
Injuries of the Skin

Gary E. Friedlaender, M.D.
Professor and Chief of Orthopaedic Surgery, Yale University School of Medi-
cine; Chief of Orthopaedic Surgery, Yale-New Haven Hospital, New Haven,
Connecticut; Consultant Orthopaedic Surgeon, West Haven Veterans Admin-
istration Hospital, West Haven, Connecticut
Allografts in the Upper Extremity

John A. Furrey, M.D.
Milton S. Hershey Medical Center; Hershey, Pennsylvania
Injuries to the Skin

Richard H. Gelberman, M.D.
Associate Professor, Orthopaedic Surgery, University of California, San Diego,
San Diego Medical Center; Veterans Administration Hospital; Children's Hos-
pital & Health Center; San Diego, California
Cerebral Palsy

Dale Glasser, M.S., O.T.R.
Research Coordinator, Department of Orthopaedic Surgery, Memorial Sloan-
Kettering Cancer Center (position paid for by a grant from the Greenwall Foun-
dation), New York, New York
Tumors of the Upper Extremity

John S. Gould, M.D.
Professor of Orthopaedic Surgery and Chief, Section of Hand Surgery, University of Alabama at Birmingham; Active Staff, University of Alabama Hos-
pitals; The Children's Hospital of Alabama; Consulting Staff, Veterans Administration Hospital; Lloyd Nolan Hospital; Eye Foundation Hospital; Courtesy
Staff, Cooper Green Hospital; Birmingham, Alabama
Injuries to and Developmental Deformities of the Elbow

William P. Graham, III, M.D.
339 Governor Rd., Hershey, Pennsylvania
Injuries to the Skin

Paul P. Griffin, M.D.
Professor, Harvard Medical School; Orthopedic Surgeon in Chief, The Chil-
dren's Hospital; Boston, Massachusetts
Injuries to the Forearm

Brian Hurson, M.D.
Orthopaedic Surgeon, James Connolly Memorial Hospital, Blanchardstown,
Dublin, Ireland
Tumors of the Upper Extremity

Frederick Kaplan, M.D.
Assistant Professor of Orthopaedics, Assistant Director of McKay Laboratory of Orthopaedic Research, University of Pennsylvania School of Medicine; Director of Division of Metabolic Bone Diseases, Department of Orthopaedic Surgery, Hospital of the University of Pennsylvania; Director of the Skeletal Dysplasia Clinic, Children's Hospital of Philadelphia, Philadelphia, Pennsylvania
Heritable and Endocrine Disorders of Connective Tissue Metabolism

William B. Kleinman, M.D.
Associate Professor of Orthopaedic Surgery, Indiana University School of Medicine; Attending Surgeon, The Indiana Center for Surgery and Rehabilitation of the Hand; Director of Congenital Hand Deformities Clinic, The Riley Hospital for Children, Indiana University Medical Center; Consultant in Hand Surgery, Indianapolis Veterans Administration Hospital, Indianapolis, Indiana
Fractures, Ligamentous Injuries to the Hand

Joseph M. Lane, M.D.
Professor, Orthopaedic Surgery, Cornell Medical School; Attending Orthopaedic Surgeon, Memorial Sloan-Kettering Cancer Center, Department of Orthopaedic Surgery; Attending Orthopaedic Surgeon, The Hospital for Special Surgery; Chief, Metabolic Bone Disease Service, New York City, New York
Tumors of the Upper Extremity

Joseph P. Leddy, M.D.
Clinical Associate Professor of Orthopaedic Surgery, University of Medicine and Dentistry of New Jersey, Rutgers Medical School; Chief, Hand Surgery Service; Chief, Orthopaedic Surgery at St. Peter's Medical Center, New Brunswick, New Jersey. Attending Orthopaedic Surgeon, Middlesex General University Hospital and Princeton Medical Center; Consultant, McCosh Infirmary, Princeton University, Princeton, New Jersey; Hurtado Health Center, Rutgers University, New Brunswick, New Jersey
Infections of the Upper Extremity

James J. Leyden, M.D.
Professor, Dermatology, University of Pennsylvania School of Medicine, Philadelphia, Pennsylvania
Dermatologic Disorders

Ellen C. Maitin, M.D.
Chief of Upper Extremity Surgery, Medical College of Pennsylvania, Philadelphia, Pennsylvania
Congenital Anomalies

James W. May, Jr., M.D.
Associate Clinical Professor of Surgery, Harvard Medical School; Chief, Division of Plastic and Reconstructive Surgery and Hand Surgical Service, Department of General Surgery, Massachusetts General Hospital, Boston, Massachusetts
Replantation and Elective Microsurgery

Richard R. McCormack, Jr., M.D.
Assistant Professor of Clinical Surgery, Cornell University Medical School; Assistant Attending Surgeon (Orthopaedics), Department of Orthopaedic Surgery, The Hospital for Special Surgery; Assistant Attending Surgeon (Orthopaedics), The New York Hospital; Part-time Attending Surgeon (Orthopaedics), Memorial Sloan-Kettering Cancer Center, New York, New York
Tumors of the Upper Extremity

A. O. Narakas, M.D.
Associate Professor, Medical School of the University of Lausanne; Chief Surgeon of the Clinic Longeraie for Reconstructive Surgery of Hand, Upper Limb and Peripheral Nerves; Attending Reconstructive and Peripheral Nerve Surgeon of the University Hospital (CHUV), Lausanne; Lausanne, Switzerland
Injuries to the Brachial Plexus

Robert J. Neviaser, M.D.
Professor and Associate Chairman, Department of Orthopaedic Surgery, George Washington University School of Medicine; Director, Hand and Upper Extremity Service, George Washington University Medical Center; Washington, D.C.
Injuries to and Developmental Deformities of the Shoulder

Kurt M. W. Niemann, M.D.
Professor, Orthopaedic Surgery; Director, Division of Orthopaedic Surgery, University of Alabama at Birmingham; Attending Physician, University Hospital and Children's Hospital; Birmingham, Alabama
Injuries to and Developmental Deformities of the Elbow

A. Lee Osterman, M.D.
Assistant Professor, Orthopaedic Surgery, University of Pennsylvania; Chief, Orthopaedic Hand Surgery Service, Children's Hospital of Philadelphia; Attending Physician, Veterans Administration Hospital, Philadelphia; Presbyterian Hospital, Graduate Hospital; Philadelphia, Pennsylvania
Replantation and Elective Microsurgery

Clayton A. Peimer, M.D.
Associate Professor, Orthopaedic Surgery; Clinical Assistant Professor, Anatomical Sciences; Clinical Assistant Professor, Rehabilitation Medicine; State University of New York at Buffalo; Chief, Division of Hand Surgery, Department of Orthopaedics, Millard Fillmore Hospital and the Erie County Medical Center; Buffalo, New York
Principles of Emergency Care

Martin A. Posner, M.D.
Associate Clinical Professor, Orthopaedic Surgery, Mt. Sinai School of Medicine; Chief of Hand Service, Hospital for Joint Diseases, Orthopaedic Institute, Lenox Hill Hospital, and Mt. Sinai Hospital; New York, New York
Upper Limb Prostheses

Robert C. Savage, M.D.
Clinical Instructor in Surgery, Division of Plastic Surgery, Harvard Medical School; Active Staff, Department of Surgery, Faulkner Hospital; Associate Staff, Department of Surgery, Massachusetts General Hospital; Courtesy Staff, Department of Surgery, New England Deaconess Hospital, Boston, Massachusetts;

Active Staff, Department of Surgery, Mt. Auburn Hospital, Cambridge, Massachusetts
Replantation and Elective Microsurgery

Lawrence H. Schneider, M.D.
Clinical Professor of Orthopaedic Surgery, Jefferson Medical College of Thomas Jefferson University; Attending Orthopaedic Surgeon, Thomas Jefferson University Hospital, Philadelphia, Pennsylvania; Consultant, Upper Extremity Service, Elizabethtown Hospital for Children and Youth, Elizabethtown, Pennsylvania
Injuries to Tendons

Ann H. Schutt, M.D.
Associate Professor, Physical Medicine and Rehabilitation, Mayo Graduate School, Mayo Clinic; Consultant, Physical Medicine and Rehabilitation, Pediatric Rehabilitation, Hand Rehabilitation, St. Mary's Hospital; Rochester, Minnesota
Arthrogryposis Multiplex Congenita

Barry P. Simmons, M.D.
Assistant Professor of Orthopedic Surgery, Harvard Medical School; Chief, Hand Surgery Service, Brigham and Women's Hospital & Children's Hospital; Boston, Massachusetts
Injuries to and Developmental Deformities of the Wrist and Carpus; Injuries to and Developmental Deformities of the Elbow

Foreword

It is a great privilege to contribute a foreword to this excellent and badly needed book. The plethora of books published on hand surgery continues to keep pace with the rapid developments in this field. However, up to this time, the immature hand had not received proper attention. *The Pediatric Upper Extremity: Diagnosis and Management* ably fills this void.

This book successfully blends the pertinent basic sciences involved in both the biological and functional development of the upper limb. It covers the whole field of care of the growing limb and gives practical yet sensitive advice on the handling of children and their equally frightened parents. This work truly meets the caveat that it quotes: "It is important to realize the pediatric patient is not just a little adult." The book is well and appropriately illustrated and supplies very helpful and up-to-date references to further reading.

Doctor Bora has gathered together a group of colleagues all of whom are acknowledged experts in their particular field. The resultant work has a delightful evenness of style that is unusual in a multi-authored book—a result no doubt of the skills and practice of my editorial colleague Bill Bora!

ADRIAN E. FLATT

Preface

Twenty years ago I established an upper extremity clinic at Children's Hospital of Philadelphia, and my experience in treating these children generated the impetus for this book. The authors of specific chapters have been chosen because of their expertise in a particular area. Their text includes the recommendations they prefer for treatment as well as the recommendations of other authors experienced in the field. I want to emphasize that this selected treatment does not replace nature's method of repair but only assists the repair process to improve the basic response of tissue to injury and disease so that the restoration of function will be maximum. Hopefully, the material presented here gives the reader information that will improve the accuracy of diagnosis and the choice of treatment and will provide a stimulus for the reader to find better ways to care for children in the future.

F. William Bora, Jr.

Acknowledgments

I am indebted to my parents, Frank and Marie Bora, and to the efforts of my teachers at all levels. The contributing editors and the house staff of the Hand Service of the University of Pennsylvania have made a major contribution to the manuscript. The valuable assistance of the Saunders staff, led by Suzanne Boyd, was greatly appreciated, and my secretaries, Lycie Benjamin and Terry Hunter, have supported the effort throughout.

Contents

PART I

Growth and Development

CHAPTER ○ 1

Embryology of the Upper Extremity

F. WILLIAM BORA, JR.
PAUL J. CARNIOL

THE ORGANOGENIC PERIOD

At birth the child has already passed through the most important period of growth and development, which starts with a single cell, a zygote, that weighs 0.005 mg. The weight of the embryo increases 27,500 times each week during the first 8 weeks and 90 times each week during the remainder of fetal development. During the first week, the single cell zygote undergoes cellular division as it passes down the fallopian tube to be imbedded in the uterine wall. During the following 7 weeks, cellular differentiation occurs, establishing the individual organ systems. This period is called the organogenic period; at its conclusion, a shift from cellular differentiation to cellular growth occurs as the fetus develops. After 8 weeks the fetus enters a period of 32 weeks in which the size and definition of the formed structures increase.

At 4 weeks, the embryo is 4.2 mm in length, and at this time the upper limb bud appears on the ventral lateral body wall, between the fifth and seventh cervical somites, as a mesodermal swelling with an ectodermal cap (Fig. 1–1).[2] In the fetus during the fourth week, mesoblast cells form capillary networks with drainage channels as the upper extremities develop in a proximal-to-distal sequence. This vascular formation initiates cellular differentiation and arm bud development. The most active differentiation occurs in the mesoderm under the epithelial cap (Fig. 1–2).[7] During the fifth week, indistinguishable bone and muscle precursors appear. The arm bud grows in a caudal direction, and a constriction that separates the future hand and forearm appears. Nerves from the spinal column begin to invade the arm bud mesenchyme and are directed to specific areas of the mesoderm that are destined to become skeletal muscle. Much of the remaining areas of mesoderm that are not innervated become skeletal precursors. This fact emphasizes the importance of the neural influence in determining early tissue differentiation (Fig. 1–3).[7] Digital swellings from the hand disc also appear at 6 weeks, the three central swellings appearing first, followed by the border digits.

G. M. Edelman[3,4] has identified a cell surface molecule in the embryos of vertebrates that plays a role in the morphogenetic movements involved with early inductive interactions and with the shaping of organ rudi-

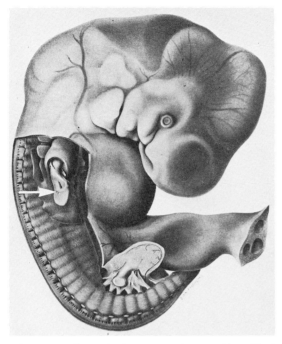

Figure 1–1. The arm bud appears on the ventral lateral body wall between the fifth and seventh cervical somites at four weeks. (From Bardeen CR, Leurs W. American Journal of Anatomy, with permission.)

ments. These cell adhesion molecules (CAMs) are glycoproteins that are present in regions in which inductive events are known to occur. In the notocord and the apical ridge of the limb bud, for example, one specific type (called N-CAM) has been demonstrated to appear and to be modulated in a defined sequence over short periods of develop-

mental time. The mechanisms that control expression and modulation of these CAMs and their relationship to the mechanisms of cytodifferentiation are currently being investigated.

During the seventh week, joint cavities and individual muscles and muscle groups appear. Also, at this time the digital clefts develop, and the thumb becomes distinguishable as a separate entity. During the eighth week, recession of the digital webbing, the final act of structural differentiation that individualizes thumb and fingers, occurs. Thus, in the first 8 weeks of development, specific structures are defined; in the following 32 weeks the growth of these structures takes precedence.

EMBRYONIC LIMB DEVELOPMENT

The limbs appear as slight elevations from the ventral lateral body wall at the fourth week, upper limb buds preceding lower limb buds by one week. The tissues of the limb bud are derived from the somatic mesoderm of the lateral plate and the ectoderm. At 6 weeks the three chief divisions of the upper and lower limbs are marked by furrows— upper arm, forearm, and hand; thigh, leg, and foot (Fig. 1–4). The limbs are first directed dorsally, nearly parallel to the long axis of the trunk. Each limb presents two surfaces and two borders. Of the surfaces, one, the future flexor surface of the limb, is directed

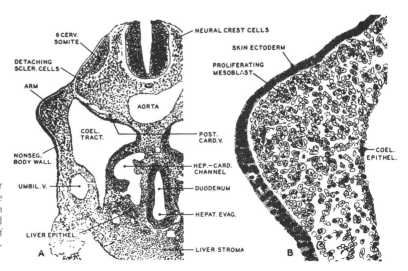

Figure 1–2. In the arm bud under an epithelial cap, there is active mesoderm proliferation. (From Streeter GL. Contrib Embryol 33:152, 1949, with permission of the Carnegie Institution of Washington.)

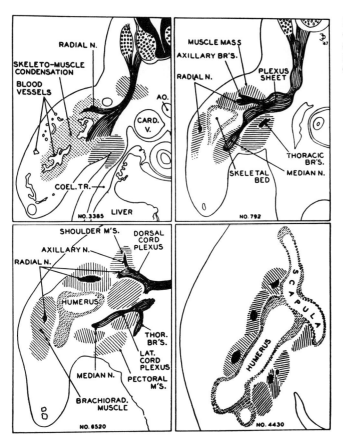

Figure 1–3. Mesoderm innervated by nerves becomes muscle; other mesoderm areas are precursors of bone. (From Streeter GL. Contrib Embryol 33:153, 1949, with permission of the Carnegie Institution of Washington.)

ventrally; the other, the extensor surface, is directed dorsally. The preaxial border is directed forward, or cephalad; the post-axial border is directed backward, or caudad.

The preaxial limb mass is derived from the anterior limb bud segments, the posterior axial limb mass from the posterior segments of the limb bud. The preaxial muscles (radial and tibial borders) are innervated by upper nerve segments of the brachial and lumbosacral plexus, and the postaxial muscles (the ulnar and fibular borders) by nerve segments from the lower brachial and lumbosacral plexus. At 7 weeks the limbs undergo a rotation through 90 degrees around their long axis, their rotation centered at the limb girdles (Fig. 1–5).[6] The upper limb rotates outward and forward, and the lower limb inward and backward. As a consequence of this rotation, the preaxial (radial) border of the forearm is directed laterally, and the preaxial (tibial) border of the hind limb medially; thus, the flexor surface of the forelimb is turned forward, and that of the hindlimb

backward. This rotation, which occurs after innervation of the limb, explains the dermatome arrangement in the adult (Fig. 1–6).[6] Causes of congenital anomalies affecting the upper limb during its most rapid development (5 to 8 weeks) may also affect other structures developing during that time, such as the heart, the eye, the nose, and the blood.

UPPER EXTREMITY FUNCTION IN CHILDHOOD

After birth and during the first year of life, upper extremity function is directed to extremity positioning and hand movement. At 4 weeks the infant holds its hands in tight fists and clenches them on contact. Initially, progress is slow, but at 8 weeks the baby opens its hands on seeing a toy. Four weeks later (at 12 weeks) the baby can hold objects briefly as the ulnar digits dominate grasp. During the following weeks, the infant begins

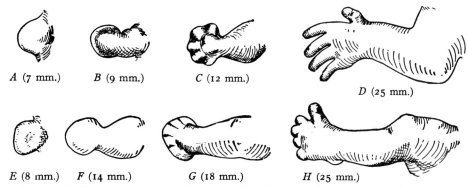

Figure 1–4. Stages in development of human limbs between the fifth and eighth weeks. *A* to *D*, the hand; *E* to *H*, the foot. (Reprinted from Arey LB. Developmental Anatomy, 7th ed. Philadelphia, WB Saunders, 1980:210, with permission.)

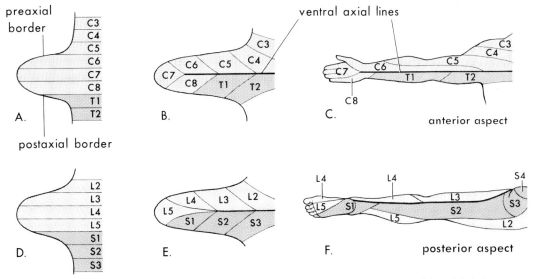

Figure 1–5. At 7 weeks (*A*), the limbs rotate in opposite directions around their long axis; the upper limbs rotate laterally, or outward, and extend ventrally; the lower limbs rotate medially, or inward, (*B* and *C*). Later, at about 8 weeks, the arms and legs are bent, the elbows pointing caudad, or downward, and the knees cephalad, or upward. (Reprinted from Moore K. The Developing Human: Clinically Oriented Embryology, 3rd ed. Philadelphia, WB Saunders, 1982:367, with permission.)

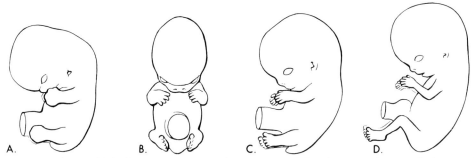

Figure 1–6. Limb rotation occurs after innervation and explains the dermatome arrangement of the adult limb. (Reprinted from Moore K. The Developing Human: Clinically Oriented Embryology, 3rd ed. Philadelphia, WB Saunders, 1982:368, with permission.)

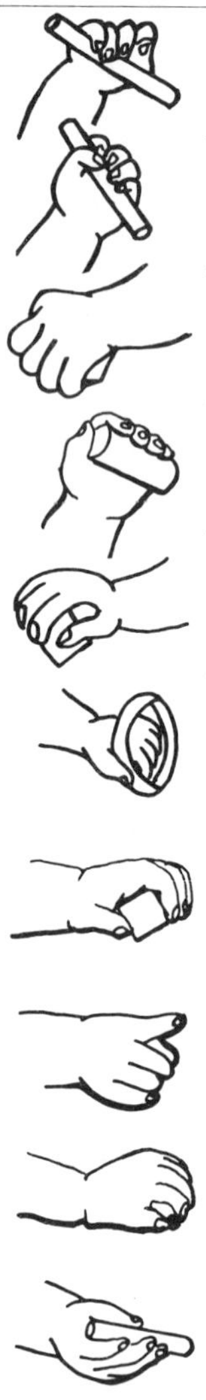

Age (weeks)	Description	Stimulation
12	Reflexive, ulnar side strongest; no reaching before eye contact.	Place objects in hand; hang toys in crib to stimulate eye contact and tracking.
16	Mouthing of fingers and mutual fingering; retains object placed in hand; no visually directed grasp until both hand and object in field of vision.	Toys hanging within swiping reach; toys on floor within visual field and hand reach.
20	Primitive squeeze, raking; fingers only; no thumb nor palm involved; immediate approach and grasp on sight.	Toys of varied textures, colors, sizes, shapes, and weights.
24	Palmar or squeeze grasp; still no thumb participation; eyes and hands combine in joint action.	Place toys in different positions and distances so eyes and hands must search.
28	Radial-palmar or whole-hand grasp; radial side stronger; thumb begins to adduct; unilateral approach; transfer from one hand to the other.	Toys that can be picked up and transferred by one hand; must be washable and safe (mouthing).
32	Inferior scissors or superior-palm grasp; known as monkey grasp because thumb is adducted, not opposed.	Toys with smaller and thinner circumferences, to strengthen thumb adductor.
36	Radial-digital or inferior forefinger grasp; fingers on radial side provide pressure on object; thumb begins to move toward opposition by pressing toward PIP joint of forefinger; finer adjustment of digits.	More pliable materials, including sand, clay, yarn, tissue paper, tape, and many types of finger food for self-feeding and exploration.
40	Inferior-pincer grasp; thumb moves toward DIP joint of forefinger; poking finger, inhibition of other four digits; beginning of voluntary release.	Many small objects with a variety of shapes to examine and palpate; toys with holes and indentations to poke and explore.
44	Neat pincer or forefinger grasp with slight extension of wrist.	Tiny objects to pick up and drop, such as dry cereal.
52	Opposition or superior-forefinger grasp; wrist extended and deviated to ulnar side for efficient prehension; release smooth for large objects, clumsy for small objects.	Toys that provide repeat motions of release, such as blocks and container, both becoming gradually smaller.

Drawings and descriptions based upon those of Gesell, Halverson, and Perlmutter.

Figure 1–7. Functional development of the upper extremity (prehension). (From Erhardt RP. Sequential levels in the development of prehension, Chart 1, AJOT. Reprinted with the permission of the American Occupational Therapy Association, Inc., copyright 1974, *The American Journal of Occupational Therapy*, Vol. 28, No. 10, p. 594.)

reaching for objects and at 5 months exhibits a primitive grip using only the fingers. Thumb adduction, a motion that dominates hand function for several successive weeks, develops at 28 weeks. At 36 weeks thumb adduction–index finger pinch is first used. Now, children reach, extending their arms for toys, and at 9 months, they can touch one toy against another. Thumb opposition and voluntary release develops between 9 and 12 months, and by one year infants can pick up large objects. At 18 months children have the ability to pile blocks with the upper extremities, and at 3 years they can stack as many as ten blocks (Fig. 1–7).[5] Also, at 3 years children can shift handedness, can use the subdominant hand, and can button and unbutton clothing. At 4 years they can throw a ball overhead, and they can use scissors, attempting to cut in a straight line.

At 5 years children begin to use their hands more than their arms for catching a ball, but they often miss; by 6 years, as efficiency in using tools increases, they can cut, paste, and hammer. At 6 years they grip a pencil tightly and close to the tip, using heavy pressure. Children at this age also can use both hands, but with unequal pressure, in playing the piano. At 8 years they handle tools less tensely, and performance is more graceful. At 9 years children become interested in increasing their strength and enjoy lifting things. They have essentially mastered control of their upper extremities by this time.

References

1. Arey LB. Developmental Anatomy, 7th ed. Philadelphia, WB Saunders, 1980:210.
2. Bardeen CR, Leurs W. Am J Anat, 1:35, 1901.
3. Edelman GM. Cell adhesion molecules. Science 219:450–457, 1983.
4. Edelman GM. Cell adhesions and morphogenesis: The regular hypothesis. Proc Natl Acad Sci 81:1460–1464, 1984.
5. Erhardt RP. Sequential levels in development of prehension. Am J Occup Ther, 28:592–596, 1974.
6. Moore KL. The Developing Human: Clinically Oriented Embryology, 3rd ed. Philadelphia, WB Saunders, 1982:367–368.
7. Streeter GL. Developmental horizons in human embryos. Contrib Embryol 33:152–153.

CHAPTER ○ 2

Biology of the Growth Plate

CARL T. BRIGHTON

Growth in length of mammalian long bones is confined in large measure to platelike structures at the ends of the bones. The structures, termed growth plates, are peripheral extensions of the primary centers of ossification that arise in the midportion of the cartilaginous anlage of the bone-to-be during early fetal life. Originally, the primary center of ossification grows and expands centrifugally in all directions. However, as the primary center of ossification continues to expand, endochondral bone growth soon becomes confined to the two platelike structures that are oriented toward each end of the bone, the growth plates (Fig. 2–1).

As growth continues, the growth plates progressively grow away from each other. At a rather definite time in each end of each long bone, in each species of animal, a secondary center of ossification appears. This center, termed the epiphysis, likewise grows and expands centrifugally in all directions, but at a much slower rate than the primary center. As the distance between the growth plate and the epiphysis gradually decreases, the portion of the epiphysis that faces the growth plate closes and becomes sealed with condensed bone termed the terminal bone plate or simply the bone plate.[7, 8] The epiphysis thereafter assumes a somewhat flattened hemispheric appearance and slowly fills out the remaining end of the long bone.

In the hand the carpal bones each develop from a primary center of ossification only—that is, these bones do not have epiphyses or secondary centers of ossification. The short tubular bones of the hand, the metacarpals and phalanges, each develop only one epiphysis or secondary center of ossification, The second, third, fourth, and fifth metacarpals each develop an epiphysis distal to the primary center of ossification, whereas the first metacarpal and all the phalanges each develop an epiphysis proximal to the primary ossification center.

ORGANIZATION OF THE GROWTH PLATE

The typical, fully developed growth plate in any given mammalian long bone consists of various tissues acting together as a unit to perform a specialized function and, as such, is an organ. The specialized function, of

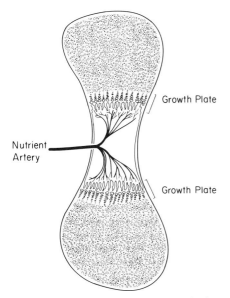

Figure 2–1. Drawing depicting the two growth plates of a typical tubular bone toward the end of fetal life. Each growth plate is a peripheral extension of the original primary center of ossification that arose in the midportion of the cartilaginous anlage of the bone-to-be early in the fetal period.

course, is longitudinal growth. The tissues comprising the growth plate are cartilage, bone, and fibrous tissue. Based on the tissue content alone, the growth plate may be divided anatomically into three different components: a cartilagenous component, itself divided into various histologic zones; a bony component, the metaphysis; and a fibrous component surrounding the periphery of the plate, consisting of the groove of Ranvier and the perichondrial ring of LaCroix (Fig. 2–2). The means by which the growth plate synchronizes chondrogenesis with osteogenesis, or interstitial cartilage growth with appositional bone growth, at the same time that it is growing in width, bearing a load, and responding to local and systemic forces and factors is a fascinating phenomenon of which the key features are only beginning to be understood at the present time. In this chapter we discuss the biology of the growth plate in light of those processes that are known.

Blood Supply of the Growth Plate

Each of the three components of the growth plate has its own distinct blood supply (Fig. 2–3).[14, 55] The epiphyseal artery supplies the

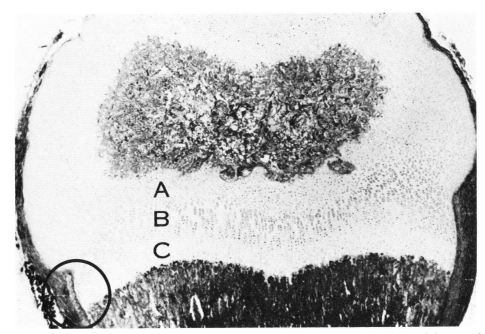

Figure 2–2. Photomicrograph of the distal femur of a 14-day-old rat showing the growth plate and the secondary bony epiphysis. A, reserve zone. B, proliferative zone. C, hypertrophic zone. The black ring at the left encircles the ossification groove and the perichondrial ring. Hemotoxylin and eosin (H & E) stain; × 500. (Reprinted from Brighton CT. AAOS. Instructional Course Lectures, Vol. 24. St Louis, CV Mosby, 1974:106, by permission.)

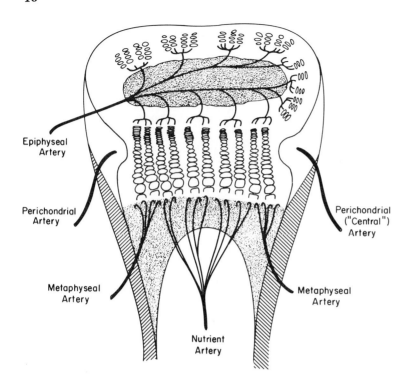

Figure 2–3. Drawing showing the blood supply of a typical fully developed growth plate. (Reprinted from Brighton CT. Clin Orthop 136:24, 1978 by permission.)

epiphysis or the secondary center of ossification, which is not part of the growth plate. Small arterial branches arise at right angles to the main epiphyseal artery in the secondary center of ossification and pass through small cartilage canals in the reserve zone to terminate at the top of the cell columns in the proliferative zone.[55] Each small arterial branch from the epiphyseal artery arborizes in rakelike fashion to supply the top portion of from four to ten cell columns. The proliferative zone, therefore, is well supplied with blood. None of the arterial branches from the epiphyseal arteries penetrate the cartilage portion of the growth plate beyond the uppermost part of the proliferative zone; that is, no vessels pass through the proliferative zone to supply the hypertrophic zone.

The metaphysis is richly supplied with blood both from terminal branches of the nutrient artery and from the metaphyseal arteries. The nutrient artery supplies the central region of the metaphysis, supplying perhaps as much as four fifths of the metaphysis, whereas the metaphyseal vessels supply only the peripheral regions of the metaphysis. Terminal branches from the nutrient and metaphyseal arteries pass vertically toward the bone-cartilage junction of the growth plate and end in vascular loops or capillary tufts just below the last intact

transverse septum at the base of the cartilage portion of the plate. The vessels turn back at this level, and venous branches descend to drain into several veins that eventually terminate in the large central vein of the diaphysis.[35, 40] All[15] or most[3] of the vascular loops are closed, and microhemorrhages from the vascular loops probably do not occur. No vessels penetrate the bone-cartilage junction beyond the last intact transverse septa; that is, no vessels pass from the metaphysis into the hypertrophic zone.

The fibrous peripheral structures of the growth plate, the groove of Ranvier and the perichondrial ring of LaCroix, are richly supplied with blood from several perichondrial arteries.

The three components of the growth plate, then, have their own distinct vascular supplies. Whereas the metaphysis and fibrous peripheral components have an abundant blood supply, only the proliferative zone of the cartilage portion of the growth plate is adequately supplied with blood. There are no vessels whatsoever in the hypertrophic zone in the fully developed growth plate, so that zone is entirely avascular. This avascularity of the hypertrophic zone has important implications for chondrocyte metabolism and matrix calcification.

After this brief outline of the vascular anatomy of the growth plate, a detailed description of each of the component parts of the plate follows.

Growth Plate Cartilage

The cartilage portion of the growth plate begins at the top of the reserve zone and ends with the last intact transverse septa at the bottom of the cell columns in the hypertrophic zone. The cartilage portion of the growth plate has been divided into various zones according to either morphology or function (Fig. 2–4). The reserve zone begins just beneath the secondary bony epiphysis and, in turn, is followed by the proliferating zone and the hypertrophic zone. The hypertrophic zone is sometimes further subdivided into the zones of maturation, degeneration, and provisional calcification.

Reserve Zone

The reserve zone lies immediately adjacent to the secondary bony epiphysis. Several different terms have been applied to this zone, including resting zone, zone of small-sized cartilage cells, and germinal zone. However, as described below, these cells are not resting and are not small in comparison with the cells in the proliferative zone, and they are not germinal cells. They appear to be storing lipid and other materials that are perhaps held in reserve for later nutritional require-

ments. If that possibility is true, the term *reserve zone* may not be inappropriate. In any event, the cells in the zone are spherical in outline, exist singly or in pairs, are relatively few when compared with the number of cells in other zones, and are separated from each other by more extracellular matrix than are cells in any other zone. As stated earlier, the cells in the reserve zone are approximately the same size as the cells in the proliferative zone.[13] The cytoplasm exhibits a positive staining reaction for glycogen. Electron microscopy reveals these cells to contain abundant endoplasmic reticulum, a clear indication that they are actively synthesizing protein. They contain more lipid bodies and vacuoles than do cells in other zones (Fig. 2–5)[13] but contain less glucose-6-phosphate dehydrogenase, lactic dehydrogenase, malic dehydrogenase, and phosphoglucoisomerase.[28] The zone also contains the lowest amount of alkaline and acid phosphatase,[29] total and inorganic phosphate, calcium, chloride, potassium, and magnesium.[57]

The matrix in the reserve zone contains less lipid,[23] glycosaminoglycan, protein polysaccharide, moisture, and ash[34] than the matrix in any other zone. It exhibits less incorporation of ^{35}sulfur than any other zone and also shows less lysozyme activity than the other zones.[50] In addition, the reserve zone matrix contains the highest content of hydroxyproline of any zone in the plate.[23] Collagen fibrils in the matrix exhibit random distribution and orientation. Vesicles are

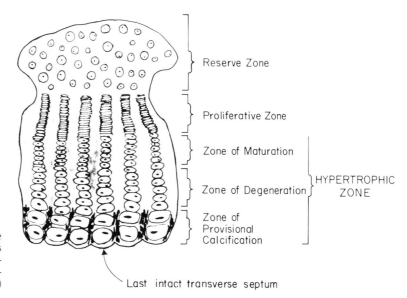

Figure 2–4. Drawing depicting the various zones of the cartilaginous portion of the growth plate. (Reprinted from Brighton CT. Clin Orthop 136:24, 1978 by permission.)

Reserve Zone

Proliferative Zone

Zone of Maturation

Zone of Degeneration

Zone of Provisional Calcification

HYPERTROPHIC ZONE

Last intact transverse septum

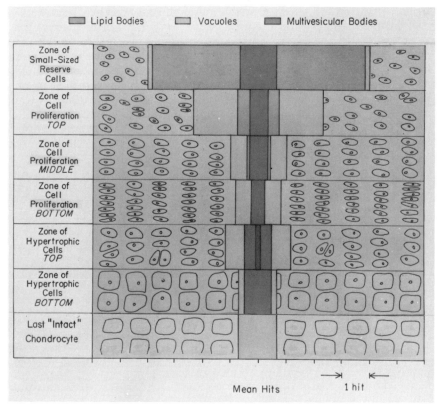

Figure 2–5. Graph showing content of cytoplasmic components of the various zones of the growth plate. (Redrawn from Brighton CT. J Bone Joint Surg [Am] 55:778, 1973, by permission.)

also seen in the matrix, but they are fewer in number here than in other zones. The matrix shows a positive histochemical reaction for the presence of a neutral polysaccharide or an aggregated proteoglycan (Fig. 2–6).

Oxygen tension measurements of the extracellular space in the different zones of the growth plate reveal that pO_2 is low (20.5 ± 2.1 mmHg) in the reserve zone.[7] This must mean that the blood vessels that pass through this zone in cartilage canals to arborize at the top of the proliferative zone do not actually supply the reserve zone itself.

The chondrocytes in the reserve zone do not proliferate or do so only sporadically.[24, 46] Therefore, the zone is not a germinal layer containing the so-called mother cartilage cells. As a matter of fact, the function of the zone is not clear. As previously stated, the high lipid body and vacuole content may mean storage of these materials for later nutritional requirements, and in this sense, the function of the zone is storage.

Proliferative Zone

The spherical single or paired chondrocytes in the reserve zone give way in the proliferative zone to flattened chondrocytes that are aligned in longitudinal columns with the long axis of the cells perpendicular to the long axis of the bone. The cytoplasm stains positively for glycogen. Electron microscopy shows the chondrocytes to be packed with endoplasmic reticulum.[13, 19] Point-counting analysis reveals the cytoplasmic area occupied by endoplasmic reticulum to increase from 14.9% at the top of the zone to 40.1% at the bottom of the zone.[13] Biochemical analyses reveal the zone of proliferation to contain the highest content of hexosamine,[18, 23] inorganic pyrophosphate,[31] sodium, chloride, and potassium.[57] The proliferative zone shows the highest incorporation of [35]sulfur of any zone in the growth plate, and it also has the highest level of lysozyme activity.[50]

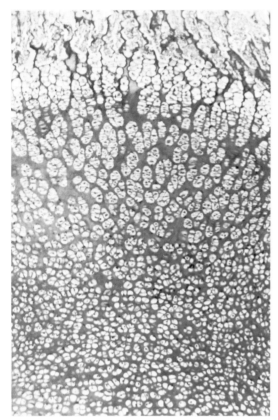

Figure 2–6. Microradiograph of 21-day-old rat costochondral junction. Hyaline cartilage is at the top, followed by the reserve zone, the proliferative zone, the hypertrophic zone, and the developing trabeculae of the metaphysis. The matrix has been stained blue in the hypertrophic zone, indicating an acid mucopolysaccharide or a disaggregated proteoglycan. Periodic acid-Schiff (PAS) alcian blue stain; × 80.

Tritiated thymidine autoradiographic studies have indicated that the chondrocytes in the proliferative zone are, with few exceptions, the only cells in the cartilage portion of the growth plate that divide.[24] The top cell of each column is the true "mother" cartilage cell for each column, and it is the beginning, or the top, of the proliferating zone that is the true germinal layer of the growth plate. Longitudinal growth in the growth plate is equal to the rate of production of new chondrocytes at the top of the proliferating zone multiplied by the maximum size of the chondrocytes at the bottom of the hypertrophic zone.[50] Kember[24] showed that the average number of new chondrocytes produced daily in each column in the growth plate of the proximal tibia in the rat was five.

Because the average diameter of the chondrocyte at the bottom of the hypertrophic zone is about 30μ, the rate of growth from that particular growth plate is about 150μ divisions per day. Kember[25] further calculated that each division of a top cell in a cell column contributes 29 cells. This means each division of a top cell eventually contributes 0.9 mm of longitudinal growth to the rat tibia (29 × 30 = 870μ). Forty to 50 top cell divisions would be required for the complete growth of the rat tibia. These principles (but not the absolute numbers) presumably hold true for all mammalian growth plates.

The matrix of the proliferating zone contains collagen fibrils, distributed at random, and matrix vesicles, confined mostly to the longitudinal septa. The matrix shows a positive histochemical reaction for a neutral mucopolysaccharide or an aggregated proteoglycan.

Oxygen tension is higher in the proliferating zone (57.0 ± 5.8 mmHg) than in any of the other zones of the growth plate.[7] This circumstance is due to the rich vascular supply present at the top of the zone, as previously described. Considering the relatively high oxygen tension present in the proliferating zone coupled with the presence of glycogen in the chondrocytes in that zone, it is apparent that aerobic metabolism with glycogen storage is occurring.

The function, then, of the proliferative zone is twofold: (1) matrix production, and (2) cellular proliferation. The combination of those two functions equals linear or longitudinal growth. It is a paradox that whereas this chondrogenesis, or cartilage growth, is solely responsible for the increase in linear growth of any given long bone, the cartilage portion of the plate itself does not increase in length. This circumstance, of course, is due to the vascular invasion that occurs from the metaphysis, with the resultant removal of chondrocytes at the bottom of the hypertrophic zone—events that in the normal growth plate exquisitely balance the rate of cartilage production.

Hypertrophic Zone

Whereas in the proliferative zone chondrocytes are flattened, in the hypertrophic zone they are spherical and greatly enlarged. These changes in cell morphology are quite abrupt, and one can usually tell the end of

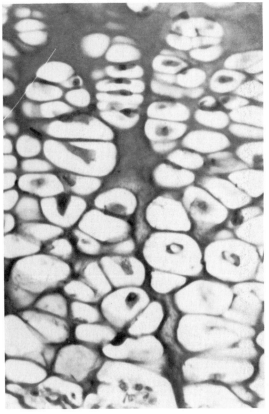

Figure 2–7. Photomicrograph of the hypertrophic zone of the 21-day-old rat costochondral junction. The PAS-positive cytoplasm of the chondrocytes in the top half of the zone indicates the presence of glycogen. Note that the cytoplasm abruptly becomes PAS-negative in the middle of the zone, indicating the absence of glycogen. PAS/alcian blue stain; × 480.

the proliferative zone and the beginning of the hypertrophic zone with an accuracy of from one to two cells. By the time the average chondrocyte reaches the bottom of the hypertrophic zone, it has enlarged some five times over its size in the proliferative zone.[13] The cytoplasm of the chondrocytes in the top half of the hypertrophic zone stain positively for glycogen (periodic acid-Schiff [PAS] reaction coupled with diastase digestion), but near the middle of the zone, the cytoplasm abruptly loses all glycogen stainability (Fig. 2–7).[12, 43] On light microscopy the chondrocytes in the hypertrophic zone appear vacuolated. Toward the bottom of the zone, such vacuolation becomes extensive, nuclear fragmentation occurs, and the cells appear nonviable. At the very bottom of each cell column in the hypertrophic zone, the lacunae

appear empty and are devoid of any cellular content.

On electron microscopy the chondrocytes in the top half of the hypertrophic zone appear normal and contain the full complement of cytoplasmic components (Fig. 2–8).[13, 21] However, in the bottom half of the zone, the cytoplasm contains holes that occupy over 85% of the total cytoplasmic column.[13] Obviously, it is holes, not vacuoles, that account for the "vacuolation" seen on light microscopy. Electron microscopy also shows that glycogen is abundant in the chondrocytes in the top half of the zone, diminishes rapidly in the middle section, and disappears completely from the cells in the bottom portion. The last cell at the base of each cell column is clearly not viable and shows extensive fragmentation of the cell membrane and the nuclear envelope, with loss of all cytoplasmic components except a few mitochondria and scattered remnants of endoplasmic reticulum. Obviously, the ultimate fate of the hypertrophic chondrocyte is death.

Electron-dense granules are seen in mitochondria in electron micrographs of growth plate chondrocytes.[36, 37] These granules are not removed by microincineration;[39] hence they must be mineral. They have been shown by direct analysis to have the characteristic x-ray spectra of calcium and phosphorus,[56] and their highest concentration in chondrocytes is in the hypertrophic zone in the normal growth plate and are absent or greatly diminished in number in the rachitic growth plate.[38] Histochemical localization of calcium at the ultrastructural level in the growth plate shows the mitochondria and cell membranes of chondrocytes in the top half of the hypertrophic zone to be loaded with calcium (Fig. 2–9).[8, 9] Toward the middle of the zone, mitochondria rapidly lose calcium, and at the bottom of the zone, both mitochondria and cell membranes are totally devoid of calcium. All of these cited studies provide circumstantial evidence that mitochondrial calcium may be involved in cartilage calcification.

Biochemical analyses of the hypertrophic zone indicate that this region, or at least the upper three-fourths of it, is active metabolically. Of all the zones it contains the highest amounts of alkaline phosphatase, acid phosphatase, glucose-6-dehydrogenase, lactic dehydrogenase, malic dehydrogenase, and phosphoglucoisomerase;[28, 29] total and in-

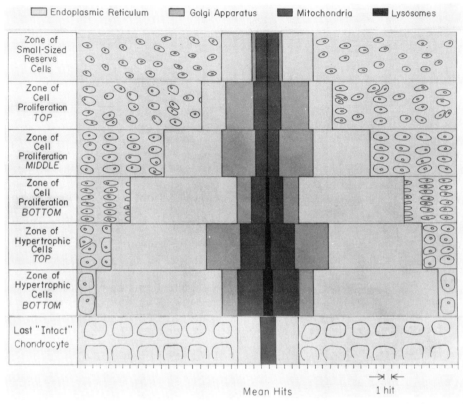

Figure 2–8. Graph showing content of cytoplasmic components of the various zones of the growth plate. (Redrawn from Brighton CT. J Bone Joint Surg [Am] 55:778, 1973, by permission.)

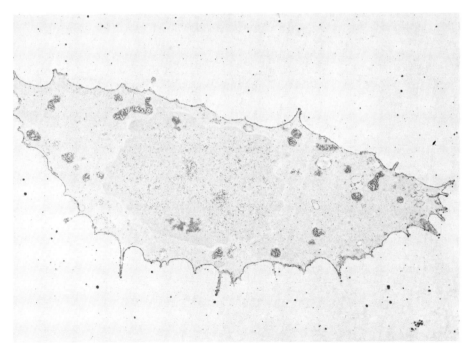

Figure 2–9. Electron micrograph of a cell from the top portion of the hypertrophic zone of the 21-day-old rat costochondral junction stained with potassium pyroantimonate (× 8000). Note that the black antimony-calcium complex is located primarily in mitochondria and the cell membrane.

organic phosphate, calcium, and magnesium;[58] moisture and ash; and lipid.[23] It has the lowest content of hydroxyproline[23] and hexosamine.[18]

Oxygen tension in the hypertrophic zone is low (24.3 ± 2.4 mmHg). No doubt this low pO_2 tension is due to the avascularity of the zone.

It may be well at this point to summarize the metabolic events occurring in the cartilage portion of the growth plate or, more correctly, in the proliferative and hypertrophic zones (Fig. 2–10).[10] In the proliferative zone, oxygen tension is high, aerobic metabolism occurs, glycogen is stored, and mitochondria form adenosine triphosphate (ATP). Mitochondria can form ATP and store calcium, but they cannot do both in the same place at the same time.[32] That is, ATP formation and calcium accumulation are alternative processes and do not occur simultaneously. In the proliferative zone, the energy requirements for matrix production and cellular proliferation are high and mitochondria form ATP. In the hypertrophic zone, oxygen tension is low; anaerobic metabolism occurs; and glycogen is consumed until, near the middle of the zone, all is depleted. At the top of the hypertrophic zone the mitochondria

switch from forming ATP to accumulating calcium.[8] Why this switch occurs at this level in the growth plate is not entirely clear. However, both the formation of ATP and the accumulation of calcium are active processes requiring energy.[34] Such energy comes from the respiratory chain in the mitochondria. ATP formation requires in addition the presence of adenosine diphosphate (ADP), whereas calcium accumulation does not. It may be that in the hypertrophic zone there simply is not enough ADP present to provide for significant ATP formation. In any event, mitochondria in the top half of the hypertrophic zone accumulate calcium and do not form ATP.

In the bottom half of the hypertrophic zone, as already stated, glycogen is completely depleted. In this area of low oxygen tension, there is no other source of nutrition to serve as an energy source for the mitochondria. Because uptake and retention of calcium by mitchondria are active processes requiring energy,[33] as soon as the glycogen supplies of the chondrocytes are exhausted, the mitochondria release calcium. This released calcium may play a role in matrix calcification.

Another noteworthy feature of growth

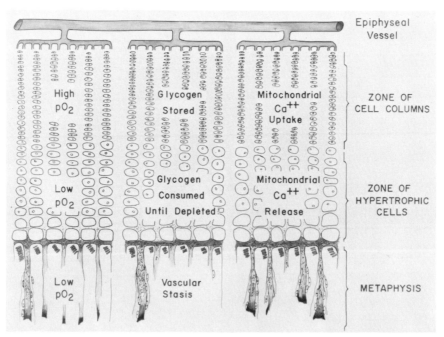

Figure 2–10. Drawing of the growth plate showing the relative oxygen tensions in the various zones in the left-hand column, the change in glycogen storage and utilization in the center column, and the role of mitochondria in the right-hand column. (Reprinted from Brighton CT. J Bone Joint Surg [Am] 60:637, 1978, by permission.)

plate metabolism is the fact that the glycerol-phosphate shuttle is absent throughout all the zones of the cartilaginous portion of the plate.[11] In most normal cells, the conversion of glucose to pyruvate via the glycolytic cycle causes the constant oxidation of cytoplasmic NADH (the reduced form of nicotinamide adenine dinucleotide) through the action of the cytoplasmic enzyme glycerol phosphate dehydrogenase. The glycerol phosphate so formed readily penetrates mitochondrial membranes, thus bringing about a shuttle (the glycerol-phosphate shuttle) of reducing equivalents from cytoplasmic NADH to the intramitochondrial respiratory chain (Fig. 2–11). In the growth plate chondrocytes, as demonstrated in Fig. 2–12, there is a lack of cytoplasmic glycerol phosphate dehydrogenase. Dihydroxyacetone phosphate cannot

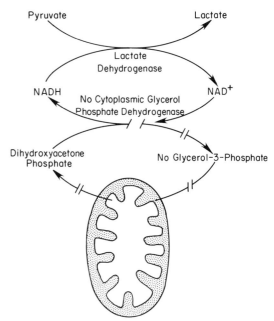

Figure 2–12. Drawing depicting the lack of the glycerol phosphate shuttle in growth plate chondrocytes. Since there is no glycerol phosphate dehydrogenase, no glycerol phosphate is formed and cytoplasmic NADH is oxidized by pyruvate via lactate dehydrogenase to form lactate. This lactate will form even in the presence of ample oxygen concentrations. (Redrawn from Brighton CT. J Bone Joint Surg [Am] 65:664, 1983, by permission.)

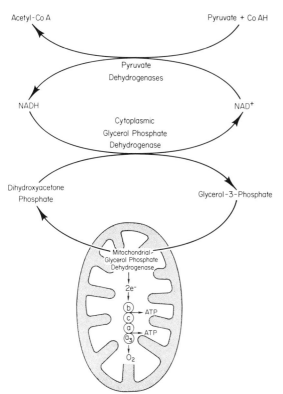

Figure 2–11. Drawing depicting the glycerol-phosphate shuttle as it exists in most cells. Note that dihydroxyacetone phosphate, an intermediary product of the glycolytic cycle, is reduced by NADH and cytoplasmic glycerol phosphate dehydrogenase to form glycerol phosphate. The glycerol phosphate readily penetrates the mitochondria and shuttles electrons from cytoplasmic NADH to the intramitochondrial respiratory chain. (Reprinted from Brighton CT. J Bone Joint Surg [Am] 65:664, 1983, by permission.)

form glycerol phosphate; instead, it reenters the glycolytic cycle to eventually form pyruvate. Cytoplasmic NADH, instead of being oxidized by dihydroxyacetone phosphate via glycerol phosphate dehydrogenase, is oxidized by pyruvate via lactate dehydrogenase to form lactate. Thus, lactate accumulates in the presence of ample oxygen concentration (aerobic accumulation) even though the Krebs cycle (tricarboxylic acid cycle) and electron transport are proceeding at normal rates.

The matrix of the hypertrophic zone, unlike the other zones, shows a positive histochemical reaction for an acid mucopolysaccharide or a disaggregated proteoglycan (Figs. 2–6 and 2–7). Electronic microscopy reveals that there are progressive decreases in the length of proteoglycan aggregates and in the number of subunits of the aggregates in the matrix from the reserve zone through the hypertrophic zone.[16] The distance between the subunits increases at the same time.

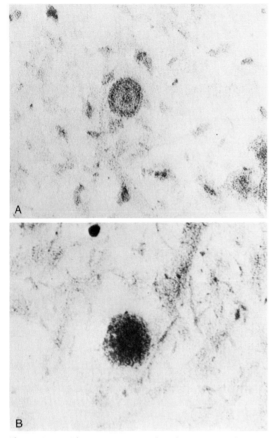

A

B

Figure 2–13. Electron micrographs of matrix vesicles from the top portion of the hypertrophic zone. The matrix vesicle in *A* was stained conventionally, and the matrix vesicle in *B* picture was stained for calcium with potassium pyroantimonate (no calcium stain complex is shown here; × 240,000).

It is speculated by some that the large proteoglycan aggregates with tightly packed subunits may inhibit mineralization or the spread of mineralization, whereas the smaller aggregates with widely spaced subunits at the bottom of the hypertrophic zone may be less effective in preventing mineral growth.[16] Lysozyme may be involved in the breakup of large proteoglycan aggregates,[27, 41, 50] or lysosomal enzymes such as neutral proteases may degrade the proteoglycan.[48] In any event, it seems apparent that proteoglycan disaggregation or degradation must occur before significant mineralization can take place.[21, 22]

The initial calcification (termed seeding or nucleation) that occurs in the growth plate in the bottom of the hypertrophic zone (zone of provisional calcification) does so within

or upon matrix vesicles that are present in the longitudinal septa of the matrix[1, 4, 5, 17] (Fig. 2–13 and 2–14). Matrix vesicles are very small structures, 1000–1500 angströms in diameter, that are enclosed in a trilamellar membrane and therefore must be produced by the chondrocyte. These vesicles occur in greatest concentration in the hypertrophic zone.[4] Matrix vesicles are rich in alkaline phosphatase,[2] and this enzyme may act as a pyrophosphatase to destroy pyrophosphate, another inhibitor of calcium phosphate precipitation.[17] Matrix vesicles begin to accumulate calcium at the same level in the middle of the hypertrophic zone at which mitochondria begin to lose calcium (Fig. 2–15 and 2–16),[8, 9] which is circumstantial evidence indicating that mitochondrial cal-

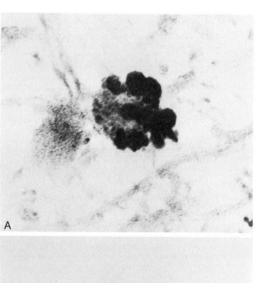

A

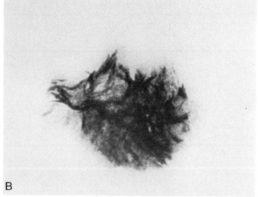

B

Figure 2–14. Electron micrographs of matrix vesicles from the middle and the bottom of the hypertrophic zone. The matrix vesicle in *A* is from the middle of the hypertrophic zone and exhibits a large clumplike calcium stain complex either upon or within the vesicle. The matrix vesicle in *B* is from the bottom of the hypertrophic zone. Note that the typical crystal formation of hydroxyapatite is present within or upon the matrix vesicle; × 240,000.

cium is involved in the initial calcification occurring in the growth plate. The initial calcification in the matrix vesicles may be in the form of amorphous calcium phosphate,[42] but this process rapidly gives way to hydroxyapatite crystal formation. With crystal growth and confluence, the longitudinal septa become calcified. This calcification of the matrix occurs in the bottom portion of the hypertrophic zone, a region frequently called the zone of provisional calcification.

The calcification just described makes the

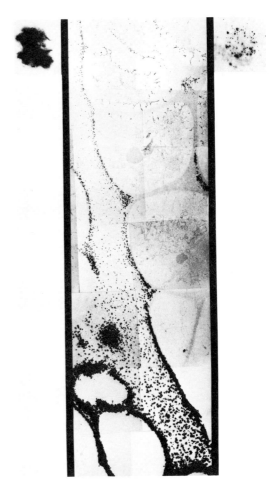

Figure 2–16. Montage of electron micrograph of the lower half of the hypertrophic zone shown in Figure 2–15 (Reprinted from Brighton CT. Clin Orthop 100:411, 1974, by permission.)

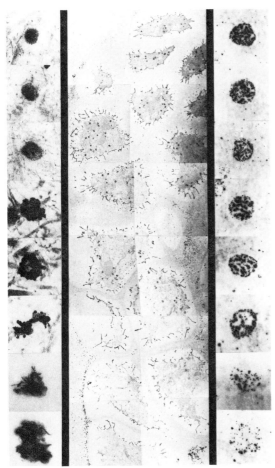

Figure 2–15. Montage of electron micrographs of the upper half of the hypertrophic zone. The antimony-calcium complex is predominantly intracellular at the top of the zone but becomes progressively more extracellular farther down. The inserts on the right are of mitochondria in chondrocytes at corresponding levels in the zone; note the gradual loss of antimony-calcium complex the farther down the zone the mitochondrion is located. The inserts on the left are of matrix vesicles at corresponding levels in the zone; note the gradual accumulation of the antimony-calcium complex the farther down the zone the vesicle is located. (Reprinted from Brighton CT. Clin Orthop 100:411, 1974, by permission.)

intercellular matrix relatively impermeable to metabolites. Diffusion coefficients of the various zones of the growth plate have been measured, and the hypertrophic zone has the lowest diffusion coefficient in the entire growth plate,[53] which is due primarily to its high mineral content. This circumstance suggests that as calcification occurs, diffusion of nutrients and O_2 to the hypertrophic chondrocyte is decreased, anaerobic glycolysis with glycogen consumption occurs until all the glycogen is depleted, mitochondria release calcium, nucleation occurs in the matrix vesicles, and calcification of the matrix occurs. Thus, a cycle is established that ultimately results in the death of the hypertrophic chondrocyte (Fig. 2–17).

The functions of the hypertrophic zone

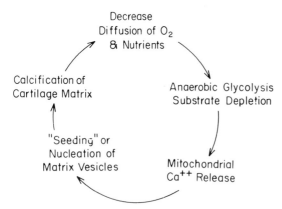

Decrease
Diffusion of O_2
& Nutrients

Calcification of
Cartilage Matrix

Anaerobic Glycolysis
Substrate Depletion

"Seeding" or
Nucleation of
Matrix Vesicles

Mitochondrial
Ca^{++} Release

Figure 2–17. Drawing showing events in the hypertrophic zone relating matrix calcification to decreased P_{O_2}, glycogen metabolism, and mitochondrial calcium release. (Redrawn from Brighton CT. J Bone Joint Surg [Am] 60:638, 1980, by permission.)

seem clear: (1) to prepare the matrix for calcification and (2) to calcify the matrix. Although these processes are complex biophysical phenomena, it is evident from the studies previously cited that we are beginning to unravel the mechanisms and factors controlling matrix calcification.

METAPHYSIS

The metaphysis begins just distal to the last intact transverse septum at the base of each cell column of the cartilage portion of the growth plate. The metaphysis ends in the region in which narrowing or funnelization of the bone end ceases—that is, the place at which the wider metaphysis meets the narrower diaphysis.[47] In the first part of the metaphysis, just distal to the cartilage portion of the plate, the oxygen tension is low (19.8 ± 3.2 mmHg).[7] The low oxygen tension and the rouleaux formation of the red cells frequently seen just distal to the last intact transverse septum[6] indicate that this is a region of vascular stasis (Fig. 2–18). A flocculent, electron-dense material present within the lumen of vascular sprouts invading the transverse septa may also indicate the presence of circulatory stasis within these vessels.[49] In addition, high levels of phosphoglucoisomerase, an enzyme active in anaerobic metabolism, are found in this region and are compatible with vascular stasis.[28]

With light microscopy, in the first part of the metaphysis, the first lacuna distal to the last intact transverse septa at the base of each column of cells is either empty or else contains one or more red cells. With electron microscopy, capillary sprouts or loops lined by a layer of endothelial and perivascular cells can be seen to invade the base of the cartilage portion of the plate.[49] Cytoplasmic processes from these cells push into the transverse septa and, presumably through lysosomal enzyme activity, degrade and remove the nonmineralized transverse septa. At this same level in the metaphysis, the longitudinal septa are partially or completely calcified. Osteoblasts—plump, oval-shaped cells with eccentric nuclei—line up along the calcified bars. Between the osteoblasts lining the calcified bars and the capillary sprouts are seen osteoprogenitor cells, with little cytoplasm but with a prominent nucleus in an ovoid-to-spindle shape.[26] This region in the me-

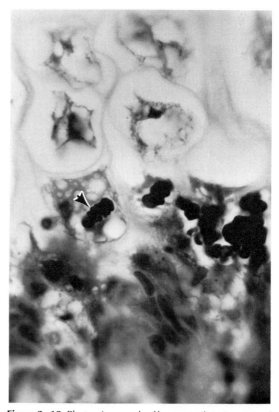

Figure 2–18. Photomicrograph of bone-cartilage junction of growth plate of the distal femur of a 24-day-old rat showing rouleaux formation of red blood cells (black arrow) just below the last intact transverse septum of a cell column at the base of the hypertrophic zone. Rouleaux formation of the red blood cells indicates vascular stasis. H & E stain; × 500. (Reprinted from AAOS Instructional Course Lectures, 24:113, 1974.)

taphysis of vascularized calcified cartilage, in which little or no bone formation occurs on the calcified bars, is termed the primary spongiosa.[39]

A short distance (within a cell or two) farther down the calcified longitudinal septa, the osteoblasts begin laying down bone (termed endochondral ossification—that is, bone formation within or upon cartilage). The farther into the metaphysis, the more bone is formed on the calcified cartilage bars. At the same time, these bars gradually diminish in thickness until they disappear altogether. This region in which bone is laid down on calcified cartilage bars is termed the secondary spongiosa.[39] Still farther into the metaphysis, the fibrous bone that originally was formed is replaced with lamellar bone. This gradual replacement of the calcified longitudinal septa with newly formed fibrous bone and of fibrous bone with lamellar bone is termed internal, or histologic, remodeling.[31] Large, irregularly shaped cells with foamy, eosinophilic cytoplasm and one or more nuclei containing several nucleoli can be seen evenly distributed throughout the entire metaphysis except in the primary spongiosa. These osteoclasts are also seen subperiosteally around the outside of the metaphysis at the place it diminishes in diameter to meet the diaphysis. This narrowing, or funnelization, of the metaphysis is termed external, or anatomic, remodeling.[31]

The functions of the metaphysis are (1) vascular invasion of the transverse septa at the bottom of the cartilaginous portion of the growth plate, (2) bone formation, and (3) remodeling, both internal and histologic (removal of calcified cartilage bars; replacement of fibrous bone with lamellar bone); and external or anatomic (funnelization of the metaphysis).

FIBROCARTILAGENOUS PERIPHERAL STRUCTURE

Encircling the typical long bone growth plate at its periphery are a wedge-shaped groove of cells termed the ossification groove and a ring, or band, of fibrous tissue and bone termed the periochondrial ring (Fig. 2–19). Ranvier,[45] the first to describe these structures, concentrated on the cells in the groove, so the groove is now named for him. La-Croix[30] studied the perichondrial ring in de-

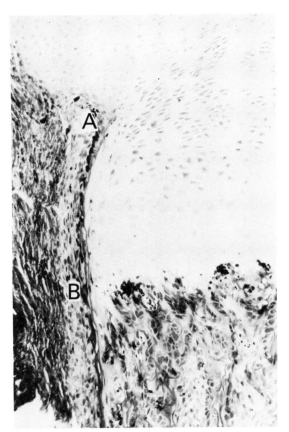

Figure 2–19. Photomicrograph of the periphery of the distal femoral growth plate of a 24-day-old rat showing the ossification groove of Ranvier (A) and the perichondrial ring of LaCroix (B) H & E stain; × 100. (Reprinted from AAOS Instructional Course Lectures, Vol 23 St. Louis, CV Mosby, 1974:107, by permission.)

tail, and this structure frequently is called by his name. Although the ossification groove and the perichondrial ring are different parts of the same structure, they have different functions, and for that reason alone, it is advantageous to consider them as separate and distinct entities.

The ossification groove contains round-to-ovoid cells that, on light microscopy, seem to flow from the groove into the cartilage at the level of the beginning of the reserve zone. For that reason, and because these cells avidly incorporate tritiated thymidine, it seems that the function of the groove of Ranvier is to contribute chondrocytes to the growth plate for the growth in diameter, or latitudinal growth, of the plate.[55] In a recent definitive study using electron microscopy and autoradiography, three different groups of cells were identified in the ossification groove: (1) a group of densely packed cells that seemed to be progenitor cells for the osteoblasts that form the bony band in the perichondrial ring; (2) a group of undifferentiated cells and fibroblasts that contribute to appositional chondrogenesis, hence to growth in width of the growth plate; and (3) fibroblasts amid sheets of collagen that cover the groove and firmly anchor it to the perichondrium of the hyaline cartilage above the growth plate.[51]

The perichondrial ring is a dense fibrous band that encircles the growth plate at the bone-cartilage junction; in it collagen fibers run vertically, obliquely, and circumferentially.[44] The ring is continuous at one end with the group of fibroblasts and collagen fibers in the ossification groove and continuous at the other end with the periosteum and subperiosteal bone of the metaphysis. In rodents, rabbits, and dogs, the innermost layer of the perichondrial ring consists of bone, which may or may not be attached to the subperiosteal bone of the metaphysis. This cylindrical sheath of bone may not be present in all species at all ages in all growth plates. Whether or not bone is present in the perichondrial ring, there is no doubt that the perichondrial ring provides mechanical support for the otherwise weak bone-cartilage junction of the growth plate.[46, 51]

The function, then, of the ossification groove is to provide chondrocytes for the growth in width of the growth plate, and the function of the periochondrial ring is to act as a limiting membrane that provides mechanical support to the growth plate.

References

1. Ali SY. Analysis of matrix vesicles and their role in calcification. Fed Proc 35:169, 1975.
2. Ali SY, Sajdera SW, Anderson HC. Isolation and characterization of calcifying matrix vesicles from epiphyseal cartilage. Proc Natl Acad Sci 67:1513, 1970.
3. Anderson CE, Parker J. Invasion and resorption in endochondral ossification. An electron microscopic study. J Bone Joint Surg (Am) 48:899, 1966.
4. Anderson HC. Vesicles associated with calcification in the matrix of epiphyseal cartilage. J Cell Biol, 41:59, 1969.
5. Bonucci E. Fine structure and histochemistry of calcifying globules in epiphyseal cartilage. Z Zellforsch 103:192, 1970.
6. Brighton CT. Clinical problems in epiphyseal plate growth and development. A.A.O.S. Instructional Course Lectures, vol 23. St. Louis, Mosby, 1974:3.
7. Brighton CT, Heppenstall RB. Oxygen tension in zones of the epiphyseal plate, the metaphysis, and diaphysis. An in vitro and in vivo study in rats and rabbits. J. Bone Joint Surg (Am) 53A:719–728, 1971.
8. Brighton CT, Hunt RM. Mitochondrial calcium and its role in calcification. Clin Orthop 100:406, 1974.
9. Brighton CT, Hunt RM. Histochemical localization of calcium in growth plate mitochondria and matrix vesicles. Fed Proc 35:143, 1976.
10. Brighton CT, Hunt RM. The role of mitochondria in growth plate calcification as demonstrated in a rachitic model. J Bone Joint Surg (Am) 60:630, 1978.
11. Brighton CT, Lackman RD, Cuckler JM. Absence of the glycerol phosphate shuttle in the various zones of the growth plate. J Bone Joint Surg 65A:663, 1983.
12. Brighton CT, Ray RD, Soble, LW, et al.: In vitro epiphyseal plate growth in various oxygen tensions. J Bone Joint Surg 51A:1383, 1969.
13. Brighton CT, Sugioka Y, Hunt RM. Cytoplasmic structures of the epiphyseal plate chondrocytes. Quantitative evaluation using electron micrographs of rat costochondral junctions with special reference to the fate of hypertrophic cells. J Bone Joint Surg 55A:771, 1973.
14. Brookes M. The blood supply of bone. An approach to bone biology. New York, Appleton-Century-Crofts, 1971.
15. Brookes M, Landon DN. The juxta-epiphyseal vessels in the long bones of fetal rats. J Bone Joint Surg 46B:336, 1964.
16. Buckwalter JA, Rosenberg L. Proteoglycan aggregate structure in mineralizing cartilage. Trans Orthop Res Soc 6:38, 1981.
17. Felix R, Felisch H. Role of matrix vesicles in calcification. Fed Proc 35:169, 1976.
18. Greer RB, Janicke, GH, Mankin HJ. Protein-polysaccharide synthesis at three levels of the normal growth plate. Calcif Tissue Res 2:157, 1968.
19. Holtrop ME, The ultrastructure of the epiphyseal plate. I. The flattened chondrocyte. Calcif Tissue Res 9:131, 1972.
20. Holtrop ME. The ultrastructure of the epiphyseal plate. II. The hypertrophic chondrocyte. Calcif Tissue Res 9:140, 1972.
21. Howell DS. Current topics of calcification. J Bone Joint Surg 53A:250, 1971.
22. Howell DS, Pita JC, Marquez JF, et al. Demonstration of macromolecular inhibitor(s) of calcification and nucleation factor(s) in fluid from calcifying sites in cartilage. J Clin Invest 48:630, 1969.
23. Irving JT, Wuthier RE. Histochemistry and biochemistry of calcification with special reference to role of lipids. Clin Orthop 56:237, 1968.
24. Kember NF. Cell division in endochondral ossification: a study of cell proliferation in rat bones by the method of tritiated thymidine autoradiography. J Bone Joint Surg 42B:824, 1960.
25. Kember NF. Cell population kinetics of bone growth: the first ten years of autoradiographic studies with tritiated thymidine. Clin Orthop 76:213, 1971.
26. Kimmel DB, Jee WS. A quantitative histologic analysis of the growing long bone metaphysis. Calcif Tissue Int 32:113, 1980.
27. Kuettner KE, Guenther JL, Ray RD. Lysozyme in preosseous cartilage. Calcif Tissue Res 1:298, 1968.
28. Kuhlman RE. A mitochemical study of the developing epiphyseal plate. J Bone Joint Surg 42A:457, 1960.
29. Kuhlman RE. Phosphates in epiphyseal cartilage and their possible role in tissue synthesis. J Bone Joint Surg 47A:545, 1965.

30. LaCroix P. The organization of bone. New York, McGraw-Hill, 1951.
31. LaCroix P. The internal remodeling of bones. *In* Bourne GH, ed. The Biochemistry and Physiology of Bone, 2nd ed., vol 3. New York, Academic Press, 1971:120.
32. Lehninger AL. Biochemistry. The Molecular Basis of Cell Structure and Function. New York, Worth, 1970:401.
33. Lehninger AL, Carafoli E, Rossi CS. Energy-linked ion movements in mitochondrial systems. Adv Enzymol 20:259, 1967.
34. Lindennbaum A, Kuettner KE. Mucopolysaccarides and mucoproteins of calf scapula. Calcif Tissue Res 1:53, 1967.
35. Marneffe R. de: Recherches morphologiques et expérimentales sur la vascularisation osseuse. Acta Chir Belg 50:469–488, 568–599, 681–704, 1951.
36. Martin JH, Matthews JL. Mitochondrial granules in chondrocytes. Calcif. Tissue Res 3:184, 1969.
37. Martin JH, Matthews JL. Mitochondrial granules in chondrocytes, osteoblasts, and osteocytes. Clin Orthop 68:273, 1970.
38. Matthews PL, Martin JH, Sampson HW, et al. Mitochondrial granules in the normal and rachitic rat epiphysis. Calcif Tissue Res 5:91, 1970.
39. McLean FC, Urist MR. Bone. An introduction to the physiology of skeletal tissue, 2nd ed. Chicago, University of Chicago Press, 1961.
40. Morgan JD. Blood supply of the growing rabbit's tibia. J Bone Joint Surg 41B:185, 1959.
41. Pita JC, Howell DS, Kuettner K. Evidence for a role of lysozyme in endochondral calcification during healing of rickets. *In* Slavkin HC, Greulich RC, eds. Extracellular Matrix Influences of Gene Expression. New York, Academic Press, 1975:721.
42. Posner AS. Crystal chemistry of bone mineral. Physiol Rev 49:760, 1969.
43. Pritchard JJ. A cytological and histochemical study of bone and cartilage formation in the rat. J Anat 86:259, 1952.
44. Rang M. The growth plate and its disorders. Baltimore, Williams & Wilkins, 1969:94.
45. Ranvier L. Quelques faits relatifs au développement du tissu osseux. C R Acad Sci (Paris) 77:1105, 1873.
46. Rigal WM. The use of tritiated thymidine in studies of chondrogenesis. *In* LaCroix P, Budy AM, eds. Radioisotopes and Bone. Oxford, Blackwell Scientific Publications, 1962:197.
47. Rubin P. Dynamic classification of bone dysplasias. Chicago, Year Book Medical Publishers, 1964.
48. Sapolsky AI, Howell DS, Woessner JF, Jr. Neutral proteases and cathepsin D in human articular cartilage. J Clin Invest 53:1044, 1974.
49. Schenk RK, Wiener J, Spiro D. Fine structural aspects of vascular invasion of the tibial epiphyseal plate of growing rats. Acta Anat 69:1, 1968.
50. Schmidt A, Rodergerdts U, Buddecke E. Correlation of lysozyme activity with proteoglycan biosynthesis in epiphyseal cartilage. Calcif. Tissue Res 26:163, 1978.
51. Shapiro F, Holtrop ME, Glimcher MJ. Organization and cellular biology of the perichondrial ossification groove of Ranvier: a morphological study in rabbits. J Bone Joint Surg 59A:703, 1977.
52. Sissions HA. Experimental study on the effect of local irritation on bone growth. *In* Mitchell JS, Holmes BF, Smith CL, eds. Progress in Radiobiology. Proceedings, International Conf. on Radiobiology, 4th. Edinburgh, Edinburgh, Oliver and Boyd, 1955:436.
53. Stambaugh JE, Brighton CT. Diffusion in the various zones of the normal and the rachitic growth plates. J Bone Joint Surg 62A:740, 1980.
54. Sutfin LV, Holtrop ME, Ogilvie RE. Microanalysis of individual mitochondrial granules with diameters less than 1000 angströms. Science 174:947, 1971.
55. Tonna EA. The cellular complement of the skeletal system studied autoradiographically with tritiated thymidine (H³TDR) during growth and aging. J Biophys Biomed Cytol 9:813, 1961.
56. Trueta J, Morgan JD. The vascular contribution to osteogenesis. I. Studies by the injection method. A zonal analysis of inorganic and organic constituents of the epiphysis during endochondral calcification. Calcif Tissue Res 4:20, 1969.
57. Wuthier RE. A zonal analysis of inorganic and organic constituents of the epiphysis during endochondral calcification. Calcif Tissue Res 4:20, 1969.

C H A P T E R ○ 3

Congenital Anomalies of the Upper Limb

F. WILLIAM BORA, Jr.
PAUL J. CARNIOL
E. C. MAITIN

GENETICS OF CONGENITAL DEFORMITIES

One of every 626 newborn infants has a congenital anomaly of the upper extremity.[31] Most of these deformities are minor and do not hinder upper extremity function, but one of ten is associated with a significant functional deficit[17] or a cosmetic deformity that makes the afflicted child subject to peer criticism. These anomalies can affect one or more systems; those most commonly involved are the musculoskeletal, cardiovascular, craniofacial, and neurologic systems.[14, 40, 45, 49, 60–62, 83, 85, 100, 111, 141] Care of these patients and management of their multiple problems require a coordinated effort by the pediatrician, geneticist, hand therapist, hand surgeon, and any other specialists who are involved. Congenital disorders have a genetic or environmental etiology and may be caused by one gene, multiple genes, or chromosomal abnormalities. Single gene disorders follow mendelian patterns of inheritance: autosomal dominant, autosomal recessive, or sex-linked. Autosomal dominant disorders are determined by a single gene, and the characteristics are expressed when only one gene in a pair is affected. Males and females have an equal chance of being affected, and the clinical expression of genetically inherited anomalies can be altered by the penetrance of the gene. If an individual is genetically heterozygous for the autosomal dominant trait, it will be clinically present in at least one of the parents of an affected baby. Several types of brachydactyly are transmitted as autosomal dominant traits.

Autosomal recessive disorders are expressed only when both genes in a pair are affected; the patient is homozygous for that trait. Both parents of the affected baby must carry the gene coding for the anomaly, but neither need have the anomaly. Males and females are equally affected. A few examples of these disorders are Morquio's syndrome, Hurler's syndrome, and radial club hand. Sex-linked genes on the X chromosome may be either dominant or recessive. In females with two X chromosomes, the gene pair may be either heterozygous or homozygous. Expression of the gene in the female will then follow a pattern similar to that of autosomal dominant and recessive genes.

Males have only one X chromosome. Thus, if a trait is present on this chromosome in a

Table 3–1. **Classification of Congenital Anomalies**

I. Failure of Formation
   A. Transverse
      1. Extremity levels
      2. Phocomelia
   B. Longitudinal
      1. Radial club
      2. Cleft
      3. Ulnar club
   C. Failure to Differentiate
      1. Simple syndactyly
      2. Complex syndactyly
   D. Intrinsic Finger Abnormalities
      1. Camptodactyly
      2. Clinodactyly
      3. Delta phalanx
      4. Kirner deformity
      5. Symphalangism
      6. Brachydactyly
   E. Thumb Anomalies
      1. Deficient components
         a. Hypoplasia
         b. Pouce flottant
         c. Absent thumb
      2. Additional components
         a. Triphalangeal thumb
         b. Polydactyly
      3. Disturbance of functional components
         a. Absent muscle-tendon units
         b. Trigger thumb
      4. Pollex varus
II. Duplication—Polydactyly
III. Overgrowth
   A. Gigantism
   B. Neurofibromatosis
   C. Vascular
IV. Constriction Bands

male, the gene will be expressed clinically as determined by its penetrance. These genes cannot be passed from father to son because of their X linkage, but they can be passed from father to daughter or from mother to either male or female children. Duchenne muscular dystrophy is transmitted by X-linked genes. Some upper extremity anom-

alies are due to abnormalities in the sex chromosomes or in other chromosomes. In Turner's syndrome, 40 XO, there is a short fourth metacarpal. In Down's syndrome, trisomy 21, the hands are small and clinodactyly of the small finger is caused by an abnormal middle phalanx.

Several classifications of upper extremity congenital deformities have been described.[48, 69, 77, 124, 135, 136] We prefer the classification reported in Table 3–1.

FAILURE OF FORMATION

Transverse Deficiencies

Extremity Levels

Transverse deficiencies, usually called congenital amputations, can occur at multiple levels and are classified by the level of the amputation (Fig. 3–1). Parts distal to the level affected are either rudimentary or absent, and proximal parts are frequently abnormal. The amputation stump can have a variety of contours, is usually well padded, and may have rudimentary digits attached (Fig. 3–2).

Birch-Jensen reports that one of every 20,000 newborns has a transverse forearm defect and that one of every 270,000 newborns has a transverse arm defect. Although many of these defects do not have a genetic origin, there is a small group of syndromes associated with congenital amputations that are inherited (Table 3–2). Several other anomalies occur in association with these amputations, which include club foot, meningocele, radial head dislocation, radioulnar synostosis, and spina bifida.[142, 143]

Table 3–2. **Syndromes With Transverse Upper Extremity Defects**

Syndrome	Congenital Defect	Mechanism of Inheritance
Hemidysplasia with psoriasis (ichthyosiform erythrodermia)[45]	Amelia; transverse defects of long bones; aplasia of fingers or toes; cardiac, renal, or central nervous system malformations	Unknown
Terminal defects with scalp defects[2]	Transverse toe and finger defects; midline scalp defects	Autosomal dominant
Splithand-splitfoot[109]	Absent middle and/or terminal phalanges of the second, third, and fourth fingers	Autosomal dominant
Acheiropody[147]	Absent radius and ulna, sometimes with one finger present; absent fibula; short tibia; thin conical ends to the extremities	Autosomal recessive

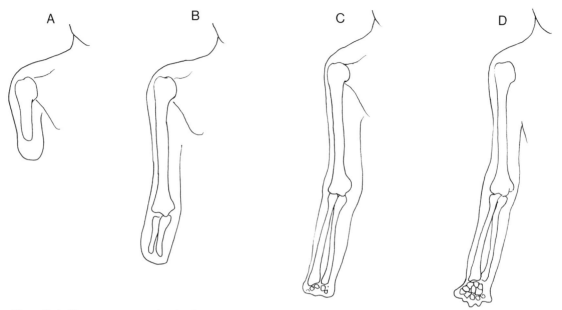

Figure 3–1. The more common levels of transverse amputation: A, midarm; B, proximal forearm; C, wrist; D midhand.

Treatment. Surgical therapy rarely improves function, but prosthetic devices may be helpful.[4, 39, 74] A nonactivated device that fits the deficient limb is recommended at 6 months, and when the child becomes more coordinated (18 months), an active prosthesis with a shoulder harness is ordered.

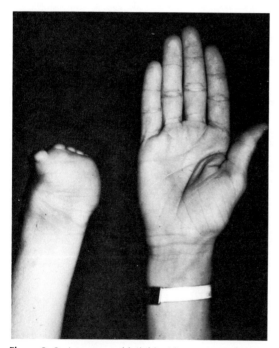

Figure 3–2. A ten-year-old child with a congenital amputation of the phalanges and the metacarpals on the left. The right hand is normal.

The Krukenberg procedure can be beneficial for two groups of patients with amputations at the wrist level: (1) blind patients with bilateral amputations, and (2) those with unilateral amputations who live in underdeveloped regions for which prostheses are not available. In this procedure, the radius and ulna are distally separated, so their tips can be used in a pincer fashion to hold objects.[101, 134]

Two longitudinal incisions are made that are joined over the amputated end distally. The incision on the flexor side of the forearm is slightly radial, and the incision on the extensor surface of the forearm is slightly ulnar. The forearm muscles are separated into two groups. The radial halves of the flexor digitorum superficialis, extensor digitorum communis, flexor carpi radialis, extensor carpi radialis brevis, extensor carpi radialis longus, brachioradialis, palmaris longus, and pronator teres are attached to the radius. The ulnar halves of the flexor digitorum superficialis, flexor carpi ulnaris, and extensor carpi ulnaris are attached to the ulna. The interosseous membrane is divided along the ulna, protecting the interosseous artery and nerve as well as the distal radial and ulnar growth plates. Motion occurs at the radiohumeral and proximal radioulnar joint.

Local flaps are used wherever possible. Skin grafts are used for coverage of skin deficits. A bulky immobilizing dressing is applied that holds the distal radius and ulna at least 6 cm apart. A long-arm plaster splint is applied and left in place for a total of 2 weeks but changed 1 week after surgery.

After 2 weeks, the cast is removed. The patient is started on a training program. This emphasizes pronation-supination of the radius against the ulna, and abduction-adduction of the radius against the ulna. The radial abductors are the brachioradialis, extensor carpi radialis brevis, extensor carpi radialis longus, and the biceps. The adductors are the pronator teres, supinator, flexor carpi radialis, and the radial components of the flexor digitorum superficialis.

The ulna is abducted by the extensor carpi ulnaris, the ulnar part of the extensor digitorum communis, and the triceps. The ulna is adducted by the flexor carpi ulnaris, brachialis, anconeous, and the ulnar components of the flexor digitorum superficialis.

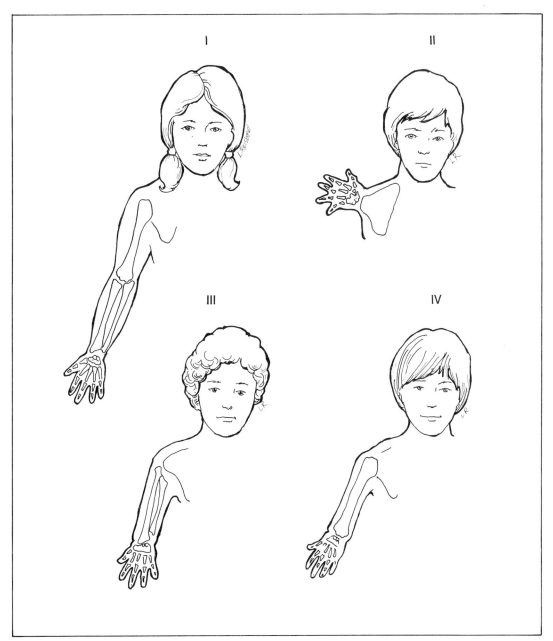

Figure 3–3. Clinical types of phocomelia compared with normal development: *I*, normal; *II*, complete phocomelia; *III*, proximal phocomelia; *IV*, distal phocomelia.

Phocomelia

Phocomelia is a severe form of transverse deficiency in which there is a proximodistal developmental failure. There are three types of phocomelia: complete, proximal, and distal (Fig. 3–3). In complete phocomelia, the upper extremity proximal to the hand is absent, and the hand articulates with the glenoid. Patients with proximal phocomelia have no arm, and the hand articulates with the forearm, which articulates with the glenoid. In distal phocomelia, the forearm is absent, and the hand articulates with the arm, which articulates with the glenoid.

This rare congenital anomaly can involve the upper or lower extremities or both. During the late 1950s and early 1960s, phocomelia became prevalent in Europe as the result of maternal thalidomide ingestion. In Germany, 60% of the babies conceived by women who took thalidomide between the thirty-eighth and fifty-fourth days after conception developed a form of phocomelia.[140]

In Great Britain,[51] "thalidomide babies" often had, besides phocomelia, preaxial defects that included radial club hand or hypoplasia of the radius, thumb, and index finger. Patients in this group had an ulna, and the humerus was normal, hypoplastic, or absent. Children with proximal agenesis of the humerus also had absence of the shoulder joint.[51] Thalidomide also affected other systems and has been reported to cause depression of the nasal bridge, coloboma, microtia, deafness, hyperhydrosis, and cryptorchidism.

Treatment. The surgical treatment of phocomelia is limited. Bone transfers and grafts can be used to provide stability and length, and tendon transfers can be used to improve joint motion. Most patients, however, derive the greatest benefit from limb training and prostheses.[51]

Longitudinal Deficiencies

Radial Club Hand

Radial club hand is a preaxial upper extremity defect that consists of several abnormalities, including a short forearm and radial deviation of the hand at the wrist. It occurs in one of every 30,000 births. Saunders,[120] using chick embryos, created the deformity by excision of the apical ectoderm.

Radial club hand can occur as an isolated upper extremity defect or in association with other congenital disorders. These may be genetically or nongenetically determined. The associated genetic syndromes are described in Table 3–3. The Vater complex is not genetically determined, and children with these defects have a unilateral radial defect associated with malformations of the spine, lung, kidney, face, and gastrointestinal tract. Radial club hand can also result from maternal thalidomide ingestion.

This upper extremity deformity has been described by several authors[21, 58, 75, 76, 103, 104, 116] and includes anomalies of bones, nerves, muscles, and joints. In the untreated adult, the hand has an abnormal perpendicular relationship to the forearm and has functional and aesthetic disadvantages (Fig. 3–4).

In Lamb's study of 117 affected limbs, 101 had no thumb, and 5 had a small thumb.[75] The other fingers had limited metacarpophalangeal and interphalangeal joint motion, which resulted in diminished power of grip. In one study of 24 patients, 83% had absent radial wrist extensors, and the remainder had ineffective radial wrist extensors.[21] Abnormalities of the carpus, especially those of the trapezium and scaphoid, have been reported.[76, 103, 104, 116] Short forearms are the

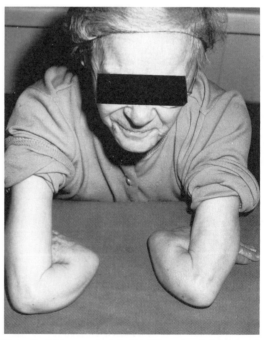

Figure 3–4. Untreated adult with bilateral radial club hands. (Reproduced from Bora FW Jr et al. J Bone Joint Surg [Am] 63:743–744, 1981, with permission.)

Table 3–3. **Syndromes With Radial Defects**

Syndrome	System	Congenital Defect	Inheritance
Holt-Oram	Musculoskeletal	Radial aplasia; proximal radioulnar synostosis; thumb hypoplasia or aplasia; proximal humerus defect	Autosomal dominant
	Cardiovascular	Atrial septal defects	
Nager (acrofacial dysostosis)[83, 96]	Musculoskeletal	Radial and thumb hypoplasia or absence; radioulnar synostosis; triphalangeal thumbs	Autosomal dominant and sporadic
	Craniofacial	Hypoplastic mandible; antimongoloid slant of palpebral fissures; small auricles; narrow external auditory canals; conductive deafness;	
Ladd[60] (lacrimoauriculo dentodigital syndrome)	Musculoskeletal	Radial defects; thumb triphalangy or duplication; clinodactyly; syndactyly;	Unknown
	Craniofacial	Cupped external ears; lacrimal duct stenosis; dental anomalies	
Fanconi's	Musculoskeletal	Radial and thumb hypoplasia or aplasia; thumb duplication	Unknown
	Integumentary	Diffuse brown pigmentation or vitiligo	
	Craniofacial	Microphthalmos; strabismus; deafness	
	Hematologic	Anemia; polymorpholeukocyte and thrombocyte deficiencies; generalized poor growth; cardiac and renal defects	
Thrombocytopenia and radial aplasia	Musculoskeletal	Radius aplasia; Humeral and ulnar absence or hypoplasia; small finger mesobrachyphalangy and clinodactyly; tibial torsion with genu varum	Autosomal recessive?
	Cardiovascular	Tetralogy of Fallot	
	Craniofacial	Narrow external auditory canals	
Craniosynostosis with radial aplasia	Musculoskeletal	Radial hypoplasia and aplasia; thumb hypoplasia	Autosomal recessive
	Craniofacial	Craniosynostosis	
	General	Short stature	

result of the radial bone defect that varies from partial to complete absence and an ulna that averages 60% of its expected growth.[21] The ulna may be bowed, and the humerus may be short.

Abnormal elbow motion further complicates extremity function and usually results in stiffening of the elbow in an extended position.[75] In such cases, centralization of the hand is not indicated because the hand can touch the face and body more easily in the radial position. If satisfactory elbow motion can be developed by conservative or surgical methods, centralization of the hand over the forearm may then be considered for treatment of the wrist deformity. A posterior elbow capsulotomy and transfer of the triceps,[26] the latissimus dorsi, or another shoulder muscle have been recommended to provide elbow flexion in such cases.

Treatment

Hypoplasia of the Radius. In this deformity, the proximal and distal epiphyses of the radius are present, but the radius is short. In addition, the forearm is short, the ulna is thick, and there is a radial bow. Radial deviation of the hand should be treated conservatively with stretching casts and dynamic orthoplast splints that pull the hand into a straight position over the forearm. In some cases, the surgical release of tight fascial structures, the brachioradialis, the extensor carpi radialis longus, and the extensor carpi radialis brevis may be required to decrease the deformity. Tendon transfers that involve movement of the extensor carpi radialis longus to the ulnar border of the wrist help balance the muscle forces to keep the hand straight.

Absence of the Radius. Partial or total absence of the radius causes radial deviation of the hand. There are differing opinions about whether any treatment of this deformity is justified. Several methods of surgical correction have been described: soft tissue release of the radial side of the forearm, replacement of the missing radius by a bone graft, osteotomy of the bowed ulna, and arthrodesis of the wrist at the end of the growth

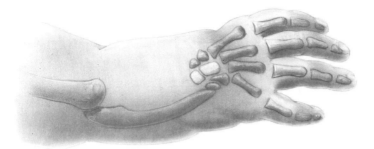

Figure 3–5. The drawing shows the central carpi, the lunate and the capitate (light shade), which may be partially or totally removed to provide a slot for the distal ulna for hand centralization. (Redrawn from Bora FW Jr. J Bone Joint Surg [Am] 52:966–979, 1970, by permission.)

period. None of these procedures has been satisfactory, although replacement of the missing radius by a vascularized fibula graft has been performed and may become the treatment of choice in the future. However, at present, centralization of the carpus over the distal ulna is the treatment of choice. In cases of recurrent deformity, tendon transfers are indicated.

Recommended Procedure. When treating a patient with radial club hand, the surgeon applies corrective casts soon after the child is born to stretch the tight soft tissue structures on the radial side of the wrist. Once this is accomplished, the hand should be centralized over the end of the distal ulna, which is done during the child's first year. The steps for this surgical procedure include exposure of the carpus and distal end of the ulna through a dorsal S-shaped incision from the midmetacarpal area to the midforearm. The distal ulnar epiphysis is freed from surrounding soft tissues, with care taken to preserve the extensor carpi ulnaris and the extensor digiti minimi tendons in their fibro-osseous canals on the dorsum of the distal ulna. The surgeon can achieve proper placement of the hand over the distal ulna by removing carpal structures to provide a slot for

placement of the ulna in the carpus (Fig. 3–5). A smooth Kirschner wire that transfixes the long finger metacarpal to the distal ulna maintains the position. It is best to place the Kirschner wire through the center of the distal ulna so that asymmetric epiphyseal plate injury is avoided. The dorsal radial carpal ligament, which one must incise longitudinally in order to expose the osseous structures, is repaired. The upper extremity is placed in a palm to axilla cast, with the elbow flexed at 90° to prevent cast slippage. The cast and Kirschner wires are removed at 6 weeks in the physician's office, and an orthoplast splint that holds the hand over the end of the ulna is worn by the child at night for 6 to 12 months, depending on the severity of the case. Bayne[13] has reported hand centralization accomplished by a shortening osteotomy of the ulna. Surgical placement of the distal ulna to the radial carpal side of the carpus also has been reported to result in alignment of the hand and forearm.

The surgeon may perform tendon transfers to prevent recurrence of the deformity. The superficialis tendons to the long and ring fingers, the hypothenar muscles, and the extensor carpi ulnaris are the units most frequently available. Active flexion of the digits

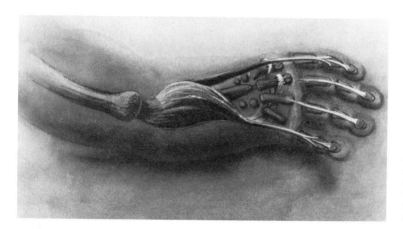

Figure 3–6. A drawing showing the superficialis tendons from the long and ring fingers used as transfers to support the hand over the ulna. (From Bora FW Jr. J Bone Joint Surg (Am) 52:966–979, 1970, by permission.)

stabilizing the fingers distal to the proximal interphalangeal joint with the wrist, metacarpophalangeal joints, and interphalangeal joints in maximum extension will determine whether the superficialis has satisfactorily developed to be transferred. If a superficialis tendon is selected, it is exposed by a volar incision over the proximal interphalangeal joint and divided, with its insertion and a 1-inch segment left attached to soft tissue (Grayson's or Cleland's ligament) so that hyperextension of the joint is prevented. A short, transverse incision is made over the volar aspect of the forearm, and the superficialis tendon is identified and pulled proximally into the forearm. If the superficialis tendons to both the long finger and the ring finger are selected, they are passed subcutaneously around the ulnar side of the forearm and inserted around the shaft of the metacarpals of the index finger and long finger and are then sutured to themselves, with tension holding the wrist in maximum extension and ulnar deviation (Fig. 3–6). Following the skin closure, a palm to axilla cast is applied, and the wrist is held in its new position, with the elbow at a right angle for 1 month. Thereafter, a night splint that holds the wrist in maximum extension and ulnar deviation is used for 6 months. If superficialis tendons are not available, one can detach the origin of the hypothenar muscles from the carpus and attach it proximally to the ulna or tighten the extensor carpi ulnaris by moving it to a more distal position along the shaft of the metacarpal. The value of tendon transfers appears to be that they complement centralization; when patients are treated with both these surgical maneuvers, arthrodesis may be avoided. Power pinch and grip are more satisfactory in these surgically treated patients than in untreated patients.

Evaluation of Treatment. It is difficult to compare treated patients with untreated ones in terms of anatomic (forearm) length and functional (digital) power on the basis of daily activities because all the untreated patients adapt to their deformity out of necessity. Untreated patients, however, wear clothes without buttons and shoes without laces and use eating utensils with bulky handles. Although untreated patients adapt satisfactorily to dressing, hygiene, and feeding, it should be pointed out that they are more limited than treated patients, who are capable of opening doors, buttoning their clothing, and performing similar tasks. The

important objective of surgical treatment of radial club hand is maximization of forearm length and of digital motion and power. The best postoperative results occur in children who are treated early (Fig. 3–7). These procedures are beneficial to the child when performed during his preschool years, but results are not as satisfactory when the child

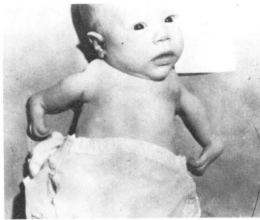

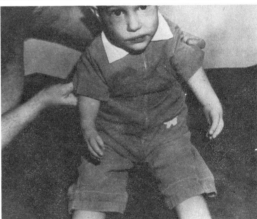

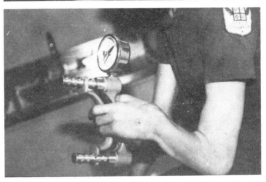

Figure 3–7. Long-term follow-up of a child treated with centralization and tendon transfers. The same child at one year, 4 years, and 17 years. (From Bora FW Jr et al. J Bone Joint Surg [Am] 63:741–745, 1981, by permission.)

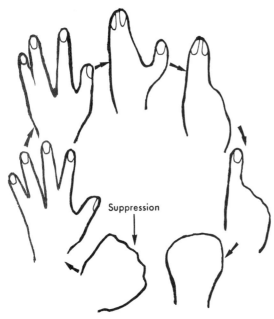

Figure 3–8. A theory of the suppression of hand formation. (Redrawn from Maisels DB. Br J Plast Surg 23:269–281, 1970, by permission.)

is treated between 5 and 10 years. After the child reaches 10 years of age, he has adapted to his activities, and surgery is therefore rarely indicated.

Cleft Hand Deformity

Central defects are commonly described as cleft, split, or lobster hands. Birch-Jensen reports that they occur in one of every 90,000 births.[18] Cleft hand has a variable inheritance and can occur sporadically as an autosomal recessive or as an autosomal dominant trait. When the anomaly involves an absence of the central rays and all extrem-

ities are involved, it is often inherited as an autosomal dominant trait.[36, 66] Maisel has proposed a centripetal theory of suppression in which the deformity can range from a developing hand plate that is suppressed and present as a simple cleft hand with no absent tissue to an extreme anomaly involving total suppression of all digits. According to Maisel, intermediate deformities present as absence of the long finger ray, with or without radial ray suppression[84] (Fig. 3–8).

Other congenital defects can occur in association with cleft hands. The associated musculoskeletal defects include cleft foot, syndactyly, tibial ray defects, ipsilateral hypoplasia of the upper extremity, and absence of the pectoral muscles.[43] Head and neck defects also are associated, including cataracts, hearing loss, cleft lip, and cleft palate.[118]

The deformity is frequently bilateral. It has been divided into two main types.[139] Patients with one type present with a ray deficiency of the phalanges of the long finger and in some cases with absence of the metacarpal, which results in absence of the entire ray. These patients have a deep central cleft that divides the hand into radial and ulnar components (Fig. 3–9). In the lobster claw, a variant of this type of deformity, bony elements and the central ray are missing (Fig. 3–10). The other type of cleft hand deformity is less common. With these defects, skeletal structures of the long finger are present but are fused with the bony elements of the adjacent fingers. Some patients have additional bony elements (e.g., six metacarpals).

Treatment. Most children with cleft hand have simple defects with excellent function and require no surgery. In some children, the defect is a simple central separation, and cleft closure positions the fingers in a more

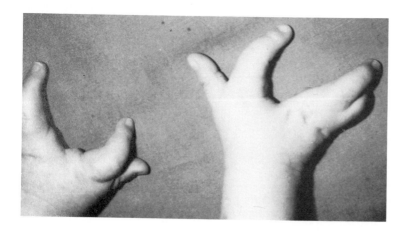

Figure 3–9. Bilateral cleft hands.

Figure 3–10. Bilateral lobster claw hands.

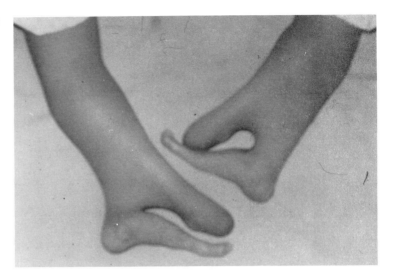

normal relationship. Barsky reported his method of raising a diamond-shaped flap from the base of one finger to be mobilized to cover the proximal web of the digits after they are drawn together (Fig. 3–11). The flap at the base of the radial digit is connected to the transverse incision at the ulnar digit by an incision in the web space. The metacarpals are held together by a strong fascial loop or strong sutures placed around the metacarpals or anchored through drill holes in the metacarpals. In some cases, there is a tendency for the metacarpals to swing back to their original position. When this occurs, an osteotomy of the metacarpal is required. In such cases, Flatt recommends keeping the periosteum intact after the osteotomy to hold the fragments in position for bone healing.[49] Kelikian and Doumanian advise using a rectangular flap from the palmar skin to bridge the gap between the bases of the separated fingers.[70] Streli recommends moving the index finger to the long finger to decrease the cleft space.[132]

For cleft hand deformities in which a thumb and index finger syndactyly compromise pinching and hand function, Snow and Littler[125] have reported osteotomizing the base of the index metacarpal and moving it to the long finger rudimentary base (Fig. 3–12). An E-shaped incision is made on the dorsal aspect of the hand over the base of the

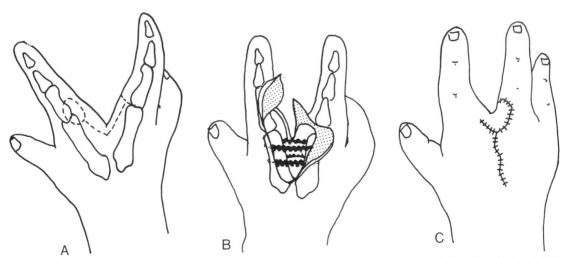

A   B   C

Figure 3–11. Surgical steps for the treatment of cleft hand (From Barsky AJ. J Bone Joint Surg [Am] 46:1707–1719, 1969, with permission.)

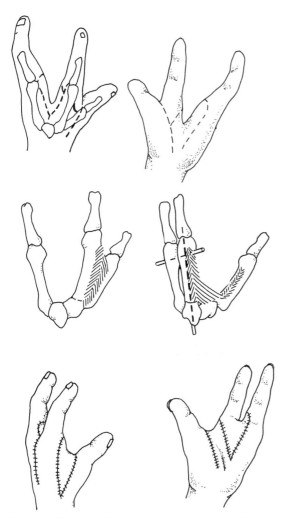

Figure 3–12. Surgical steps for the treatment of cleft hand. (From Flatt AE. The Care of Congenital Hand Anomalies. CV Mosby, 1977:275–279, with permission.)

In patients with cleft hand deformities in which pinch is compromised because of a thumb–index finger syndactyly, Miura and Komada[95] have also described osteotomizing the index finger at its base and transposing it to the long finger position by fixing it to the vestigial long finger metacarpal base with K-wires. This frees the thumb and improves opposition. A linear incision begins on the radial side of the ring finger and runs to the ulnar side of the index finger across the cleft space. A curved incision is added around the base of the index finger in line, permitting creation of the new thumb web. After the index metacarpal is osteotomized at its base, the distal fragment is transposed to the long finger metacarpal base and fixed with K-wires. To secure the new position of the index finger, the surgeon places an additional internal wire between the shaft of the index finger metacarpal and the shaft of the ring finger metacarpal. Transfer of the first dorsal interosseous with the index metacarpal assists pinch (Fig. 3–13). With the Littler-Snow and Miura-Komada procedures, the hands are casted for 6 weeks postoperatively. Casting the hand for 1 month protects isolated soft tissue procedures in which fasciae, tendon grafts, or areas of local tissue are used to hold separated metacarpals together.

metacarpals of the index finger and ring finger. This incision is extended volarly, forming a racquet-shaped cut around the base of the index finger, with the "handle" extending down to the palm. After the skin incisions are made, fibrous bands between the metacarpals are released, and origins of the first dorsal interosseous are divided and mobilized from bony attachments. The index metacarpal is osteotomized at its base, transferred to the long finger base, and fixed with K-wires between the index finger and the third metacarpal to maintain its new position. The skin is sutured between the ring and index fingers and the thumb in its abducted position. If local flaps do not completely cover the defect, a split-thickness skin graft is used to complete skin coverage.

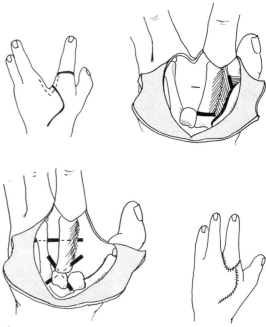

Figure 3–13. Surgical steps for the treatment of cleft hand. (From Miura T et al. Simple method for reconstruction of the cleft hand with an adducted thumb. Plast Reconstr Surg 64:65–67, 1979, by permission.)

Table 3–4. **General Syndromes With Associated Ulnar Defects**

Syndrome	Congenital Defect	Inheritance
Goltz (focal dermal hyperplasia)	Ulnar defect; split hand or foot; syndactyly; long bone defects; skin atrophy or papillomas of the lips, anus, or vulva; mental retardation; microphthalmia, coloboma of the iris	X-linked dominant
Splithand with ulnar aplasia	Cleft hand with ulnar hypoplasia or aplasia; cleft foot deformity	Autosomal dominant
Ulnar defect with mammary gland aplasia	Ulnar defect; aplasia or camptodactyly of the little finger; postaxial hexadactyly	Unknown

Functional position in deformities of the interphalangeal joints may be improved by a simple fusion. Occasionally, border digits have good passive motion but lack motor function. Wrist flexors, wrist extensors, digital flexors, and digital extensors may be present and used for tendon transfers. In severe suppression deformities in which only one digit is present, a toe to hand transfer reported by Reed provides a second digit for pinching.[114] This requires microsurgical anastomosis of the arteries and nerves, and suture of the toe tendons to the hand tendons is required. Barsky used an iliac bone graft and a tube pedicle for a second digit. However, as follow-up studies showed, the grafted bone resorbed, and the tube pedicle lacked reliable sensibility. The procedure reported by Reed has proved more reliable than that reported by Barsky.

Ulnar Club Hand

Ulnar club hand is less common than radial club hand and cleft hand deformities.[104] The majority of patients with this defect have unilateral upper extremity involvement.[23, 73, 106]

Most cases of ulnar club hand are sporadic, lacking an obvious cause. There are a few genetic syndromes, however, in which there are associated ulnar defects (Table 3–4).

The ulnar club hand presents with ulnar shortening, radial bowing, and digital abnormalities in over 50% of the patients.[23] Absence of the small and ring finger metacarpals as well as deformities of the pisiform, lunate, triquetrum, and capitate can occur. The ulna may be totally or partially absent; when present, it may be ankylosed to the humerus. The deformity may also present with a radial humeral synostosis, and dislocation of the radial head occurs in 50% of these extremities[23] (Fig. 3–14). A fibrocartilaginous anlage connecting the ulna to the carpus restrains wrist motion and may produce a radial bowing.[28] Unlike patients with radial club hand, patients with this deformity have surprisingly good function (Fig. 3–15). Less than one third of patients have fixed ulnar deviation at the radiocarpal joint, and

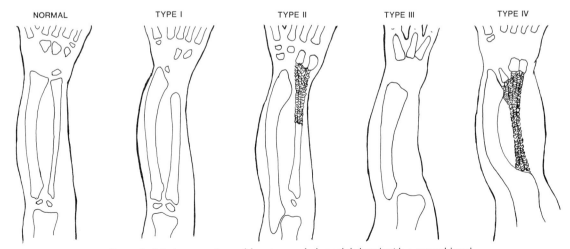

Figure 3–14. A comparison of four types of ulnar club hand with a normal hand.

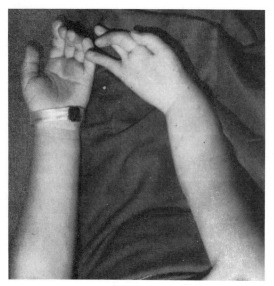

Figure 3–15. A child with an ulnar club hand with a short forearm, three fingers, a thumb, and with good hand function. This child was treated with fusion of the proximal ulna to the distal radius—a one-bone forearm.

the majority are able to bring their hands into a neutral position.

Treatment. The deformity and the age of the patient when first seen help determine treatment. If the child is seen early, treatment consists of long-arm, serial casts that stretch the tight ulnar structures. Mild deformities may be corrected in 6 months. Resistant de-

formities have a fibrocartilaginous anlage that, when recognized, should be surgically excised. The anlage is approached through an ulnar incision along the wrist and forearm, with care taken to protect the ulnar artery and nerve. The entire anlage need not be excised, but removal of at least 50% of the tissue is necessary, and after closure the wrist is placed in maximum radial deviation in a long-arm cast for 1 month. Night splints are then used for 3 to 6 months for maintenance of the corrected position.

Untreated children seen after 1 year of age present with an ulnar deviated hand caused by the fibrocartilaginous anlage, and radial head dislocation also may be present. In these children, it is important for the surgeon to excise the anlage to prevent further deformity. If the radial head is in place, no other treatment is indicated. If the radial head is dislocated and there is good forearm rotation, no additional treatment is recommended in the type II deformity. If the radial head is dislocated and there is limited forearm rotation, the surgeon should create a one-bone forearm by excising the proximal radius and fusing the remaining distal radius to the proximal ulna for stabilization (Fig. 3–16). If it is not clear whether the exchange of forearm rotation for forearm stability is wise in a child, it is better for one to wait until the child is older before performing the procedure. The incision for a one-bone fore-

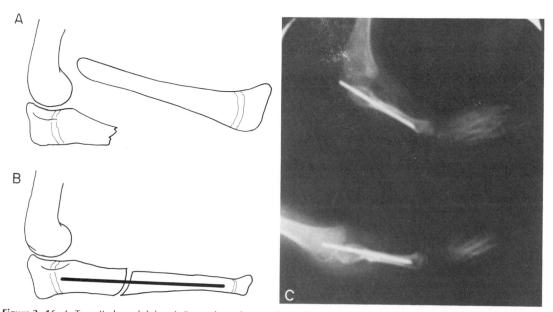

Figure 3–16. *A,* Type II ulnar club hand; *B,* one-bone forearm formed by excision of proximal radius and fusion of remaining distal radius to proximal ulna; *C,* x-ray of "one-bone forearm."

arm is posterior, which exposes the radius and ulna, and care is taken to protect the posterior interosseous nerve. After the ends of the radius and ulna are freshened, sufficient proximal radius is excised so that the bones can be brought into alignment, after which they are fixed with an intramedullary pin, a compression plate, or an external fixation device. In children over 10 years of age, an iliac bone graft is used to promote union. A long-arm cast is applied until bone union occurs. Bone union usually requires 10 weeks and must be documented by x-ray. When radiohumeral synostosis is present, the surgeon must excise the ulnar anlage to prevent increased radial bowing and excessive deviation of the distal radial epiphysis. Older children with radiohumeral synostosis may have a deformity at the humeral level. In these patients, an osteotomy through the humerus can improve the extremity alignment. In older untreated children, the hand is deviated in an ulnar position, radial bowing is pronounced, and the radial head is dislocated. In these patients, the anlage is resected so that progressive deformity is prevented, but creation of a one-bone forearm for improvement of stability compromises forearm rotation and is not indicated unless the child can define an activity in which stability is more important than rotation.

Failure of Differentiation

Syndactyly

Syndactyly is failure of differentiation of tissue between the digits. Soft tissue webbing involving part of the finger length is *incomplete syndactyly*; soft tissue webbing extending to the fingertips is *complete syndactyly*; syndactyly involving the soft tissue and bone is *complex syndactyly*.

Syndactyly occurs between the sixth and eighth week of fetal development. The deformity occurs as a spontaneous intrauterine event or from a genetically determined trait. Syndactyly is often an autosomal dominant trait with variable penetrance when present by itself, but it has also been classified by geneticists into five phenotypical groups.[141]

Type 1 Syndactyly. Patients with this anomaly usually have a simple skin web between the long and ring fingers. It may be complete or incomplete. Their toes also may have syndactyly.

Type 2 Syndactyly. Patients with this abnormality have a web between the long and ring fingers. Within this web there is a duplication of the bony structure of the ring finger. The toes also may be affected.

Type 3 Ring-Small Syndactyly. Patients with this deformity have complete simple syndactyly between the ring and small fingers. Occasionally, there is complex syndactyly resulting from distal phalangeal fusion. The small finger is usually short owing to absence of the middle phalanx.

Type 4 Hass Type Syndactyly. Patients with this anomaly have simple syndactyly involving all the digits, including the thumb. Occasionally, there are a sixth metacarpal and a sixth phalanx.

Type 5 Syndactyly. This is a rare type of syndactyly between the long and ring fingers. There is an associated fusion between the third, fourth, and fifth metacarpals. The toes are similarly affected.

Syndromes Associated with Syndactyly. Syndactyly can also occur in variable association with a syndrome or as a component of a syndrome. These syndromes are described in Tables 3–5 and 3–6.

Incidence. Syndactyly occurs in one of

Table 3–5. **Syndromes That May Be Associated With Syndactyly**

A. Chromosomal syndromes
  1. Trisomy 13
  2. Trisomy 18
  3. Trisomy 21
  4. Triploidy
  5. Deletion of the short arm of chromosome 5
B. Craniofacial syndromes
  1. Aglossia adactylia
  2. Möbius syndrome
  3. Familial static ophthalmoplegia
  4. Glossopalatine ankylosis; microglossia and limb anomalies
  5. Hypertelorism and syndactyly
  6. Hanhart's syndrome (micrognathia and limb anomalies)
  7. Oculomandibulofacial syndrome
  8. Retinal dysplasias
C. Cutaneous syndromes
  1. Focal dermal hypoplasia
  2. Popliteal pterygium syndrome
  3. Bloom's syndrome (short stature, molar hypoplasia, facial telangiectatic erythema)
  4. Ectrodermal dysplasia
D. Other syndromes
  1. Silver's syndrome
  2. Cornelia de Lange's syndrome
  3. Prader-Willi syndrome
  4. Lysinemia
  5. Congenital heart disease and syndactyly

Table 3–6. **Syndromes in Which Syndactyly Is a Consistent Component**

Syndrome	Components	Inheritance
Poland's syndactyly	Unilateral synbrachydactyly; aplasia of the sternal head of the pectoralis major; absent nipple and breast tissue[63, 62]; auxillary webbing	Sporadic
Apert's	Craniosynostosis; hypertelorism; exophthalmos; mild mental retardation; depressed nasal bridge; complex syndactyly; mitten hand; ankylosing proximal interphalangeal and distal interphalangeal joints	Autosomal Dominant
Chotzen's cephalodactyly	Hypertelorism; exophthalmos; parrot beak nose; hypoplasia of the maxilla; craniosynostosis; syndactyly; often, thumb and little finger involvement	Autosomal dominant
Waardenburg's	Acrocephaly; orbital and facial asymmetry; cleft palate; abnormal ears; strabismus; thin, long, pointed nose; brachydactyly; simple syndactyly; occasional bifid terminal phalanx	
Pfeifer's	Acrocephaly; short broad thumbs; proximal phalanx thumb, triangular or trapezoidal; simple syndactyly	Autosomal dominant
Summit's	Acrocephaly; variable hand and foot deformities	Autosomal recessive
Noack's	Acrocephaly; enlarged thumbs; duplication of the great toe; syndactyly of the fingers and toes	
Carpenter's	Acrocephaly; mandibular hypoplasia; flat nasal bridge; brachydactyly; simple ring finger–long finger syndactyly; preaxial hand and foot polydactyly; mental retardation	Autosomal recessive
Oculodentodigital	Microphthalmia; microcornea; glaucoma; thin nose; hypoplastic alae; small teeth; enamelogenesis imperfections; ring finger–small finger syndactyly	Autosomal dominant
Orofaciodigital (syndrome I)	Hyperplastic frenula; cleft tongue; grooved mandibular and alveolar processes; abnormalities of lower incisors and other teeth; cleft palate; medial cleft lip; hypoplastic malar bones; simple syndactyly	X-linked dominant; lethal to males
Orofaciodigital (syndrome II)	Lobulate tongue; midline cleft lip; high arch or cleft palate; hypertrophied frenulum; mandibular hypoplasia; syndactyly	Autosomal recessive
Acropectoral-vertebral dysplasia	Carpal synostosis; tarsal synostosis; duplication of postaxial toes; toe syndactyly; prominent sternum; spina bifida occulta; mental retardation; craniofacial anomalies; thumb–index finger syndactyly	Autosomal dominant

every 2000 to 2500 births. Boys are more commonly affected than girls, and there is often bilateral involvement. Syndactyly most frequently involves the ring finger and long finger; the thumb and index finger are the least often involved. This may be due to the earlier development of the thumb.

Treatment

Timing of Surgical Correction. In simple syndactyly, fingers of unequal length should be separated so that a flexion-rotation deformity is prevented. Thumb–index finger syndactyly should be separated at 6 months, and ring finger–small finger syndactyly (Fig. 3–17) should be corrected prior to 1 year. Children with complex syndactyly often require multiple surgical procedures, which should be performed early so that progres-

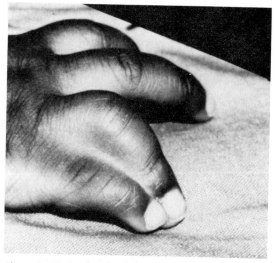

Figure 3–17. Syndactyly of the ring and small fingers. The shorter small finger restricts joint motion of the longer finger, and separation is recommended prior to one year.

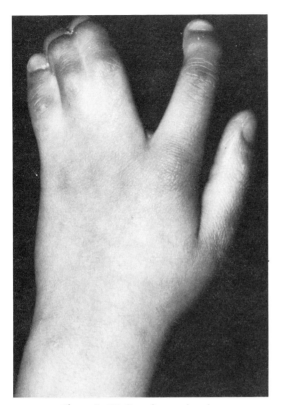

Figure 3–18. Complex syndactyly.

sive bone deformity is prevented and so that separation will be completed prior to school age (Fig. 3–18).

Flatt reported that when separation of simple syndactyly was performed in children younger than 18 months, postoperative scar-ring caused flexion and rotational deformities of the separated digits.[49] We also have observed this complication and therefore postpone simple syndactyly separation of the digits with similar length (long and ring fingers) until the preschool years. We release complex syndactyly during the first year because bone involvement limits joint motion and increases deformity as the child grows. Functional hand patterns are established by 24 months,[55] so children with syndactyly should be encouraged to use the involved hand during the first 20 months to learn digital patterns during that period.

Correction of Simple Syndactyly. The method used for separation of simple syndactyly depends on the extent of the web. When only web space deepening is required, a local flap procedure may suffice, but simple incomplete (Fig. 3–19) and complete (Fig. 3–20) syndactyly require local flaps and skin grafting for coverage. For separation of simple syndactyly, we recommend using a broad dorsal rectangular flap for web space coverage, first described by Bauer and coworkers[12] (Fig. 3–21). All incisions are drawn with a pen or methylene blue. The dorsal flap should include two thirds of the proximal phalanx length and extend proximally to the level of the metacarpal head. A zigzag incision from the distal end of the flap

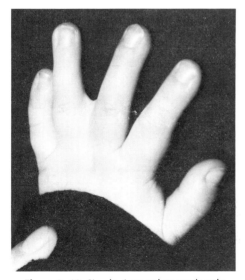

Figure 3–19. Simple, incomplete syndactyly.

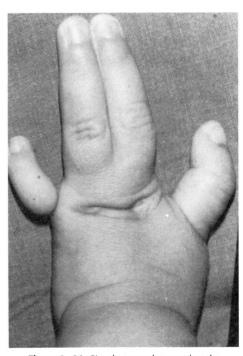

Figure 3–20. Simple, complete syndactyly.

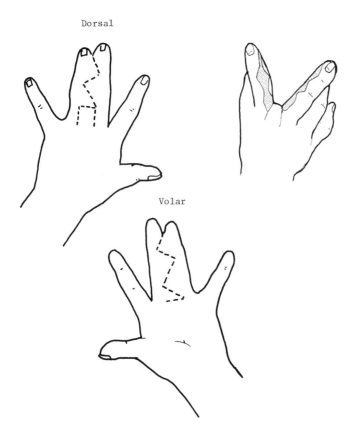

Dorsal

Volar

Figure 3–21. The technique using a rectangular flap to cover the web space when separating simple syndactyly.

to the fingertips helps lessen postoperative linear scar contracture. On the volar surface, a transverse incision is placed at the line of the new web space level, which is connected by a zigzag incision in the volar skin to the distal end of the skin web. Another technique involves volar and dorsal "V" flaps that cover the web base (Fig. 3–22).

The surgeon should take care to identify and preserve the neurovascular bundles. If the digital nerves divide distal to the level of the planned web space, intraneural separation of the proper nerve fascicles preserves nerve continuity and permits deepen-

ing of the web. Artery separation requires special consideration. Flatt[49] recommends establishing the web at the level of the digital vessels rather than dividing the vessels. Dobyns[38a] reports that ligation of one artery to a digit is occasionally indicated to make separation easier but is justified only if the other digital vessel to that finger is observed to be functioning at surgery. The skin flaps elevated to separate the web should be placed on the sides of the divided fingers without tension. We recommend using full-thickness skin grafts taken from the inguinal crease to cover deficient skin areas. Skin that

1   2   3

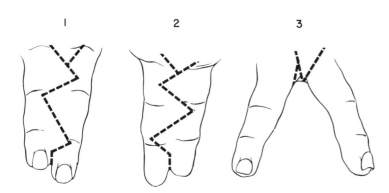

Figure 3–22. Use of volar and dorsal V-flaps to cover the web space in separating simple syndactyly.

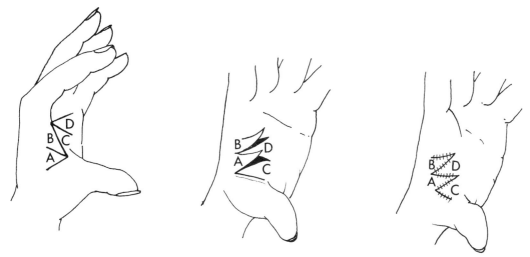

Figure 3–23. Four-flap Z-plasty for deepening the thumb web. (From Flatt AE. The Care of Congenital Hand Anomalies. CV Mosby, 1977:64, with permission.)

will become hair-bearing at puberty should be avoided. Prior to placing the grafts, the surgeon should release the tourniquet and achieve hemostasis to prevent hematoma from separating the grafts from the recipient bed. The grafts should be sutured in position without tension on the graft or the flaps.

Deepening the thumb–index finger web can be achieved with the four-flap Z-plasty technique.[161] (Fig. 3–23) or the double Z-plasty and V-Y advancement.[60] Both techniques involve the multiple Z-plasty principle to increase the thumb–index finger web. In the former technique, a total of four flaps are used; in the latter, five flaps are required. We prefer the four-flap Z-plasty. Each of the flaps in this technique has a broad base and tapers toward the tip, increasing the chance of flap survival.

Correction of Complex Syndactyly. Complex syndactyly involves fusion of the phalanges as well as skin webbing (Fig. 3–24) and often occurs in association with other congenital anomalies. These may involve other systems or proximal muscles of the upper extremity. When other systems are involved, corrective surgery for syndactyly will need to be coordinated with treatment of the other medical problems. Common associated upper extremity defects include neurovascular deficiencies, digital hypoplasia, concealed polydactyly, and musculoskeletal anomalies besides fusion. These associated problems will make improvement of hand function more difficult.

We agree with Flatt[49] that in patients with complex syndactyly, restoration of the skeleton of the hand should be achieved first. If

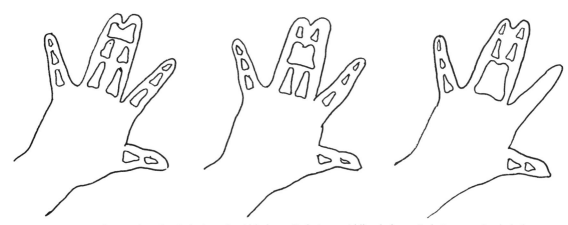

Figure 3–24. Complex syndactyly: *A*, fusion, distal phalanx; *B*, fusion, middle phalanx; *C*, fusion, proximal phalanx.

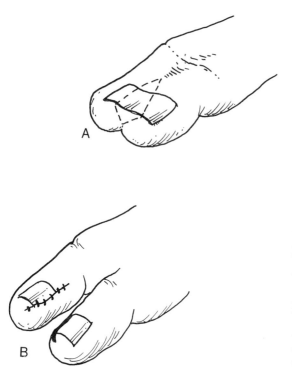

Figure 3–25. The release of "joined" fingernails in the syndactyly abnormality. (From Dobyns JH et al. *In* Green DP, ed. Operative Hand Surgery, Vol. 1. Churchill Livingstone, 1982:291, with permission.)

there is a concealed polydactyly, the extra phalanges should be removed. Fused, angled, or rotation bone deformities should be corrected by osteotomy. One must take care during all procedures to protect the neurovascular bundles because they may be anomalous or absent on one side of a digit. If tendons have abnormal insertions or are missing, tendon transfers may be required for finger motion. Cojoined fingernail deformities are first corrected by removal of a central strip of nail. After longitudinal excision of pulp, the skin edge is sutured to the nail edge (Fig. 3–25). This narrows the nails to a normal width and permits independent distal phalanx motion. In these cases, the distal phalanx is separated when first seen, which permits independent distal phalanx motion and makes separation of the rest of the web easier at a later date.

Synostosis

Synostosis, another anomaly of differentiation, will be discussed in detail elsewhere in this book. It has been observed in the elbow

(see Chap. 12), the radius and ulna (see Chap. 12), the carpals (see Chap. 10), and the metacarpals, earlier in this Chapter.

Intrinsic Digital Anomalies

Camptodactyly

Camptodactyly is a nontraumatic, painless flexion deformity of the proximal interphalangeal joint that has an insidious onset and is gradually progressive until fully developed (Fig. 3–26).[90] The metacarpophalangeal and the distal interphalangeal joints are not involved. The little finger is most frequently involved, but the other fingers can be affected. Patients often present with functional or cosmetic complaints.

Camptodactyly is inherited as an autosomal dominant trait with variable penetrance but may appear sporadically.[6, 82, 97] Girls are affected more often than boys.[34, 123] The etiology of camptodactyly is not known. Several mechanisms have been proposed, including flexor tendon contracture, flexor tendon sheath contracture, collateral ligament contracture, volar plate contracture, ab-

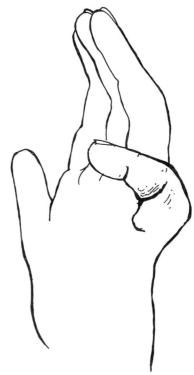

Figure 3–26. Camptodactyly: flexion deformity of the PIP joint.

normalities of the lumbricales and interossei, vascular abnormalities, phalangeal abnormalities, and flexion-extension imbalance at the proximal interphalangeal joint.

Camptodactyly may be clinically apparent at birth[99] or at a later age.[3,6] The deformity undergoes the greatest change during the growth spurt and may progress until the patient is 20 years old.[123] The flexion contracture deformity ranges from 10° to over 90° with an average of 50°.[44]

Treatment. Children with camptodactyly are initially treated with stretching exercises. One series[44] reported 20% of the patients improved with a conservative program of exercises and static and dynamic splinting. Even though the results of conservative therapy are limited, surgery also has mixed success. Smith and Kaplan[123] reported that tenotomy of the flexor digitorum sublimis improved the flexion contracture in four of 12 selected patients who preoperatively could extend the proximal interphalangeal joint with the wrist flexed. After the flexor tenotomy, the patients were casted with the proximal interphalangeal joint in maximum extension for 3 to 6 months. The transfer of the flexor superficialis through the lumbrical canal to the extensor apparatus also has been reported to improve finger function[37] by decreasing the flexor deformity of the proximal interphalangeal joint. Flatt[49] reports that in patients with deformity of the proximal phalanx, a wedge osteotomy through the neck of

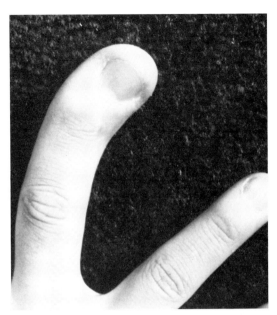

Figure 3–28. Clino- and macrodactyly of the long finger.

the proximal phalanx improves finger alignment. The base of the wedge is dorsal, and after osteotomy the phalangeal fragments are fixed with a K-wire (Fig. 3–27). This procedure changes but does *not* increase the range of proximal interphalangeal joint motion, and finger flexion is decreased in exchange for increased extension. This procedure is indicated in selected cases of flexion deformities of 75° or greater. If a volar skin defect is present after tendon, ligament, or bone correction, it is covered by a skin graft or flap.

Clinodactyly

Radioulnar deviation of a digit is called clinodactyly. The small finger is most often involved, but any finger can be affected. Involvement is often bilateral, and the genetic pattern has been reported to be sporadic or autosomal dominant.[112]

Unequal growth plate development or an abnormal interphalangeal ligamentous development can cause clinodactyly, and the deformity may be accompanied by macrodactyly (Fig. 3–28), brachydactyly, or a short middle phalanx.

Treatment. Although this deformity rarely causes a functional problem, patients may request surgical correction because of its appearance. Stretching exercises and splints do *not* help, but a wedge osteotomy with pin fixation through the abnormal phalanx

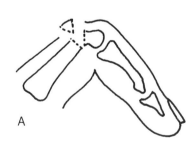

A

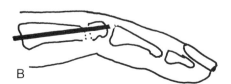

B

Figure 3–27. The steps in osteotomizing the neck of the proximal phalanx in cases where bone deformity contributes to the flexion deformity in camptodactyly: *A*, removal of dorsal-based wedge; *B*, K-wire fixation of fragments.

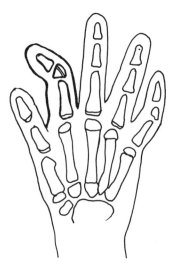

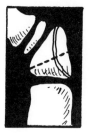
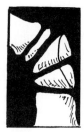
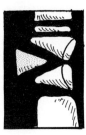

Figure 3–30. A drawing of open-wedge osteotomy with bone graft for the correction of a delta phalanx. (From Flatt AE. The Care of Congenital Hand Anomalies. CV Mosby, 1977:159, with permission.)

Figure 3–29. An abnormal C-shaped epiphysis in a delta phalanx. (From Flatt AE. Care of Congenital Hand Anomalies. CV Mosby, 1977:157, with permission.)

straightens the finger and has been used in some cases. The corrected finger, the adjacent finger, and the wrist are casted until the bone heals, usually 6 weeks after surgery.

Delta Phalanx

Delta phalanx is an abnormally shaped bone in the finger (it can occur at the metacarpal level) that resembles a triangle, or the Greek letter delta. The abnormal phalanx, however, is usually trapezoidal rather than triangular, causing deviation of the digit towards the shorter side of the abnormal bone. This abnormality occurs in tubular bones with a longitudinally positioned, C-shaped epiphysis in place of the usual transverse epiphysis (Fig. 3–29).[49] The abnormally shaped growth plate is responsible for the progressive angulation associated with growth. The thumb usually angles in an ulnar direction, the index finger may angle in either direction, and the postaxial digits angle radially. Delta phalanx may be associated with other congenital anomalies in the upper extremity, including polydactyly,[158] triphalangeal thumb,[159] and cleft hand.[8] Although the etiology of delta phalanx is unclear, this deformity has been reported to be a manifestation of polydactylism[152] or a form of complex syndactyly.[122]

Treatment. This bone deformity does not respond to exercises or splinting. The treatment of significant angulation that causes functional impairment is surgical. Proce-

dures that have reportedly improved finger alignment are the opening wedge osteotomy, in which iliac bone is used; the reverse wedge osteotomy, in which local bone is used; and the closing wedge osteotomy. In the opening wedge osteotomy,[67, 122] a bone graft is used to fill the osteotomy site, offsetting the angulation. When there is an associated polydactyly, the bone from the excised parts can be used as a bone graft source. These are fixed in place with K-wires that pass through the osteotomized bone, the graft, and the adjacent phalanges (Fig. 3–30). Alternatively, a reverse wedge osteotomy can be used as advocated by Carstam[28] and Flatt.[49] In this technique, a wedge of bone is taken from the center of the delta phalanx and then placed in the opposite position to reverse the angulation. This is fixed in place with K-wires (Fig. 3–31). In a closing wedge, bone is resected from the midlevel of the delta phalanx, with the base of the edge on the long side of the digit and the angle on the short side. After bone removal, the remaining fragments are placed together and fixed with a K-wire (Fig. 3–32). Flatt[49] recommends hand tools rather than power tools for the osteotomy because the former instruments are less likely to injure the growth

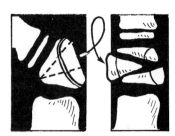
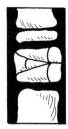

Figure 3–31. A drawing of a reverse-wedge osteotomy for the correction of a delta phalanx. (From Flatt AE. The Care of Congenital Hand Anomalies. CV Mosby, 1977:160, with permission.)

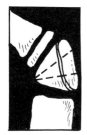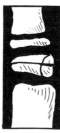

Figure 3–32. A drawing of a closing-wedge osteotomy for correction of a delta phalanx.

plate in these small bones. If the delta phalanx is small, simple excision followed by pin fixation of the digit in a straight position is recommended.

Kirner's Deformity

Kirner's deformity presents as a painless swelling and progressive curvature of the terminal phalanx of the small finger (Fig. 3–33). X-rays show a palmar curvature of the distal phalanx with growth plate widening and delayed epiphyseal closure. The deformity is usually bilateral and is not apparent until 8 to 12 years of age. Conservative therapy is not effective, and surgery is reserved for severe cases.

Treatment. Surgical correction is accomplished with multiple wedge osteotomies, as described by Carstam and Eiken.[27] The surgeon approaches the distal phalanx with a midlateral incision, preserving the tactile volar skin surface. Two osteotomies are made through the phalanx, with the dorsal periosteum left intact to act as a hinge for the bone fragments. The fragments of the distal phalanx are then held straight by K-wire fixation (Fig. 3–34).

Symphalangism

Symphalangism was first reported in 1916 by Harvey Cushing,[35] who used the term to describe a stiff proximal interphalangeal joint. Later, it was reported by others that the distal interphalangeal joint also can be involved with short fingers, a combination known as symbrachydactylism.[50] As reported by Cushing and subsequent investigators, symphalangism is an autosomal dominant trait.[127, 133] Distal symphalangism involving the distal interphalangeal joints with brachydactyly of the middle phalanx is a distinct genetic disorder that is also inherited as an autosomal dominant trait.[20]

Symphalangism is present at birth and therefore is readily distinguishable from acquired joint ankylosis. Failure of the joint cavity to develop normally, which causes joint immobility, occurs at the eighth week of fetal development. X-rays show bony fusion or a narrow joint space.

This disorder can be divided into three types: true symphalangism, symbrachydactylism, and symphalangism with other anomalies. Flatt[49] reports that true symphalangism is uncommon and involves one or more stiff fingers. The affected digit is slightly shorter and more slender than normal fingers. Transverse skin creases over the

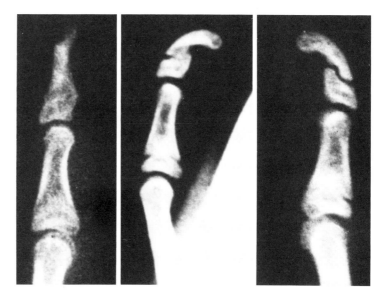

Figure 3–33. X-ray of Kirner's deformity, a volar curvature of the distal phalanx.

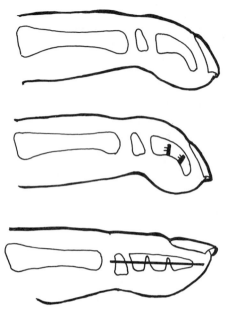

Figure 3–34. Drawing of surgical steps for the correction of Kirner's deformity. *A*, the deformity; *B*, the osteotomies that keep the dorsal periostium intact; *C*, K-wire fixation of the fragments. (From Carstam N et al. J Bone Joint Surg [Am] 52:1665, 1970, with permission.)

affected joint are absent, and the joint is usually fixed in a straight position. Symbrachydactylism, the most common type, involves a short middle phalanx and varying stiffness of the distal interphalangeal and proximal interphalangeal joints. Anomalies found in association with symphalangism include syndactyly, brachyphalangia, acrophalangia, Apert's syndrome, Poland's syndrome, foot anomalies, cleft palate, facial paralysis, hip dislocation, hearing loss, Möbius' syndrome, dysplasia epiphysealis multiplex, and gargoylism.[50]

   Treatment. Treatment of symphalagism is directed toward fixing the joint in a more functional position or improving joint motion. Conservative therapy has not been successful. Surgery also has been reported to fail. Only Palmieri[105] has reported some success, using silicone joint implants to obtain 50° range of motion for symphalangism of the proximal interphalangeal joints in four patients. Fortunately, patients often adapt to the loss of flexion with symphalangism. Arthrodesis of the joint in a more functional position has been successful in improving finger function. This is reserved for selected children who are at least 10 to 15 years old, so that if growth is arrested by surgery, finger length will remain reasonable for function and appearance.

Brachydactyly

Brachydactyly is a short finger due to shortening of the metacarpal or phalanges. The number of bones is usually normal, and the affected finger has satisfactory function. There are many variations of brachydactyly, which are distinguished according to the finger and the bones involved as well as the extent of the shortening. Brachydactyly is often inherited independently as a dominant trait. It also occurs in association with several congenital abnormalities, including Poland's syndrome, Holt-Oram syndrome, Cornelia de Lange's syndrome, Bloom's syndrome, Silver's syndrome, trisomy, and Treacher Collins syndrome.

   Treatment. Although osteotomy, external devices, and bone grafts can lengthen fingers, they do not significantly improve motion. Techniques reported to lengthen digits may be indicated in selected patients.

Thumb Anomalies

Thumb anomalies can be separated into four groups, subdivided as follows:
A. Deficient components
   1. Hypoplasia
      a. First-degree: slim thumb
      b. Second-degree: lax metacarpophalangeal joint
      c. Third-degree: hypoplastic metacarpal
   2. Pouce flottant
   3. Absent thumb
B. Additional components
   1. Triphalangeal thumb
   2. Polydactyly
C. Disturbance of functional components
   1. Absent muscle or tendon units
   2. Trigger thumb
D. Pollex varus

Deficient Components

There are several variants of thumb deficiencies, including hypoplasia, pouce flottant, and absent thumb; this classification is modified from that reported by Blauth.[19]

Thumb Hypoplasia

The normal thumb extends to the level of the proximal interphalangeal joint of the index finger. Hypoplasia of the thumb may be the result of underdevelopment of bone or soft tissue or both and can occur as an isolated deformity or in association with other congenital defects. The upper extremity defects include brachydactyly and preaxial deficiencies. The preaxial abnormalities include malformation of the thenar muscles, the trapezium, and the scaphoid.

First-degree thumb hypoplasia appears as a slim thumb with hypoplasia of the abductor pollicis brevis and opponens. Function is normal or has minimal impairment. In *second-degree thumb hypoplasia*, there are poor thenar muscles, a tight thumb web, and a lax metacarpophalangeal joint. Anomalies of muscle, nerve, tendon, and joint also are present. Function is weak. In *third-degree thumb hypoplasia*, there are partial metacarpal absence and poor or absent thenar muscles. Tendon, nerve, and vessle structures also are anomalous. Function is poor.

Treatment. The surgical objectives for the treatment of thumb hypoplasia depend on the deformity. Moderate tight thumb web contracture in second-degree hypoplasia is helped by a Z-plasty release with or without a skin graft. Severe tight thumb web contractures require fascial release and skin cover by a distal flap. If the thumb metacarpophalangeal joint is lax, thenar muscles are usually hypoplastic, requiring a tendon transfer. The transferred tendon should be sutured into the joint capsule to improve joint stability.

"Pouce Flottant": Fourth-degree Hypoplasia

The "pouce flottant" is a short, unstable thumb that contains a hypoplastic proximal and distal phalanx and has an absent or rudimentary metacarpal.[10] It is attached to the radial side of the hand by a slender skin pedicle and lacks intrinsic and extrinsic muscles (Fig. 3–35). The thumb is positioned more distally than normal, and the surgical replacement of the metacarpal rarely produces a functional digit for opposition. Excision and pollicization constitute the recommended treatment. The soft tissue of the pouce flottant can be retained and used for skin coverage in the pollicization procedure.

Pollicization. Pollicization of an index fin-

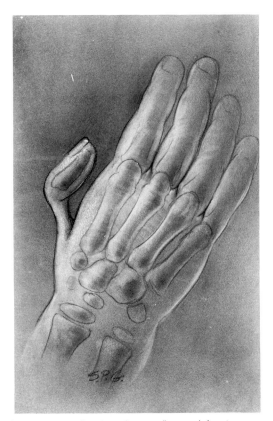

Figure 3–35. A drawing of pouce flottant deformity.

ger with a floating thumb allows the surgeon the luxury of using the extra skin provided by the hypoplastic thumb as a source for skin coverage during the procedure. There may be a number of other anatomic anomalies associated with this deformity.[41] Besides a neural ring circling the common digital artery, there may be only one digital artery to the index finger. This anomaly must be recognized so that the artery will be carefully protected during transposition. Flatt[49] has reported that the operation can be done in one or two stages: The vestigial thumb can be amputated first, with pollicization performed later, or both procedures can be done at the same time. We prefer to do both procedures simultaneously so that tissue elements from the amputated thumb can be used to replace deficient tissues during the pollicization procedure.

Absent Thumb: Fifth-degree Hypoplasia

Absence of the thumb is not a common congenital anomaly of the upper extremity. It can occur as an isolated defect or in association with other congenital anomalies. These include thalidomide embryopathy, Holt-Oram syndrome, Fanconi's syndrome, trisomy-18, Rothmund-Thompson syndrome, and Treacher Collins syndrome.

The absent thumb causes a functional and aesthetic deficit that should be corrected. A toe to thumb transfer and a soft tissue toe (wraparound flap) to thumb over a bone graft flap[98] have been described. These tech-niques require microvascular and digital nerve repairs and may become the preferred methods in the future. At present, they re-quire a few hours of surgical time and a mi-crovascular team, and they are technically demanding. Pollicization is a reliable tech-nique and produces a functional thumb with an acceptable appearance.[7,24,25,30,79–81,115,157]

Pollicization. Numerous techniques for pollicization have been reported. We rec-

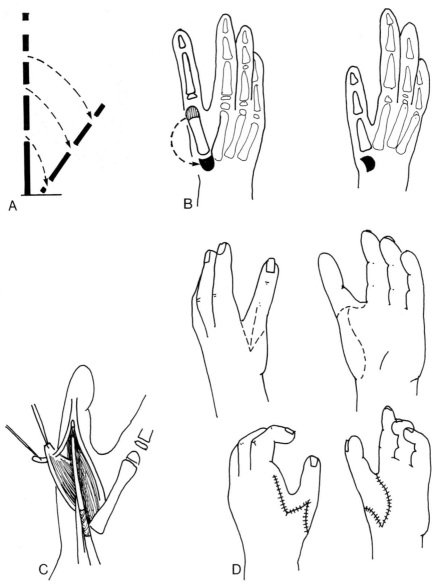

Figure 3–36. Drawings of the surgical steps for pollicization as recommended by Buck-Gramcko for children born without a thumb: *A*, the concept of shortening an index finger to a thumb; *B*, shortening the metacarpal, arresting the metacarpal growth plate, and placing the metacarpal head to prevent CMC joint hyperextension. *C*, intrinsic muscles of the index finger are attached to the lateral bands of the metacarpophalangeal (MCP) joint. The extensor communis is fixed to the base of the proximal phalanx (the new metacarpal), and the extensor indicis proprius is shortened; *D*, incisions and flaps at closing. (From Buck-Gramcko D. J Bone Joint Surg [Am] 53:1605–1617, 1971, with permission.)

ommend the pollicization procedure described by Buck-Gramcko.[24] The important concepts in modifying an index finger to a thumb are (1) shortening, (2) proper positioning, (3) adequate stability and motion, and (4) acceptable sensibility. Shortening is accomplished by metacarpal bone resection so that the distal interphalangeal joint of the index finger becomes the interphalangeal joint of the new thumb, the proximal interphalangeal joint of the index finger becomes the metacarpophalangeal joint of the thumb, and the metacarpophalangeal joint of the index finger becomes the carpometacarpal joint of the thumb (Fig. 3–36A). Epiphysiodesis of the metacarpal head growth plate of the transposed index metacarpal is important for preventing the transposed digit from increasing its length and becoming too long for satisfactory function during the growth period. The digit position should be in 120° of rotation and angulated 40° in palmar abduction for satisfactory pinch.

This operative technique has five basic steps: (1) planning and development of skin flaps; (2) skeletal shortening of the metacarpal including arrest of the growth plate and placement of the cartilaginous metacarpal head so that it is 70° to the palmar side of the base of the metacarpal, a position that prevents hyperextension at the carpometacarpal joint level (Fig. 3–36B); (3) protection of the neurovascular pedicle for viability and satisfactory sensibility; (4) identification and release of extrinsic and intrinsic muscles for transfer; and (5) attachment of these muscles to the newly positioned index finger for maximum stability and movement of the joints (Fig. 3–36C).

The incisions used to develop flaps for pollicization of the index finger are shown in Figure 3–36D. The surgeon identifies the neurovascular pedicles and frees the bundle between the index finger and long finger by ligating the artery on the radial side to the long finger. The common digital nerve is separated into its proper fascicular components for the distance required to prevent tension on the nerve after index transposition. A neural ring has been reported around the artery[41] (Fig. 3–37). In such cases, the ring is carefully split so that nerve fascicles can be mobilized to permit transposition and so that there will be no angulation of the artery after transposition. Veins must be mobilized and left intact so that an outflow channel will be preserved.

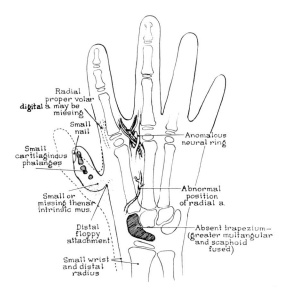

Figure 3–37. Anatomical abnormalities of the congenital hand reported by Edgerton. If the digital artery penetrates the digital nerve, the nerve can be mobilized by neurolysis to free the artery for transportation. (From Edgerton MT et al. J Bone Joint Surg [Am] 47:1453–1455, 1965, with permission.)

After the soft tissues have been dissected and prepared for transfer, the growth plate at the distal end of the metacarpal is incised and cartilage is removed. The surgeon identifies the base of the metacarpal and cuts the bone at this level, leaving a small stump, after which he removes the diaphysis of the metacarpal. The metacarpal head is then rotated 70° so that the proximal phalanx is brought into a position of hyperextension in relation to the metacarpal head, and the head is fixed to the base of the index metacarpal with K-wires and 2-0 sutures. This position prevents hyperextension of the joint.

Experience has shown that stability is important for proper function and is accomplished by intrinsic and extrinsic tendon attachment to the pollicized thumb. The extensor digitorum communis is severed at the metacarpophalangeal joint, and its end is sutured to the base of the former proximal phalanx, becoming an abductor pollicis longus. The extensor indicis serves as the extensor of the new metacarpophalangeal and interphalangeal joints (previously the proximal interphalangeal and distal interphalangeal joints of the index finger) ie. the new extensor pollicis longus. Occasionally, this tendon may have to be shortened and resutured by end-to-end anastomoses. Mobilization of the palmar and dorsal interosseous

to the index finger is done carefully to preserve neurovascular supply. The dorsal interosseous is placed to the volar radial side
of the new thumb, becoming the abductor
pollicis brevis. The deeper palmar interosseous is attached to the dorsal ulnar side of
the new thumb, becoming the adductor pollicis. These intrinsic muscles are attached to
the respective lateral bands of the transposed
index finger at the level of the metacarpophalangeal joint in the digit's new position.

After skin closure with small absorbable
sutures (5-0), a long-arm thumb spica is applied, and a drain is placed near the base of
the metacarpal. The hand is elevated for 48
hours, the vascular status of the pollicized
index finger is carefully inspected every 4
hours, and observations are recorded. The
cast is removed after 1 month, and hand
function is improved by play activities.

Triphalangeal Thumb

There are three types of triphalangeal thumb,
an anomaly that involves an extra phalanx
between the proximal and distal phalanges.
Type I involves a delta-shaped middle phalanx, which is usually angulated toward the
index finger and rarely in a radial direction.[93] (Fig. 3–38A). In type II, there is a trap-
ezoidal-shaped middle phalanx with angulation in the opposable direction (Fig. 3–
38B). Type III appears as a normal thumb
with increased length and without angulation (Fig. 3–38C).

Boys and girls are affected equally and

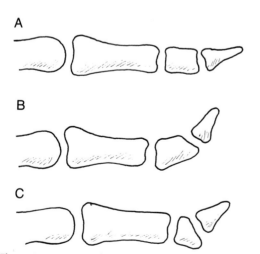

Figure 3–38. Types of the triphalangeal thumb: *A*, type I;
B, type II; *C*, type III. (From Flatt AE. The Care of Congenital
Hand Anomalies. CV Mosby, 1977:112, with permission.)

87% have bilateral involvement.[53, 159] In
some families, thumb triphalangism is inherited as an autosomal dominant trait.[113,
137] Triphalangeal thumb also occurs in association with other congenital anomalies,
which include several cardiac defects, such
as the Holt-Oram syndrome, atrial septal defect, ventricular septal defects, transposition
of the great vessels, anomalous coronary arteries, and patent ductus arteriosus.[46, 61, 62,
113] Lobster claw feet,[108] Fanconi's pancytopenia syndrome,[1] Blackfan-Diamond anemia,[37, 91] hypoplastic anemia,[100] and trisomy
13–15[110] also are associated with this thumb
malformation.

Surgical Treatment

Type I. If the middle phalanx is small and
delta-shaped, it is excised, and the distal and
proximal phalanges are fixed with a K-wire
and a thumb spica for 1 month. Large delta-
shaped phalanges are osteotomized with a
pie-shaped piece removed from the middle
of the phalanx with the base on the long side.
After the wedge is closed, the fragments are
pinned and held until bone healing occurs.

Type II. Thumb hyperphalangism causes
excessive length and angular deviation, making pinching weak and awkward. Removal
of the abnormal middle phalanx was first
proposed by Beatson in 1897[93] and has also
been reported by other surgeons.[32, 88] Removal of the phalanx has been reported to
make the thumb unstable.[121] We prefer the
technique of shortening the bone through the
abnormal middle phalanx, thus preserving
the joints and correcting the angulation. The
bone fragments are fixed with a K-wire and
a thumb spica until healing occurs. The extrinsic tendons adapt to this decrease in
thumb length.

Type III. A thumb with normal length in
the plane of the other fingers should be
moved into an opposable position. Barsky[9,
10] recommended metacarpal shortening and
rotation to a more functional position with
fixation of the fragments with K-wires (Fig.
3–39). A thumb spica is applied until bone
healing occurs.

Mild thumb web contractures can be released by a four-flap Z-plasty,[161] as described
in the section on syndactyly. In some cases,
a rotational flap will be required to release
the thumb web so that the thumb can be
placed in functional opposition.

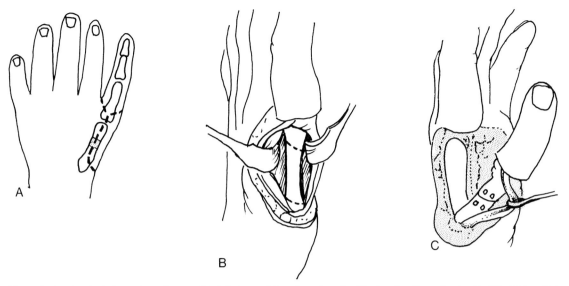

Figure 3–39. Surgical shortening of a type III triphalangeal thumb as described by Barsky. (From Barsky AJ. Clin Orthop Rel Res 15:101, 1959, with permission of JB Lippincott Company.)

Thumb Polydactyly

Polydactyly is one of the two most common congenital anomalies of the upper limb. Thumb polydactyly occurs in eight of every 100,000 births. Wassel[151] has separated this defect into seven types, based on the skeletal involvement (Fig. 3–40).

Type I: Bifid distal phalanx
Type II: Duplication distal phalanx
Type III: Duplication distal phalanx, bifid proximal phalanx
Type IV: Complete duplication proximal phalanx and complete duplication distal phalanx
Type V: Duplication proximal and distal phalanges, bifid metacarpal
Type VI: Duplication metacarpals, proximal and distal phalanges
Type VII: Thumb duplication and triphalangism of the thumb

Thumb polydactyly often occurs as an isolated congenital defect. Type IV is the most common. Thumb polydactyly, however, can occur with congenital defects involving other systems, including the cardiovascular, nervous, hematopoietic, and musculoskeletal systems.[145]

The thumbs of these patients frequently have functional impairment because they are not in a good position for opposition and have ligamentous instability of the metacarpophalangeal joint or an angular deformity in a radial direction.

Surgical Treatment. Patients with type I or type II polydactyly can be treated with a modification of the Bilhaut-Cloquet procedure,[15] which was described in 1890. The central part of each of the duplicated distal phalanges is excised, and the remaining "outer" portions are re-approximated in the midline. It is important that bone be removed into the distal interphalangeal joint so that when the radial and ulnar portions that remain are brought together the distal phalanx has a normal contour (Fig. 3–41). This technique preserves the collateral ligaments of the interphalangeal joint and is preferred when the two distal phalanges are of equal size (Fig. 3–42). If one of the distal phalanges is small, it is excised, but soft tissue attachments are preserved and are sutured to the larger phalanx so that they will act as a stabilizing collateral ligament on the operated side.

Treatment of more complex thumb polydactyly must be individualized according to the particular deformity. Osteotomy will straighten angular and rotational deformities, and growth plate arrest can be used to improve bone alignment during the growth period.

Retained phalanges must have tendons attached or tendons transferred to provide joint motion. Whenever possible, the ulnar collateral ligament—a structure important to pinch stability—should be preserved. Ligaments can be transferred with bone frag-

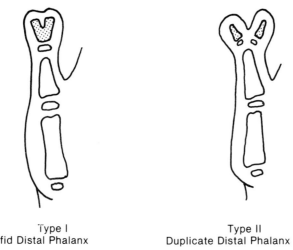

Type I
Bifid Distal Phalanx

Type II
Duplicate Distal Phalanx

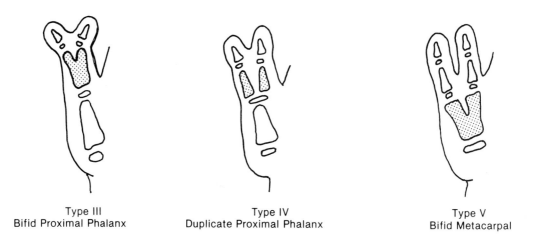

Type III
Bifid Proximal Phalanx

Type IV
Duplicate Proximal Phalanx

Type V
Bifid Metacarpal

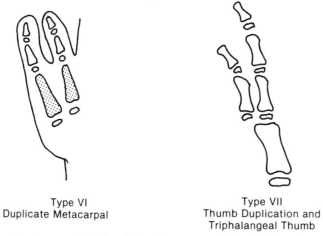

Type VI
Duplicate Metacarpal

Type VII
Thumb Duplication and
Triphalangeal Thumb

Figure 3–40. Wassel's classification of thumb polydactyly. (From Wassel AD. Clin Orthop Rel Res 64:175, 1969, with permission of JB Lippincott Company.)

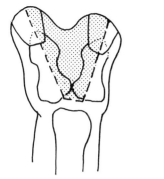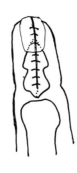

Figure 3–41. The Bilhaut-Cloquet procedure for thumb polydactyly excises the central quarter of the articular surface of the conjoined bases of the two distal phalanges. The bones are then brought together with periosteal sutures. (From Dobyns JH et al. *In* Green D, ed. Operative Hand Surgery, Vol. 1. Churchill Livingstone, Inc., 1982:291.)

ments, or tendon grafts can be used to reconstruct ligaments if collateral ligament excision is necessary during the reconstructive procedure. Suture of the retinacular extensions of the intrinsic muscles are important to joint stability and should be attached to the phalanges that are retained. Skin, nail, or nail bed cover, if deficient in the preserved bone, may be obtained from the amputated parts, which should therefore be evaluated for this possible use before being discarded.

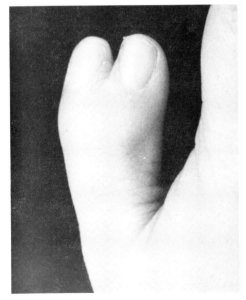

Figure 3–42. Bifid thumb showing distal phalanges of equal size.

Disturbance of Functional Components

Absent Muscle or Tendon Units

Congenital muscle and tendon abnormalities of the thumb are not common, but if present, thumb extension, flexion, and opposition may be deficient. Embryologically, they result from a primary failure of muscle and tendon development or from deficient nerve innervation.

Deficiencies of the thumb extensors are most commonly found in the thumb-clutched hand. This defect can involve absence or hypoplasia of the extensor pollicis brevis[8, 9] or the extensor pollicis longus.[102, 163] Thumb extensor defects can also occur as an isolated anomaly,[8, 89, 163] with extensor defects of the other fingers,[33, 154, 156] or without the thumb-in-palm deformity.[87] Details of the thumb-clutched hand and the treatment of thumb extensor defects are described in the discussion of pollex varus (see further on).

Absence of the flexor pollicis longus and median innervated thenar intrinsic muscles was first described in 1895.[52] This defect involves an adducted thumb due to loss of abduction from the pull of the abductor pollicis brevis. In addition to the adduction contracture, there is flattening of the thenar eminence. Patients with this anomaly have significant impairment of opposition, fine pinch, key pinch, and grasp. Strauch and Spinner also found that these patients had instability of the ulnar collateral ligament.[130]

Treatment. To treat this defect, the surgeon must release the thumb web contracture and perform a tendon transfer to provide abduction. Mild contractures can be released by a four-flap Z-plasty, as described for syndactyly. If the contracture is tight, a flap release may be necessary for restoration of the web. Three flaps have been described by Flatt: the thumb flap[129] (Fig. 3–43A), the sliding flap[49] (Fig. 3–43B), and the transposition flap[49] (Fig. 3–42C). We prefer the transposition flap.

Two tendon transfers have been described to provide opposition function: transfer of the superficialis of the ring finger and transfer of the abductor digiti quinti. The steps required to transfer the abductor digiti quinti (Fig. 3–44) include release of its insertion and mobilization of the muscle so that it can be passed under the thenar skin and attached to the abductor pollicis brevis tendon inser-

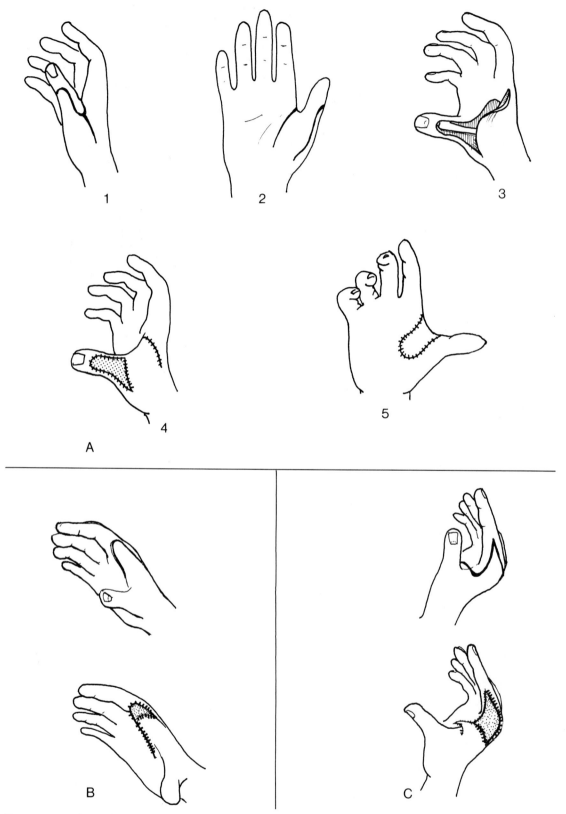

Figure 3–43. Release of the thumb web contracture: *A*, the thumb flap; *B*, the sliding flap; *C*, the transposition flap. (From Flatt AE. The Care of Congenital Hand Anamalies. CV Mosby, 1977:70–71, with permission.)

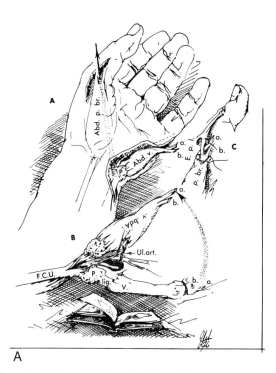
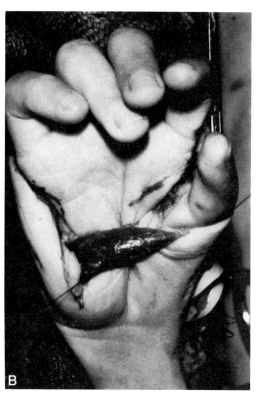

Figure 3–44. *A* and *B*, Transfer of the abductor digiti quinti for thumb opposition. (From Strauch B, Spinner MB. J Bone Joint Surg [Am] 58:115–118, 1976, by permission.)

tion at the metacarpophalangeal joint of the thumb. This transfer provides thumb abduction and bulk to the thenar region. Care must be taken to prevent kinking of the neurovascular bundle at the proximal base of the abductor digiti quinti at the time of the transfer.

In some cases, we use the ring finger superficialis tendon to create motor opposition, a method reported by Strauch and Spinner.[130] The superficialis tendon is divided in the finger, withdrawn into the forearm, redirected through a slip of the flexor carpi ulnaris, which serves as a pulley. The tendon is then passed subcutaneously under the thenar skin to be inserted on the thumb. The more ulnar portion of the tendon is used to reinforce the ulnar collateral ligament. The radial portion is attached in the insertion of the abductor pollicis brevis (Fig. 3–45).

Malpositions of the flexor pollicis longus also have been described. These include anomalous tendon slips to the flexor digitorum profundus,[78] to the extensor pollicis,[119] and to the transverse carpal ligament.[68, 94] Treatment of these tendon anomalies is necessary only if function is impaired. In such cases, treatment consists of

transfer of the tendon for restoration of joint motion.

Trigger Thumb

Congenital trigger thumb is an uncommon anomaly, but, when seen, is the most common digit involved.[38] The thumb is held in flexion at the interphalangeal joint. Pain is produced by passive extension; there also is a palpable click with extension. The majority of patients with this anomaly have bilateral involvement. Triggering results when the flexor pollicis longus glides through a constricted pulley of the flexor tendon sheath at the level of the metacarpophalangeal joint. Dinham and Meggit[38] found that 31% of patients with this defect recovered spontaneously within 12 months of the diagnosis. Thus, one should not consider surgical release of the flexor tendon sheath in children for at least 1 year to allow for the possible spontaneous restoration of tendon gliding.

Treatment. Surgical treatment consists of release of the flexor sheath constriction, a procedure that is recommended if resolution does not occur after 1 year.

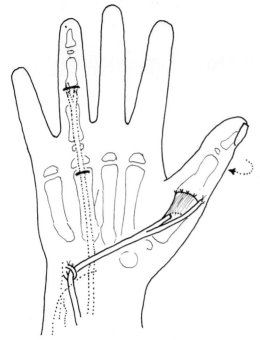

Figure 3–45. Tendon transfer for thumb opposition using the ring finger superficialis tendon. (From Strauch B et al. J Bone Joint Surg [Am] 58:115–118, 1975, with permission.)

Pollex Varus: Congenital Clasped Thumb

All neonates hold their thumb in the flexed and adducted position until 3 months of age, at which time the normal baby then begins to move its thumb,[54] but the baby with pollex varus continues to hold its thumb in its palm.[156] Congenital trigger thumbs should be differentiated from pollex varus. Weckesser and colleagues[154] have divided pollex varus disorder into four groups. Type I is an extension deficiency that is due to hypoplasia or absence of the extensor pollicis brevis[9] or the extensor pollicis longus.[163] Patients with type II have an extensor deficiency with a flexion contracture and may also have a flexion deficiency. The adduction contracture in patients with type III is due to skeletal hypoplasia and instability of the metacarpophalangeal joint. The extensor tendons and thenar muscles as well as the abductor pollicis longus are absent.[102] Patients who have other deformities causing pollex varus are by exclusion assigned to the type IV group.

    Treatment. Children with congenital clasped thumb[153] should be treated with serial stretching casts for at least 6 months so that remodeling of tight soft tissue and de-velopment of hypoplastic muscles and tendons can occur. Most patients will respond to this treatment without surgery. If the deformity persists, release of the tight soft tissue structures on the flexor surface of the thumb by a four-flap Z-plasty or by use of a dorsal rotation flap with or without a skin graft is recommended. If intrinsic muscles are tight, their lengthening is indicated, and in some cases joint capsule release is required. The extensor mechanism must be inspected during the procedure and, if absent, the extensor indicis proprius is used for transfer. The extensor indicis proprius is divided proximal to its insertion into the extensor hood of the index metacarpophalangeal joint, pulled back in the forearm through a separate incision, passed subcutaneously to the dorsal aspect of the proximal phalanx of the thumb, and sutured to the rudimentary tendon of the extensor pollicis brevis or attached through drill holes in the dorsal cortex of the proximal phalanx of the thumb. The soft tissue release and the tendon anastomosis are protected in a thumb spica for 6 weeks, with the thumb in the abducted and extended position. The surgeon may also replace a nonfunctioning or absent extensor pollicis longus by a tendon transfer, using the superficialis to the ring finger,[33] the extensor carpi radialis longus,[163] or the extensor carpi ulnaris[71] if the extensor indicis proprius is not available. In this situation, the superficialis of the ring finger is preferred because the other motors require a tendon graft to reach the thumb distal phalanx. The superficialis tendon is released from its insertion on the volar aspect of the ring finger through a chevron-shaped incision on the volar aspect of the proximal interphalangeal joint. The insertion is divided so that a centimeter of tendon is left, which is then sutured to the surrounding soft tissue to prevent hyperextension of the proximal interphalangeal joint of the ring finger after transfer. The tendon is pulled back into the forearm through a separate incision and passed through the interosseous membrane, then passed subcutaneously to the dorsal aspect of the distal phalanx of the thumb. The tendon is attached to the distal insertion of the extensor pollicis longus if this muscle is present; if the muscle is absent, the tendon is passed into drill holes in the dorsal cortex of the distal phalanx. The tendon anastomosis is protected by a cast, with the thumb held in extension and abduction for 6 weeks.

POLYDACTYLY

Polydactyly is a common hand anomaly that occurs in all races, but it has been reported most frequently among blacks, affecting one in 100 black children.[14] Polydactyly can be separated into three groups by the location of the affected fingers: preaxial, central, and postaxial. Preaxial polydactyly has the highest incidence among whites, and postaxial polydactyly is most common among blacks (Fig. 3–46).

Stelling and Turek have divided polydactyly into three groups.[126, 150] In type I polydactyly, there is an extra soft tissue mass without any supporting skeletal elements. Type II polydactyly consists of a relatively normal-appearing extra digit articulating with an enlarged or bifid phalanx or metacarpal. In type III polydactyly, there is an additional digit with its own metacarpal.

The mode of inheritance varies with the type of polydactyly. The anomaly can occur as an isolated defect or in association with other anomalies. Preaxial polydactyly is often sporadic,[16, 29, 160] but occasionally a definite pattern of inheritance is established. When it occurs with triphalangeal thumb, toe preaxial polydactyly, or tibial deficiencies, the pattern is autosomal dominant. It also is inherited with tuberous sclerosis as an autosomal dominant trait and with acro-cephalopolysyndactyly as an autosomal dominant or an autosomal recessive trait.

Preaxial polydactyly is described with the thumb anomalies. Central polydactyly can involve the index, long, or ring fingers, which present as a polysyndactyly. The extra digital components are contained in a complex syndactyly fusion.

Central polydactyly of the index finger is often inherited as an autosomal dominant trait,[65, 138, 141] as is polysyndactyly of the ring and long fingers.[56, 86, 158]

Postaxial polydactyly is more frequently associated with congenital syndromes than is preaxial polydactyly. These syndromes include chromosomal abnormalities (trisomy 13 and trisomy 18); bone dysplasias (Ellis–van Creveld syndrome—autosomal recessive, infantile thoracic dystrophy of Jeune, and achondroplasia); and atrial septal defect. The related ophthalmologic syndromes are Laurence-Moon-Bardet-Biedl syndrome (mental retardation, obesity, genital dysmorphism, retinitis pigmentosa, ulnar polydactyly—autosomal recessive), Biemond's syndrome (iris coloboma, hypogenitalism, mental retardation, postaxial syndactyly—autosomal recessive); anophthalmia, microphthalmia, and postaxial syndactyly (autosomal recessive); and retinal dysplasia.

The cutaneous syndromes associated with postaxial syndactyly are focal dermal hypoplasia with skin defects and skeletal, ocular, and oral anomalies (dominant inheritance); nail hyperplasia polydactyly and brachydactyly; and Bloom's syndrome (facial telangiectatic erythema, decreased stature, and malar hypoplasia). The orofacial syndromes include cleft lip and palate with postaxial polydactyly; acrofacial dysostosis (postaxial hexadactyly, mandibular cleft, abnormal teeth—autosomal dominant); and Merckel's syndrome (microcephaly, cleft palate, postaxial hexadactyly, abnormal teeth—autosomal recessive).[117]

Treatment. The anatomy of duplicated parts may be abnormal with variable neurovascular bundles and hypoplastic or absent flexor and/or extensor tendons. Joint anomalies occur frequently. One common example consists of two fingers articulating with an enlarged metacarpal. Surgical correction of polydactyly should be completed in the preschool years, and one must assess duplicated digits by clinical examination and x-ray to determine which digits are most functional.

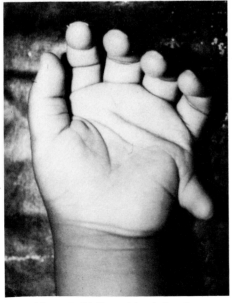

Figure 3–46. Postaxial polydactyly.

Most cases of type I (Sterling and Turek) polydactyly present with extra soft tissue without skeletal elements. The duplicated parts are frequently tied off by ligature soon after birth and allowed to become gangrenous and fall off. If a rudimentary metacarpal or phalanx is left behind, it may require a formal excision. In older children, removal of the "floppy extra digit" is recommended. Central polydactyly involves the index, long, and ring fingers and is complex in that bone abnormalities are present. Flatt and Wood[50] have observed that in these cases, a three-fingered hand is frequently more functional than one in which four fingers have been preserved because most of the fingers are stiff and nonfunctioning after multiple operative procedures. There is a wide variation in anatomic structures, and care must be taken at surgery to preserve the arteries, nerves, and tendons of the retained digits. It is important to preserve or replace collateral ligaments if they are resected during metacarpophalangeal or proximal interphalangeal joint surgery.

In cases involving articulation of two phalanges with the same metacarpal, the phalanx to be amputated should be excised by 1 year so that angular deformities are prevented. This eliminates the need for corrective osteotomies later. In central polydactyly with syndactyly, the abnormal phalanges and metacarpals should be excised by 1 year. Neurovascular bundles must be preserved, and if tendons are absent in the retained phalanges tendon transfers may be required for joint motion. Skin grafts are rarely required for closure. Unpredictable neurovascular arrangements may create postoperative problems leading to necrosis, and it is important that parents be warned of this possible complication before surgery. In older children with angular deformities, osteotomy of the phalanx or metacarpal or fusion of a finger joint may improve finger alignment.

Treatment of Postaxial Polydactyly. In type I polydactyly, the extra digit, which consists of soft tissue alone, can be tied off at its base soon after the patient's birth. In type II polydactyly, there are soft tissue and bone in the accessory digit; if the extra digit is amputated, important structures must be preserved and transferred to a retained digit. For example, if the ulnar collateral ligament and abductor digiti quinti are attached to the accessory digit, they must be preserved after amputation and attached to the preserved

small finger. After these procedures are performed, the metacarpophalangeal joint is held in 30° flexion by a K-wire to protect the soft tissue repair. The K-wire is removed at 3 weeks.

GIGANTISM (Macrodactyly)

Macrodactyly is the disproportionate enlargement of a digit (Fig. 3–47). This is a rare defect that accounts for only 1% or less of congenital hand anomalies and should be distinguished from other disorders that can cause finger enlargement. In macrodactyly, there is enlargement of osseous, neural, vascular, adipose, and cutaneous elements. Other causes of finger enlargement include hemangiomas, lymphangiomas, arteriovenous fistuale, polyostotic fibrous dysplasia, and osteoid osteoma. The index finger is the most frequently involved digit. Multiple digit involvement is more common than isolated single digits.[11]

The etiology of macrodactyly has not been proved. It may be due to a digital nerve abnormality[148] or neurofibromatosis.[22, 42, 64, 85] Other causes that have been proposed but that remain unproved include an abnormal

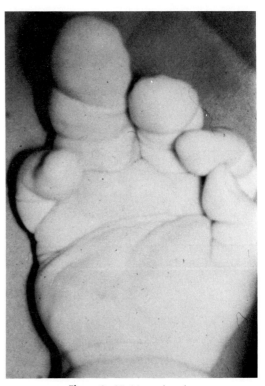

Figure 3–47. Macrodactyly.

blood supply and an abnormal hormonal mechanism.[64]

Two different growth patterns are associated with macrodactyly. In one, the involved digit is disproportionately larger at birth and thereafter grows at the same rate as the other fingers. In the other, the finger appears normal at birth but then grows to a disproportionately large size.

The involved digit is characterized by enlarged phalanges and by increased subcutaneous fat and adipose tissue surrounding other structures.[146] An enlarged arterial lumen[146] and thickened flexor sheath[92] also have been demonstrated. There is early joint stiffening, and radiographically evident degenerative joint changes may be present.[149] The digital nerves are enlarged by adipose or fibrous infiltration. The epineurium is also thicker than normal. These changes have also been observed proximally in the median and ulnar nerves.[5, 146] Digits with problem macrodactyly are unattractive, stiff, and angulated. Their size and malalignment impair the function of the noninvolved digits.

The surgical objective is improvement of function by control of the size of the digit. Children with this anomaly require skin, fat, and bone resection when the involved finger prematurely achieves adult length. In such

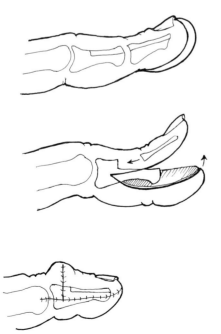

Figure 3–48. Tsuge's technique for shortening finger with preservation of nail. (From Dobyns JH et al. *In* Green DP, Operative Hand Surgery, vol 1. Churchill Livingstone, Inc, 1982:418, with permission.)

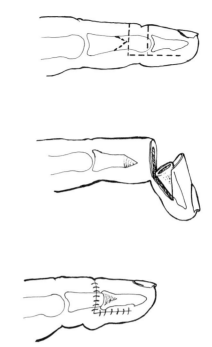

Figure 3–49. Barsky's technique of fusion of the distal interphalangeal joint and soft tissue excision decreases finger length. (From Dobyns JH et al. *In* Green DP, ed. Operative Hand Surgery, vol 1. Churchill Livingstone, Inc, 1982:418, with permission.)

cases, epiphysiodesis by curettage or drilling of the growth plate is recommended for arrest of bone growth when the finger is adult size. If the child presents with a digit larger than adult size, soft tissue resection and bone-shortening procedures may be necessary.

Tsuge[148] has devised a method involving a dorsal flap that preserves the nail. The flap is elevated with the skin, soft tissue, nail, nail matrix, and the underlying dorsal portion of the distal phalanx. The remainder of the distal phalanx is removed. A portion of the dorsum of the distal part of the middle phalanx is removed to correspond to the preserved segment of the distal phalanx. The distal phalanx flap is then attached to the middle phalanx. This often leaves a dorsal skin bulge that may resolve or be revised at a second procedure (Fig. 3–48).

Barsky[11] has accomplished shortening of the finger by fusing the distal interphalangeal joint. Angular deformity, if present, can be corrected, and redundant dorsal skin can be excised at the time of surgery (Fig. 3–49).

Narrowing of these digits may also require separate debulking of soft tissue (Figure 3–50, A and B). This should be done only one side at a time, with care taken to preserve

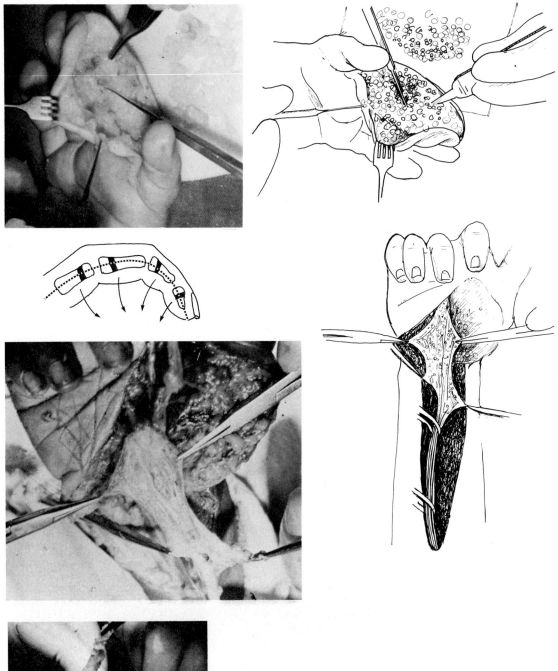

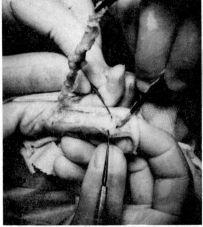

Figure 3–50. Reduction of soft tissue bulk: *A* and *B*, defatting the fingers; *C*, epiphysiodesis of the phalanx; *D* and *E*, neurolysis of the median nerve; *F*, neurectomy of the digital nerve.

distal blood supply. As previously noted, if the child's finger is of adult size, epiphysiodesis of the phalanges by the surgical destruction of the growth plate may be indicated (Fig. 3–50C). In cases of macrodactyly with median nerve enlargement, neurolysis of the median nerve has been shown to arrest progressive digit enlargement (Fig. 3–50, D and E). At times, removal of one digital nerve may be required to decrease soft tissue bulk (Fig. 3–50F). In such cases, preoperative testing of nerve function is necessary for assessment of the sensibility of both sides of the digit. The sensibility on the side of the large nerve in macrodactyly is usually abnormal, and resection of the digital nerve does not significantly alter finger sensation. The result is best if the contralateral side of the digit has a normal nerve and normal sensibility. Nerve resection in digits with bilateral abnormal nerves and sensibility is rarely indicated.

CONGENITAL CONSTRICTION BANDS

Constriction bands can cause upper extremity defects, facial clefts, and abdominal grooves. These constrictions occur in one of every 15,000 births[107] and probably develop as a result of amniotic banding.[47] This may be due to excessive uterine muscle contraction and hemorrhage.[72] A germ plasm defect also has been proposed as a possible etiology.[131] Upper extremity constriction bands occur sporadically, and their genetic cause is unknown.

Often there are other congenital anomalies that present with the constriction band. In the upper extremity, these include brachydactyly, camptodactyly, symphalangism, synbrachydactyly, and syndactyly. At least 40% of patients with these defects have other congenital anomalies that do not affect the upper extremity.[144] These include club foot, cleft lip, cleft palate, and cranial defects.

Proximal to the constriction band the affected part is usually normal, but median and ulnar nerve dysfunctions have been reported to be associated with the defect.[155] Distal to the band, the remainder of the part may be malformed or absent. Lymphedema can occur in these distal parts. Patterson[107] separates patients with this anomaly into four groups (Fig. 3–51). Members of the first group have mild grooving. Those in the second group have a circular constriction band with an enlarged soft tissue deformity of the distal part. In the third group, patients have fusion of the distal extremity components that can vary from mild to complete acrosyndactyly. Those in the fourth group have complete transverse amputations. Surgical treatment varies depending on the extent of the involvement. The release of constriction bands is best staged by partial excision and Z-plasty closure (Fig. 3–52). Only one side of the constricted digit should be released because the swelling from surgery may im-

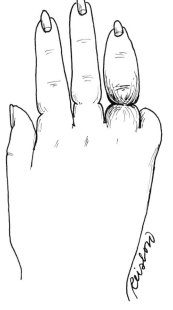

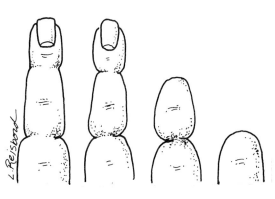

Figure 3–51. The four types of constriction bands: A, grooving, constriction, fusion of, distal parts, and amputation.

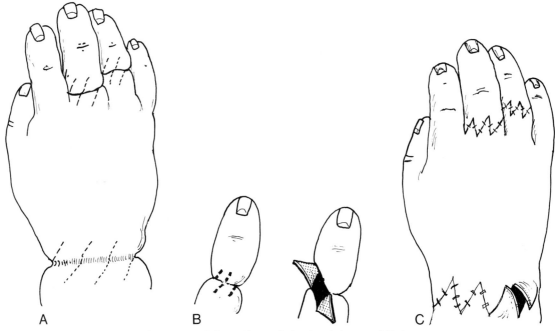

Figure 3–52. Release of constriction hands by staged Z-plasty.

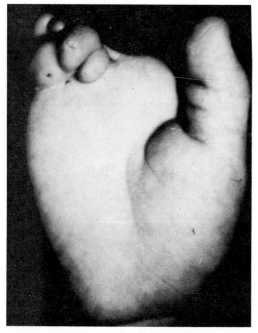

Figure 3–53. Acrosyndactyly.

pair the digital vessel flow, and if both sides are released the tissue distal to the surgery may be lost. Lymphedematous soft tissue, if present, should be thinned from the Z-plasty flaps at surgery. Skin grafts may be required to supplement the Z-plasty release.

Separation of acrosyndactyly (Figs. 3–53 and 3–54) should be started by 6 months of age. Multiple procedures are usually performed so that risk to the blood supply to the distal parts is minimized. Often, the neurovascular bundles are close to the constriction, making their separation and preservation difficult. Local flaps should be developed for covering the web between the finger to be separated, and skin grafts are used for covering areas of skin deficit at the time of separation. Osteotomy, which may be necessary for correction of angulation, should be performed as a delayed procedure after the skin and subcutaneous tissue have healed. Severe constrictions may require amputation, but if more than one digit is involved the distal tissue may be used for transfer rather than being discarded.

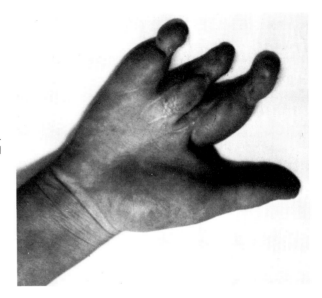

Figure 3–54. Four procedures were required to separate the acrosyndactyly in Figure 3–52 to give the hand better ability to function.

References

1. Aase JM, Smith DW. Congenital anemia and triphalangeal thumbs. J Pediatr 74:471–474, 1969.
2. Adams RH, Oliver CP. Hereditary deformities in man due to arrested development. J Hered 36:3, 1965.
3. Adams W. On congenital contraction of the fingers and its association with "Hammer-Toe"; its pathology and treatment. Lancet 2:111–114, 165–168, 1891.
4. Aitken GT. Management of severe bilateral upper limb deficiencies. Clin Orthop 37:53, 1964.
5. Allende BT. Macrodactyly with enlarged median nerve associated with carpal tunnel syndrome. J Plast Reconstr Surg 39:578, 1967.
6. Ashley LM. The inheritance of streblomicrodactyly. J Hered 38:93–96, 1947.
7. Aston JW, Lankford LL. Use of THW, mobile skin flaps in pollicization of the index finger. Plast Reconstr Surg 62:870–872, 1978.
8. Barsky AJ. Congenital anomalies of the hand. J Bone Joint Surg 33A:35, 1951.
9. Barsky AJ. Congenital Anomalies of the Hand and Their Surgical Treatment. Springfield, IL, Charles C Thomas, 1958.
10. Barsky AJ. Congenital anomalies of the thumb. Clin Orthop 15:96–110, 1959.
11. Barsky AJ. Macrodactyly. J Bone Joint Surg 49A:1255–1266, 1967.
12. Bauer TB, Tondra JM, Trusler HM. Technical modification in repair of syndactylism. Plast Reconstr Surg 17:385, 1956.
13. Bayne Loui G. Personal communication. Atlanta, Georgia, 1983.
14. Bergsma D. Birth Defects. Atlas and Compendium. Baltimore, Williams & Wilkins, 1973.
15. Bilhaut M. Guerision d'un pouce bifide per un nouveau procede operatoire. Congr Fr Chir 4:576, 1890.
16. Bingle GJ, Niswander JD. Polydactyly in the American Indian. J Hum Genet 27:91–99, 1975.
17. Birch-Jensen A. Congenital Deformities of the Upper Extremities. Odense, Denmark, Andelsbogrykkeriet, 1949:15–16.
18. Birch-Jensen A. Congenital Deformities of the Upper Extremities. Odense, Denmark, Andelsbogtrykkeriet, 1949:15–36.
19. Blauth W, Schneider-Sickert F. Congenital Deformities of the Hand. New York, Springer-Verlag, 1976:120–121.
20. Bloom AR. Hereditary multiple ankylosing arthropathy. Radiology 29:166, 1937.
21. Bora FW Jr, Nicholson JT, Cheema HM. Radial meromelia. The deformity and its treatment. J Bone Joint Surg 52A:966–978, 1970.
22. Boyes JG. Macrodactylism—a review and proposed management. Hand 9:172–180, 1977.
23. Broudy AS, Smith RJ. Deformities of the hand and wrist with ulnar deficiency. J Hand Surg 4:304–315, 1979.
24. Buck-Gramcko D. Pollicization of the index finger. J Bone Joint Surg 53:1605–1617, 1971.
25. Buck-Gramcko D. Thumb reconstruction of digital transposition. Orthop Clin North Am 8:329–342, 1977.
26. Carroll RE, Hill NA. Triceps transfer to restore elbow flexion. J Bone Joint Surg 52A:239–244, 1979.
27. Carstam N, Eiken O. Kirner's deformity of the little finger. J Bone Joint Surg 52A:1663–1665, 1970.
28. Carstam N, Theander G. Surgical treatment of clinodactyly caused by longitudinally bracketed diaphysis (delta phalanx). Scand. J Plast Reconstr Surg 9:199–20, 1975.
29. Castilla E, Paz J, Mutchinick O, et al. Polydactyly: a genetic study in South America. Am J Hum Genet 25:405–412, 1973.
30. Chase RA. Atlas of Hand Surgery. Philadelphia, WB Saunders, 1973.
31. Conway H, Bowe J Jr. Congenital deformities of the hands. Plast. Reconstr Surg 18:286–290, 1956.
32. Cotta N, Jager M. Die operative behandlung der angeborenen daumenfehlbildung einschlieblich der daumenaplasie. Arch Orthop Unfallchir 62:339–358, 1977.
33. Crawford HH, Horton CE, Adamson JE. Congenital aplasia or hypoplasia of thumb and finger extensor tendons. J Bone Joint Surg 48A:82–91, 1966.

34. Currarino G, Waldman I. Camptodactyly. Am J Roentgenol 92:1312–1321, 1964.
35. Cushing H. Hereditary ankylosis of the proximal phalangeal joints. Genetics 1:90, 1916.
36. David TJ. The differential diagnosis of the cleft hand and cleft foot malformations. Hand 6:58–61, 1974.
37. Diamond LR, Allen DM, Magill FB. Congenital (erythroid) hypoplastic anemia: a 25-year study. Am J Dis Child 102:403, 1961.
38. Dinham JM, Meggitt DF. Trigger thumbs in children. J Bone Joint Surg 56B:153–155, 1974.
38a. Dobyns JH. Congenital hand deformities. In Green DP. Operative Hand Surgery, vol 1. Edinburgh, Churchill Livingstone, 1982:291.
39. Downie GR. Limb deficiencies and prosthetic devices. Orthop Clin North Am 7:465, 1976.
40. Duchenne GB. Physiology of Motion. Demonstrated by Means of Electrical Stimulation and Clinical Observation and Applied to the Study of Paralysis and Deformities. Philadelphia, JB Lippincott, 1949.
41. Edgerton MT, Synder GB, Webb WL. Surgical treatment of congenital thumb deformities. J Bone Joint Surg 47A:1453–1474, 1965.
42. Edgerton MT, Tuerk DB. Macrodactyly (digital gigantism), its nature and treatment. In Littler SW, Cramer LM, Smith JW (eds). Symposium on Reconstructive Hand Surgery, vol. 9. St Louis, CV Mosby, 1974:157.
43. Engber WD. Cleft hand and pectoral aplasia. J Hand Surg 6:574–577, 1981.
44. Engber WD, Flatt AE. Camptodactyly: an analysis of sixty-six patients and twenty-four operations. J Hand Surg 2:216–224, 1977.
45. Falek A, Health CW, Ebbin AJ Jr, McCean WR. Unilateral limb and skin deformities with congenital heart disease in two siblings: a lethal syndrome. J Pediatr 73:910, 1968.
46. Ferber C. A Contribution to the three-phalangia of the thumb. Orthop 83:55–64, 1952.
47. Field JH, Kaag DO. Placental studies on the development of congenital constricting bands and congenital amputation of the fingers. J Bone Joint Surg 55:874, 1973.
48. Flatt AE. A test of a classification of congenital anomalies of the upper extremity. Surg Clin North Am 50:509–516, 1970.
49. Flatt AE. The Care of Congenital Hand Anomalies. St. Louis, CV Mosby, 1977:51.
50. Flatt AE, Wood VE. Rigid digits or symphalangism. Hand 7:197–214, 1975.
51. Fletcher I. Review of the treatment of thalidomide children with limb deficiency in Great Britain. Clin Orthop 148:18–25, 1980.
52. Fromont. Anomalies musculaires multiples de la main. Absence du flechisseur propre du pouce; l'eminence thenar; lombricaux supplementaires. Bull Soc Anat de Paris 70:395–401, 1895.
53. Gates RR. Human Genetics. New York, MacMillan, 1946:413.
54. Gesell A. An Atlas of Infant Behavior, vol. 1. New Haven, Yale University Press, 1934:243–249.
55. Gesell A, Halverston HM, Thompson H, et al. The First Five Years of Life: A Guide to the Study of the Preschool Child. New York, Harper & Row, 1940.
56. Goodman RM. A family with polysyndactyly and other anomalies. J Hered 56:37, 1965.
57. Green DP. Operative Hand Surgery. Edinburgh, Churchill Livingstone, 1982.
58. Helkel HVA. Aplasia and hypoplasia of the radius. Studies on 64 cases and on epiphyseal transplantation in rabbits with the imitated defect. Acta Orthop Scand (Suppl) 391:1, 1959.
59. Hirshowitz B, Karev A, Rousso M. Combined double Z-plasty and Y-V advancement for thumb web contracture. Hand 7:291, 1975.
60. Hollister DW, Klein SH, DeJager HJ, et al. Lacrimo-auriculo-dento-digital (Ladd) syndrome. Birth Defects 10(5):153, 1974.
61. Holmes LB. Congenital heart disease and upper extremity deformities. A report of two families. N Engl J Med 272:437, 1965.
62. Holt M, Oram S. Familial heart disease with skeletal malformations. Br Heart J 22:236, 1960.
63. Hoover GH, Flatt AE, Weiss MW. The hand and Apert's syndrome. J Bone Joint Surg 52A:878–892, 1970.
64. Inglis K. Local gigantism (a manifestation of neurofibromatosis): its relation to general gigantism and to acromegaly. Am J Pathol 26:1059, 1950.
65. James JIP, Lamb DW. Congenital abnormalities of the limbs. Practitioner 191:159–172, 1963.
66. Jaworska M, Popiolek J. Genetic counseling in lobster-claw anomaly: discussion of variability of genetic influence in different families. Clin Pediatr 7:396–399, 1968.
67. Jones GB. Delta phalanx. J Bone Joint Surg 46B:226–228, 1964.
68. Kawai M, Shiraoka K, Yoshida K, et al. Congenital malposition of the flexor pollicis longus. Orthop Surg (JAP) 27:1484–5, 1976.
69. Kay HW, Day HJB, Henkel HL, et al. A proposed international terminology for the classification of congenital limb deficiencies. Orthop Pros Appl J 28:33–48, 1974.
70. Kelikian H. Congenital Deformities of the Hand and Forearm. Philadelphia, WB Saunders, 1974:467–489.
71. Kelikian H. Congenital Deformities of the Hand and Forearm. Philadelphia, WB Saunders, 1974:555–565.
72. Kino Y. Clinical and experimental studies of the congenital constriction band syndrome, with an emphasis on its etiology. J Bone Joint Surg 57A:636–643, 1975.
73. Knavel AB. Congenital malformation of the hand. Arch Surg 25:1.282, 1932.
74. Kritter AE. The bilateral upper extremity amputee. Orthop Clin North AM 3:419, 1972.
75. Lamb DW. The treatment of radial club hand, absent radius, aplasia of the radius, hypoplasia of the radius, radial paraxial hemimelia. Hand 4:22–30, 1972.
76. Lamb DW. Radial club hand. J Bone Joint Surg 59A:1–13, 1977.
77. Lenz W. Genetics and limb deficiencies. Clin Orthop 148:9–17, 1980.
78. Linburg RM, Comstock BE. Anomalous tendon slips from the flexor pollicis longus to the flexor digitorum profundus. J Hand Surg 4:79–83, 1979.
79. Littler JW. The neurovascular pedicle method of digital transposition for reconstruction of the thumb. Plast Reconstr Surg 12:303–319, 1953.
80. Littler JW. Founder's lecture on making a thumb: one hundred years of surgical effort. J Hand Surg 1:35–51, 1976.

81. Littler JW. Reconstruction of the thumb in traumatic loss. In Converse JM (ed). Reconstructive Plastic Surgery, vol. 6, 2nd ed. Philadelphia, WB Saunders, 1977:3350–3367.

82. Littman A, Yates JW, Treger A. Camptodactyly: a kindred study. JAMA 206:1565–1567, 1968.

83. Lowry RB. The Nager syndrome (acrofacial dysostosis): evidence for autosomal dominant inheritance. Birth Defects 13:(3c) 195, 1977.

84. Maisels DO. Lobster claw deformities of the hand. Hand 2:79, 1970.

85. McCarroll HR. Clinical manifestations of congenital neurofibromatosis. J Bone Joint Surg 32A:601, 1950.

86. McClintic BS. Five generations of polydactylism. J Hered 26:141, 1935.

87. McMurtry RY, Jochims JL. Congenital deficiency of the extrinsic extensor mechanism of the hand. Clin Orthop 125:36–39, 1977.

88. Milch H. Triphalangeal thumb. J Bone Joint Surg 33A:692–697, 1951.

89. Miller JW. Pollex varus. A report of two cases. Univ Hosp Bull Ann Arbor 10:10, 1944.

90. Millesi H. Camptodactyly. pp. 175–177. In Littler JW, Cramer LM, Smith JW (eds). Symposium on Reconstructive Hand Surgery. St. Louis, CV Mosby, 1974.

91. Minagi H, Steinbach HL. Roentgen appearance of anomalies associated with hypoplastic anemias of childhood. Am J Roentgenol Radium Ther Nucl Med 97:100, 1966.

92. Minkowitz S, Minkowitz F. A morphological study of macrodactylism: a case report. J Pathol Bacteriol 90:323, 1965.

93. Miura T. Triphalangeal thumb. Plast Reconstr Surg 58:587–594, 1976.

94. Miura T. Congenital anomaly of the thumb—unusual bifurcation of the flexor pollicis longus and its unusual insertion. J Hand Surg 6:613–615, 1981.

95. Miura T, Komada T. Simple method for reconstruction of the cleft hand with an adducted thumb. Plast Reconstr Surg 64:65–67, 1979.

96. Mohinder AM. Congenital radioulnar synotosis and congenital dislocation of the radial head. Orthop Clin 7:375–383, 1976.

97. Moore WG, Messina P. Camptodactylism and its variable expression. J Hered 27:27–30, 1936.

98. Morrison WA, O'Brien BM, MacLeod AM. Thumb reconstruction with a free neurovascular wraparound flap from the big toe. J Hand Surg 5:575–583, 1980.

99. Murphy DP. Familial finger contracture and associated familial knee-joint subluxation. JAMA 86:395–397, 1928.

100. Murphy S, Lubin B. Triphalangeal thumbs and congenital erythroid hypoplasia: report of a case with unusual features. J Pediatr 81:987–989, 1972.

101. Nathan PA, Trung NB. The Krukenberg operation: a modified technique avoiding skin grafts. J Hand Surg 2:127, 1977.

102. Neviaser RJ. Congenital hypoplasia of the thumb with absence of the extrinsic extensors, abductor pollicis longus, and thenar muscles. J Hand Surg 4:301–303, 1979.

103. O'Rahilly R. Radial hemimelia and the functional anatomy of the carpus. J Anat 80:179–183, 1946.

104. O'Rahilly R. Morphological patterns in limb deficiencies and duplications. Am J Anat 89:135–193, 1956.

105. Palmieri TJ. The use of silicone rubber implants arthroplasty in treatment of true symphalangism. J Hand Surg 5:242, 1980.

106. Pardini AG Jr. Congenital absence of the ulna. J Iowa Med Soc 57:1106, 1967.

107. Patterson TJS. Congenital ring constrictions. Br J Plast Surg 14:1–31, 1961.

108. Phillips RS. Congenital split foot (lobster claw) and triphalangeal thumb. J Bone Joint Surg 53:247–257, 1971.

109. Portter EL, Nadelhoffer L. A familial lobster claw deformity of the feet and hands in a mother and two children. J Hered 38:331, 1947.

110. Poznanski AJ, Gall JC Jr, Stern AM. Skeletal manifestations of the Holt-Oram syndrome. Radiology 94:45–53, 1970.

111. Poznanski AK, Garn SM, Holt JF. The thumb in the congenital malformation syndromes. Radiology 100:115–129, 1971.

112. Poznanski AK, Pratt GB, Manson G, Weiss L. Clinodactyly, camptodactyly, Kirner's deformity and other crooked fingers. Radiology 93:573–582, 1969.

113. Qazi QH, Smithwick EM. Triphalangy of thumbs and great toes. Am J Dis Child 120:255–257, 1970.

114. Reed DA. Reconstruction of the thumb. J Bone Joint Surg 42B:444–465, 1960.

115. Reid OAC. Pollicization—an appraisal. Hand 1:27–31, 1969.

116. Riordan DC. Congenital absence of the radius. J Bone Joint Surg 37A:1129–1140, 1955.

117. Ruby L, Goldberg MJ. Syndactyly and polydactyly. Orthop Clin North Am 7:361–374, 1976.

118. Rudiger RA, Haase W, Passarge E. Association of ectrodactyly, ectodermal dysplasia, and cleft lippalate. Am J Dis Child 120:160–163, 1970.

119. Salama R., Weisman SL. Congenital bilateral anomalous band between flexor and extensor pollicis longus tendons. Hand 7:25–26, 1975.

120. Saunders JW Jr. The proximo-distal sequence of origin of the parts of the chick wing and the role of the ectoderm. J Exp Zool 108:363–403, 1948.

121. Schrader E. Three-jointed thumbs, case. Fortschr Geb Roentgenstr 40:693, 1929.

122. Smith RJ. Osteotomy for "delta-phalanx" deformity. Clin. Orthop 123:91–94, 1977.

123. Smith RJ, Kaplan EB. Camptodactyly and similar atraumatic flexion deformities of the proximal interphalangeal joints of the fingers. J Bone Joint Surg 50A:1187–1203, 1968.

124. Smith RJ, Lipke RW. Treatment of congenital deformities of the hand and forearm. N Engl J Med 300:344–349, 1979.

125. Snow JW, Littler JW. Surgical Treatment of Cleft Hand. Transactions of the International Society of Plastic and Reconstructive Surgery, 4th Congress. Rome, Excerpta Medica Foundation, 1967:888–893.

126. Stelling F. The upper extremity. In Ferguson AB (ed). Orthopaedic Surgery in Infancy and Childhood. Baltimore, Williams & Wilkins, 1963.

127. Strasburger AK, Hawkins MR, Eldridge R, et al. Symphalangism: genetic and clinical aspects. Bull Johns Hopkins Hosp 117:108–127, 1965.

128. Straub LR. Congenital absence of ulna. Am J Surg 109:300–305, 1965.

129. Strauch B. Dorsal thumb flap for release of adduction contracture of the first web space. Bull Hosp Joint Dis 36:34–39, 1975.

130. Strauch B, Spinner M. Congenital anomaly of the thumb: absent intrinsics and flexor pollicis longus. J Bone Joint Surg 58A:115–118, 1976.

131. Streeter GL. Focal deficiencies in fetal tissues and their relation to intra-uterine amputation. *In* Contributions to Embryology, no. 126, vol. 22. Washington, DC, Carnegie Institution of Washington, 1930:1–44.

132. Streli R. Behandlung der spalthand durch syndaktylisierung, eine neve einfache methode. Handchirurgie 2:104–109, 1969.

133. Suguira Y, Inagaki Y. Symphalangism with carpal and tarsal bone fusions. Jpn J Hum Genet 5:117, 1960.

134. Swanson AB. The Krukenberg procedure in the juvenile amputee. J Bone Joint Surg 46:1540, 1964.

135. Swanson AB. A classification for congenital limb malformations. J Hand Surg 1:8–22, 1976.

136. Swanson AB, Barsky AJ, Entin MA. Classification of limb malformations on the basis of embryological failures. Surg Clin North AM 48:1169–1178, 1968.

137. Swanson AB, Brown KS. Hereditary triphalangeal thumb. J Hered 53:259–265, 1962.

138. Tada K, Kurisaki E, Yonenobu K, et al. Central polydactyly—a review of 12 cases and their treatment. J Hand Surg 7:460–465, 1982.

139. Tada, K., Yonenobu K., Swanson AB. Congenital central ray deficiency in the hand — a survey of 59 cases and subclassification. J Hand Surg 6:434–441, 1981.

140. Taussig HB. A study of the German outbreak of phocomelia: the thalidomide syndrome. JAMA 180:1106, 1962.

141. Temtamy SA, McKusick VA. Synopsis of hand malformations with particular emphasis on genetic factors. Birth Defects 5:125–184, 1969.

142. Temtamy, SA, McKusick VA. Absence deformities as isolated malformations. Birth Defects 14:36, 1978.

143. Temtamy SA, McKusick VA. Absence deformities as a part of syndromes. Birth Defects 14:73, 1978.

144. Temtamy SA, McKusick VA. Digital and other malformations associated with congenital ring constrictions. Birth Defects 14:547, 1978.

145. Temtamy SA, McKusick VA. Polydactyly. Birth Defects 14:364, 1978.

146. Thorne FL, Posch JL, Mladick RL. Megalodactyly. Plast Reconstr Surg 41:232–239, 1968.

147. Toledo SPA, Saldania PH. A radiological and genetic investigation of acheirpody in a kindred including six cases. J Genet Hum 17:81, 1969.

148. Tsuge K. Treatment of macrodactyly. Plast Reconstr Surg 39:590–599, 1967.

149. Tuli SM, Khanna NN, Sinha GP. Congenital macrodactyly. Br J Plast Surg 22:237, 1969.

150. Turek SL. Orthopaedic Principles and Their Application. Philadelphia, JB Lippincott, 1967.

151. Wassel HD. The results of surgery for polydactyly of the thumb: a review. Clin Orthop 64:175–193, 1969.

152. Watson HK., Boyes JH. Congenital angular deformity of the digits. Delta phalanx. J Bone Joint Surg 49A:333–338, 1967.

153. Weckesser EC. Congenital flexion, adduction deformity of the thumb (congenital clasped thumb). J Bone Joint Surg 37A:977, 1955.

154. Weckesser EC, Reed JR, Heiple KG. Congenital clasped thumb (congenital flexion—adduction deformity of the thumb). J Bone Joint Surg 50A:1417–1428, 1968.

155. Weeks PM. Radial, median, and ulnar nerve dysfunction associated with a congenital constricting band of the arm. Plast Reconstr Surg 69:333–336, 1982.

156. White JW, Jensen WE. The infant's persistent thumb-clutched hand. J Bone Joint Surg 34A:680, 1952.

157. White WF. Pollicization for the missing thumb, traumatic or congenital. Hand 1:23, 1969.

158. Wood VE. Treatment of central polydactyly. Clin Orthop 74:196–205, 1971.

159. Wood VE. Treatment of the triphalangeal thumb. Clin Orthop 120:188–200, 1976.

160. Woolf CM, Woolf RM. A genetic study of polydactyly in Utah. Am J Hum Genet 22:75–88, 1970.

161. Woolf RM, Broadbent TR, The four-flap Z-plasty. Plast Reconstr Surg 49:48, 1972.

162. Yonenobu K, Taba K, Tsuyuguchi Y. Apert's syndrome—a report of five cases. Hand 14:317–325, 1982.

163. Zadek I. Congenital absence of the extensor pollicis longus of both thumbs. Operation and cure. J Bone Joint Surg 16:432–434, 1934.

PART II

Injury and Deformity

Principles of Emergency Care

CLAYTON A. PEIMER

GENERAL PRINCIPLES

The management of acute upper extremity injury in the child follows the same principles as for the adult. A thorough history, careful examination, x-rays, and appropriate ancillary studies will lead to an accurate diagnosis—the first step in effective treatment.[1] The ease of case management and accessibility of information, however, vary inversely with the age of the patient, and there may not be a direct relationship to the severity of the injury sustained. The physician must deal with the fears of the child as well as the fears and guilt of the parents. Special sensitivity and additional time and consideration are required to elicit physical and historical data and to gain the trust of the patient and family.

Children are not normally used to being independent and self-sufficient. In times of crisis they have even greater need for the presence and comfort of their usual custodians (typically, parents). In most circumstances, examination and treatment will proceed far better if performed in the presence of those adults on whom the child relies. The trust of both the child and the adult must be gained before a meaningful dialogue can occur. It is important that the parents and child understand what data are being sought and the reasons for procedures or examinations proposed. Some young children will respond well to simple explanations and directions, whereas others react more positively if their parents act as mediators. It is usually better to deal directly with adolescents, while simultaneously interacting indirectly with their parents. The physical examination should be demonstrated on the uninjured side first to help eliminate the child's fear of the unknown. Once the situation is carefully assessed and trust is gained, examination and treatment can usually proceed in a routine fashion.

Severe Injury

In any serious injury, the vascularity of the limb or injured part must be established first. Distal pulse palpation and wrist or digital Doppler examination can determine the arterial status in many cases. Fingertip temperature probes are valuable but generally are not available in the emergency department; subjective assessment of tip warmth can be unreliable. Examination for pulp turgor or intumescence can be easily done and the injured digit compared with adjacent digits or those on the opposite hand (Fig. 4–1). If the fingertip has not been directly traumatized, nailbed color is often an excellent reflection of vascular perfusion. Capillary refill can be checked by stroking the paronychial tissues with the edge of a paper clip and comparing the findings with uninjured digits.

Certain serious injuries will unquestionably need immediate operative treatment and are best handled in the emergency area with minimal manipulation and examination. In these situations, no benefit is gained from repeatedly viewing and redressing multiple unstable metacarpal fractures, soft tissue avulsions, or other painful and extensive open injuries. A thorough but rapid inspection and application of a temporary dressing to cover the wound and limit blood loss provide data sufficient to establish the urgency of treatment. The patient can be sent for x-ray, have blood samples drawn, and be started on IV antibiotics. Communicating to the parents a general description of the seriousness of the injury as well as an estimate of the operative time and treatment needs will allow them to assist in caring for their child. They will understand that a detailed examination is best deferred until the child is anesthetized and a bloodless field can be established in the operating room.

Child Abuse

Dealing with the confused and agitated injured child and his parents can be very demanding but is less worrisome than meeting a traumatized youngster who is sullen and withdrawn even in the presence of his parents. In these circumstances or, conversely, when the parents appear overly concerned about a small injury, the possibility of child abuse must be suspected, even in the best socioeconomic situations.[4] With battered children, there will often be discrepancies in the history offered by different family members or from the same person to different examiners, or the story may be altogether inconsistent with the injuries found. The abused child is quiet and fearful, does not spontaneously seek reassurance from his parents, but may respond dramatically to expressions of caring from the medical staff. An unusual or unreasonable number, type, or distribution of skeletal and soft tissue lesions should arouse suspicion. Each hospital or local health system has established child protective and investigative services that should be contacted. It is the physician's legal and moral responsibility to report cases of suspected child abuse.[3]

Physical Assessment

Once a conscientious effort has been made to soothe the child and his parents, evaluation may proceed. It is unusual for the younger child to be able to provide an accurate description of the mechanism of injury, and it should be remembered that parental information is often second- or third-hand. Assessment will therefore depend in largest measure on the physical examination. Observation and inspection, sometimes from a distance of several paces, provides valuable

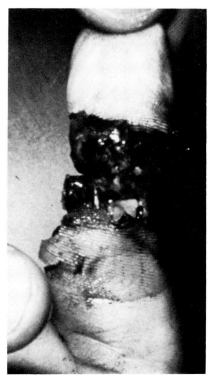

Figure 4–1. This devascularized thumb tip has lost its normal pulp turgor, compared with the proximal segment and other tips.

information that might otherwise be unobtainable. A small child with a wrist laceration who is offered a coin or key from the examiner's hand or from his parents will spontaneously provide data regarding thenar and intrinsic muscle function, tendon continuity, and possibly sensibility as well. Any physical maneuvers and manipulations still required should be explained and demonstrated on the uninjured side. The parts of the examination likely to cause discomfort are best deferred until last.

Sensibility should be assessed early in the examination process. In children old enough to cooperate, it may be reliably established using only a paper clip (never a pin). The methods of sensibility determination[1] with a paper clip are "edge/no edge," which is the equivalent of "sharp/dull" testing in the adult (Fig. 4–2 A and B). In the older child, findings may be confirmed by modified "two-point discrimination," which is designed to determine the presence of nerve function rather than to quantitate the response (Fig. 4–2C). Loss of normal pulp moisture (anhydrosis) is detected by lightly stroking the child's fingertip with one's own; this can aid in confirming a peripheral nerve injury. If a serious question of nerve injury remains even after careful examination and if the trauma was sufficient to have produced a nerve lesion, the use of the scalpel as a diagnostic tool is justifiable conservative management. Primary or delayed primary treat-

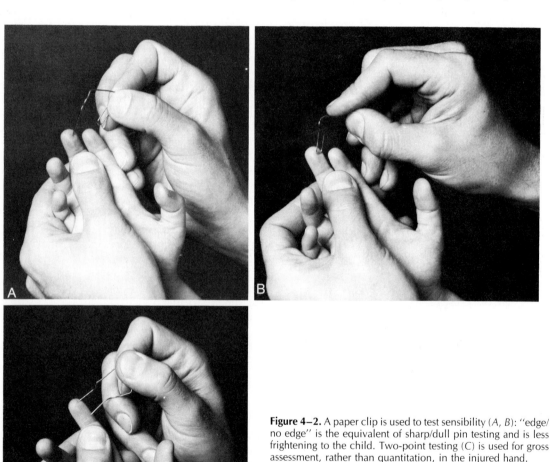

Figure 4–2. A paper clip is used to test sensibility (A, B): "edge/no edge" is the equivalent of sharp/dull pin testing and is less frightening to the child. Two-point testing (C) is used for gross assessment, rather than quantitation, in the injured hand.

ment of nerve injuries is a reasonable standard of care, but overlooking the possibility of nerve division is not.[7, 14] When doubt exists or when nerve lesions are diagnosed, the child should be referred for definitive care.

Careful inspection and indirect examination will also provide diagnostic information in most tendon injuries. The resting position of the hand and a knowledge of topographic anatomy with reference to the site of injury tell the examiner whether normal flexor and extensor tone is present. In the completely uncooperative or unconscious child, tendon disruption can be checked using either of two methods. The presence of flexor continuity is easily verified by squeezing the muscles about the distal third of the volar forearm (Fig. 4–3 A and B). This maneuver will produce involuntary flexion of all fingers if tendons and muscles are intact. A lack of response in any finger suggests disruption. Pressure over the distal flexor carpi radialis muscle produces this same involuntary flexion response limited to the thumb interphalangeal (IP) joint if the flexor pollicis longus (FPL) is intact (Fig. 4–3C).

Musculotendinous units normally exert a static (viscoelastic) effect on the digits to which they are connected, known as tenodesis. Passive wrist dorsiflexion increases flexor tenodesis, and palmar flexion diminishes the flexor effect while increasing extensor tenodesis tone (Fig. 4–4 A and B). A loss of the symmetric passive digital response with this maneuver is easily observed (Fig. 4–4C). The cooperative child can obviously assist, with some encouragement, by attempting to actively flex or extend the injured part. If, after all attempts, one is still unsure of the diagnosis, wound exploration under appropriate anesthesia may be necessary. Tendon injuries are not true emergencies, however, and if someone experienced in treating hand problems is not available, the wound should be cleansed and closed so that a delayed primary repair can be performed.[2, 6, 8]

Roentgenographic Evaluation

Except for obviously trivial injuries, the hand must be x-rayed as part of the complete evaluation. Our protocol is to obtain the history of injury (however indefinite) and inspect the area of maximal complaint before sending the patient for x-rays, and then (finally) to perform the actual physical examination. In the child with open epiphyses, similar views of the uninjured extremity are essential. We recommend x-rays in four projections (PA or AP, lateral, and both obliques), especially in cases of multiple digital injuries or when manipulating a painful finger will only negatively prejudice the subsequent physical evaluation. Whenever possible, of course, individual fingers should be x-rayed; for this purpose, dental films or flexible, thin paper cassettes are very helpful. X-rays will not only disclose bone and joint injuries but may be the only means to demonstrate retained foreign material following open laceration. Lead aprons or shields must be provided for the child and accompanying parent during x-ray examinations.

Anesthesia and Sedation

The specific injuries and the attitude of the patient will determine the timing and type of anesthetic required. If, despite all attempts at gaining the child's confidence, he remains seriously uncooperative, it may be appropriate to use some sedation in addition to local anesthetic; one thereby avoids the risks of general anesthesia in a child who is not NPO. In instances in which sedation is used, it is essential to monitor the child closely; if that is not possible, the use of any systemic depressants is absolutely contraindicated. We use a "sedative cocktail" intramuscularly, administered on a weight/volume calculation, which consists of analgesics and tranquilizers (Table 4–1).

Local anesthetics can be administered as regional nerve blocks at the elbow for the ulnar nerve; at the wrist for the radial sensory, median, and ulnar nerves; or in the interdigital webs for common digital nerves. In no case, however, should epinephrine be mixed with the anesthetic solution, since it will cause a zone of permanent fibrosis within the nerve if it is directly infiltrated with the solution.[13] Epinephrine about the digital vessels can also cause local (digital) circulatory embarrassment due to prolonged vasospasm. The maximum local anesthetic dose is 5 mg per kg body weight. Because lidocaine is rapidly metabolized and its effects may last only 20 to 30 minutes, we prefer to use carbocaine, which also has a rapid onset but remains effective for about 2 hours.

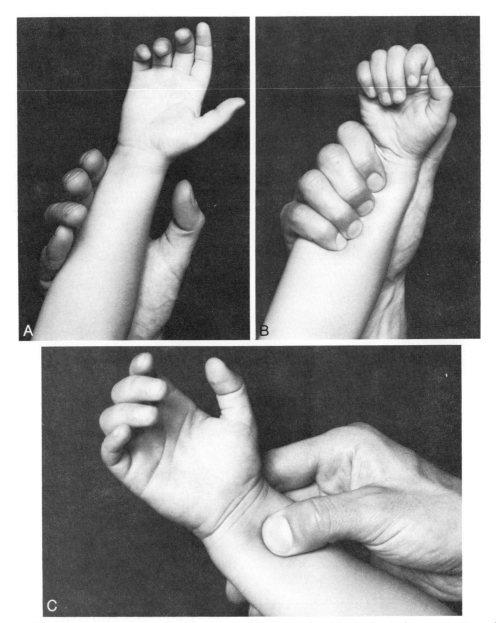

Figure 4–3. Flexor mechanism continuity is verified by squeezing the muscles of the distal volar forearm (*A, B*): involuntary finger flexion results if intact. The same result produced in the thumb IP joint by pressure over the flexor carpi radialis area (*C*).

An equal mixture of lidocaine and carbocaine, or of lidocaine and etidocaine, can also be useful. Etidocaine alone is not generally recommended, since 25 to 45 minutes may be required after injection for the onset of adequate anesthesia. In actual practice, 2 to 5 ml of anesthetic solution is needed for a major mixed nerve block at the wrist or elbow in a child, and 1 to 3 ml for each common digital nerve in a web space.

The technique of metacarpal block (i.e., "digital") anesthesia is quite simple and reproducible if the common digital nerves are injected just palmar to the metacarpal heads, where they lie in a loose, areolar plane (Fig. 4–5). It is usually sufficient to deposit anesthetic about the area of the nerves and not probe for a Tinel response, since the fluid readily diffuses about this space. The so-called digital ring block technique should be

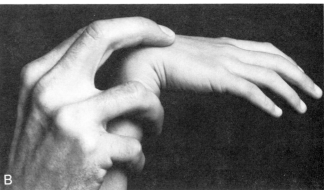

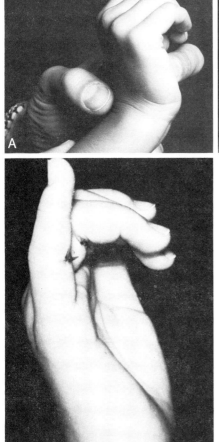

Figure 4–4. Intact muscle-tendon units have a (static) viscoelastic affect on joints (tenodesis). *A,* Passive wrist dorsiflexion increases flexor tenodesis. *B,* Palmar flexion relaxes the flexors while increasing extensor tone. *C,* Loss of symmetrical digital response is obvious in this child with flexor tendon lacerations at PIP joint level.

avoided, since the circumferential constriction effect of the anesthetic volume may embarrass circulation in an already injured finger. It is also rather difficult to block the proper digital nerves within a finger because they lie in the osteocutaneous sheath formed by Grayson's and Cleland's ligaments and must be virtually impaled to be properly anesthetized.

Finally, it may be helpful to secure the position of the younger child with a "papoose board" or by wrapping him in a sheet. Even the sedated youngster may move about during a procedure, and a moving target is an unwelcome challenge for even the most skilled surgeon.

Tetanus Prophylaxis and Antibiotics

Tetanus is most likely to occur following dirty lacerations, crush injuries, burns, and puncture wounds. Although most children in the United States have had a complete and current immunization series, there are a certain number for whom there is merely a vague history of immunization or for whom there may be no record of prophylaxis. According to United States Public Health Service recommendations,[17] clean, minor

Table 4–1. **Sedative-Analgesic Cocktail (IM)**

Demerol 2 mg/kg*
Phenergan 1 mg/kg
Thorazine 0.5 mg/kg

* Maximum dose equivalent of 20 kg body weight for all medications.

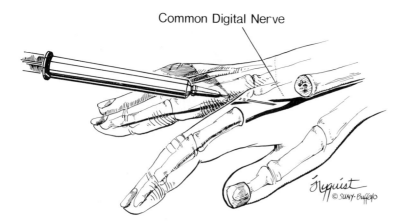

Common Digital Nerve

Figure 4–5. Digital anesthesia is accomplished by injecting the common digital nerves proximal and palmar to the metacarpal heads, where the solution can diffuse about the loose, areolar plane. Skin is entered through the interdigital webs.

wounds require no tetanus toxoid if the patient has had a complete series or a booster, or both, within the past decade. If the child has not had any immunizations, the series should be started in the Emergency Room and completed subsequently. A dirty wound or burn requires the use of a tetanus toxoid if a booster has not been given within 5 years (presuming a complete series). Dirty wounds in the child with no reliable history of immunization deserve both tetanus toxoid and 250 IU of tetanus immune globulin (human) administered into a site distant from the toxoid booster.

Cleansing is the single most important prophylactic maneuver for wound decontamination, bacterial reduction, and prevention of infection. Wound cleansing and debridement are, quite simply, the most effective antimicrobial treatment available. Dirty, open wounds and compound fractures may also benefit from broad-spectrum antibiotic coverage during the first 48 to 72 hours. The drug chosen should include effective staphylococcocidal medication. We routinely use one of the cephalosporins initially.[5]

Specific Injuries

Once an accurate diagnosis is established, the exact treatment plan can be formulated. Primary repair is a reasonable goal as long as the proposed treatment does not pose an increased risk to the patient. Certain problems can be effectively treated in an emergency area, depending on the nature of the injuries as well as on the hospital facilities and instruments available. What is reasonable or appropriate in one hospital setting may be clearly contraindicated in another. Only a very few hand injuries are true emergencies

requiring urgent, immediate surgery. Those problems with the most serious functional complications, such as tendon and nerve loss, do best when treated by an experienced surgeon under safe, semi-elective anesthetic control.[2, 6, 8, 14] The experience and judgment of the surgeon determines what is best in an individual case. Adequate planning and the use of sedation, local anesthesia, and fine hand instruments allow the primary treatment of many injuries in the (outpatient) emergency surgery area. A pneumatic arm tourniquet is required to perform hand surgery; digital tourniquet bands are contraindicated in children. Following treatment, the patient may be discharged or admitted for antibiotics and observation, depending on the circumstances.

Fingertip Amputations. The most common mechanism of pediatric fingertip loss is a crush amputation, typically in a door edge but also from garden equipment, snow blowers, or bicycle chains. If a skin bridge remains (incomplete amputation), it is essential that viability of the distal segment be determined prior to definitive treatment; this is best done following local anesthetic block and scrub. If the part is clearly or even marginally viable, it should be reattached with a minimum number of fine, nonreactive sutures (absorbable sutures for young children). The so-called composite grafts of complete tip amputations, which include skin, fat, nail, and some of the distal phalanx, rarely survive. If hope is substituted for good judgment, the procedure may serve only to delay definitive treatment or complicate wound care. Complete tip amputations in children under 10 years of age rarely require a skin graft, since secondary epithelialization occurs rapidly in the wound that has been adequately cleansed

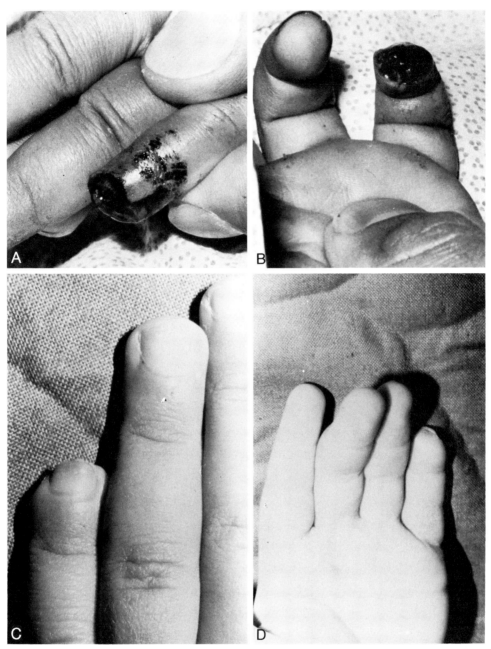

Figure 4–6. *A, B,* This crush amputation through the distal phalangeal tuft in the little fingertip of a 4-year-old child was treated by cleansing and dressings. *C, D,* The result, 10 weeks after injury, is an acceptable appearance.

(Fig. 4–6). Even a few millimeters of exposed, protruding bone will not require coverage by a local flap, as in the adult, but can also be left to heal secondarily. At most, the defect should be reduced in size by the use of absorbable sutures in the exposed subcutaneous fat, or by removing a few millimeters of excessive, exposed bone. This kind of wound is generally redressed after 5 days,

when the child may be started on Band-aid dressings and soaks.

Fingernail and Nailbed Injuries. The combination of a significant subungual hematoma and distal phalangeal fracture means that a nailbed laceration is present (Fig. 4–7).[18] Under appropriate anesthesia, the nail must be removed and the matrix repaired with 6-0 Dexon or Vicryl sutures; the nail is

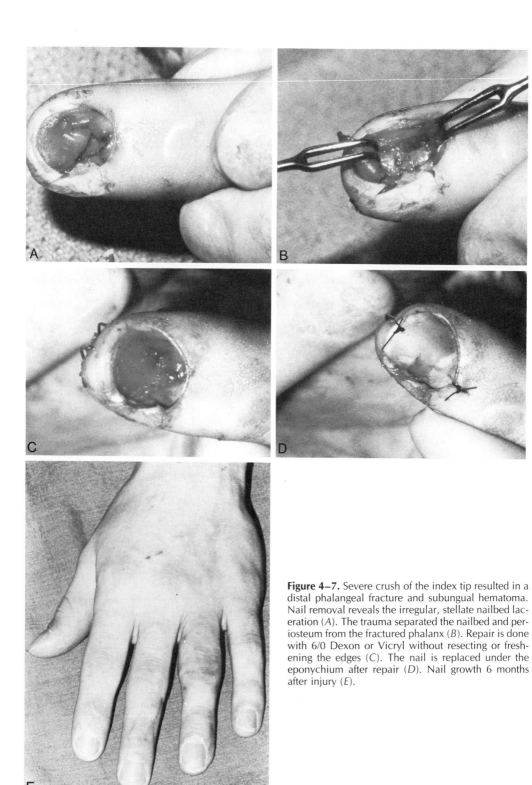

Figure 4–7. Severe crush of the index tip resulted in a distal phalangeal fracture and subungual hematoma. Nail removal reveals the irregular, stellate nailbed laceration (*A*). The trauma separated the nailbed and periosteum from the fractured phalanx (*B*). Repair is done with 6/0 Dexon or Vicryl without resecting or freshening the edges (*C*). The nail is replaced under the eponychium after repair (*D*). Nail growth 6 months after injury (*E*).

then replaced under the eponychium. If the nail has been lost, a piece of nonadherent gauze (Adaptic or Xeroform) can be substituted to temporarily separate the eponychial tissues from the germinal matrix. Proper primary treatment of nailbed injuries will give a near-uniform good result, but those ignored initially are most difficult to correct secondarily. The common, but very painful, simple subungual hematoma without serious distal phalangeal fracture can be relieved by making a hole in the nail with a heated paper clip and evacuating the blood.[6, 18]

Tendon Lacerations. Flexor tendon injuries should be treated in the operating room by primary or delayed primary technique. The final result will depend on the technique and experience of the treating surgeon.[2, 6, 8] In the best circumstances, management of flexor tendon injuries in the child is a significant challenge, and although the biology of tendon healing in children is more forgiving than in adults, the structures are considerably smaller, making their repair more difficult. With adequate instruments and assistance, many extensor tendon lacerations can be repaired in an outpatient Emergency Operating Room. Details of these techniques will be found in Chapter 6.

Nerve Injuries. Open wounds near a peripheral nerve require the exclusion of a partial or complete nerve laceration in every case. Nerve repairs are best done under magnification and with fine, minimally reactive sutures.[6, 14] Primary or delayed primary nerve repair is the treatment of choice and is best done in the operating room with adequate optics, illumination, and assistance.

Skeletal Injuries. Phalangeal and metacarpal fractures are common. Diagnosis of a fracture, dislocation, or fracture-dislocation is difficult by inspection, and x-rays in four planes, with comparison views of the opposite hand, are essential in most injuries. Examination requires inspection of the finger in *both* flexion and extension to determine the angulation and rotation of the fragments. The use of local anesthesia may be necessary in order to (actively or passively) position the finger for proper evaluation of alignment. Closed manipulation may be facilitated by applying tincture of benzoin to the fingers of both physician and patient to aid in traction. Aluminum splints in children are essentially useless for fractures and dislocations; plaster splint immobilization should be used to maintain fracture reduction. Pressure splints

and buddy-taping of fingers to "maintain" reduction of unstable fractures are unacceptable. Unstable or irreducible fractures and dislocations require operative treatment and internal fixation with wires or screws. Some fractures are difficult to visualize on initial x-rays (e.g., scaphoid); when doubt exists, plaster splint immobilization and referral for re-evaluation within 7 to 10 days are recommended.

Wringer Injuries. Washing machine wringer injuries to small children have become less common but continue to occur.[12] The arm is caught and compressed as soft tissue layers are drawn into the rollers. The child may be trapped for some time (usually at elbow level), and a parent or sibling may even reverse the device to extricate the child, doubling the crush. Because the effects of a wringer injury may not be apparent immediately, most patients should be hospitalized for 48 to 72 hours of close observation. Problems can range from partial- and full-thickness skin loss to fractures, compartment syndromes, or severe neurovascular compromise. We favor the use of a bulky dressing (rather than a pressure dressing) and elevation of the extremity in a splint. Specific injuries that develop are treated later; the treatment is described in other chapters.

Thermal and Electrical Burns. Palmar burns and glove-distribution (immersion) burns are unusual, especially if bilateral, and should raise the question of child abuse as a possible contributing factor.[9, 15] Frostbite is also a thermal injury and should be treated by rapid rewarming of the affected part in very warm, but not hot, water (104 to 111°F, or 40 to 44°C).[11] Electrical burns require careful initial evaluation and reinspection or debridement after 3 to 5 days. Small areas of skin loss are treated by gentle cleansing, application of Silvadene cream, an occlusive dressing, and a plaster splint. An office or clinic follow-up visit after 2 days is important for wound inspection and care. Hospitalization is required for many thermal and electrical injuries, and the reader is referred to Chapter 5 for a complete discussion.

Animal and Human Bites. All bite wounds are seriously contaminated injuries and should be regarded as potential major problems. X-rays should always be obtained to rule out fractures and to demonstrate retained tooth fragments. Human and animal bites can be equally dangerous. They should be vigorously cleansed and never closed primarily.[5, 10] Aggressive parenteral antibiotic coverage and hospitalization for a minimum of 24 to 48 hours are essential. Following animal bites, rabies must be excluded by retrieval of the animal or immunization of the child.

Infections. Bacterial contamination is a serious problem in all open injuries.[5] Established infection must be treated with appropriate local and systemic measures. Closed-space infections, such as felons, paronychial abscesses, and tenosynovitis, require drainage as well as antibiotics; treatment details are found in Chapter 20.

Major Part Amputation and Replantation. Children should always be considered as potential candidates for digital or limb replantation or revascularization (see Chapter 8).[16] The child's biologic potential for recovery makes functional salvage a possibility in situations in which amputation and prosthetic fitting would be more appropriate for the adult. Each part must be carefully evaluated; often vessels must be examined under the microscope before a replantation-feasibility decision can be made. The proximal limb is dressed sterilely, with a pressure wrap, if required, to avoid clamping bleeding vessels.

Since prolonged warm ischemia time can prevent successful revascularization, it is important to efficiently and rapidly process the patient and parts for surgery or interhospital transfer. Desiccation of amputated parts is avoided by wrapping them in a saline- or Ringer's-moistened gauze. The gauze and part are then put in a small plastic bag, and the bag is placed on a bed of ice for cooling. The amputated part is never floated in an iced solution; neither should dry ice be used. When there is a delay in transferring the patient because of cardiovascular or other complications, it is wise to consider transporting the iced amputated parts first, separately, and allowing the long surgical process to start without delay. A replantation candidate should never actually be transferred, however, without direct clearance and acceptance by the treating microsurgical team (even microsurgeons go on vacations). If they are already doing a replantation procedure and cannot accept the patient, they will assist in referral to another center.

Splints and Dressings

Operative repairs and reduced fractures and dislocations require adequate protective splints and dressings. To minimize later pain, the dressing layer against the wound should be an open-mesh, nonadherent material, such as Adaptic. Dressings may be voluminous and uniformly mildly compressive but never occlusive. Fingertips should be left in view to allow assessment of digital circulation. The limb should be kept elevated. There is rarely an indication for a circumferential plaster cast, and in most situations casts are contraindicated in the fresh injury.

Digital problems in the young child usually require a splint that extends above the elbow to secure immobilization of the injury

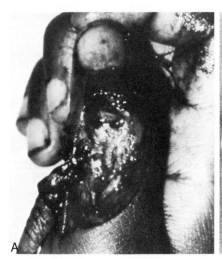
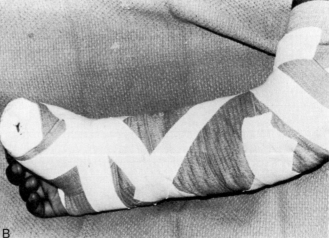

Figure 4–8. *A,* Dorsal thumb skin avulsion in a 6-year-old child required skin graft coverage. *B,* The thumb was immobilized with an above-elbow plaster "sugar-tong" U-splint.

(Fig. 4–8). We use a padded plaster "sugar-tong" splint in almost all circumstances.

Parents and guardians should receive written instructions regarding arm elevation, swelling, the signs of possible circulatory embarrassment, and follow-up care. Complaints of increasing pain should be taken seriously, and telephone reports from worried parents must be investigated immediately by an experienced surgeon.

Acknowledgement. The author thanks John A. Nyquist, Associate Medical Illustrator, State University of New York at Buffalo, for his work.

References

1. American Society for Surgery of the Hand. The Hand: Examination and Diagnosis, 2nd ed. New York, Churchill Livingstone, 1983:2–48, 103–106.
2. Bora FW. Profundus tendon grafting with unrepaired sublimis function in children. Clin Orthop Rel Res 71:118, 1970.
3. Curran WJ. Failure to diagnose battered child syndrome. N Engl J Med 296:795, 1975.
4. Ellerstein NS. The role of the physician. In Ellerstein NS (ed). Child Abuse and Neglect. A Medical Reference. New York, John Wiley & Sons, 1981:1–10.
5. Fitzgerald RH, Thompson RL. Cephalosporin antibiotics in the prevention and treatment of musculoskeletal sepsis. J Bone Joint Surg 65 (A):1201, 1983.
6. Flatt AE. The Care of Minor Hand Injuries, 4th ed. St. Louis, CV Mosby Co, 1979.
7. Grabb WC. Median and ulnar nerve suture. An experimental study comparing primary and secondary repair in monkeys. J Bone Joint Surg 50 (A):964, 1968.
8. Herndon JH. Tendon injuries in children. Orthop Clin North Am 7:717, 1976.
9. Jewett TC Jr, Ellerstein NS. Burns as a manifestation of child abuse. In Ellerstein NS (ed). Child Abuse and Neglect. A Medical Reference. New York, John Wiley & Sons, 1981:185–196.
10. Linscheid RL, Dobyns JH. Common and uncommon infections of the hand. Orthop Clin North Am 6:1063, 1975.
11. Mills WJ Jr. Frostbite: A method of management including rapid rewarming. Northwest Med 65:119, 1966.
12. McCulloch JH, Boswick JA, Jonas R. Household wringer injuries: A three year review. Trauma 13:1, 1973.
13. Oune L. Peripheral nerve blocks. Am Soc Surg Hand Newsletter 15, 1980.
14. Spinner M. Injuries to the Major Branches of Peripheral Nerves of the Forearm, 2nd ed. Philadelphia, WB Saunders, 1978.
15. Stone NH, Rinaldo L, Humphrey CR, et al. Child abuse by burning. Surg Clin North Am 50:6, 1970.
16. Urbaniak JR. Replantation. In Green DP (ed). Operative Hand Surgery. New York, Churchill Livingstone, 1982: 811–817.
17. U. S. Public Health Service. Morbid Mortal Wkly Rep 34, 27, 1985.
18. Zook EG. Fingernails. In Green DP (ed). Operative Hand Surgery. New York, Churchill Livingstone, 1982:895–908.

CHAPTER ○ 5

Injuries to the Skin

RICHARD S. FOX
WILLIAM P. GRAHAM, III
JOHN A. FURREY

Soft tissue injuries in children heal more quickly and with less disability than comparable injuries in adults. When major upper extremity injuries occur in children, growth as well as function may be affected. (Fig. 5–1). Delayed deformity, caused by soft tissue injuries that affect bone growth, can be minimized by appropriate treatment.

TREATMENT PRINCIPLES FOR LACERATIONS AND CRUSHING INJURIES

The fat padding of the small child's hand protects deep structures from most lacerations (Fig. 5–2). Deep longitudinal lacerations over digital flexor creases may cause hypertrophic scars, and in such cases primary Z-plasty or split skin graft or both help to minimize contractures.[6, 7, 12, 13] Occasionally, a delayed Z-plasty or a full-thickness graft is required to revise a volar flexion contracture as the child matures. In more severe soft tissue injuries in which skin viability is in doubt, the injection of 5 to 20 ml of 25 percent fluorescein (depending on the size of the child) prior to examination under a Wood's lamp is of value in determining what tissue should be excised.[24, 32, 38, 46] When the injury causes tissue loss, the treatment alternatives are delayed closure, early allografting, or immediate closure with skin grafts or flaps. For the wringer injury, early excision (within 24 hours) and resurfacing by a moderately thick (1/18,000 inch) split-thickness skin graft (Fig. 5–3) is recommended. Skin graft may be harvested from avulsed tissue or from other body areas. The donor site should not be the anterior or lateral thigh, but a concealed area, such as the buttock region or femoral crease.

Skin Loss

Considerable thought is required in planning flaps for children, since they are more active than adults and spontaneously free themselves of dressings. For coverage of an extensive soft tissue defect, the axillary (Fig. 5–4) and the groin flaps are recommended, and in selected cases free flaps may be indicated. The free-flap technique is technically difficult in young children and is best used in those over 10 years of age.

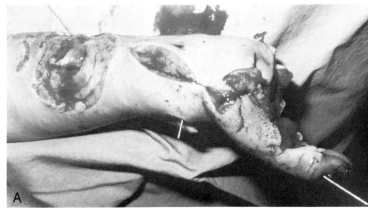
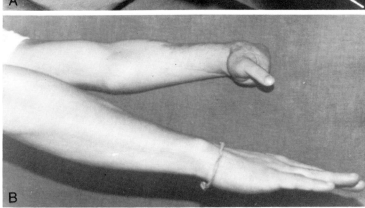

Figure 5–1. *A,* Severely injured left upper extremity in a 6-year-old boy who was run over by a power mower. *B,* Nine years after the injury there is a marked discrepancy in growth in the two limbs.

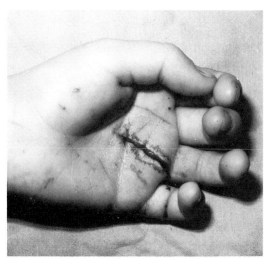

Figure 5–2. Typical palmar laceration of a child who fell on a piece of broken glass.

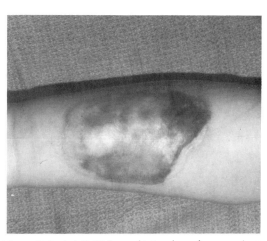

Figure 5–3. A full thickness friction burn from a wringer injury. No deep structures were injured and coverage was by a split thickness skin graft.

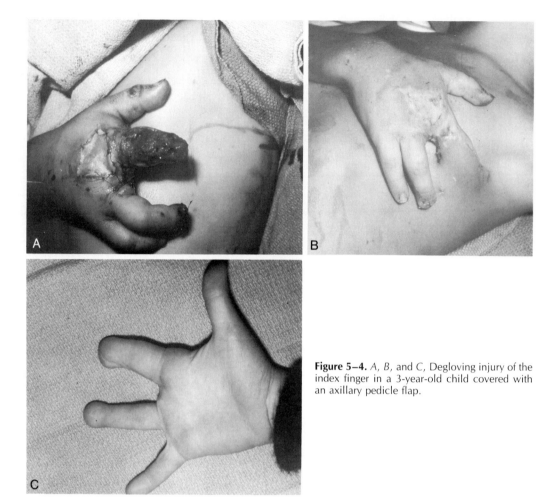

Figure 5–4. *A, B,* and *C,* Degloving injury of the index finger in a 3-year-old child covered with an axillary pedicle flap.

FINGERTIP INJURIES

Children explore their environment with their fingers, and fingertip injuries are common in this age group. Many of these injuries are manageable by dressing changes, with a good prognosis for recovery. If the injury includes the nail matrix and the nail bed, a permanent deformity (Fig. 5–5) will occur unless it is repaired. In these cases the repair of the nail structures with fine absorbable sutures (6° Dexon) (Fig. 5–6), with a tourniquet and under general anesthesia, improves the result and eliminates the trauma of suture removal in young children.

Digital pad lacerations and minor avulsions heal spontaneously when covered with nonadherent dressings. Fingertip injuries with a moderate loss of tissue that are treated with split-thickness skin coverage heal faster and more predictably than do those healed with full-thickness graft (Fig. 5–7).[10, 36, 39–41] The replacement of avulsed tissue may be disappointing because of mechanical damage to the amputated part. Thenar and palmar flaps are not recommended because small hands are difficult to immobilize over the time required for the flap to be vascularized by the recipient bed.

Exposed bone and tendon are frequently present in extensive fingertip injuries, and in these cases flap coverage is indicated. The following five flap techniques are available, and each has its advantages and disadvantages.

Local Advancement. Exposed bone is resected so that remaining viable skin can cover the fingertip. This requires shortening of the finger but provides skin cover of good texture and sensibility.

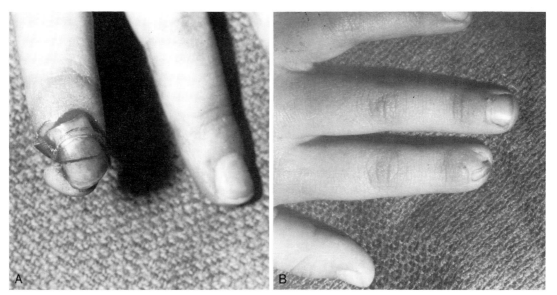

Figure 5–5. *A,* Crushing avulsion injury, to fingertip of a 3-year-old girl (caused by a car door). *B,* Appearance of nail and digital tip six months later.

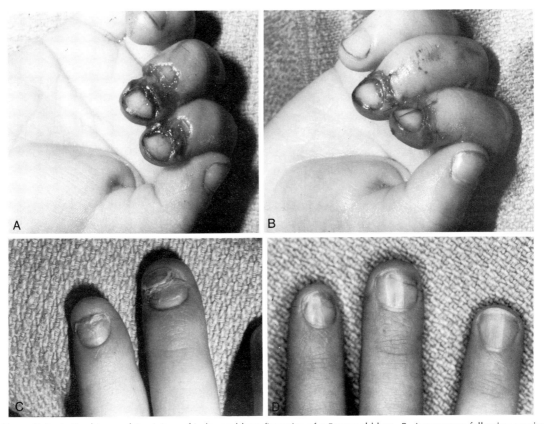

Figure 5–6. *A,* Crushing avulsing injury of index and long fingertips of a 5-year-old boy. *B,* Appearance following precise repair and anatomical reinsertion of nail plate into cleft. *C,* Appearance of nails three months after injury. *D,* Final appearance seven months after injury.

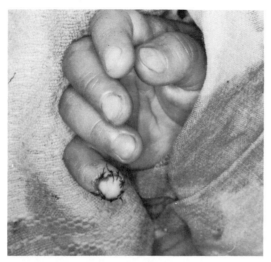

Figure 5–7. Thick split-thickness graft obtained from groin crease to repair an avulsed fingertip.

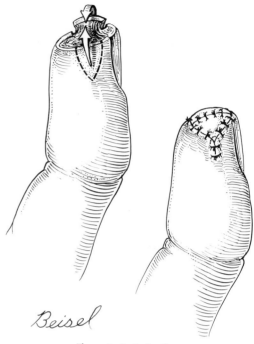

Figure 5–9. Kutler flap.

Kleinert-Atasoy.[1] A volar skin and subcutaneous pedicle is developed and advanced distally to cover the tip. The V-shaped donor defect is closed in a Y shape on the tactile pulp (Fig. 5–8).

Kutler.[23] Two skin-subcutaneous flaps are developed on the radial and ulnar borders of the digits and advanced to cover the exposed bone. The donor defects are closed in a V-Y fashion (Fig. 5–9). A disadvantage is a midline scar on the sensate tip.

Moberg Flap.[35, 45] Radial and ulnar axial incisions mobilize a volar soft tissue flap to cover the exposed bone at the end of the digit (Fig. 5–10). In the thumb and fingers, advancement is limited to 1.0 to 1.5 cm. Care must be taken to protect the digital vessels, or flap necrosis may occur.

Cross-Finger Flap.[4, 21, 47] A full-thickness skin flap is raised over the dorsal aspect of the middle phalanx (rarely, the proximal

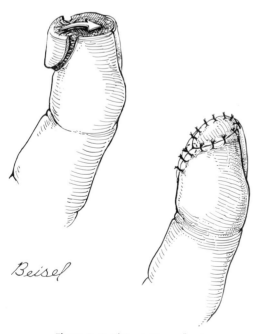

Figure 5–8. Kleinert Atasoy flap.

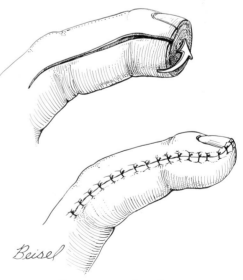

Figure 5–10. Moberg flap.

phalanx) of an adjacent digit and sutured over the damaged fingertip. The donor defect is covered with a split-thickness skin graft. It is difficult to get young children to accept the immobilization time that is necessary for this procedure to be successful. It works best in children over 10 years of age. We have observed scarring on the dorsum of the donor digit in the early postoperative period, but this usually remodels with time.

NAIL AND NAIL BED

Injuries to the nail bed are repaired under magnification with fine sutures (6° Dexon), so that the nail bed can provide support for new nail growth. To accomplish this, much of the nail may have to be removed, but it is inadvisable to remove the nail from the germinal matrix (see the following section). Injuries that displace fragments of the dorsal cortex must be reduced in order to provide a flat surface for the nail bed, which prevents a hooked-nail deformity. Deformities of the nail from old injuries to the nail bed may require excision and resurfacing with a split-thickness skin graft. If a hooked-nail deformity has occurred, the treatment objective is to restore a flat bone platform for the nail bed. This may require resecting the injured nail bed and making the bone support level by using a small bone graft from the iliac crest.[48]

GERMINAL NAIL MATRIX

Repair of lacerations to the germinal matrix and to the eponychial fold should be performed with fine absorbable sutures or deformity of the nail will occur. If there was a complete avulsion of the nail at the time of injury to the eponychium, the eponychial fold must be kept open with lubricated gauze to accommodate the nail as it grows from the germinal matrix. An injured germinal matrix may produce an abnormal nail, such as nail horns. This injury is best treated by resection of the scar tissue between the functioning matrix tissue and its repair.[20] In selected patients, particularly young females, transfer of the germinal matrix from the toe has been recommended.[3, 31, 43] Injuries with extensive damage to the nail, nail bed, nail matrix, and distal phalanx may necessitate amputation. In these cases, we preserve the cartilage covering the middle phalanx, which gives better support to the overlying soft tissue than a cancellous bone end.[49]

BURNS

The majority of burns in children are due to contact with hot surfaces, and most heal with cleaning and bandaging of the area (Fig. 5–11). More severe burns are caused by hot water or clothing fire, but, fortunately, fire-

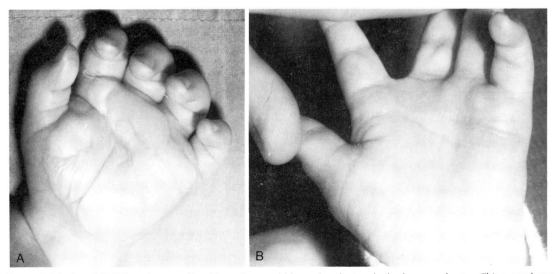

Figure 5–11. A and B, Palmar burns suffered by a 2 year-old-boy when he touched a kerosene heater. This wound was treated with dressings alone.

proof pajamas, electrical safety measures, and housing codes have decreased these injuries. Burns are occasionally the result of abuse by a parent or guardian (Fig. 5–12).[26]

We recommend that partial-thickness burns be cooled with ice saline for 24 hours, at which time it is easier to decide whether excision and grafting or topical antibacterial therapy is the best treatment. Third-degree burns with exposed tendon, bone, and joint require flap coverage. In some of these cases, transarticular stabilization with Kirschner wires may be helpful in maintaining joint position when grafting or flap coverage is required.[8, 25] Early postburn therapy includes carefully designed splints to keep joints in functional positions and to prevent contractures (Fig. 5–13).[19] Jobst gloves as well as compressive garments help to reduce hypertrophic scarring and contracture.[11] Unsatisfactory results after conservative therapy may require surgical correction. Z-plasty and split-skin grafting are helpful for the treatment of burn syndactyly. Scar excision with split-thickness skin grafting may be required for burns on the dorsum of the hand. Boutonnière deformity after skin and extensor tendon damage may develop even with good splinting (Fig. 5–14); in these cases, joint releases and skin grafts or flaps are required for coverage before tendon reconstruction.

Flap Coverage

Burns, avulsions, explosions, and wringer injuries may require flap coverage, and we find the axillary and groin flaps to be the most satisfactory in children. Axial pattern flaps survive well and permit a liberal amount of tissue to be raised for transfer because they are vascularized by a perforating artery in its subcutaneous tissue.

Groin Flap

The superficial circumflex iliac artery arises 2.5 cm distal to the inguinal ligament and branches laterally from the common femoral artery, giving arterial support to the groin flap. The flap consists of skin and subcutaneous tissue and should be raised on the ipsilateral side of the hand to be resurfaced. The flap dimensions can be up to 10 cm by 25 cm. Children tolerate postoperative extremity immobilization in a soft dressing satisfactorily.

Axillary Flap

Based on the direct cutaneous perforators from the internal mammary artery, the axillary flap may be raised as a unipedicle or bipedicle flap. It is usually thicker than the groin flap and after attachment to the extremity defect, immobilization is by a sling and swathe. Attaching the hand to the upper chest has a significant advantage in that it facilitates personal hygiene and maintains the hand in an elevated position, which minimizes postoperative edema.

We prefer to wait 14 to 21 days before dividing these flaps, although earlier division has been reported. If there is any doubt about flap survival, it is best to divide the dominant vessel within the pedicle at 2 to 3 weeks and then the pedicle itself a week later. The transverse scapular[14] and the radial forearm flap[37]

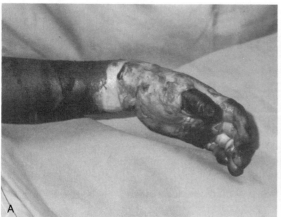 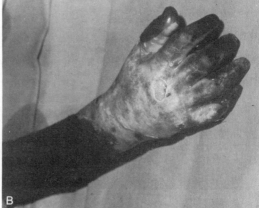

Figure 5–12. Circumferential burns from immersion of child's hands in hot water as punishment by a parent.

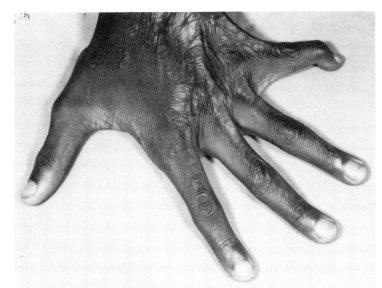

Figure 5–13. Multiple dorsal and ulnar contractures following an early childhood burn.

have been reported to be used as *free* flaps to cover defects in children. In children, however, free flaps are rarely indicated because vessel repair is technically difficult and the results unpredictable.

Forearm Coverage

Loss of skin and soft tissue in the forearm are satisfactorily covered with split-thickness skin grafts. Deeper defects necessitating repair or replacement of tendons, nerves, and vessels require flap coverage, and we prefer the axillary or groin flaps previously mentioned. Soft tissue loss in the proximal forearm is best covered by a random flap from

the thorax or abdomen, because it is difficult to maintain the upper extremity in the required position long enough for the axillary or groin flap to be vascularized.

Defects including soft tissue, muscle, and bone are best covered by a musculocutaneous flap. Proximal forearm defects are best covered by a latissimus dorsi pedicle flap[44] and distal forearm defects by a superiorly or inferiorly based rectus abdominis musculocutaneous flap.[29] For isolated defects around the elbow the anconeus flap is useful for small defects, but the tensor fascia lata or pectoralis major musculocutaneous flap[27] is recommended if the defect is large. Deep defects in the wrist have been reported to be covered by the abductor digiti minimi musculocuta-

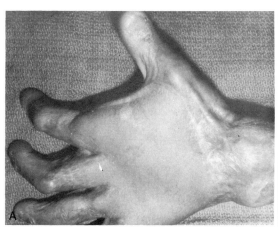
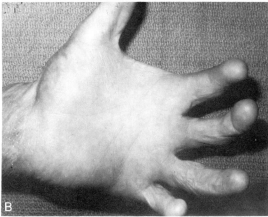

Figure 5–14. A and B, Rarely do hand burns in children require flap coverage as proved necessary in this young boy with a deep dorsal burn.

neous flap,[34] but in young children it is small and the donor defect unattractive. Musculolocutaneous flaps have a good blood supply and survive well but do have donor defect problems. A soft tissue defect and muscle weakness occur after the lattissimus dorsi flap, and a soft tissue defect and herniation may occur after the rectus abdominis flap.

Tissue Expansion

The clinical application of tissue expansion is developing[28] and will play a major role in the coverage of extremity defects in the future. In this technique, a tissue expander is inserted subcutaneously and inflated with saline intermittently. This space-occupying device stretches the skin to produce extra soft tissue, which can be transferred in a delayed procedure.

Z-Plasty

The Z-plasty is a valuable tool for the treatment of syndactyly or contractures resulting from injuries such as burns. An incision in the line of the contracture is interrupted by incisions divergent at 60 degree angles, making the shape of a Z. The flap positions are reversed at closure. The flaps must be large enough to allow for wound contraction, or deformity will recur. Z-plasties are not recommended in children who have extensive damage to local soft tissue, because the surgical manipulation of skin with a tenuous dermal blood supply produces skin necrosis.

COLD INJURY

Deformity and growth disturbance of the distal phalanx are complications of multiple exposures to cold. There are reports that the application of nitroglycerin ointment to the exposed digit for 1 to 7 days following the cold insult may reduce the small blood vessel damage and help prevent these deformities.[15]

DIRT AND FOREIGN BODIES

The impregnation of foreign material usually occurs in the skin of the palm or the dorsum

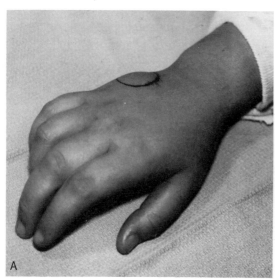
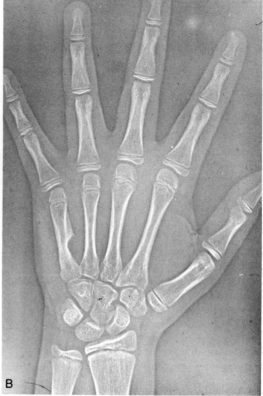

Figure 5–15. A, Marked dorsal swelling after penetrating injury of dorsal aspect of hand in a fall in a field. B, "Scalloping" of fifth metacarpal from pseudotumor due to retained grass fragments.

of the hand. It frequently is a complication of children who fall off bicycles. Removal of the material within 72 hours of the injury prevents its incorporation into the pigment of the dermis. Under anesthesia (local or general, depending upon the age and maturity of the child), scrub brushes, toothbrushes, or dermabrasion are used according to the physician's preference. Dirt particles are removed with a No. 11 scalpel blade or an 18-gauge needle under loupe magnification. Foreign bodies around gliding structures, such as joints or tendons, should be removed because motion is likely to be impaired by the foreign body and the tissue reaction it provokes (Fig. 5–15). Foreign bodies of plant origin are capable of producing marked reaction (pseudotumors) that can produce bony deformities not unlike those of cellular tumors (Fig. 5–15). In general, foreign bodies in the hands of children should be removed in the hospital and not in the office.

References

1. Atasoy E, Ioakimidis E, Kasdan MD, et al. Reconstruction of amputated finger tip with triangular volar flap: New surgical procedures. J Bone Joint Surg 52A:921, 1970.
2. Bossley CJ. Terminal digit amputations. J Bone Joint Surg 57B:257, 1975.
3. Buncke HJ Jr, Gonzalez RI. Fingernail reconstruction. Plast Reconstr Surg 30:452, 1962.
4. Cohen BE, Cronin BD. An innervated cross finger flap for fingertip reconstruction. Plast Reconstr Surg 72:688, 1983.
5. Conolly WB. Spontaneous healing of hand wounds. Aust NZ J Surg 44:393, 1974.
6. Davis JS. Present evaluation of the merits of the Z-plasty operation. Plast Reconstr Surg 1:26, 1946.
7. Dingman RO. Some applications of the Z-plasty procedure. Plast Reconstr Surg 16:246, 1955.
8. Evans EB, Larson DO, Alleston S, et al. Prevention and correction of deformity after severe burns. Surg Clin North Am 50:1361, 1970.
9. Fox CL. Use of silver sulfadiazine in burned patients. In Lynch JB, and Lewis SR (eds). Symposium on the Treatment of Burns. St Louis, CV Mosby, 1973.
10. Frazier TG, Graham WP. Finger tip injuries. Penn Med 74:51, 1971.
11. Fujimari R, Hiramoto M, Ofufi S. Sponge fixation method for treatment of early scars. Plast Reconstr Surg 42:322, 1968.
12. Furnas DW, Fischer GW. The Z-Plasty: Biomechanics and mathematics. Br J Plast Surg 24:144, 1971.
13. Gibson T, Kenedi RM. Biomechanical properties of skin. Surg Clin North Am 47:279, 1967.
14. Gilbert A, Teot L. The free scapular flap. Plast Reconstr Surg 69(4):601–604, 1982.
15. Graham WP III, Furrery JA, Manders EK. Treatment of frostbite with nitroglycerin paste. Proceedings, Northeastern Society of Plastic Surgeons, Philadelphia, Sept, 1984.
16. Holm A, Zachariae L. Fingertip lesions: An evaluation of conservative treatment vs free skin grafting. Acta Orthop Scand 45:382, 1974.
17. Illingworth CM. Trapped fingers and amputated fingers in children. J Pediat Surg 9:853, 1974.
18. Janzekovic Z. A new concept in early excision and immediate grafting of burns. J Trauma 10:1103, 1970.
19. Johnson CJ, Graham WP III. Use of thermoplastic splints in the treatment of burned hands. Plast Reconstr Surg 41:399, 1969.
20. Johnson RK. Nail plasty. Plast Reconstr Surg 47:275, 1971.
21. Joshi DB. A sensory cross finger flap for use on the index finger. Plast Reconstr Surg 58:210, 1976.
22. Ketchum LD. Skin flaps. In Green DP, ed. Operative Hand Surgery. New York, Churchill Livingstone, 1982:1315–1345.
23. Kilgore ES, Graham WP III. The Hand, Surgical and Non-Surgical Management. Philadelphia, Lea & Febiger, 1977:280.
24. Kutler W. A new method for finger tip amputation. JAMA 133:29, 1947.
25. Lange K, Boyd LJ. The use of fluorescein to determine the adequacy of circulation. Med Clin North Am 26:943, 1942.
26. Larson DL, Abston S, Evans EB, et al. Techniques for decreasing scar formation and contractures in the burned patient. J Trauma 11:807, 1971.
27. Luce E, Gottlieb S. The pectoralis major island flap for coverage in the upper extremity. J Hand Surg 7(2):156, 1982.
28. Lung RJ, Davis TS, Graham WP, et al. Burns as a manifestation of the battered child syndrome. Clin Res 24(5):622A, 1976.
29. Manders EK, et al. Soft tissue expansion: Concepts and complications. Plast Reconstr Surg 74(4):493–507, 1984.
30. Mathes SJ, Nahai F. Upper extremity—reconstruction. In Mathes SJ, and Nahai F (eds.) Clinical Applications for Muscle and Musculocutaneous Flaps. St Louis, CV Mosby, 1982:620–633.
31. May JW, Bartlett S. The groin flap in pediatric hand reconstruction. Proceedings, Thirty-fifth Annual Meeting of the American Society for Surgery of the Hand. Atlanta, Feb 4–6, 1980.
32. McCash CR. Free nail grafting. Br J Plast Surg 8:19, 1955.
33. McCraw JB, Myers B, Shanklin KD. The value of fluorescein in predicting the viability of arterialized flaps. Plast Reconstr Surg 60:710, 1977.
34. McGregor RA, Jackson RT. The groin flap. Br J Plast Surg 25:3, 1972.
35. Millard TM, Stott WG, Kleinert HE. The abductor digiti minimi muscle flap. Hand 9:82, 1977.
36. Moberg E. Aspects of sensation in reconstructive surgery of the upper extremity. J Bone Joint Surg 46A:817, 1964.
37. Mosher JF. Split thickness hypothenar grafts for skin defects of the hand. Hand 9:45, 1977.
38. Muhlbauer W, Herndl E, Stock W. The forearm flap. Plast Reconstr Surg 70:336–342, 1982.
39. Myers MB. Prediction of skin sloughs at the time of operation with the use of fluorescein dye. Surgery 51:158, 1962.
40. Patton HS. Split skin grafts from hypothenar area for fingertip avulsions. Plast Reconstr Surg 43:426, 1969.
41. Porter RW. Functional assessment of transplanted

skin in volar defects of the digits. J Bone Joint Surg 50A:955, 1968.

42. Salaman JR. Partial thickness skin grafting of fingertip injuries. Lancet 1:705, 1967.

43. Salter RB, Harris WR. Injuries involving the epiphyseal plate. J Bone Joint Surg 45A:586, 1963.

44. Schiller C. Nail replacement in fingertip injuries. Plast Reconstr Surg 19:521, 1957.

45. Silverston JS, Nahai F, Jurkiewicz MJ. The latissimus dorsi myocutaneous flap to replace a defect on the upper arm. Br J Plast Surg 31:29, 1978.

46. Snow JW. The use of a volar flap for repair of finger tip amputations: a preliminary report. Plast Reconstr Surg 40:163, 1967.

47. Stein MR, Parker CW. Reactions following intravenous fluorescein. Am J Ophthalmol 72:861, 1971.

48. Thomson HG, Sorokolet WT. The cross finger flap in children. A follow up study. Plast Reconstr Surg 39:482, 1967.

49. Verdan C. The Nail. New York, Churchill Livingstone, 1981:93–101.

50. Whitaker LA, Graham WP III, Riser WH, et al. Retaining the articular cartilage in finger tip amputations. Plast Reconstr Surg 49:542, 1972.

CHAPTER ◦ 6

Injuries to Tendons

LAWRENCE H. SCHNEIDER

The treatment of tendon injuries in children parallels the treatment recommended for adults. There are, however, some different problems in the treatment of children that warrant special consideration in their care. For example, it is difficult, at times, to make the correct diagnosis in the injured child. Because the structures are smaller, their surgical repair is more exacting; after surgery, children are more difficult to immobilize and rehabilitation is less predictable.[28] On the positive side, children heal quickly and rarely develop joint contractures unless their joints have sustained direct injury. They are seldom involved in the economic and legal problems that tend to impair the recovery process in many adults.

DIAGNOSIS OF TENDON INJURY

The recognition of tendon injury is best made by the posture of the involved fingers at rest and with hand motion. The patient examiner can often make a diagnosis on seeing one finger more flexed than the others, suggesting an extensor tendon injury, or an extension posture of a finger, indicating a flexor tendon injury (Fig. 6–1). Also helpful is the use of techniques to stimulate withdrawal of the fingers into flexion or extension, thereby testing tendon continuity. The examiner must be wary of a patient using the adjacent fingers (trapping) to flex a finger with a flexion tendon injury, a substitution technique that develops in old injuries. Difficulty in diagnosis may justify exploratory surgery on some occasions.

EXTENSOR TENDON INJURIES

Some authors[9, 63] now recognize that extensor injuries can produce poor functional results similar to those that occur after flexor tendon injuries. The treatment of extensor tendons therefore requires the anatomic knowledge, decision making, and attention to detail that is needed for the successful treatment of flexor tendon injuries. I repair extensor tendons with 4-0 Dacron suture and the skin with 5-0 absorbable suture.

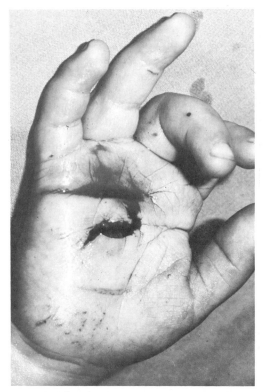

Figure 6–1. In the hand at rest, the extended posture of the ring and little fingers in association with the palmar wound strongly suggests interruption of the flexor tendons to those fingers.

Extensor Tendon Anatomy

The long extensor tendons of the fingers in the forearm include the extensor digitorum, the extensor indicis, and the extensor digiti minimi. These pass beneath the extensor retinaculum and join the tendons of the intrinsic muscles, the interossei and lumbricals, to form the dorsal apparatus at the MP joint. The long extensors are the prime extensors of the MP joint through the sagittal bands of the extensor hood mechanism. Distally through a complex linkage, the long extensors and the intrinsics form the extensor mechanism of the fingers (Fig. 6–2). This mechanism, along with the retinacular ligament system, control extension in the fingers.[16, 22, 26, 27, 37, 47, 76, 77]

Acute Extensor Tendon Injury. Because the extensor tendons in the fingers have interconnections, retraction does not occur, and injuries, if seen early, can often be treated nonoperatively by splinting. Injuries seen late more frequently require surgery and

have poorer results, making an early diagnosis important.[12]

Injuries at the Distal Interphalangeal Joint (Mallet Injury)

This injury results from a strong flexion force applied at the extended fingertip, with resultant stretching or tearing of the extensor tendon. Commonly seen in sport activities, it has been called baseball finger or drop finger. Swelling about the joint may, early on, mask injury to the tendon, causing a delay in seeking treatment. Most of these tendon ruptures are closed injuries, but some are caused by a laceration at the level of the DIP joint (Fig. 6–3). After injury, close observation of the finger will show an inability to fully extend the distal joint. Although the mallet finger usually occurs without bone injury, x-ray studies of the finger may show avulsion of bone from the dorsal base of the distal phalanx of varying size, up to a complete separation of the epiphyseal plate.

Treatment of Acute Injury

I recommend maintenance of the finger in extension for 6 weeks.[19] In children, this usually requires the application of some unremovable device, such as a finger cast.[74] It is important that the finger be held straight (zero degrees) for 6 weeks; otherwise, healing is disrupted and it is necessary to start the 6-week period over again. Although many different splint devices have been marketed for the treatment of this lesion, in children the cast technique is recommended. The most frequent cause of failure is premature removal of the device. In older children the PIP joint should be included in flexion, in order to keep the device on (Fig. 6–4). In younger children, I use a hand cast that extends above the wrist. The open mallet finger is treated by wound closure, followed by immobilization for 6 weeks. An alternative technique for external splinting is the placement of a fine Kirschner wire longitudinally down the medullary canal of the distal phalanx, across the joint (at zero degrees), and into the proximal portion of the middle phalanx. This internal fixation technique is particularly recommended for a hand with multiple open injuries requiring surgery.

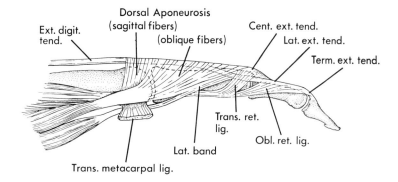

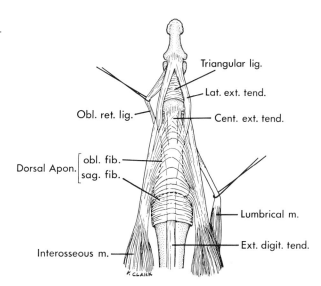

Figure 6–2. Anatomy of the extensor system in the fingers.

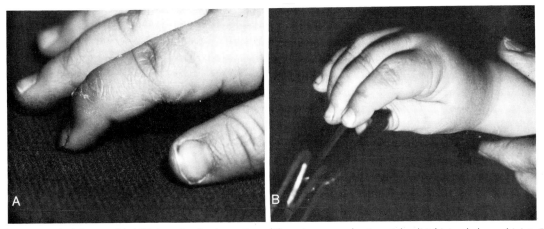

Figure 6–3. *A*, A 2-year-old child 4 weeks after laceration of the extensor mechanism at the distal interphalangeal joint. *B*, Full extension was recovered by casting in extension for six weeks.

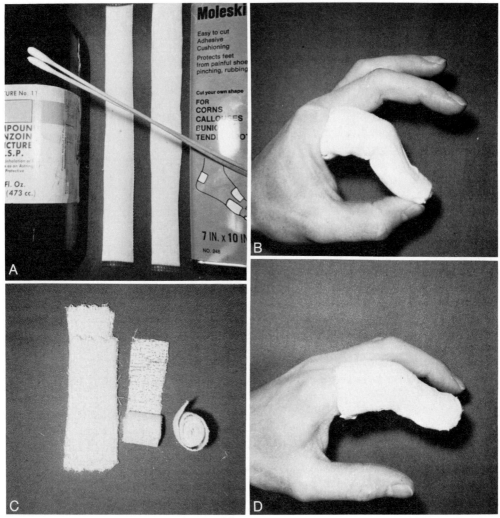

Figure 6–4. Cast technique. *A*, Materials include padded adhesive tape and a liquid skin adherent. *B*, The padded adhesive is applied in strips to the finger. If the patient is old enough, he or she can be shown the position to adopt while the plaster is setting. *C*, Fast-setting plaster is precut in ¾-inch widths. *D*, The completed cast.

Whatever form of immobilization is used, placement of the DIP joint in hyperextension should be avoided, for it can cause an area of skin necrosis over the DIP joint.

The widely displaced epiphyseal avulsion is not a true tendon injury but requires open reduction, with gentle replacement of the fragment with its attached tendon. The placement of a Kirschner wire (0.028 inch in the younger child) will serve to hold the fragment until healing occurs (usually 4 weeks) (Fig. 6–5).[86]

Several operative procedures have been reported for the treatment of the extensor tendon injury at this level.[18, 78] These procedures are not indicated in the acute closed tendon injury in the child, and open surgery

is recommended only for the epiphyseal separation, as previously mentioned.

Chronic Extensor Injury at the Distal Interphalangeal Joint Level

It is not uncommon for the mallet injury to go unrecognized in the young child. If mobility and full passive extension are present, I treat these old injuries by 6 weeks of uninterrupted extension, regardless of the time elapsed since injury. This may require the use of a fine longitudinal Kirschner wire when the patient cannot comply with the casting program.

When the joint has a fixed flexion contracture of 20 degrees, stretching spring

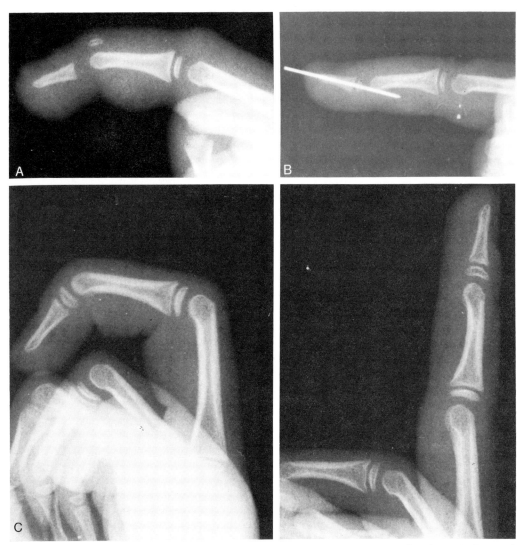

Figure 6–5. *A*, A widely displaced mallet fracture is represented in this child by epiphyseal avulsion. *B*, Open reduction with Kirschner-wire fixation. *C*, Result 2 years later.

splints are helpful but passive stretching followed by the application of a nonpadded plaster is more successful. This technique is repeated with weekly cast changes until a neutral position (zero degrees) is achieved, which usually requires 6 to 8 weeks.

When a patient has not responded to the conservative procedures described, I have found it was usually due to improperly applied or unsupervised splinting or a failure of the patient to cooperate in the program. Rarely is operative shortening of the extensor mechanism required in these chronic injuries.[18] In the few instances in which open repair was done, I shortened the healed but lengthened extensor mechanism either by

reefing the tendon or by cutting, then overlapping and suturing, the tendon. The finger is then immobilized for 6 weeks. There may be difficulty in regaining flexion in these joints after surgery, but extension is usually full. Because of the importance of full flexion of the ulnar fingers for power grip, the exchange of flexion for extension by surgery is rarely indicated in the ring and small digits.

Aftercare in Mallet Finger Injury. Assuming adequate immobilization has been carried out, the aftercare period is directed to regaining flexion. If active flexion exercises fail, blocking exercises are added. This technique stabilizes the middle phalanx while the patient actively flexes the distal joint.

Most young people need no formal exercise program after closed treatment.

Boutonnière Injuries (Extensor Mechanism Disruption at the Proximal Interphalangeal Joint Level)

Injury to the extensor mechanism of the finger at the level of the PIP joint presents with swelling and tenderness over the dorsum of the joint. Loss or weakness of extension is present, and occasionally there is a small chip fracture where the central slip has been avulsed.

Stretching or laceration of the central slip creates a tendon defect that is gradually enlarged by flexion of the PIP joint with pushing of the head of the proximal phalanx through the defect (Fig. 6–6). This force gradually displaces the lateral bands more laterally, and the bands begin a volar migration around the head of the proximal phalanx with stretching of the triangular ligament.[49] In the immediate postinjury period the lateral bands can extend the PIP joint; however, this effect is lost, for as the flexion deformity of the PIP joint increases, the lateral bands migrate volar to the axis of PIP motion, and they become flexors of the joint. Increased tension on the lateral bands by their volar position causes extension of the DIP joint. The DIP joint extension position is correctable early but becomes fixed if not treated.

Treatment of Extensor Injury at the Proximal Interphalangeal Joint

Acute injuries can be satisfactorily treated by splinting the PIP joint in extension for 6 to 8 weeks. While various splints[18] will do this, they are unreliable in children. I recommend

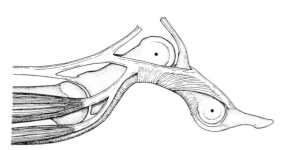

Figure 6–6. Pathology of the boutonnière deformity (after Tubiana).

a small finger cast (Fig. 6–7), leaving the distal joint free for active motion. This cast is applied after the skin is painted with an adherent and a layer of moleskin tape is applied to the finger. One-inch wide strips of a fast setting plaster are then placed over the moleskin. The PIP joint is kept at zero, but the DIP joint is not included so that active motion is possible. This motion prevents lateral band adhesions and is helpful in preventing DIP joint extension deformities. I use this conservative method in late cases if the PIP joint is not fixed in flexion. The useful time limit of conservative management is not known,[75] and I suspect that it is longer than practiced. The open laceration can be similarly treated after skin suture, with the PIP joint splinted straight for 6 weeks. At times, the placement of an oblique fine Kirschner wire transfixing the joint at zero degrees is recommended for noncompliant children.

Chronic Boutonnière Injury

Patients presenting late are also treated with casting for 6 to 8 weeks. If contracture has occurred, they are treated with stretching exercises combined with splints and finger casts. Once the finger is straight, it is held straight for an additional 6 weeks. Surgical repair is rarely necessary, but if conservative therapy fails, operative treatment may be indicated.

Surgical Technique (Fig. 6–8). A curvilinear incision through the skin on the dorsum of the PIP joint exposes the central slip, which is usually healed but is too long to be effective. The intervening scar is removed, and an anatomic repair as advocated by Elliott[18] is carried out. The central slip is visualized and freed along its deep (bone) surface of adhesions to the proximal phalanx. The central tendon is shortened by a reefing stitch, by removing a small segment of the central tendon and doing an end-to-end repair, or by transecting the central slip proximal to the insertion overlapping the segments and repairing them with 5-0 Dacron suture. It is surprising how little shortening is needed to make extension satisfactory (as little as 3 mm in the adult). Advancement of the central slip by this technique relieves the tension on the lateral bands and allows distal joint flexion. If the lateral bands are fixed volar to their normal position at the PIP joint, the transverse retinacular ligaments are released at surgery to free the bands so that

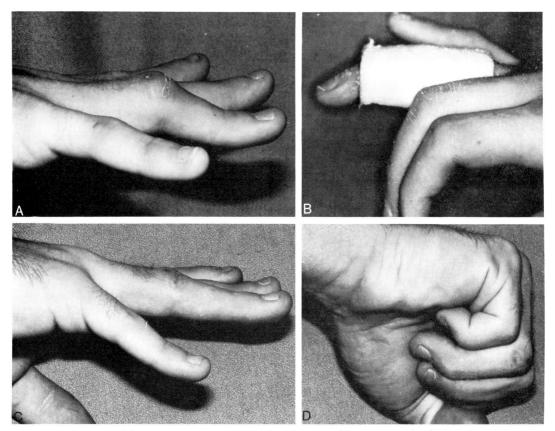

Figure 6–7. Boutonnière deformity, conservative treatment. *A*, A 15-year-old patient 4 weeks after laceration at the PIP joint has a 35-degree drop at the joint. *B*, A finger cast is applied for 6 weeks. The DIP joint is left free for active exercise. *C* and *D*, Range of extension and flexion at 3 months.

they can migrate to their normal dorsal position; however, they are not sutured to one another or to the central tendon. After the PIP joint is fixed in zero degrees extension with a Kirschner wire, the patient is instructed in DIP joint motion postoperatively to promote lateral band motion. The finger is kept in extension for 6 weeks, although the wire may be removed at 4 weeks. At 6 weeks, active flexion exercises are started, with blocking exercises added if progress is slow. The problem becomes one of regaining flexion at the PIP joint.

In fixed boutonnière deformities, transection of the central tendon over the middle phalanx, as described by Dolphin[11] and attributed to Fowler, is helpful in increasing DIP flexion. This technique is especially helpful in older children who have reasonable PIP function but are troubled most by the loss of flexion at the DIP joint. When transection is performed proximal to the insertion of the oblique retinacular ligaments, there will still be some active extension pos-

sible at the DIP joint, but flexion at this joint will be markedly improved. In long-standing cases it may be necessary to add a dorsal capsulotomy at the DIP joint.

Lacerations at the Metacarpophalangeal Joint Level and the Dorsum of the Hand

Injuries at this level will result in loss of active extension at the MP joint. Tendon interconnections and paratenon attachments will mask the significance of the underlying tendon injury, so that careful examination is indicated where there is any hint of tendon dysfunction. This may be as subtle as a minimal loss of full extension at the MP joint. There may even be full extension in the presence of a complete lesion, but the examiner should be able to pick up weakness of that extension if resistance is applied to the finger in the cooperative child. When a decision

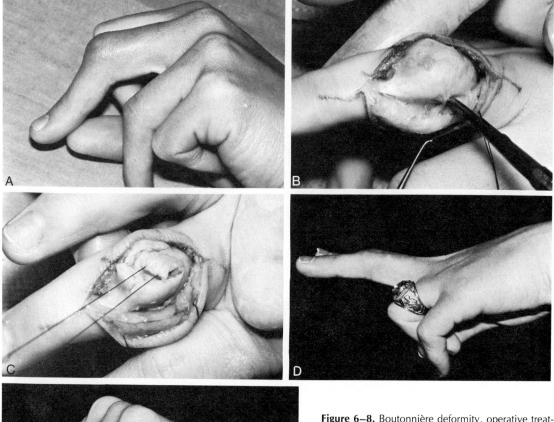

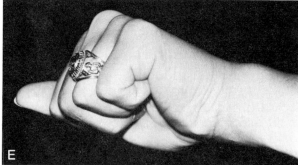

Figure 6–8. Boutonnière deformity, operative treatment. *A*, A girl aged 16, six months after injury, with full passive motion at the PIP joint. *B*, At surgery, the contracted transverse retinacular ligament is seen holding the lateral bands volarly. These contracted bands are released to allow the lateral bands to assume a more dorsal position. *C*, The central slip, having been reconstituted by scar tissue in a lengthened condition, is shortened by 3 mm. *D* and *E*, Extension and flexion one year later.

cannot be made or when definitive care is not available, it is appropriate to close the skin and splint the wrist and fingers in extension and refer the patient for later examination. Delayed repair within the next 2 to 3 weeks is a reasonable procedure in injuries at this level and may even be more pertinent in an "untidy" wound. Closure of the wound would not apply in the case of an infected wound or a wound inflicted by a human tooth.

Repair Technique (Fig. 6–9)

A vertical curvilinear surgical approach is used, combining, where possible, the wound of injury. The tendon ends are reapproxi-

mated with any of the end-to-end tendon sutures. I prefer the grasping-type suture described by Kessler,[38] but the criss cross suture[9] will do as well. After skin repair, the hand is immobilized in extension at the wrist and MP joints for 4 weeks. In the young child, it is best to include the interphalangeal joints, in extension, in the dressing.

Lacerations of the Extensor Tendons at the Dorsum of the Wrist and Distal Forearm Levels

Diagnosis will depend on recognition of the loss of extensor function at the MP joint level. End-to-end repair is carried out as described for the MP joint level. At the wrist the surgeon should try to leave a segment of transverse retinaculum, away from the repair site, or even dorsal fascia to prevent bow-stringing of the tendons in the postrepair period. Prognosis is generally good at this level (Fig. 6–10).

Lacerations of the Extensor Pollicis Longus

Diagnosis of laceration of this tendon is not always simple. While the main function of this tendon is to provide extension to the IP joint of the thumb, the thumb intrinsic muscles, by virtue of their insertions into the MP hood mechanism, can also perform this function. In the cooperative patient, the examiner may find full, but weak, extension at the IP joint and must test further by having the patient adduct the thumb dorsal to the plane of the palm while extending the IP joint. In this position, the extensor pollicis longus, if intact, should be palpable across the dorsum of the hand. Lacerations of this tendon should be repaired at all levels when wound conditions permit. After repair, the thumb and wrist must be protected in splint or cast, in extension, for 4 weeks prior to the insti-

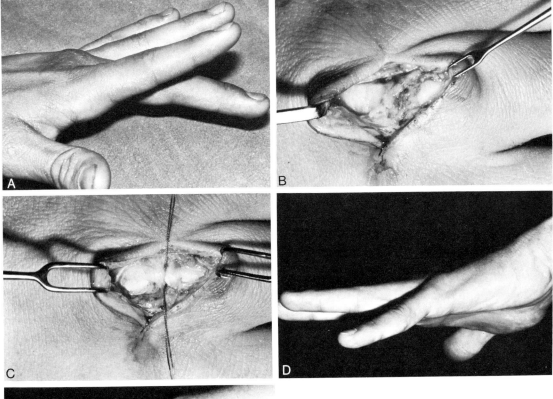

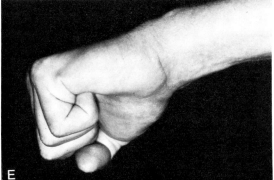

Figure 6–9. Laceration at the MP joint 4 weeks earlier had left this patient with an extension deficit at the joint. *B,* At surgery, reparative scar tissue is seen in the tendon defect. *C,* A Kessler suture is used to join the tendon ends. *D* and *E,* Full extension and flexion were recovered.

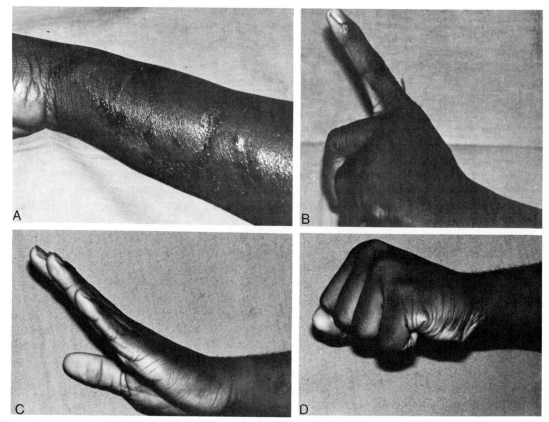

Figure 6–10. *A,* Multiple lacerations of the forearm resulted in severance of the extensor digitorum tendons to the long, ring, and little fingers as well as to the extensor digiti minimi, as shown in *B. C* and *D* show recovery 4 months after repair.

tution of active motion exercises. In chronic lesions, secondary repair may be possible; if this is not feasible, tendon transfer using the extensor indicis[71] is an excellent procedure.

Extensor Tendon Reconstruction

When early direct repairs of the long extensor tendons either have not been carried out or have been unsuccessful, it may rarely be necessary to perform tendon grafting or tendon transfer to restore extensor function to the hand. Tendon grafts using palmaris longus or any of the other donor tendons can be utilized. The technique by which the distal portion of a divided tendon is sutured to an adjacent intact tendon is well proved.[64] Use of the extensor digiti minimi, extensor indicis, or wrist motor is also helpful as a transfer in reconstruction of irreparable long extensor injuries.

Extensor Tenolysis. When recovery of gliding function has not been satisfactory, owing to the formation of adhesions, and when hand therapy measures have been ap-

plied without success, one may be justified in offering extensor tenolysis.[23, 70] The functional deficit should be significant enough to justify the procedure, and elapsed time without improvement should be more than 3 months. Extensor lysis may have to be combined with capsular (joint) releases and can be even more extensive than the original repair itself. After this surgery, a hand therapy program is essential for a successful result. Fortunately, tenolysis is rarely needed in young patients.

FLEXOR TENDON INJURIES

Anatomy of the Flexor Tendon System (Fig. 6–11)

This section is concerned with the nine tendons derived from the flexor muscles that are in the volar compartment of the forearm, i.e., the flexor digitorum superficialis, the flexor digitorum profundus, and the flexor pollicis

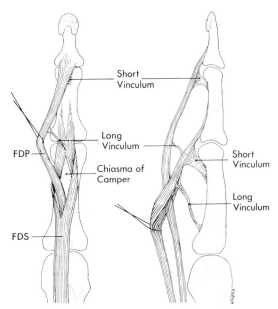

Figure 6–11. Anatomy of the flexor system in the finger. (From Schneider LH. Flexor Tendon Injuries. Boston, Little, Brown, 1985, with permission.)

tendons will provide efficient joint motion. This area, where two tendons are held closely together within an unyielding compartment, is the most difficult in which to obtain satisfactory results after tendon injury and has been designated as "no-man's land" by Dr. Bunnell.[8] Dissection studies[13, 30] have shown that the retinaculum can be divided into five heavier annular bands and three finer cruciform ligaments. Doyle and Blythe also studied the flexor retinaculum in the thumb.[14] Within the retinaculum in the finger as well as under the carpal ligament in the carpal canal, the long flexor tendons are enveloped in a double-layered synovial sheath (Fig. 6–13). These layers are in contact at the ends of the synovial sheath, but along the length of this sheath they are connected by folds of fine tissue called mesotenon. Within the flexor retinaculum, condensations of the mesotenon form the

longus. Also of importance are the supportive tissues of these tendons, the synovial sheaths, and the fibrous retinacular system.[37]

The flexor muscles at the distal one third of the forearm provide tendons, two for each finger and one for the thumb. The flexor digitorum superficialis tendons terminate at the middle phalanges and act to flex the proximal interphalangeal joints. It is noted that the flexor superficialis becomes flattened and divides into a radial and an ulnar band that encircle the flexor profundus and then reunite dorsal to it. This area is known as the chiasma of Camper (Fig. 6–11).[37] The flexor profundus and flexor pollicis longus insert at the base of the distal phalanges and principally flex the distal interphalangeal joints of the fingers and the interphalangeal joint of the thumb.

The Flexor Retinaculum in the Finger (The Pulley System in the Fingers and Thumb) (Fig. 6–12)

The fibrous retinaculum, which begins at the neck of the metacarpal and ends at the distal interphalangeal joint, is reinforced along its course at areas designated as pulleys. This structure holds the flexor tendon close to the bone, preventing bowstringing so that the

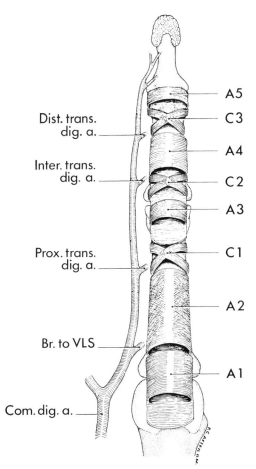

Figure 6–12. The flexor retinaculum in the finger. (From Schneider, LH. Flexor Tendon Injuries. Boston, Little, Brown, 1985, with permission).

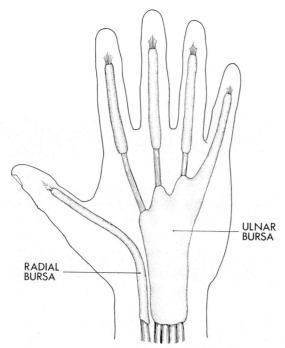

Figure 6–13. The flexor synovial sheath. (From Schneider LH. Flexor Tendon Injuries. Boston, Little, Brown, 1985, with permission.)

vincula, which carry blood vessels to the tendons (Fig. 6–11).[10, 30, 41, 56, 57]

Flexor Tendon Zones—Level of Injury in the Flexor Tendon

The actual level of injury to the tendon in relation to its surrounding tissues is of significance, especially in estimating prognosis. Treatment itself is not determined by the level of injury if one subscribes to direct repair of flexor tendon injuries at all levels,[39, 83, 84] although some do adhere to the technique of secondary tendon grafting in zone 2 injuries.[6] It is important to identify the level of the injury so that the results of the various repair techniques can be more accurately compared.

Flexor Tendon Zones

For practical purposes I have found useful the division of the flexor system into five zones (Fig. 6–14).[40]

Zone 1. From the distal phalanx to the middle of the middle phalanx. This zone is distal to the insertion of the flexor profundus, so a wound here will injure only the flexor profundus.

Zone 2. The "no-man's land" of Bunnell is delineated to a large degree by the extremes of the flexor retinaculum. From the midportion of the middle phalanx proximally to the neck of the metacarpal. Depending on the position of the fingers during wounding, and the direction and nature of the wounding force, lacerations here can sever either one or both of the flexor tendons.

Zone 3. The palm. Proceeds proximally from the metacarpal neck to the distal edge of the carpal ligament. Injuries here affect both flexor tendons or the superficialis.

Zone 4. The carpal canal. This zone underlies the transverse carpal ligament, and its landmarks are the same. On the skin the proximal limit would correspond to the volar wrist crease. Injury to the main trunk of the median nerve or its branches greatly complicates recovery of hand function at this level. A synovial sheath invests the flexor tendons as they pass through the carpal canal.

Zone 5. The distal forearm. This zone extends proximally from the radiocarpal joint (the volar wrist crease) to the musculotendinous juncture of the long flexor tendons. In addition to the long flexor tendons of the fingers and thumb, the wrist flexors will also be injured at this level. Injury here is fre-

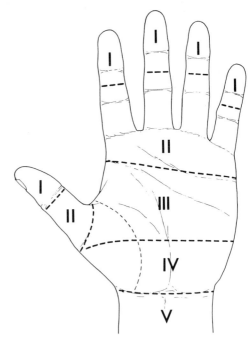

Figure 6–14. Flexor tendon zones. (From Schneider LH. Flexor Tendon Injuries. Boston, Little, Brown, 1985, with permission.)

quently accompanied by major nerve injury, which will have great bearing on the functional result.

Flexor Tendon Zones in the Thumb

The flexor tendon system in the thumb presents a simpler anatomic arrangement in that there is only one flexor tendon and the thumb has one less phalanx. The flexor system of the thumb has also been divided into zones.

Zone 1. At the insertion of the flexor pollicis longus.

Zone 2. From the neck of the proximal phalanx to the neck of the metacarpal. This zone coincides with the flexor retinaculum of the thumb.

Zone 3. The level of the thenar muscles, to the distal edge of the carpal canal.

Zone 4. The carpal canal.

Zone 5. Proximal to the radiocarpal articulation to the level of the musculotendinous juncture.

Flexor Tendon Healing

The mechanism by which flexor tendons heal after injury and repair is not completely clear. The question concerns itself with the part (if any) that the tendon plays in its own healing process. Does the tendon heal by reparative growth emanating from the cut tendon ends (intrinsic healing), or is the tendon completely passive in the healing process, which is carried out through the activities of the surrounding tissues (extrinsic healing)? Or do both processes occur simultaneously? For background material, readers would be served well to study the works of Mason and Shearon,[54] Mason and Allen,[53] and Lindsay[44] as well as the classic works of Potenza.[59] This last author, working with dogs, concluded that there was a lack of active participation of the cut tendon in the healing process. Healing transpired through the activity of the surrounding fibrous tissues, which invaded the repair site, supplying vascular inflow and cells necessary for the heal-

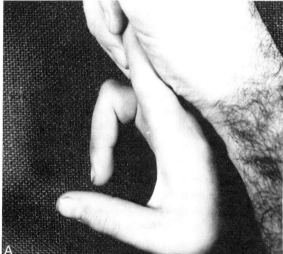
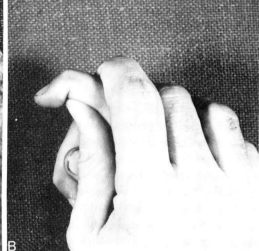
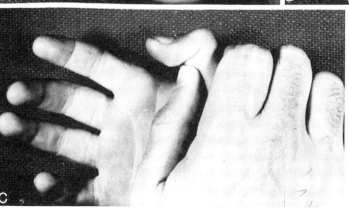

Figure 6–15. Direct testing of tendon function. *A,* The flexor digitorum superficialis. With the examiner holding the other fingers in complete extension and thus preventing profundus action, the integrity of the flexor superficialis can be demonstrated. *B,* The flexor profundus is the only flexor of the distal joint. *C,* Active flexion of the IP joint of the thumb proves the continuity of flexor pollicis longus.

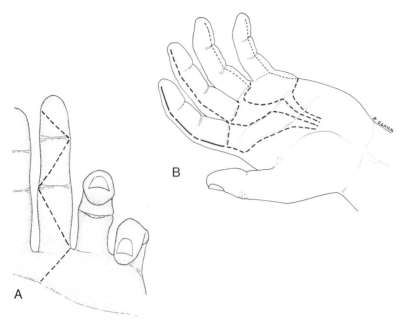

Figure 6–16. Incisions used in flexor tendon surgery. *A,* The volar zigzag. *B,* The midaxial, with palmar extensions.

ing process but forming adhesions in the process. For the tendon to glide in the postrepair period, a remodeling process was deemed necessary in the late healing phase. It was pointed out by Potenza[59] and others[44] that gentle technique was necessary to limit the number and density of these obligatory adhesions so that the adhesions necessary for healing would be as pliable as possible and more responsive to postoperative exercise designed to re-establish the gliding planes necessary for return of flexor tendon function.

Chiefly because of Potenza's work, the theory of a passive role for the flexor tendon in healing was dominant until the 1970s. At that time, prompted by the questions raised by Furlow[24] and the work of Matthews and Richards,[55] the question again arose. Are adhesions a normal and necessary accompanying feature of tendon healing, or could they be a phenomenon related to the trauma to the surrounding tissues created by the injury and the surgical repair? Couldn't these adhesions be a response to local ischemia or lack of nutrition at the injury site? Succeeding years brought further reports[50] suggesting that tendons could heal without the intercession of vascular (and binding) adhesions. These exciting studies emphasized the importance of a synovial nutritional system that worked along with a vas-

cular system to supply the metabolic needs of the tendon in health or injury.[52] Nutrition for the tendon through the synovial fluid route brings forth a possibility for a repaired tendon to heal without the need for adhesions and with a potential for maintenance of its gliding function. This creates a more optimistic picture for tendon injury in the most difficult area for success, the zone 2 lesion, where this synovial healing system would be expected to be active. The concept of sheath closure over a repair in the difficult zone 2 has now been expounded to take advantage of this system.[17] Preservation of as much of the uninjured sheath system as possible is now advocated both in early and in late repair in an effort to utilize this repair potential.[45]

Obviously, all is not settled in these questions of tendon healing mechanisms.[60] I believe that the tendon can heal without the need for vascular adhesions, although the quality of that healing has not been completely tested. In the acute injury, the question as to the origin of the healing cells (whether from the tendon itself or from extrinsic sources) is still rightfully in dispute. Nevertheless, in the observed clinical situation, adhesions do form, invading the tendon surface and the repair site with resultant restriction of gliding, thereby reducing the effectiveness of the repair. In the zone 2 injury in particular, gentle techniques reduce the density and quantity of the adhesions formed. At this time, it seems that closure of the sheath in zone 2 at the time of primary or delayed direct repair, to take advantage of synovial nutritional mechanisms, is a reasonable course to follow. Many surgeons, including this writer, are following the example of Kleinert and Lister and coworkers[45, 46] by using this technique at the time of repair in zone 2.

In an effort to hinder formation of tendon adhesions associated with healing, experimentors have utilized drugs that interfere with biosynthesis of collagen. These include beta-aminoproprionitrile[58] and cishydroxyproline.[4] There is still no proof of their safety at this time, studies now being done may provide a chemical adjuvant that would be practical for clinical use.

Diagnosis

The diagnosis of flexor tendon injury can be very difficult to make in young children. The following techniques are helpful in clarifying the injury.

1. *Finger position*. Observation of the posture that the fingers adopt. There is a normal cascade of the fingers when the flexors are intact, with the fingers seen in more flexion as one proceeds from index to little finger (see Fig. 6–26). This will be more useful if the patient is relaxed; loss of this cascade is obvious when a patient is under general anesthesia. If one finger appears persistently to be in more extension than expected, one must suspect a flexor injury and proceed accordingly (see Fig. 6–1).

2. *The squeeze test*. In a lesion distal to the forearm this maneuver may be of value.

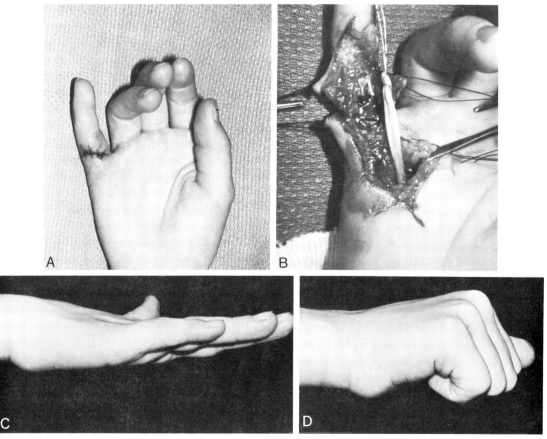

Figure 6–17. Zone 1 injury. *A*, Although the skin laceration in this 10-year-old child is seen overlying zone 2, the finger was in flexion at the time of injury, resulting in a zone 1 tendon injury (as seen in *B*). *C* and *D*, Extension and flexion 6 months after delayed repair.

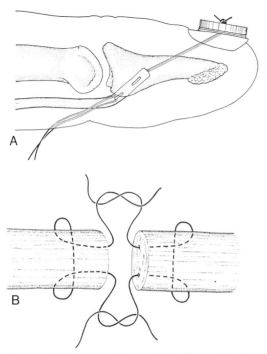

Figure 6–18. Suture techniques. *A,* The Bunnell distal juncture to bone. *B,* The Kessler suture for end-to-end repair.

Pressure on the forearm will demonstrate flexor motion distally at the fingers when the flexor tendons are intact. This test will be false negative in partial lacerations or where synovial interconnections from intact flexors give weak continuity.

3. *Tenodesis effect.* Tenodesis effect through motion of the wrist may give a clue to tendon disruption. The examiner passively extends the wrist, and fingers with severed flexor tendons will not go into a flexed posture but will remain extended, whereas fingers with intact flexors will tend to assume a more flexed position.

4. *Active motion examination.* There really is no substitute for direct testing of the tendon in question (Fig. 6–15). Unfortunately, this test may not be possible in a child who is not able to cooperate. The flexor profundus being the only flexor at the DIP joint, testing for full flexion at this joint proves its continuity. The flexor digitorum superficialis is more difficult to test, as its function at the PIP joint is overlapped by that of the flexor profundus. Because of a common origin of the four profundus muscles in the forearm, the superficialis function of a finger can be isolated through restraint of the pro-

fundi by completely extending all the other fingers. The independently functioning superficialis, if intact, can then be demonstrated by the presence of full flexion at the PIP joint of the finger being tested. It should be noted that this test may not be applicable in the index finger of patients with independence of function of the profundus or those with a poorly developed superficialis in the little finger.[2]

The Level of the Skin Wound in Relation to the Tendon Injury. The actual level of the tendon laceration is dependent on the angle of the cutting instrument and the position of the fingers when the wound occurred. If the finger is injured in flexion, the laceration of the tendon itself will be found distal to the skin wound. In injuries sustained in extension, the injury level on the tendon will more closely correspond to the level of injury in the skin. Therefore, a tendon injury sustained in full flexion may have a skin wound overlying zone 2, but the tendon might easily have been injured in zone 1. The level of the skin injury is not significant, but the level of tendon injury is. To be consistent in reporting the level of injury on the tendon, the repair level is noted in relation to the surrounding structures, with the finger held in extension on the operating table prior to closure of the wound.

Acute Flexor Tendon Injury

Timing of Repair.[15] I recommend direct repair of all flexor tendon injuries at all levels when wound conditions permit.[82] This is not to say that they must be treated within 6 hours of injury as was the directive in the past,[20, 21] but owing to the less restrictive time conditions of the delayed repair program, one can close the skin and plan to do definitive repair within the next 10 days. I have, however, observed my results to be satisfactory if the repair is done within 21 days of the injury.[69] At one time, early direct repair was advocated only when the lesion was located outside the difficult zone 2.[5] Because of the poorer results seen after direct repair in zone 2, most authorities recommended skin closure only and definitive repair of the zone 2 injury by secondary tendon graft.[6, 8] Now the trend has shifted to direct repair even in "no-man's land." With time restriction eased,[1, 69] the patient can have the skin closed and be referred, if indicated, to a sur-

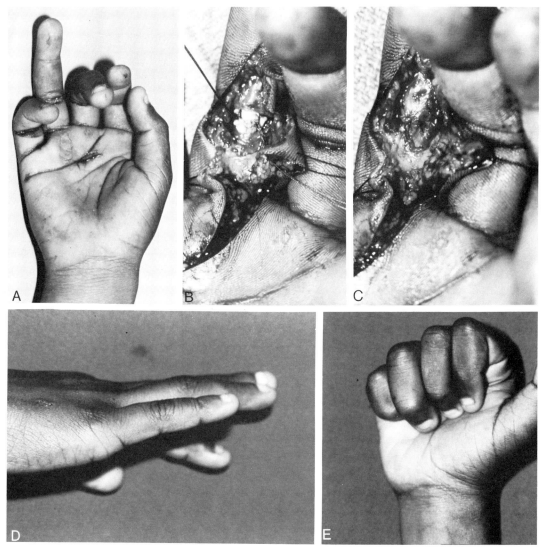

Figure 6–19. Zone 2 injury. *A,* Laceration of both flexor tendons at the PIP joint level in an 8-year-old boy. *B,* Repair through a window in the retinaculum. *C,* The sheath has been repaired using fine suture material. *D* and *E,* Result seen at 4 months.

geon versed in repair of tendon injuries. At times, because of wound conditions, a tendon graft will still be considered the better alternative, but generally, however, a direct repair, expertly carried out, offers a better chance for success than the more difficult tendon graft. In fact, primary repair in zone 2 injury was condoned for children before it received the acceptability for adults that it now enjoys.[5] It took the work of Verdan[83, 84] and Kleinert[39] to re-establish this technique, although a group of surgeons did do primary repairs, albeit with very rigid time considerations.

A series of papers concerning children[1] and adults,[39] and our series[69] published in 1977, reported that primary repairs carried out from 1 day to 21 days post injury are simpler to do and have results comparable to or better than tendon grafting.

Treatment of Acute Flexor Tendon Injuries

Incisions used in Flexor Tendon Surgery. Although the midlateral incision still has its adherents,[6] I prefer to approach the flexor

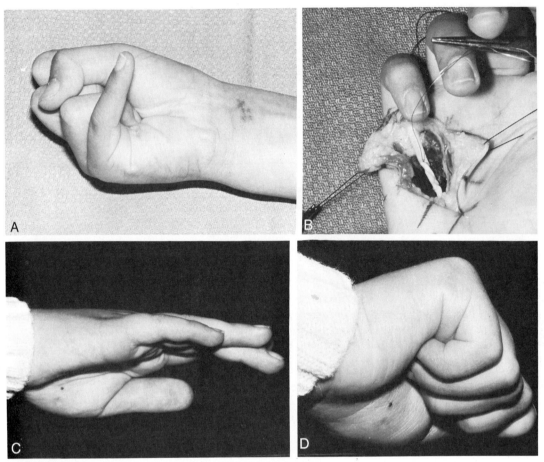

Figure 6–20. Zone 3 injury. *A,* An 8-year-old girl lacerated both flexor tendons in the midpalm region. *B,* Repair accomplished, using wire. *C* and *D,* Result several months later.

system through the zigzag incision described by Brunner[7] (Fig. 6–16).

As noted, 4-0 Dacron suture (occasionally 5-0) in the very young child is used in tendon repair. The skin is closed with absorbable suture in the young or uncooperative patient.

Treatment of Acute Flexor Tendon Injuries by Level

Zone 1 Injuries. In this region only the flexor profundus is injured, so the deficit will be in the loss of distal joint flexion. Early direct repair is offered, preferably before more than three weeks have elapsed. Results are generally good, and there is a potential for near-normal function after early repair in this zone (Fig. 6–17). If the laceration or closed rupture is exactly at the insertion, reattachment is performed to bone distal to the epiphysis (Fig. 6–18A). It should be noted that when the lesion is more proximal,

direct end-to-end repair is recommended (Fig. 6–18B), as the technique of advancement can often be underestimated and result in troublesome flexion deformities. I prefer the modified Kessler[38, 64, 66] suture technique (Fig. 6–18B). Both ends of the tendon are located; it may be necessary to lengthen the incision to find the tendon, which may have retracted into the palm. Care is taken not to add unnecessary trauma to the sheath or the chiasma. It may be difficult to pass the profundus through the superficialis decussation, and at times it may be necessary to pass the tendon around the superficialis. Although some authors have resorted to the excision of one tail of the superficialis to make room for the profundus, it is not justifiable to sacrifice an intact uninjured superficialis when repairing the profundus.

Zone 2 Injuries. Injuries at this level within the digital sheath present the greatest difficulty for the surgeon in the effort to re-

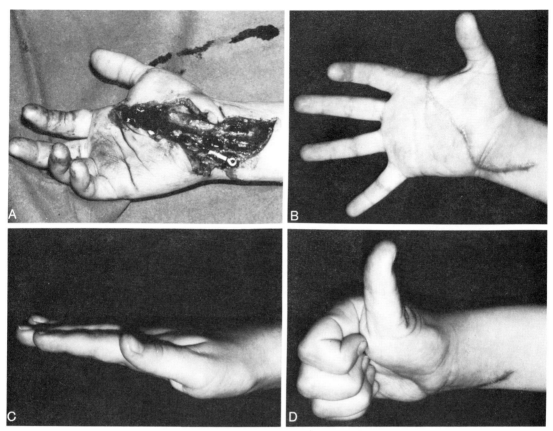

Figure 6–21. Zone 4 injury. *A,* A massive laceration at the wrist level with both flexor tendons to index and long fingers severed and with division of the FPL. *B, C* and *D,* Results of primary repair.

store active flexion to a finger. At this time, I believe that primary or early direct repair is the most satisfactory method of treatment when wound conditions allow. Although this technique is usually applied within 3 weeks, I feel that better results are obtained when the repair is carried out within the first 10 days.[69]

Surgical Technique in Zone 2 (Fig. 6–19)

The area is approached through a zigzag incision combining, where possible, the wound of injury. The skin incision is carried down to the flexor retinaculum, and this structure is exposed for 2 cm in either direction from the sheath wound. It may be possible to carry out the repair through the laceration in the retinaculum, but it may be necessary to reflect a portion to carry out the repair.[45, 66] When the tendon has retracted proximally, it is necessary to extend the skin incision and explore the retinaculum through transverse incisions. At this time both tendons, superficialis and profundus, are repaired. A one-half Kessler type suture is placed in either end of the cut tendon, preferably in the volar half of the cross section of the tendon. These are brought together and tied with the help of an assistant, and an oversew circumferential suture of 6-0 prolene is utilized. Because of the relationship of the circulation of the profundus to the superficialis, both tendons usually are repaired. When repair of the superficialis is not possible and excision is elected, the proximal portion is pulled into the wound, transected, and allowed to retract. The distal portion of the superficialis is not excised but left to provide a bed for the profundus repair. The retention of the superficialis stump makes less likely the development of a hyperextension deformity at the PIP joint, as seen in loose-jointed patients.

To take advantage of the intrinsic repair potential as well as synovial nutrition, as discussed under tendon healing, repair of the

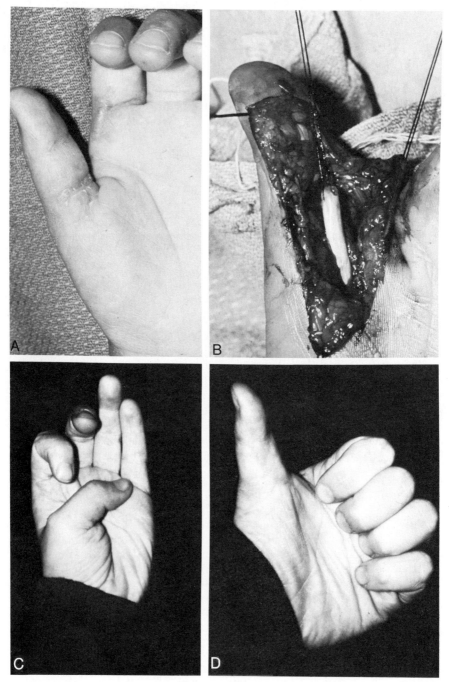

Figure 6–22. *A,* A 6-year-old boy who had lacerated his left thumb over the proximal phalanx 2 weeks prior to this photograph and had lost IP joint flexion. *B,* Direct repair of the flexor pollicis longus was performed. *C* and *D,* The range of motion obtained at 3 months, although not complete, was satisfactory.

flexor retinaculum has been advocated in the zone 2 injury. As shown by Lister,[45] closing of the sheath also allows for easier passage of the repair through the retinaculum. At times, closure of the sheath is not possible, and it may be necessary to excise a portion of the sheath to allow free passage of the repair. I have not been satisfied with my ability to successfully reconstruct pulleys using tendon or ligament material at the time of direct

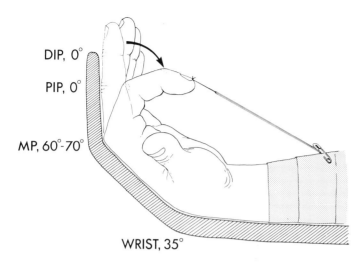

DIP, 0°

PIP, 0°

MP, 60°-70°

WRIST, 35°

Figure 6–23. Technique of early protected mobilization after flexor tendon repair. (From Schneider LH. Flexor Tendon Injuries. Boston, Little, Brown, 1985, with permission.)

tendon repair. If major pulley reconstruction is needed, I feel this is an indication for staged tendon reconstruction.[30–32]

Zone 3 Injuries

In the palm, prognosis for the tendon injury itself is relatively good (Fig. 6–20). Both tendons are repaired using the Kessler type suture. In borderline cases, in which the repair will lie under the A-1 pulley (in zone 2) in extension, the surgeon should consider excision of this pulley to convert the problem to the more favorable zone 3 lesion.

Zone 4 Injuries (Fig. 6–21)

The area is approached through a vertical curvilinear incision. The carpal ligament is completely transected and the tendons evaluated. The median nerve is identified and prepared for repair. The tendons are tagged distal and proximal with the one-half Kessler suture. Because of the unyielding nature of this compartment it is better not to repair the superficialis here; one's efforts should be directed to the repair of the profundi and the flexor pollicis longus. After completion of the tendon repairs, the nerve repairs are

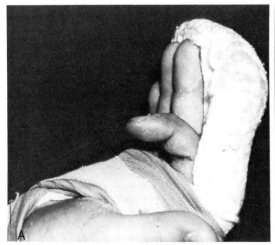
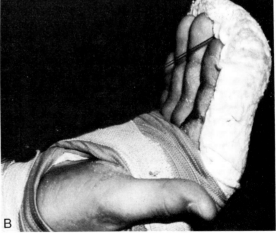

Figure 6–24. Clinical application of the mobilization technique. *A,* The index finger is passively pulled into flexion by the elastic band. *B,* The patient actively extends the finger as far as the splint allows.

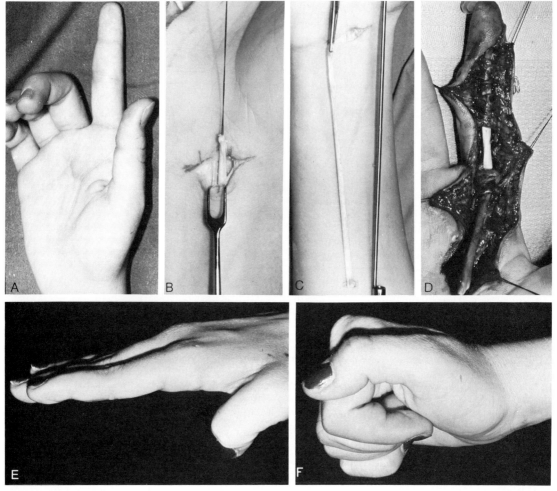

Figure 6–25. Flexor tendon graft. *A*, four months before the photograph was taken this 13-year-old girl lacerated both flexor tendons in zone 2. *B* and *C*, The palmaris longus is located at the wrist and is removed, using a tendon stripper. *D*, The graft is in place. As much uninjured retinaculum as possible is preserved. Because of scarring, retinaculum at the site of injury had to be removed. *E* and *F*, Results at about one year. Full flexion has not been recovered at the distal joint.

carried out and the skin closed. It should be noted that the carpal ligament is not repaired.

Zone 5 Injuries

This zone, in the forearm, presents the best location for tendon injury as far as recovery of tendon function is concerned. The problem is related to recovery from major nerve injuries that generally accompany tendon laceration in this area. The approach is through a curvilinear incision, which should be generous so as to properly find and identify all injured structures. As a general rule, the carpal ligament should be opened. The tendons are paired and readied for repair using the Kessler suture as before (one-half in each tendon end). These are set aside while the nerves are readied for repair. Now the tendon sutures are completed. Both flexors and the flexor pollicis are repaired at this level. No circumferential suture is necessary at this level. The wrist flexors (when injured) are also repaired at this time. The nerve suture is carried out and the skin closed.

Treatment of Flexor Pollicis Longus Lacerations (Fig. 6–22). Lacerations of this tendon are repaired directly at all levels, as long as the wound permits and less than 3 or 4 weeks have elapsed. An end-to-end repair using the Kessler suture is made, with an oversew added only in the zone 2 level. Sheath closure is also carried out in the zone 2 area.

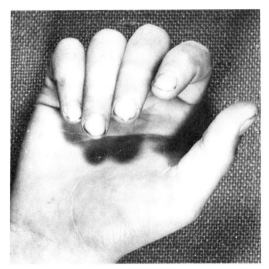

Figure 6–26. Adjusting the graft. When deciding how much tension is to be placed in a tendon graft, the surgeon should note that each finger falls into semiflexion, slightly less flexed than its ulnar neighbor and more flexed than the radially adjacent finger. The graft should be adjusted by placing the grafted finger in proper relation to its neighbor.

Not infrequently, this tendon recoils into the proximal forearm; therefore, when dealing with distal lacerations, the surgeon should be prepared to explore the distal forearm for the proximal end of the tendon.

Postoperative Care After Flexor Tendon Repair

One of the major problems facing the surgeon repairing flexor tendons in the young involves techniques of immobilization. Long-arm casts and splints have been recommended for children postoperatively, and this is reasonable. These devices do not prevent tension from occurring at the repair site, as the patient can flex isometrically and even in the absence of motion disrupt the repair. It is preferable to put the patient in a long- or short-arm posterior splint with the wrist in a flexed position of 60 or 70 degrees to weaken the power in the flexor system.

Also of use in the older child is the dynamic mobilization technique, in which an elastic band is fixed to the nail at one end and to the volar part of the dressing at the distal forearm level at the other end,[46, 68] (Fig. 6–23). This band passively flexes the finger, but the system allows active extension as far as the posterior aspect of the splint; when the finger relaxes, it is pulled, by the elastic, into flexion (Fig. 6–24). I have used this method in children as young as 6 years of age, as a means of lessening tension at the repair site and allowing some gliding to occur at the repair site. This technique requires a reliable family and frequent attendance at the office for close supervision. If it fails, troublesome flexion deformities can develop. If there is any question about reliability or attendance, the elastic band "dynamic mobilization" technique is not used. Instead, a standard posterior splint is applied with the wrist flexed, as mentioned, to about 60 to 70 degrees and the metacarpophalangeal joint flexed 70 degrees with the interphalangeal joints in extension. The repair is generally protected for 4 weeks, and then active motion exercises are begun. In the flexor tendon injury, formal hand therapy is offered even to the youngest patient, with active exercise progressing to blocking exercise at 5 to 6 weeks.

Suture of the tip of the finger to the palm has been advocated as a form of immobilization,[51] and although this will prevent extension of the finger, it will not prevent flexion (as noted earlier). I have seen a severe flexion deformity of the PIP joint develop when this technique was used.

Injuries of the Flexor Tendon (Late Treatment)

Secondary Procedures

Despite the widespread use of early repair techniques there are times when secondary procedures are needed. Examples include cases in which it was deemed judicious (or it was the surgeon's choice) to allow wound healing to occur prior to definitive treatment, or cases in which the significance of the injury was underestimated. In other instances, primary treatment may have yielded a less than satisfactory functional result, and secondary salvage procedures are indicated.

Secondary Repair of Flexor Tendon Injuries

When the time limit for primary or delayed repair techniques has elapsed (up to 3 or 4 weeks), secondary repair can be accomplished in some instances. It is rare that such a repair can be done in the zone 1 or zone 2 injury, because with time the receded muscle

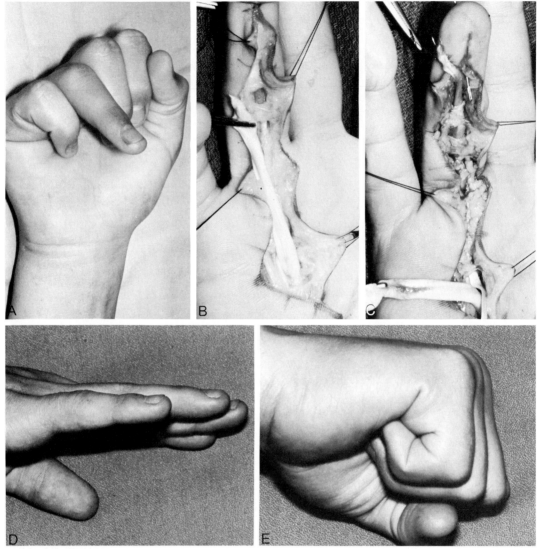

Figure 6–27. A flexor profundus graft in the presence of an intact superficialis. *A* and *B*, A 16-year-old football player had sustained a closed rupture of the profundus flexor 3 months before reporting for treatment. *C*, A palmaris longus graft is seen in the flexor system. *D* and *E*, The result, 6 months later, is excellent restoration of function.

contracts, making it impossible to withdraw the tendon out to full length. Repair would have to be carried out under increased tension, creating an unacceptable flexion deformity. Rarely, in the zone 1 injury the short vincula remains intact, holding the tendon well out in the finger and making late repair feasible. Secondary repair is often possible in zone 3, where the lumbrical origin prevents significant retraction of the profundus tendon. Zones 4 and 5 also lend themselves to secondary repair, as synovial interconnections keep the lacerated tendon in the area of injury. As a general rule, I would repair only the profundus in the usual second-

ary repair case. The technique of secondary repair, as far as suture technique is concerned, is similar to that of early repair.

Flexor Tendon Grafting in Zone 2 (Fig. 6–25)

The replacement of the injured flexor tendon system by an autogenous tendon graft is the solution offered as a secondary procedure in this difficult area of the finger. By placing the junctures distally in zone 1 and proximally in the palm (zone 3), the surgeon bypasses the area of "no-man's land." Unfortunately, tendon grafting, a difficult procedure in the

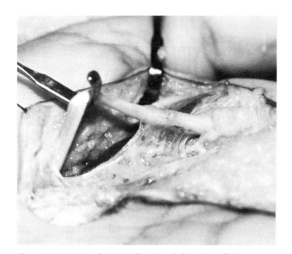

Figure 6–28. Tenolysis. Following failure to achieve movement, this tendon repair site was explored; the presence of adhesions at the site limits tendon gliding. Release of the adhesions restored function in the finger.

adult, is also quite difficult in children. The main problem I have found in very young children has been the size of available grafting material. The palmaris longus tendon can be very small, and the plantaris, when available, even smaller. These grafts take suture material very poorly. They are obtained using a tendon stripper.[68] When doing tendon grafts in children, I use the interweave techniques for the proximal juncture because of the inherent strength in their construction.[61, 80] The distal juncture preferred is one of the end-to-end suture techniques, but if there is no distal tendon stump available, I use the Bunnell[8] pull-out technique, drilling the bone distal to the epiphysis (see Fig. 6–18A). The distal juncture is completed first, and the finger is closed. Tension is set at the proximal juncture in the palm by observing the cascade of the fingers with the wrist in the straight (zero) position on the table (Fig. 6–26). The finger being grafted assumes a position of partial flexion, increasing as one proceeds in the ulnar direction.

Tendon Grafts in the Presence of an Intact Superficialis (Zone 1 Injury) (Fig. 6–27)

The use of a tendon graft in the presence of a normally functioning superficialis is a decision not to be taken lightly. Through the superficialis the finger has a great percentage of its flexion arc, and this will be risked by the procedure. If, during passing of the graft, the delicate superficialis function is reduced, the finger may very well be made worse as far as range of motion is concerned. Despite this, the procedure is probably better indicated in the supple-fingered, loose-jointed child than in the adult. It is also more strongly indicated in the power-grip, ulnar side of the hand than on the radial side, where, especially in the older child, either no treatment or stabilization of the distal joint may suffice. In 1970, Bora[3] published a series of young patients in whom the injured profundus tendon was grafted in the presence of the intact superficialis with good results. Others have advocated the use of the staged reconstructive technique for this lesion.[29, 31] In my series of carefully selected patients in whom I performed this operation, there was a need to do secondary tenolysis in the majority of cases in order to obtain the sought-after distal joint function. Now when this surgery is done, the parents are warned of this possibility..

Tendon Grafts in Zones 3, 4, and 5

It may be necessary at a secondary repair to bridge a short gap with a "bridge" or interposition graft. Usually the profundus is involved; I prefer to use the flexor superficialis as the graft, although if it is not available, the palmaris longus is usable.[61]

Tendon Transfer

In some reconstructive situations the use of flexor superficialis as a transfer to motor the irreparable profundus has been advocated. This has been especially useful as an alternative to grafting of the flexor pollicis longus[73] or in the zone 3 injury, where the proximal profundus is inadequate and a flexor superficialis is transferred to the distal profundus.[68]

Tenolysis

Tendon adhesions can occur wherever the surface of a tendon is injured.[59] Since active motion is based on the ability of the flexor tendon to glide within its bed, the formation of nonpliable adhesions often causes an inability to achieve full gliding, despite our best intentions and a vigorous postoperative program (Fig. 6–28). Some of these

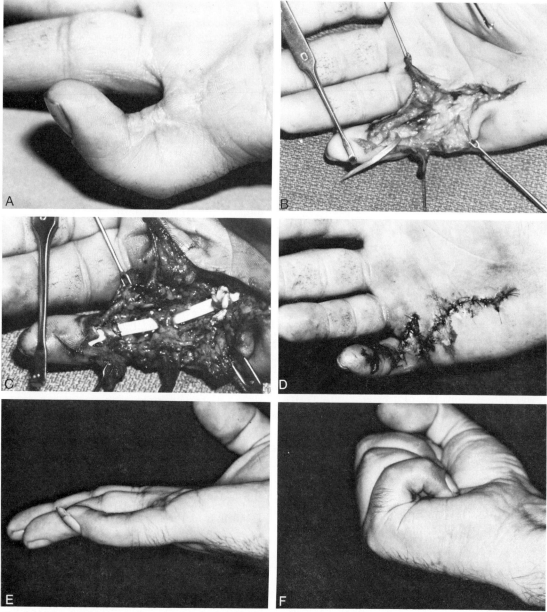

Figure 6–29. Staged flexor tendon reconstruction. This 16-year-old boy had undergone multiple failed procedures after flexor injury to his little finger. *A*, There was no active motion at the interphalangeal joints, and skin and joint contracture were evident. *B*, At stage 1, scarred tendons were removed, and the PIP joint was released. *C*, The implant is in place and pulleys have been reconstructed at A-2 and A-4 using tendon remnants. A-3 was salvaged. *D*, Z-plasty revision of the skin was used for closure. Stage 2 was accomplished 4 months later; the range of motion shown in *E* and *F* was observed 6 months after stage 2.

patients become candidates for tenolysis. This procedure involves the direct incision of restraining adhesions from the surface of the injured and repaired tendon while an attempt is made to maintain the supportive vascular and retinacular structures. In adults, using proper indications and careful technique, tenolysis will recoup a significant number of tendon repair failures.[23, 67, 68, 70, 87]

Indications for tenolysis are not absolute but include a deficiency in active range of motion and a plateau reached in the exercise program. The patient must be able to cooperate in a diligent postoperative program. This may limit the availability of the procedure to younger children. As a rule, a lysis should not be done before 3 months have elapsed from the time of repair and even longer after a tendon graft.[23] As stated, there are no absolute indications for tenolysis. What has to be considered is the significance of the functional loss in the individual patient, and this will be a difficult decision to make in the child. The presence of joint injury and neurovascular injury should also play a part in the decision-making process. A cold and insensate finger will be poor even if some degree of motion can be recovered. It should be noted that the condition may not improve after this procedure and may even be made worse.

Technique. The surgeon must be prepared to explore the involved tendon system from one end to the other. In children, general anesthesia is needed. After painstakingly freeing the tendon, the surgeon can make an incision in the distal forearm to do a "flexor-check" by pulling on the involved tendon proximally.[87] In older children, it may be possible to do the procedure under a local-sedative anesthesia[35] with their direct cooperation. While this anesthesia technique is recommended, it is rarely usable in children. In my local anesthesia series,[67] I did have one successful tenolysis in a 7-year-old. A postoperative early-motion program is essential if the gains made at the lysis are to be maintained. At times this can be facilitated by the use of an indwelling catheter, with local anesthetic instillation used for the first 5 to 7 postoperative days.[36, 70]

Staged Tendon Reconstruction (Fig. 6-29)

When the flexor tendon system is involved in heavy scarring due to the severe nature of the original injury or to failed prior surgery such that a standard one-stage tendon graft is unlikely to succeed, there may be an indication for a two-stage reconstructive procedure. In this procedure a reinforced silicone rubber tendon implant is installed as a first stage to act as a template for the reconstruction of the flexor system.[31–34, 65] At the first stage, scarred tendon remnants are excised, joint contractures released, and pulleys reconstructed as needed. The implant is placed within the flexor system, running from the distal phalanx to the distal forearm.

After stage 1, the patient enters a passive motion program in which gains made at stage 1 are maintained. In response to the implant, a pseudosheath forms that will service a tendon graft placed at stage 2. After a delay of at least 3 months, the implant is replaced by a tendon graft, which is placed with as little disruption to the newly formed sheath as possible. This procedure has been valuable in the salvage of flexor systems in children, as reported by Hunter and Salisbury.[31] It must be recognized that this is a salvage operation and should be reserved for those patients able to cooperate in a difficult multi-staged procedure. I would not recommend it in a child less than 6 years of age and would try to defer its use until the child gets older. The procedure is detailed in references 31 to 33.

Flexor tendon injuries present difficult problems both for the surgeon and for the young patient. A solid knowledge of the anatomy involved and careful attention to surgical principles and details will reward both surgeon and patient. Because direct repair is a better procedure at all ages,[82] it is more important to use this technique in children owing to the aforementioned difficulties with grafting. When injury of the flexors is diagnosed, surgical repair of both tendons, if possible, is carried out at all levels (with the possible exception of the zone 4 carpal tunnel level, where it may be better to repair only the profundus). At this time I would defer surgical reconstruction by graft in one or two stages until after the age of 6 years and even older, if possible.

References

1. Arons MS. Purposeful delay of the primary repair of cut flexor tendons in "some-man's land" in children. Plast Reconstr Surg 53:638, 1974.
2. Baker DS, Gaul JS, Williams VK, et al. The little finger superficialis—Clinical investigation of its anatomic and functional shortcomings. J Hand Surg 6:374, 1981.
3. Bora FW. Profundus tendon grafting with unimpaired sublimis function in children. Clin Orthop Rel Res 71:118, 1970.
4. Bora FW, Lane JM, Propcock DJ. Inhibitors of collagen biosynthesis as a means of controlling scar formation in tendon injury. J Bone Joint Surg, 54-A:1501, 1972.
5. Bell JL, Mason ML, Koch SL, et al. Injuries to flexor tendons to the hand in children. J Bone Joint Surg 40-A:1220, 1958.
6. Boyes JH. Operative technique of digital flexor tendon grafts. In AAOS Instructional Course Lectures, vol 10. Ann Arbor, JW Edwards, 1953.

7. Bruner JM. The zig-zag volar digital incision for flexor tendon surgery. Plast Reconstr Surg 40:571, 1967.

8. Bunnell S. Surgery of the Hand. Philadelphia, JB Lippincott, 1944.

9. Burton RI. Extensor tendons, late reconstruction. In Green DP (ed). Operative Hand Surgery. New York, Churchill Livingstone, 1982.

10. Caplan HS, Hunter JM, Merklin RJ. Intrinsic vascularization of flexor tendons. In AAOS Symposium on Flexor Tendon Surgery in the Hand. St Louis, CV Mosby, 1975.

11. Dolphin JA. The extensor tenotomy for chronic boutonnière deformity of the finger. J Bone Joint Surg 47-A:161, 1965.

12. Doyle JR. Extensor tendons—acute injuries. In Green DP (ed). Operative Hand Surgery. New York, Churchill Livingstone, New York, 1982.

13. Doyle JR, Blythe WF. The finger flexor tendon sheath and pulleys: anatomy and reconstruction. In AAOS Symposium on Tendon Surgery in the Hand. St Louis, CV Mosby, 1975.

14. Doyle JR, Blythe WF. Anatomy of the flexor tendon sheath and pulleys of the thumb. J Hand Surg 2:149, 1977.

15. Eaton RG. Hand problems in children. A timetable for management. Pediatr Clin North Am 14:643, 1967.

16. Eaton RG. The extensor mechanism of the fingers. Bull Hosp Joint Dis 30:39, 1969.

17. Eiken O, Hagberg L, Lundborg G: Evolving biological concepts as applied to tendon surgery. Clin Plast Surg 8:1, 1981

18. Elliott RA. Injuries to the extensor mechanism of the hand. Orthop Clin North Am 12:335, 1970.

19. Elliott RA. Splints for mallet and boutonnière deformities. Plast Reconstr Surg 52:282, 1973.

20. Entin MA. Flexor tendon repair and grafting in children. Am J Surg 109:287, 1965.

21. Entin MA. Flexor tendon surgery in children. In AAOS symposium on Surgery of the Hand. St Louis, CV Mosby, 1975.

22. Eyler DL, Markee JE. The anatomy and function of the intrinsic muscles of the fingers. J Bone Joint Surg 36-A:1, 1954.

23. Fetrow KO. Tenolysis in the hand and wrist. A clinical evaluation of 220 flexor and extensor tendolyses. J Bone Joint Surg 49-A:677, 1967.

24. Furlow LT. The role of tendon tissues in tendon healing. Plast Reconstr Surg 57:39, 1976.

25. Hage J, Dupuis CC. The intriguing fate of tendon grafts in small children's hand and their results. Br J Plast Surg 18:341: 1965.

26. Haines RQ. The extensor apparatus of the fingers. J Anat 85:251, 1951.

27. Harris C, Rutledge GL. The functional anatomy of the extensor mechanism of the finger. J Bone Joint Surg. 54-A:713, 1972.

28. Herndon JH. Treatment of tendon injuries in children. Orthop Clin North Am 7:717, 1976.

29. Honnor R. The late management of the isolated lesion of the flexor digitorum profundus tendon. Hand 7:171, 1975.

30. Hunter JM, Cook JF. The pulley system: Rationale for reconstruction. In Strickland JW, Steichen JB (eds). Difficult Problems in Hand Surgery. St Louis, CV Mosby, 1982.

31. Hunter JM, Salisbury RE. Use of gliding artificial implants to produce tendon sheaths. Techniques and results in children. Plast Reconstr Surg 45:564, 1970.

32. Hunter JM, Salisbury RE. Flexor tendon reconstruction in severely damaged hands. A two stage procedure using a silicone Dacron reinforced gliding prosthesis prior to tendon grafting. J Bone Joint Surg 53-A:829, 1971.

33. Hunter JM, Schneider LH. Staged flexor tendon reconstruction. In AAOS Symposium on Tendon Surgery in the Hand. St Louis, CV Mosby, 1975.

34. Hunter JM, Schneider LH. Staged flexor tendon reconstruction. In AAOS Instructional Source Lectures, vol. 26. St Louis, CV Mosby, 1977.

35. Hunter JM, Schneider LH, Dumont J, et al. A dynamic approach to problems of hand function using local anesthesia supplemented by intravenous fentanyl-droperidol. Clin Orthop 104:112, 1974.

36. Hunter JM, Seinsheimer F, Mackin EJ. Tenolysis: pain control and rehabilitation. In Strickland JW, Steichen JB (eds). Difficult Problems in Hand Surgery. St Louis, CV Mosby, 1982.

37. Kaplan EB. Functional and Surgical Anatomy of the Hand, 2nd ed. Philadelphia, JB Lippincott, 1965.

38. Kessler I. The "grasping" technique for tendon repair. Hand 5:252, 1973.

39. Kleinert HE, Kutz JE, Ashbell ST, et al. Primary repair of lacerated flexor tendons in no-man's land. J Bone Joint Surg 49-A:577, 1967.

40. Leddy JP. Flexor tendons—acute injuries. In Green DP (ed). Operative Hand Surgery. New York, Churchill Livingstone, 1982.

41. Leffert RD, Weiss C, Athanasoulis, CA. The vincula. J Bone Joint Surg 56-A:1191, 1974.

42. Lindsay WK. Hand injuries in children. Clin Plast Surg 3:65, 1976.

43. Lindsay WK, McDougall EP. Direct digital flexor repair. Plast Reconstr Surg 26:613, 1960.

44. Lindsay WK, Thomson HG. Digital flexor tendons: An experimental study. Part 1. The significance of each component of the flexor mechanism in tendon healing. Br J Plast Surg 12:289, 1960.

45. Lister GD. Incision and closure of the flexor sheath during primary tendon repair. Hand 15:123, 1983.

46. Lister GD, Kleinert HE, Kutz JE, et al. Primary flexor tendon repair followed by immediate controlled mobilization. J Hand Surg 2:441, 1977.

47. Littler JW. The finger extensor mechanism. Surg Clin North Am 47:415, 1967.

48. Littler JW. Hand, wrist and forearm incisions. In Littler JW, Cramer LM, Smith, JW (eds). Symposium of Reconstructive Hand Surgery. St Louis, CV Mosby, 1974.

49. Littler JW, Eaton RG. Redistribution of forces in correction of boutonnière deformity. J Bone Joint Surg 49-A:1267, 1967.

50. Lundborg G. Experimental flexor tendon healing without adhesion formation—a new concept of tendon nutrition and intrinsic healing mechanisms. Hand 8:235, 1976.

51. Mangus DJ. Immobilization of fingers and thumb after tendon surgery:a simple technique. Plast Reconstr Surg 58:510, 1976.

52. Manske PR, Whiteside AL, Lesker PA. Nutrient pathways to flexor tendons using hydrogen washout technique. J Hand Surg 3:32, 1978.

53. Mason ML, Allen HS. The rate of healing of tendons—an experimental study of tensile strength. Ann Surg 113:424, 1941.

54. Mason ML, Shearon CG. The process of tendon re-

pair: an experimental study of tendon suture and tendon graft. Arch Surg 25:615, 1932.

55. Matthews P, Richards H. The repair potential of digital flexor tendons. J Bone Joint Surg 56-B:618, 1974.

56. Ochiai N, Matsui T, Miyagi N, et al. Vascular anatomy of flexor tendons. J Hand Surg 4:321, 1979.

57. Peacock EE. A study of the circulation in normal tendons and healing grafts. Ann Surg 149:415, 1959.

58. Peacock EE, Madden JW. Some studies on the effect of β-aminoproprionitrile in patients with injured flexor tendons. Surgery 66:215, 1965.

59. Potenza AD. Tendon healing within the flexor digital sheath in the dog. An experimental study. J Bone Joint Surg 44-A:49, 1962.

60. Potenza AD, Herte MC. The synovial cavity as a "tissue culture in situ"; science or nonscience? J Hand Surg 7:196, 1982.

61. Pulvertaft RG. Suture materials and tendon junctures. Am J Surg 109:346, 1965.

62. Rank BK, Wakefield BR. Surgery of Repair as Applied to Hand Injuries, 2nd ed. Baltimore, Williams & Wilkins, 1960.

63. Rosenthal EA. The extensor tendons. In Hunter JM, Schneider LH, Mackin E, Callahan A (eds). Rehabilitation of the Hand, 2nd ed. St Louis, CV Mosby, 1984

64. Schneider LH. Reconstruction in chronic extensor tendon problems. In Strickland JW, Steichen JB (eds). Difficult Problems in Hand Surgery. St Louis, CV Mosby, 1982.

65. Schneider LH. Staged flexor tendon reconstruction using the method of Hunter. Clin Orthop Rel Res 171:164, 1982.

66. Schneider LH. Flexor Tendon Injuries. Boston, Little Brown, 1985.

67. Schneider LH, Hunter JM. Flexor tenolysis. In AAOS Symposium on Tendon Surgery in the Hand. St Louis, CV Mosby, 1975.

68. Schneider LH, Hunter JM. Flexor tendons—late reconstruction. In Green DP (ed). Operative Hand Surgery. New York, Churchill Livingstone, 1982.

69. Schneider LH, Hunter JM, Norris TR, et al. Delayed flexor tendon repair in no-man's land. J Hand Surg 2:452, 1977.

70. Schneider LH, Mackin EJ. Tenolysis. In Hunter JM, Schneider LH, Mackin EJ, Bell JA (eds): Rehabilitation of the Hand. St Louis, CV Mosby, 1978.

71. Schneider LH, Rosenstein RG. Restoration of extensor pollicis longus function by tendon transfer. Plast Reconstr Surg 71:533, 1983.

72. Schneider LH, Wehbe, MA. Reconstruction of flexor profundus injury by superficialis transfer. Abstracts of International Federation of Societies of the Hand. 2nd Int. Congress, Boston, 1983.

73. Schneider LH, Wiltshire D. Restoration of flexor pollicis longus function by flexor digitorum superficialis transfer. J Hand Surg 8:98, 1983.

74. Smillie IS. Mallet finger. Br J Surg 24:439, 1937.

75. Souter WA. The boutonnière deformity. A review of 101 patients with division of the central slip of the extensor mechanism. J Bone Joint Surg 49-B:710, 1967.

76. Stack HG. Muscle function in the fingers. J Bone Joint Surg 44-B:899, 1962.

77. Tubiana R, Valentin P. Anatomy of the extensor apparatus and physiology of finger extension. Surg Clin North Am 44:897, 1964.

78. Tubiana R. Surgical repair of the extensor apparatus of the fingers. Surg Clin North Am 48:1022, 1968.

79. Tubiana R. Incisions and techniques in tendon grafting. Am J Surg 109:339, 1965.

80. Urbaniak JR, Cahill JD, Mortenson RA: Tendon suturing methods: Analysis of tensile strengths. In AAOS Symposium on Tendon Surgery in the Hand. St Louis, CV Mosby, 1975.

81. Urbaniak JR, Hayes MG. Chronic boutonnière deformity—An anatomic reconstruction. J Hand Surg 6:379, 1981.

82. Vahvanen V, Gripenberg L, Nuutinen P. Flexor tendon injury of the hand in children. Scand J Plast Reconstr Surg 15:43, 1981.

83. Verdan CE. Half a century of flexor tendon surgery. Current status and changing philosophies. J Bone Joint Surg 54-A:472, 1972.

84. Verdan CE. Primary and secondary repair of flexor and extensor tendon injuries. In Flynn JE (ed). Hand Surgery, 2nd ed. Baltimore, Williams & Wilkins, 1975.

85. Wakefield AR. Hand injuries in children. J Bone Joint Surg 46-A:1226, 1964.

86. Wehbé MA, Schneider LH. Mallet fractures. J Bone Joint Surg 66-A:658, 1984.

87. Whitaker JH, Strickland JW, Ellis RK. The role of flexor tenolysis in the palm and fingers. J Hand Surg 2:231, 1977.

C H A P T E R ○ 7

Injuries to Nerves

F. WILLIAM BORA, JR.

TRANSECTION

Transection of peripheral nerves is frequent in both civilian and military populations. After continuity of a nerve is interrupted, the axons and myelin sheaths degenerate distal to the laceration (wallerian degeneration). Within 2 days of section, axonal disruption can be discerned by electron microscopy. Later, axonal fragmentation can be visualized by light microscopy of silver-stained sections. Myelin sheaths retract and form into globules of fat, and myelin and axonal fragments are phagocytized. In addition to paralysis and anesthesia in the territory innervated by the severed nerve, there is loss of the trophic influences of the nerve on muscle, joints, nails, and skin. This results in progressive atrophy of muscle, bone, and skin as well as in degenerative changes in the joints.

Nerve Regeneration Following Transection

For restoration of normal neurologic function, axons in the proximal stump of the interrupted nerve must sprout, migrate through the scar between proximal and distal stumps, and reach end-organs. Proteins required for the formation of these regenerating axons must be synthesized; this assemblage occurs chiefly in the nerve cell bodies in the anterior horns of the spinal cord and dorsal root ganglia. These proteins are transported peripherally to the axon tips, with most being carried through the axons from the nerve cell bodies at a rate of 2 to 5 mm/day in mammals, a rate comparable to the observed rate of axonal regeneration.[18] The specific protein constituting the bulk of this flow is neurotubular monomer, globular protein with a molecular weight of 60,000.[13] Most nerve cells require several months before nerve regeneration is complete (Fig. 7–1).

Ideally, after nerve section, normal neurologic function would be restored by prompt, orderly axonal outgrowth and remyelination prior to end-muscle deterioration. In practice, unfortunately, nerve regeneration is often prolonged, misdirected, and incomplete. Full return of sensory and motor trophic nerve function is rarely achieved.

Figure 7–1. The response of the nerve cell to injury. (Redrawn from Ducker TB, Kemper LG, Hayes GJ. Neurosurgery 30:272–273, 1969.)

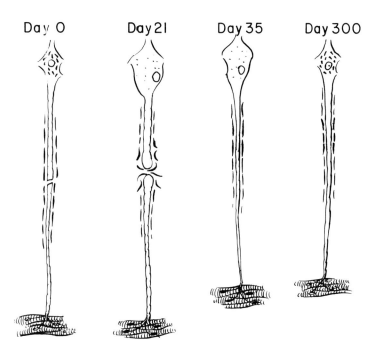

Several factors are responsible for this incomplete recovery:

1. Axons may penetrate the scar promptly but grow into the incorrect fascicle in the distal nerve stump so that they never reach the appropriate end-organs. This problem can be reduced by careful matching of nerve fascicles between the proximal and distal stumps at the time of surgical repair of a severed nerve[5] and might be further reduced by control of scar formation at the site of laceration of the nerve.

2. Axons may fail to penetrate the scar, so that a neuroma forms at the site of section. The neuroma consists of whorls and tangled masses of axonal sprouts enmeshed in fibrous tissue. Sunderland[23] has emphasized the importance of local obstruction by collagen fibrils in the scar as the chief impediment to proper axonal penetration into the distal stump. Even in optimal circumstances, the penetration through the nerve scar takes 3 to 5 weeks. Inhibition of collagen synthesis might shorten this period and reduce the size of neuromas.

3. Axons that do bridge the scar, choose the proper fascicle in the distal stump, and reach the end-organ cannot conduct impulses properly unless insulated by myelin of normal thickness over their entire length (except at the nodes of Ranvier). Schwann cells are stimulated to initiate such remyelination only when axons reach a diameter of at least one µ.[19] A Schwann cell must then revolve around an axon 20 or more times to form mature myelin. Closely matted collagen fibers prevent remyelination by restricting the size of the axons in the scar and by diminishing the mobility of the Schwann cells. Incomplete remyelination results in the persistent reduction in motor and sensory conduction velocities often found following nerve laceration.

Morphologic and Histologic Findings Following Transection

Morphologic observations by Holmes and by Saunders and Young[14, 20] suggested that, after nerve transection, the endoneurial Schwann cell tubes in the distal nerve segment become progressively blocked by deposition of endoneurial collagen and that this endoneurial fibrosis prevents regenerating axons from reaching end-organs because the diameter of the tubes is reduced. Abercrombie and Johnson[1, 2] found that the collagen content of the distal nerve segment of transected rabbit sciatic nerve increases linearly for more than 1 year after the injury and they concluded that the entire distal segment was involved. We have confirmed that collagen scar formation does occur in the distal stump of transected nerves, regardless of whether the nerves are repaired. We have found, however, that the scar is confined to the initial few millimeters below the injury and does not extend into the remainder of the distal nerve segment.

It has been suggested that one of the reasons that full muscle power fails to recover after nerve transection and regeneration is progressive fibrosis of denervated muscle, which results in permanent impairment of the mechanical properties of the muscles, despite reinnervation. Biochemical studies of denervated muscle confirm that the proportion of the muscle cross-section taken up by fibrous tissue is increased, but we have found that the total collagen content in triceps sural muscle after sciatic nerve transection in rats does not increase, even 1 year following denervation. Rather, collagen content remains constant while the muscle fibers atrophy (Pleasure and Bora, unpublished data). These observations indicate that progressive muscle fibrosis is not a major contributing factor to muscle weakness after nerve transection. Therefore, the evidence suggests that the primary problem is collagen scar formation in the motor nerve, which is confined to the region of nerve transection, and that measures limiting scar in this region might be successful in improving the prognosis of patients with nerve injuries.

Clinical Presentations of Nerve Injury

Nerve injuries present in various clinical pictures that alter function. *Neuropraxia* is a contusion of the nerve without wallerian degeneration, and functional recovery is complete 6 weeks after injury. *Axonotmesis* is a more severe injury in which wallerian degeneration occurs. The neural elements distal to the injury degenerate in axonotmesis, but the fibrous tubes, epineurium, perineurium, and endoneurium remain intact. Ultimate functional recovery usually occurs at 6 months. *Neurotmesis* is the most severe nerve injury, in which both the neural and the supporting fibrous tubes are disrupted. The treatment of neurotmesis is nerve suture. The results in children are satisfactory but in adults are guarded. If the injury creates a gap too great to be treated with mobilization and suture, nerve grafting should be considered. The results of nerve grafting are generally inferior to those of nerve suture.

Surgical Repair

Nerve Suture

Following laceration, peripheral nerve elasticity combined with an apparent precut tension creates a gap between the proximal and the distal stumps. Prior to nerve suture, a force mediated through forceps or traction sutures is required to overcome the gap. The irregular cuts causing most nerve lacerations stimulate a scar tissue response in the contiguous ends of the proximal and distal nerve stumps, which, if not block-excised prior to suture, stimulates scar tissue that obstructs axon sprout passage across the anastomosis. In clinical situations, excision of the nerve ends is usually necessary, creating a gap that must frequently be overcome by joint positioning, tension on the nerve ends, and nerve mobilization. More severe cases in which a large gap exists may require nerve grafting. After healing of the surgical repair, nerve gliding and extensibility are essential to extremity rehabilitation, including joint extension. How does a nerve, shortened and treated by mobilization and tension to overcome a gap, stretch to permit joint mobilization? An experiment in which rat sciatic nerves were used was developed to measure the biomechanical adjustments that a peripheral nerve makes to tension. Our results suggest that nerve tissue has considerable remodeling capabilities. (Fig. 7–2).[6]

Most nerve lacerations are clean and proximal to their terminal fascicular division. Two of the most important decisions to be made by the surgeon treating acute nerve lacerations are how and when to suture these multifascicular injuries. It has been reported that epineurial suture is unreliable in restoring accurate fascicular anatomy after nerve laceration and that perineurial suture gives more satisfactory results in both clinical and experimental situations.[5] Perineurial sutures are technically more difficult than epineurial sutures, demand more time, and, if not properly executed, create more intraneural scar, which obstructs axon growth.[7]

We designed an experimental study to compare the effectiveness of epineurial, perineurial, and combined epineurial and perineurial suture after laceration of the sciatic nerve in rabbits. Biochemical assays of mye-

NORMAL   IMMEDIATE   7 WEEKS

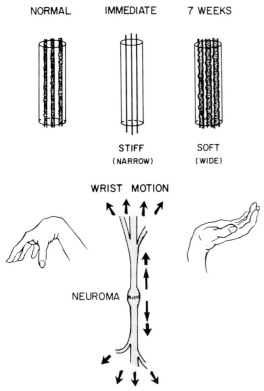

STIFF   SOFT
(NARROW)   (WIDE)

WRIST MOTION

NEUROMA

Figure 7–2. The response of the peripheral nerve tension when stretched within physiologic limits. (Redrawn from Bora FW, Richardson S, Black J. J Hand Surg 5:23, 1980.)

most rapid in this group. This experiment showed epineurial suture to give the best results, and this technique is recommended for most nerve lacerations (Fig. 7–3).

However, in nerve lacerations cut at a level where a nerve divides into its terminal fascicular branches, intraneural sutures using the internal epineurial bulk next to the perineurium are recommended for suture placement to match fascicles. For example, if the median nerve is cut at the level of the carpal canal where it divides into several fascicles, sutures using the internal epineurium more accurately align the fascicles of the proximal main trunk with the fascicles cut more distally.[6, 7, 19, 23] There are several other common situations where intraneural sutures are recommended: (1) When the ulnar nerve is cut two inches proximal to the wrist it is necessary to accurately align the main trunk and dorsal sensory division using intraneural sutures. (2) In Guyon's canal, the ulnar nerve separates into the deep motor branch, a branch to the intrinsic muscles, a hypothenar branch, and sensory branches of the small and ring fingers. Intraneural sutures are recommended when the nerve is cut at this level as well. (3) Radial nerve lacerations proximal to the elbow should be treated with separation of motor and sensory fascicle groups. In this manner axon misdirection is minimized when sprouts penetrate the distal stump. (4) Lacerations of a common digital nerve where it divides into proper digital branches at the base of the finger are also sutured by the intraneural technique (Fig. 7–4).

lin were used to determine nerve regeneration in both immediate and delayed repairs. The amount of myelin was greatest in the animals in which epineurial sutures were used, which suggests that nerve regeneration was

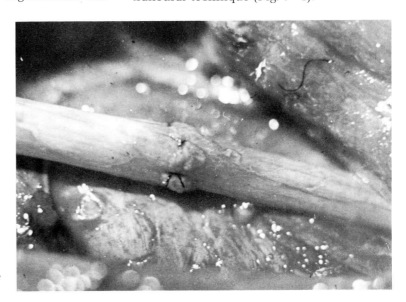

Figure 7–3. Epineurial suture in the midforearm.

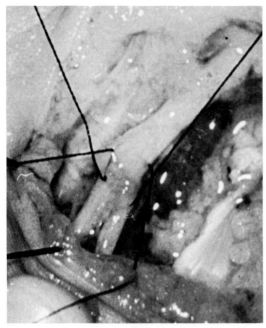

Figure 7–4. Intraneural suture of proper digital branches to the common digital trunk at the base of the finger.

Primary Versus Secondary Repair

In clinical practice, immediate repair of the nerve injury is often not possible owing to contamination of the wound and associated injuries of other tissues. Suturing must then be delayed and is best accomplished by specialized personnel with microsurgical instrumentation.

Factors that one should consider when deciding whether a nerve laceration should be repaired primarly or secondarily are (1) circumstances of the injury (a clean knife wound in a kitchen suggests primary repair; a wound in a machine shop with a large component of crush suggests secondary repair); (2) time elapsed between the injury and treatment (after 1 hour primary suture is favored; after 24 hours secondary repair is indicated); (3) character or contamination of the wound (a clean wound favors primary repair; a dirty wound favors secondary repair); (4) other injuries (a cut involving skin, nerve, or one or two tendons favors primary suture; multiple injuries—such as head, abdomen, and multiple tendon lacerations—favor secondary nerve repair); and (5) the leisure of the surgeon (a well-rested operator performs a more exact suture, and the ultimate functional result of the nerve repair reflects the technical exactness of the method of suture). The fore-

going examples are obviously at the extremes of the scale of each consideration; when injuries approach the middle of the scale, as they frequently do, each factor must be evaluated not only by itself but also in relation to all the other factors present. In general, open nerve lacerations should be repaired primarily, whereas closed nerve injuries should be observed by clinical and electrical diagnostic study until a period of time has elapsed in which one would expect end-organ reinnervation. If recovery has not occurred as expected, secondary surgery should be performed.

In general, primary suture of a nerve subjects the patient to only one operation and one hospitalization and is therefore preferable. Primary nerve suture lessens the reinnervation time of muscle and sensory receptor endorgans. Observations made in evaluations of the functional results in clinical cases as well as data from experimental situations make it clear that the main objective of a surgeon who is treating a nerve laceration is to suture the cut as soon as possible. However, if the acute injury is complicated by multiple injuries or possible infection of the wound, secondary repair is the treatment of choice. Factors favoring secondary suture are as follows: (1) The epineurium is thicker, which enables the surgeon to place sutures more accurately and holds the suture more firmly, making tying easier; and (2) the interneurial fibrosis that occurs at the cut ends after nerve laceration can be more easily assessed at secondary repair, making it easier to determine how much of the nerve one must trim at the cut ends.

Acute Skin Lacerations

Lacerations can usually be incorporated into incisions that adequately expose cut nerves for repair without causing joint contractures. After skin and subcutaneous dissection, normal nerves should be identified proximal and distal to the neuroma, after which the neuroma, including some of the surrounding scar tissue, is isolated by sharp dissection. With this technique, intact fascicles may be observed and left in continuity in partial nerve injuries, and only the injured fascicles within the neuroma resected, with the cut nerve ends sutured. With acute lacerations, there is a blood clot in various degrees of maturation between the cut ends rather than the tough fibrous tissue that is present in late nerve repair situations. After the neuroma or injured nerve ends are isolated, a No. 11 scalpel blade is used to trim the nerve to normal fascicular tissue. A moistened tongue blade is placed behind the nerve to protect other structures and to provide cutting resistance as the nerve ends are freshened. Magnification is helpful in aligning rotation, in matching fascicles, and in placing and tying sutures. The microscope is used in most upper extremity repairs, although loops may be used for epineurial repairs of large proximal nerves. The recommended suture consists of 10-0 monofilament nylon, but a large suture may be used if more strength is needed to bring nerve ends together. In many cases, two or three 7-0 nylon sutures are required to hold the nerve ends together, and after tension is overcome smaller 10-0 sutures are used to approximate the lacerated epineurial edges. Fine jeweler forceps, a nonlocking eye needle holder, and sharp nerve scissors are especially helpful in this delicate surgery. Fascicular orientation is indicated by vascular markings on the outside of the nerve and by the size of the fascicles on the proximal and distal faces of the lacerated nerve edges, especially if the cut ends have not been trimmed. If an acute, sharp laceration is clean, the surgeon can remove the blood clots between the fascicles, thereby avoiding all trimming. This technique increases the chance of good fascicular matching because axons change places within the peripheral nerve as they run from the shoulder to the fingertip, and trimming changes the fascicular patterns at the cut ends. Nerve mobilization and joint positioning help overcome moderate gaps so that nerve suture holds the nerve ends together with minimal tension. Each nerve suture provokes fibrous tissue that obstructs axon sprouting and maturation; therefore, the minimum number of stitches is recommended for nerve end repairs. Fascicular sutures require at least one suture per fascicle and, in some cases, two or three. Judgment regarding the number of sutures depends on how each fascicle lies after the placement of each suture.

Postoperative Results (Children Compared with Adults)

It is well recognized that children respond better and attain a higher functional level of activity than adults following surgery for similar conditions. Peripheral nerve surgery is a prime example of this axiom. If a median nerve laceration is sutured at the wrist in a clean wound, the result will be normal nerve function in children 10 years of age and younger. An adult of 40 years, however, will be fortunate to reach a level of 50% of normal. The reason for this disparity has been studied, and Almquist[3] reported that children have a cerebral compliance that can adjust to mixed peripheral signals, integrating them into a more normal pattern than that demonstrated by adults. Another advantage for children is that they have shorter arms than adults, so the axoplasm has less distance to travel to end-organs. Furthermore, the cross-sectional face of a child's cut nerve has a fascicular area that represents 80% of the tissue, whereas in adults the fascicular area is 60% (Fig. 7–5). This observation suggests that with surgical repair the chance of fascicular alignment is greater in children than in adults and that interfascicular fibrous tissue in adults will play a more prominent role as a producer of scar that compromises axonal penetration as well as axon and myelin maturation. The end of a cut nerve under magnification shows axonal bulging (similar to a frog's eye) in children, whereas adults have axon tissue level with—or (in older patients) even withdrawn from—the cut end of the

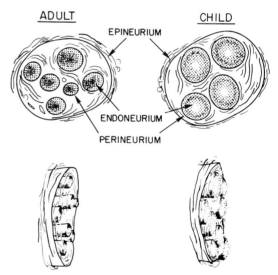

Figure 7–5. This drawing represents a comparison of cross section of peripheral nerves in the adult and the child. The fascicles represent a larger area of the cross section of the nerve in the child than in the adult, and there is more apparent axoplasm bulging from the fascicle at the laceration level in the child than in the adult.

nerve (Fig. 7–5). This suggests that nerve cells and axonal pressure in children are superior to those in adults and is probably another reason that findings after peripheral nerve laceration and repair are better in children than in adults.

Postoperative Evaluation of Cutaneous Sensibility

After nerve laceration and suture, regular evaluation of cutaneous sensibility helps evaluate the surgical result and establish a functional treatment program for the patient. Sensation should be evaluated at 6-week intervals by the following modalities:

1. *Tinel's sign.* This is the tingling sensation experienced when cutaneous percussion is made over the injured nerve to define the level to which axons have regenerated after nerve injury and its treatment. The patient determines the point of maximal sensitivity to the stimulus and experiences paraesthesias in the area of innervation distal to the injury. After axons have penetrated the neuroma, the point of percussion causing a Tinel's sign advances along the course of the nerve at approximately 1 mm/day, or 1 inch/month.

2. *Measurements of the size of the anesthetic and dysesthetic zones.* These are determined by the patient's subjective description of the quality of sensibility. From this information, a sensory mapping is obtained, which is used as a baseline to which future mappings are compared.

3. *Sensory localization.* This is determined by use of a moving-touch stimulus and a constant-touch stimulus. This method has been used to evaluate the quick and slow adapting capacities of group A beta fibers, which control the perception of touch.[11] This modality measures a pattern of sensory recovery in which moving touch is perceived and localized prior to constant touch. It helps one determine the appropriate time to institute a program of sensory re-education. Appreciation of light touch to deep pressure, through the process of localization, is tested with Frey's hairs or Semmes-Weinstein pressure-sensitive monofilaments. Fibers of varying diameters are placed against the skin. Pressure is exerted until a fiber of a specific diameter bends. Larger fibers require greater force to bend; accordingly, fibers of various diameters are used until a sensory response is elicited. This examination is a study of the patient's sensibility in which the variable is the diameter of the fiber.[24] The test provides the physician with an opportunity to chart the patient's recognition of touch. Results of these examinations and those observed when the patient is tested at subsequent visits can be compared.

The two-point discrimination test involves a two-point aesthesiometer consisting of two sharp points with a variable distance between them calibrated in millimeters. The minimum distance between two sharp points applied longitudinally that the patient can discriminate from a single applied point is recorded in millimeters within each zone. After determining the patient's two-point discriminatory abilities, the physician relates them to function by comparing the results to those obtained with the Moberg pick-up test, which measures tactile manipulation of objects.

Postoperative Sensory Re-Education

In addition to sensory evaluation, various rehabilitative programs are important in determining the results of nerve injury. Sensory re-education teaches the patient to maximize sensibility and improve hand function. Exercises help the patient relearn altered sensory impulses. Various stimuli (moving touch, constant touch, and objects of varying size and shape) are placed in contact with impaired sensory areas, and the patient is taught to reassociate the new sensation with an old activity. Sensory relearning by active motion is another modality that helps patients improve impaired sensibility. In this program, the patient manipulates blocks of various shapes and textures as well as objects used in everyday life to improve appreciation of touch localization.[12, 25]

Postoperative Activities for Muscle Strengthening

During sensory evaluation and re-education, one must be careful to prevent deformity and to strengthen weak muscles. Dynamic and functional splints prevent joint contracture, keeping joints in their functional positions while muscle imbalance improves during nerve regeneration. This procedure maximizes hand function early in the muscle recovery process, because the joints are mobile and the muscle action is delivered while the joints are in their most functional position.

Patients are also instructed in passive exercises to increase joint motion.

Postoperative treatment also includes various activities that the patient can perform to increase muscle strength (e.g., using therapeutic putty and practicing resistive muscle exercises). Progress in grip strength is measured periodically with the Jamar dynamometer. Lateral and palmer pinch exercises for individual fingers are encouraged, and digital strengths are recorded.

Periodic EMG testing can help one determine the reinnervation of paralyzed muscles by defining functioning motor unit potentials. Biofeedback may be used on surface muscles in some cases as a strengthening modality.

HEMORRHAGE, SCARRING, AND DETERIORATION OF NERVE FUNCTION FOLLOWING OTHER INJURIES

Nerve function is compromised by injuries other than transection. Bullet wounds, needle injections, and localized pressure on the skin produce hemorrhage and scarring in and around the nerves in the area of injury. Patients with such injuries who have altered nerve function should be followed carefully by repeated clinical examination and electrical diagnostic testing. If the nerve function deteriorates or does not return to an acceptable level within a reasonable period of time, surgical release should be considered. The level of the injury and the characteristics of the wound are important factors in the timing of surgery. Neurolysis, in which magnification and microsurgical techniques are used, may be helpful in such cases.

RECONSTRUCTION AFTER IRREPARABLE NERVE DAMAGE

Nerve that cannot be repaired causes muscle paralysis, which compromises extremity function. Joint motion is limited and deformities occur because of muscle imbalance. Tendon transfers balance muscle forces, which improve joint position and motion. A muscle tendon unit may be transferred to another location with its innervation and vascular supply preserved or as a free graft in which a vessel and nerve attached to the transferred muscle are sutured to a vessel and nerve in the recipient bed (see Chap. 8).

Understanding the patient's needs and selecting muscles with adequate power to transfer are important prerequisites to successful tendon transfers. Muscle power may be evaluated by the following scale before surgery: zero—paralysis; trace—palpable contraction; poor—moves the joint through a full range of motion with gravity eliminated; fair—moves the joint through a full range of motion against gravity; good—moves the joint through a full range of motion against gravity with resistance, but not equal to the contralateral side; and normal—moves a joint through a full range of motion against gravity and resistance that is equal to the contralateral normal side. After transfer, a muscle loses one grade of power; thus, a fair muscle will become a poor muscle and fail to move the joint through a full range of motion against gravity postoperatively. Only muscles with normal or good power are recommended for tendon transfers. Use of muscles that work in synchrony with those they replace makes it easier for children to learn a new function after surgery. For example, wrist extensors, finger flexors, and finger adductors as well as wrist flexors, finger extensors, and finger abductors work in synchrony. Additional prerequisites are mobile skin cover and passive joint mobility. Matching muscle–tendon units of similar amplitude (excursion) is desirable. A transferred muscle should perform only one function and should pass in a straight line. An exception, however, is the opponens transfer, which is purposely routed around a stable pulley.

When selecting a donor, one should make a list of the functional loss, make a list of the muscles that are working and available for transfer, and then choose the muscle that is best suited for the job and that gives up the least function. The transfer should be attached as close as possible to the insertion of the tendon that it is replacing. In general, flexor transfers are protected for 3 weeks and extensor transfers for 5 weeks after surgery. The patient usually wears a protective splint for an additional 2 months while sleeping.

Procedures that supplement tendon transfer function are tendon grafting (to increase tendon length), tenodesis, capsulodesis, and, occasionally, joint arthrodesis in older children.

The most common nerve injuries in children occur to the median and ulnar nerve at the wrist and to the radial nerve at the elbow. Numerous combinations of transfers have been proposed for these nerve deficits, and all have merit in the proper setting. The following tendon transfers, however, are recommended in the pediatric age group.

Median Nerve Injury at the Wrist

The functional motor loss to be restored in this injury is thumb opposition. The standard procedure, with certain modifications, is transfer of the flexor digitorum superficialis of the ring finger, as originally described by Bunnell.[8] The flexor digitorum superficialis is transected proximal to the volar plate. Superficialis tags are preserved so that swan neck deformity is avoided at the proximal interphalangeal joint. The tendon must be isolated through a separate incision in the forearm and then looped around the flexor carpi ulnaris (as close to the pisiform as possible), which acts as a pulley. The tendon is tunneled subcutaneously through the palm to the thumb metacarpophalangeal where it is divided into two slips. One tendon slip is woven into the thumb abductor tendon and the other into the extensor mechanism (see Fig. 3–44).[16]

Transfer of the extensor indicis proprius[9] through the palm or the extensor digiti minimi[21] around the ulna are useful opponens transfers when the palm, wrist, and forearm have been badly scarred. A simple transfer for opposition is that described by Camitz,[10] in which the palmaris longus tendon, harvested in continuity with the pretendinous band to the long finger, is tunneled subcutaneously and attached to the dorsum of the thumb metacarpophalangeal joint. While this transfer does not provide as much power as the previously mentioned procedures, it does give adequate palmar abduction. Littler's[15] drawing of the transfer first described by Huber uses the abductor digiti minimi for opposition (see Fig. 3–43). This is useful in hands with congenital deficient thenar musculature. The insertion of the muscle is detached, as is its origin from the pisiform, after the neurovascular pedicle has been isolated. It is held only by its attachment to the flexor carpi ulnaris and the neurovascular pedicle. The muscle is rotated and passed subcutaneously to be attached to the abductor pollicis brevis tendon. During

this maneuver, one must take care to avoid kinking the neurovascular pedicle.

Ulnar Nerve Injury at the Wrist

Weak pinch and clawing of the small and ring fingers are the result of ulnar nerve injury at the wrist. Although some of these deformities can be treated with splinting, many require surgery.

Claw deformity (extension of the metacarpophalangeal joint and flexion of the interphalangeal joints) may be significantly improved by the superficialis loop[27] and by the volar plate advancement procedures described by Zancolli.[26] In the loop procedure, the superficialis is divided proximal to its insertion, directed through an incision in the A2 pulley, and sutured to itself in the palm. This maneuver makes the superficialis a flexor of the metacarpophalangeal joint rather than the proximal interphalangeal joint. The volar plate advancement procedure attaches the volar plate more proximally by suture to the metacarpal neck. This is accomplished by passing a suture in the volar plate through a drill hole in the metacarpal neck, which is tied over a button on the dorsum of the hand. This capsulodesis tethers the metacarpophalangeal joint in flexion but is less satisfactory in younger children because the volar plate may attenuate with growth.

Pinch is weak because the adductor muscle to the thumb and abduction of the index finger by the first dorsal interosseous are paralyzed. Transfer of the extensor indicus proprius to the first dorsal interosseous restores index abduction. Adductor function to the thumb is restored by transfer of the ring finger superficialis. In children close to skeletal maturity, metacarpophalangeal fusion may be used to stabilize the thumb, which then makes the extensor pollicis brevis expendable for transfer to the first dorsal interosseous tendon for index abduction, thereby sparing the extensor indicis proprius muscle for other transfers.

Radial Nerve Injury at the Elbow

The functional motor losses to be restored in this injury are wrist extension, metacarpophalangeal joint extension of the fingers, and thumb extension and radial abduction.

Transfer of the pronator teres to the extensor carpi radialis brevis for wrist extension, the flexor carpi radialis through the interosseous membrane to the extensor digitorum communis for finger extension, and the ring superficialis through the interosseous membrane to the extensor pollicis longus for thumb extension are recommended. If the superficialis of the fourth finger is not available, the palmaris longus may be substituted. Similarly, the flexor carpi ulnaris may be substituted for the flexor carpi radialis, although this transfer has less excursion and leaves the radial wrist motors unopposed, which radially deviates the wrist.

References

1. Abercrombie M, Johnson M. Collagen content of rabbit sciatic nerve during wallerian degeneration. J Neurol Neurosurg Psychiatry 9:113, 1946.
2. Abercrombie M, Johnson M. The effect of reinnervation on collagen formation in degenerating sciatic nerves of rabbits. J Neurol Neurosurg Psychiatry 10:89, 1947.
3. Almquist E, Eeg-Olofsson O. Sensory-nerve-conduction velocity and two-point discrimination in sutural nerves. J Bone Joint Surg 52A:791–796, 1970.
4. Ballantyne JP, Jr, Campbell M. Electrophysiological study after surgical repair of sectioned human peripheral nerves. J Neurol Neurosurg Psychiatry 36:797, 1983.
5. Bora FW Jr. Peripheral nerve repair in cats: The fascicular stitch. J Bone Joint Surg 49A:659, 1967.
6. Bora FW Jr. Black J. The biochemical response to tension in a peripheral nerve. J Hand Surg 15(1):21, 1980.
7. Bora FW Jr. Pleasure DE, Didizian NA. A study of nerve regeneration and neuroma formation after nerve suture by various techniques. J Hand Surg 1(2):138, 1976.
8. Bunnell S. Opposition of the thumb. J Bone Joint Surg 20:269–284, 1938.
9. Burkhalter WE, Christensen RC, Brown PW. Extensor indicis proprius opponensplasty. J Bone Joint Surg 55A:725–732, 1973.
10. Camitz H. Surgical treatment of paralysis of opponens muscle of thumb. Acta Chir Scand, 65:77–81, 1929.
11. Dellon AL, Curtis RM, Edgerton MT. Evaluating recovery of sensation of the hand following nerve injury. Johns Hopkins Med J 139:235–243, 1972.
12. Dellon AL, Curtis RM, Edgerton MT. Re-education of sensation in the hand after injury and repair. Plast Reconstr Surg 53(3):297–304, 1974.
13. Grafstein B, McEwen BS, Shelanski ML. Axonal transport of neurotubule protein. Nature 227:289, 1970.
14. Holmes W, Young Y. Nerve regeneration after immediate and delayed suture. J Anat 77:63, 1942.
15. Littler JW, Cooley SGE. Opposition of the thumb and its restoration by abductor digiti quinti transfer. J Bone Joint Surg 45A:1389–1396, 1963.
16. Palende DD. Opponensplasty in intrinsic muscle paralysis of the thumb in leprosy. J Bone Joint Surg 57A:489, 1975.
17. Pleasure D, Bora FW Jr, Lane J, et al. Regeneration after nerve transection: effect of inhibition of collagen synthesis. Exp Neurol 45:72, 1974.
18. Pleasure DE, Mishler K, Engle WK. Axoplasmic transport of proteins in experimental neuropathies. Science 166:524, 1966.
19. Pleasure DE, Towfighi J. Onion bulb neuropathies. Arch Neurol, 26:289–301, 1972.
20. Saunders F, Young Y. The role of the peripheral stump in the control of fiber diameter in regenerating nerves. J Physiol 103:119, 1944.
21. Schneider LH. Opponensplasty using the extensor digiti minimi. J Bone Joint Surg 51:1297–1302, 1969.
22. Shantaveerappa T, Bourne G. Perineural epithelium: a new concept of its role in the integrity of the peripheral nervous system. Science 154:1464, 1966.
23. Sunderland S. Nerves and Nerve Injuries. Baltimore, Williams & Wilkins, 1968.
24. Werner JL, Omer GE. Evaluating cutaneous pressure sensation of the hand. Am J Occup Ther 24:5,347–356, 1970.
25. Wynn-Parry CB, Salter M. Sensory re-education after median nerve lesions. Hand 8(3):250–257, 1976.
26. Zancolli GA. Claw-hand caused by paralysis of the intrinsic muscles. A simple surgical procedure for its correction. J Bone Joint Surg 39A:1076–1080, 1957.
27. Zancolli GA. Structural and Dynamic Cases of Hand Surgery, 2nd ed. Philadelphia, JB Lippincott, 168–174, 1978.

CHAPTER ○ 8

Replantation and Elective Microsurgery

JAMES W. MAY, JR.
ROBERT C. SAVAGE
A. LEE OSTERMAN

Replantation

Experimental replantation began as early as 1903 with Hopfner's canine investigations.[21] Carrel and Guthrie's study of vascular anastomotic technique and limb replantation and transplantation stimulated further laboratory efforts.[9, 10, 11] Human replantation, however, was not performed until 1962, when Malt successfully reattached an arm in a 12-year-old boy.[32] It is most fortunate that the first successful replantation was performed on a child. The positive functional recovery in this case provided additional impetus to other workers in the field.[19, 31, 33] Komatsu and Tamai performed the first successful thumb replantation in 1965,[28] and, at the same time, Kleinert and associates were reporting successful revascularization of limbs and digits.[24–27] Concomitant refinements in microvascular technique and instrumentation by Buncke, Lee, Kleinert, and Kasdan solidified replantation surgery as a reality.[4–7, 25, 26, 30] Since these early replantation efforts, the treatment objective has progressed from extremity viability to extremity function.

The adaptability of children to nerve injury makes them ideal candidates for replantation efforts. Children have good nerve regeneration, tendon gliding, bone healing, and joint mobility after injury, which favorably affects the results of replantation.[1, 22, 44, 53] Jaeger and associates have reported an overall survival rate as high as 85% in a series of 60 amputated parts in children.[22] Others have reported a tissue survival rate following replantation to be worse in the pediatric group than in adults with comparable injuries.[1, 22, 44, 53] This has been our experience, but we believe it is related to the fact that in adults who have an occupation which does not require replacement of a specific part, the part is amputated so that they can return to work. In children, the injured part is revascularized or replanted because their future is uncertain. Moreover, children have vessels that are smaller and prone to spasm after anastomosis, which makes survival more unpredictable. Hesitancy to use vein grafts because of technical difficulty and additional scarring may be a secondary reason for decreased success in children. The limited cooperation of children in the postoperative phase has been reported to detract from the success of these procedures, but we believe that with appropriate sedation and immobilization this factor can be minimized.

Digital replantation has been successful in patients as young as 13 months[29] and has been accomplished in the small finger at the proximal interphalangeal joint in a 21-month-old child with a vessel diameter of 0.3 mm. Exceptional functional return has also been reported in an amputation as high as the deltoid insertion in another 21-month-old child.[46] Although technically difficult, the potential for excellent functional and cosmetic results makes replantation worthwhile and gratifying in the pediatric age group.

INDICATIONS

In general, indications for replantation in children should be broader than those recognized for adults. No replantation, however, should be attempted unless a reasonable functional result can be expected, and no replantation of the upper extremity should be performed if it endangers life because of other injuries or medical conditions.

Factors involved in the decision to replant are summarized in Figure 8–1. All thumb, multiple digit, distal forearm, hand, and midpalm amputations should be replanted if patient condition and technical considerations permit. Replantation of a single digit can be worthwhile if the amputation is clean, because the sensory return after nerve suture in children is predictably superior to that in adults. Upper arm amputations should be attempted provided the following conditions are present: (1) Other injuries do not preclude the surgical effort; (2) ischemia time is not prolonged; (3) the brachial plexus has not been avulsed; (4) muscle destruction and contamination are not excessive; and (5) there is no serious double-level injury.

In children, digital replantation distal to the distal interphalangeal joint is often technically impossible because the vessels are small, but success has been reported with arterial repair alone.[13, 29, 48, 49] Digital vessels are larger in more proximal amputations, so better survival rates can be expected.[44] In experimental situations, repair of a vessel that measures between 0.5 and 1 mm in diameter results in survival of distal tissues in 85% of cases.[16] This is the diameter of the vessels distal to the proximal interphalangeal joint, and replantation at that level yields rewarding functional results, even in single digit amputations (Fig. 8–2). Single digit replantation proximal to the proximal interphalangeal joint is controversial because at follow-up these fingers are short and have limited proximal interphalangeal joint motion because of scarring between extrinsic tendons and bone. In O'Brien's series, replantation of the long and index fingers yielded the highest survival rates, and replantation of the little finger gave the poorest.[44]

Amputations can be classified into three groups: (1) "guillotine," or sharp, amputation; (2) crush amputation; and (3) avulsion amputation. Crush and avulsion amputations are most common[22] and have a peak incidence at age 5. Guillotine amputations occur most frequently around age 15. As in adults, survival and functional recovery in children are better with guillotine and localized crush injuries than with avulsion amputations.[22]

MECHANISM AND ETIOLOGY OF INJURY

Most traumatic amputations occur on the fingers, on the palm of the hand, or around the elbow.[18] Amputations are more common in boys than girls.[18, 47] The level and type of amputation is often related to the mechanism of injury. Hand or digit amputations are most frequently caused by an axe or saw.[22] Bicycle

REPLANT RESULTS

Poor	Good
Adult	Youth
Poor Desire	Minimal Avulsion
Single Proximal Digit	Thumb, Hand, or Multi-Digit
Double Level	Short Ischemia
Systemic Disease	Experienced Team

Figure 8–1. Prognostic factors in replantation.

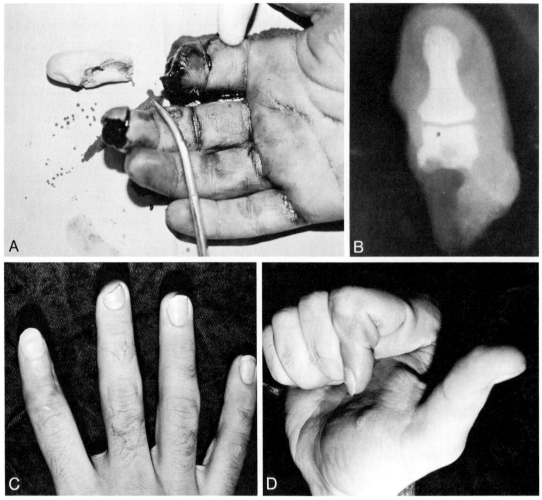

Figure 8–2. *A,* Index finger amputation distal to PIP joint in 16-year-old male. *B,* X-ray of index finger amputation through the middle phalanx. *C,* One-year postoperative result: finger extension. *D,* One year after surgery: there is good PIP flexion despite being an isolated index finger replantation.

chains and door slams usually cause crush amputations. Motor vehicle accidents, train accidents, and power tool injuries are responsible for most major limb divisions.[22, 47] Social conditions also seem to be a factor when considering pediatric amputations.[18] It has been reported that neglected children seek psychological release by playing in dangerous environments, thus increasing the risk of injury. In support of this interpretation, patients with amputations resulting from electrical injury, motorcycle accidents, train accidents, and explosions are frequently products of "broken homes" and unstable marriages. In contrast, certain types of injuries do not appear to be related to poor social conditions. Accidents involving lawn mowers, farming equipment, logging equip-

ment, and industrial machinery generally involve children from stable home environments.

PREOPERATIVE CONSIDERATIONS

The Microsurgery Team and Organization

Since the 1970s, a large number of surgeons from several disciplines have been trained in the fundamental principles of microsurgery and replantation.[40] Technical training in microsurgical techniques is important, but for optimal results, the replantation surgeon must also be fully competent in all aspects of traumatic hand surgery.[39] The organization of a team of surgeons in a referral center offers the patient a group of individuals who are available for long and tedious procedures and who can decrease ischemia time of the amputated part by prompt surgical replantation.

The replantation team must be carefully orchestrated by a leader who evaluates the case and oversees the transition from the emergency room to the operating room without excessive delay. A frank discussion with the patient and family concerning operative plans and long-term possibilities is the responsibility of the team leader, who ultimately decides what parts should be replanted, the sequence of replantation, and the division of labor among personnel. Although the leader will not place every stitch during replantation, he keeps the team running smoothly.

Emergency Care and Transportation

Although replantation centers have proliferated, many candidates have a considerable distance to travel to the referral hospital. Evaluation and initial management at the referring institution are critical to the ultimate success of the replantation effort. The patient should be carefully screened for all injuries and must have stable neurologic, respiratory, and hemodynamic function prior to transport. The replantation center should be called prior to transfer of the patient so that manpower availability can be confirmed and ample time to prepare for the patient can be ensured.

After transport of the patient, an intravenous catheter should be placed in the opposite extremity for administration of broad-spectrum antibiotics. Active and passive tetanus immunization should be given depending upon the patient's inoculation history. The stump should be irrigated with a physiologic solution and wrapped in a sterile bandage. Soaking the stump in soap solutions can increase cellular damage and should therefore be avoided.[3] Hemostasis should be obtained by direct pressure. Under no circumstances should blind hemostats or suturing be performed in the emergency room. The amputated part should be wrapped carefully in moist saline gauze and then placed in a plastic bag. The bag is then positioned in a closed, iced saline container. Avoidable tragedies have occurred from the use of formaldehyde and dry ice as preservative modalities. Because 6 to 10 hours of warm ischemia and over 24 hours of cold ischemia are tolerable, referrals from long distances can be successful.[37, 43]

Patient Evaluation

After arrival at the replantation center, evaluation of the patient and the amputated part determines the feasibility of replantation. Limited joint motion, vessel thrombosis requiring reoperation, and cold intolerance, as well as the need for secondary reconstructive procedures must be discussed with the family prior to surgery. Permission must be obtained for the use of vein and skin grafts. The amputated part is inspected and, after an x-ray, is taken to the operating room. It is important to realize the pediatric patient is not just "a little adult" and that young children have special fears and fantasies that pediatricians, clergy, social workers, and psychiatrists need to address. After this overall evaluation, including medical clearance for surgery, the child is taken to the operating room.

Anesthesia

Most children require general anesthesia except for the occasional cooperative adolescent who can tolerate regional block anesthesia. Because of the unpredictable length of replantation procedures, patients undergoing general anesthesia require careful padding of the pressure areas: occiput, sacrum, scapulae, and heels. A Foley catheter is inserted prior to the procedure, and hematocrits should be checked periodically during the procedure because blood loss can be significant. Arterial blood gases are monitored during major limb replantations so that complications of metabolic acidosis and hyperkalemia are avoided. In upper arm replantations, mannitol and sodium bicarbonate help prevent acute renal failure, which has been reported secondary to myoglobinuria.[52]

In pediatric patients, hypothermia is a constant danger, particularly in long procedures involving exposed limbs and multiple blood transfusions. Body temperature must be continuously monitored and adjusted with heating blankets and room temperature changes.

INTRAOPERATIVE CONSIDERATIONS

Steps in Operative Technique

The amputated part precedes the patient to the operating room, and each procedure begins by a thorough cleansing and irrigation of the part. Mid-lateral digital incisions are used for exposure, and dorsal and volar flaps are raised for identification of structures and facilitation of bony shortening. These incisions can be converted into Z-plasties at the conclusion of the case so that constricting scar is avoided. With loop magnification and headlight illumination, the damaged ends of all critical structures are labeled with 5-0 nylon sutures. Microclamps are avoided because they may traumatize the tissue and are easily lost in the wound.

In children, the vessels are embedded in a thicker layer of fat than in adults, making identification of these structures more difficult. In digital amputations, two or three dorsal veins are identified superficial to the extensor tendon. Both neurovascular bundles should be dissected free just lateral and volar to the flexor tendons.

After arrival in the operating room, the proximal stump is cleaned and suture-labeled by a second team of surgeons. This proximal stump labeling is performed under tourniquet control so that the surgeon does not blindly dissect these structures in a bloody field. Both neurovascular bundles and two or three dorsal veins should be identified and dissected free. A small hematoma at the end of each vein and artery may help identify these structures. In addition, milking the amputation stump may extrude a small amount of blood, making vessel identification easier. All contaminated and hopelessly traumatized tissue should be generously debrided from both the proximal and distal stumps.

Sequence of Repair

After appropriate debridement and structure labeling, repair must proceed in an orderly sequence. However, no particular sequence is mandatory, and adjustments should be made depending on the injury and ischemia time. We prefer the following sequence in most situations, taking care to ensure con-tinuous cooling of the amputated part by iced saline irrigation of each digit wrapped in gauze:

1. Bony shortening and fixation
2. Periosteal repair
3. Extensor tendon repair
4. Dorsal vein anastomosis
5. Loose dorsal skin closure
6. Flexor tendon repair
7. Arterial anastomosis
8. Neurorrhaphy
9. Volar skin closure

Venous repair prior to arterial anastomoses decreases blood loss, and tendon repair before vessel anastomosis avoids unnecessary disturbances of delicate vessel and nerve suture. We recommend neurorrhaphy after the arterial repair to avoid hematoma formation at the site of nerve repair. Hematomas form because it is impossible to locate and coagulate fine perineural vessels prior to arterial repair and release of tourniquet. In upper arm replantation, vascular repair is done immediately following bony fixation so that muscle ischemia is minimized.

Bone Shortening and Fixation

The surgeon must perform bone shortening to minimize tension on neurovascular repairs and to provide soft tissue coverage of these anastomoses. Epiphyseal growth has been demonstrated following experimental replantations, pediatric replantations, and free, microvascular joint transfers (Fig. 8–3).[17, 22, 44, 51] It is important, therefore, that joints and growth plates be preserved and not removed in a bone shortening step if the injury permits. In spite of careful management, growth plate injury is common, however, and injured growth plates and malaligned bones often show significant remodeling.[44] In fact, compensatory overgrowth of epiphyseal plates has been reported in several cases.[22]

Usually, 1 to 1.5 cm of shortening is required in digital replantation, and 2 to 4 cm is necessary at the wrist. We have shortened as much as 10 cm in upper arm replantations to prevent dead space formation after necrotic muscle excision and to close the wounds. Length discrepancy is less important in the upper extremity than in the lower extremity. The surgeon should use vein grafts generously to salvage joints or epiphyses.

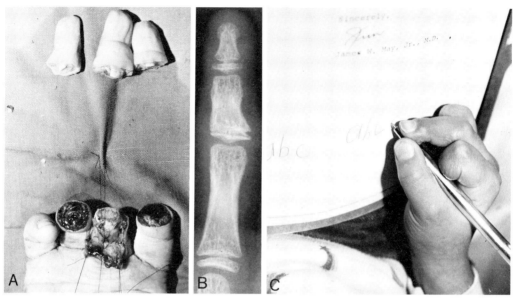

Figure 8–3. *A,* Three distal amputations in the right hand of a 4-year-old female. *B,* Three years after surgery, an x-ray shows an open epiphysis. *C,* Functional result following replantation of the middle finger.

Four techniques for bony fixation in digital replantations have been recommended: Kirschner wires, compression plating, intramedullary screws, and interosseous wiring.[8, 12, 39] We prefer interosseous wiring because it provides good bone fixation in controlling angulation and rotational deformities. After bone is shortened with a side-cutting drill, two small drill holes are made on each end of the bone, approximately 2 mm from the cut edge. No. 26 or No. 28 stainless steel wires are passed through the holes, with the loops on the volar surface and the twisted ends on the dorsal surface. When a joint is destroyed, primary arthrodesis is our preferred treatment. In the author's experience, compression plates require excessive dissection, and percutaneous Kirschner wires increase the chance of infection; however, they are indicated in certain situations. In distal digital injuries, smooth Kirschner wires are used to stabilize the bone structures and are placed through the center of the growth plate to lessen the chance of asymmetrical growth. In amputations at the wrist level, longitudinal Kirschner wires do well in children. In most major limb replantations, we favor internal A.O. compression plate fixation and have found that external fixation, such as the Hoffman, may be awkward and may make the microvascular anastomoses awkward.

Tendon Repair

Tendons are trimmed prior to suture, and the bone and tendon cuts are planned so that the tendon suture line and fracture line are staggered. In most situations, both flexor profundus and flexor sublimis are sutured when cut, because tendon gliding after primary suture is surprisingly good in children. If flexor tendons are beyond repair, silastic rods are used if the wound permits,[34] and suture or replacement of pulleys is performed if needed. The author's preferred technique for flexor tendon suture includes retrieval of the proximal end, fixation of it in the wound with a straight Keith needle, then completion of suture with Kleinert's modification of Kessler's technique.

Extensor tendons are repaired with a figure of 8 suture, and the lateral bands are sutured if they are retrievable.

Vascular Repair

Vascular exposure should be completed at the time of initial structure labeling. The proximal and distal stumps are prepared under the microscope. Arterial injuries may result in separation of the adventitia and the media and rupture of the vasa vasorum. Occasionally, small red dots are seen in the adventitia owing to a leakage of blood, resulting in the *measles sign*.[39] When separation of the media and adventitia or of the intima and media occurs, the two layers may separate into the *telescope sign* (Fig. 8–4). After trimming an amputated vessel end and irrigating the segment with heparinized saline, the surgeon should inspect the lumen for deposits of fibrin, platelets, or debris. Such deposits under high magnifications assume a *cobweb* or *cotton candy* appearance and may indicate endothelial damage.[39] These arterial changes may be observed in both the amputated part and the proximal stump.

Slow flow in the proximal vessel should be bathed in 2% lidocaine (Xylocaine) for elimination of spasm. Inadequate vessel shortening and acceptance of a sluggish flow are among the most common factors in early arterial thrombosis. The use of vein grafts decreases tension on the repair which lessens the risk of arterial thrombosis and the need for reoperation. The ipsilateral volar forearm and dorsum of the foot are the donor sites most frequently used for vein grafts. The donor choice depends on the size of the vein required. Once arteries are trimmed to healthy tissue, a vein graft of appropriate length and lumen size is harvested (Fig. 8–5). A vein graft that is too long will dilate and override the proximal and distal anastomoses, creating the *pantaloon sign*,[39] and resulting in thrombosis. Vein grafts that are too short have their lumen constricted, a situation that also increases the chance of thrombosis. Once a vein graft of proper length is chosen, it is important to reverse the graft to orient venous valves so that they do not occlude flow. After the approximating clamp is placed, the ends are irrigated with heparinized saline and signs of vessel damage are rechecked. The anastomosis is accomplished by standard microvascular techniques.[39]

Veins are repaired first so that excessive blood loss is avoided. If possible, two arteries

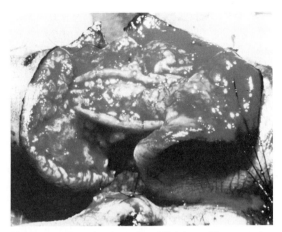

Figure 8–5. Dorsal vein graft at PIP joint, with appropriate lumen size and tension.

and veins are repaired for each digit, although a digit will survive with a single artery and vein repair. After removal of the clamps, the part should become pink, but one should remember that the reflow process sometimes takes an hour or longer, depending on the amount of previous ischemia.[38, 39] After arterial repair, the measles sign indicates layer disruption in a segment that, if left in place, becomes red and thickened, exhibiting *sausage sign*. If this repair is not revised, vessel wall dissection will, in most cases, eventually lead to thrombosis.

After any vessel repair, patency is checked by an atraumatic method such as the double forcep technique.[20] If patency testing reveals questionable flow, removal of a few sutures and inspection of the anastomosis or complete revision of the repair are preferable to agonizing about reoperation in the early postoperative period.

Nerve Repair

A careful epineurial repair with accurate fascicular alignment visualized under the microscope is our preferred technique. Primary nerve suture is recommended, but if avulsion of nerve bulk is present, primary or secondary nerve grafting may be required. The ultimate functional result achieved by replantation is, to a great degree, a reflection of the success of nerve regeneration; therefore, it is important for surgeons to be as meticulous about nerve repair as they are about vessel repair. Excessive suture material and extensive intraneural dissection should be avoided. A bipolar coagulator helps achieve hemostasis at the cut end of the nerve.

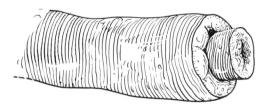

Figure 8–4. Telescope sign. Vascular injury has led to separation of the arterial wall into layers. (Reprinted from Current Problems in Surgery, 1980, by permission of Year Book Medical Publishers.)

Skin Closure

Skin closure should be performed loosely. The surgeon must be very careful during suture placement to avoid injury to the underlying anastomoses. Closure must be tension-free so that skin necrosis and venous congestion are avoided. The generous use of skin grafts is preferred to tight closure. Questionably, viable skin may be assessed by the use of intravenous flourescein. Areas that do not flouresce should be either observed closely or excised and grafted. Skin grafts, in general, do well over anastomoses.

Distant pedicle flaps and free tissue transfers are rarely necessary in replantation surgery. Occasional massive defects require flap coverage, but these large wounds are best treated initially with a biologic dressing and delayed coverage so that tissue viability can be more accurately assessed. Flap coverage is then performed after the acute swelling has subsided and the wound is free of necrotic tissue.

POSTOPERATIVE CARE AND MONITORING

Postoperatively, the wounds are covered with Neosporin ointment and loosely dressed with gauze. One must exercise great care to avoid circumferential gauze wrappings. A loose, bulky hand dressing is applied with fluff gauze. Longitudinal plaster splints are used for immobilization. Above elbow dorsal and volar splints are used to lessen the chance of the child removing the dressing, and to better immobilize the repaired structures. The limb is elevated on several pillows, and stockinette suspension is avoided because it has constricting tendencies. The outer bandage is rewrapped in 24 hours so that constriction does not occur, and the replanted parts are clearly exposed for frequent inspection.

The patient is best monitored in a unit accustomed to the care of replantation patients. The replanted part is inspected hourly under good lighting. Temperature probe monitoring, with external probe placement, is useful as an adjunct.[50]

Postoperative medication includes intravenous cephalosporin, aspirin, and low molecular weight dextran. Systemic heparinization is avoided because it is associated with postoperative bleeding complications.[45] Heparinization is occasionally indicated in distal amputations where vessels are very small and after reoperation for vascular thrombosis, but bleeding complications in pediatric patients have been more frequent than in comparable adult groups.

The first dressing change usually occurs in the operating room 1 week postoperatively, at which time appropriate cleansing and minor debridements are performed and all medications discontinued. Dressings should be changed earlier if they are hard, blood-soaked, and constricting.

Reoperation for vascular thrombosis is worthwhile and should be done promptly upon recognition. The classic sign of arterial thrombosis is pallor, whereas venous obstruction is indicated by a bluish hue. Pricking a replanted part with a small needle can be helpful when thrombosis is suspected. If bright red blood is not expressed, arterial thrombosis is likely; if dark blood extrudes, venous flow problems may exist. Thrombosis of the artery or vein quickly compromises flow of the other. Fifty percent of digital re-explorations can result in salvage if done early.[39]

Special Level Considerations

No major limb replantations should be attempted if associated trauma endangers life. In children, the mechanisms of injury frequently lead to trauma that is more significant than that occurring in adults.

Most upper arm replantations fail because of inadequate muscle debridement and bone shortening, a pitfall that produces muscle necrosis and gram-negative infections that can become life-threatening. In such cases, early "second look" procedures with appropriate debridement are essential.

Unexpected fluid requirements are frequently needed after reperfusion of the amputated limb, and mannitol and sodium bicarbonate are helpful replacements (see previous discussion of anesthesia). Fasciotomies may be helpful for massive postoperative swelling, which is common.

Replantation at the wrist level may require primary wrist fusion following shortening by resection of the proximal carpal row (Fig. 8–6). We recommend fixation by nonthreaded wires in such cases, but compression plating also is effective. Removal of the articular surface of the capitate and radius is necessary

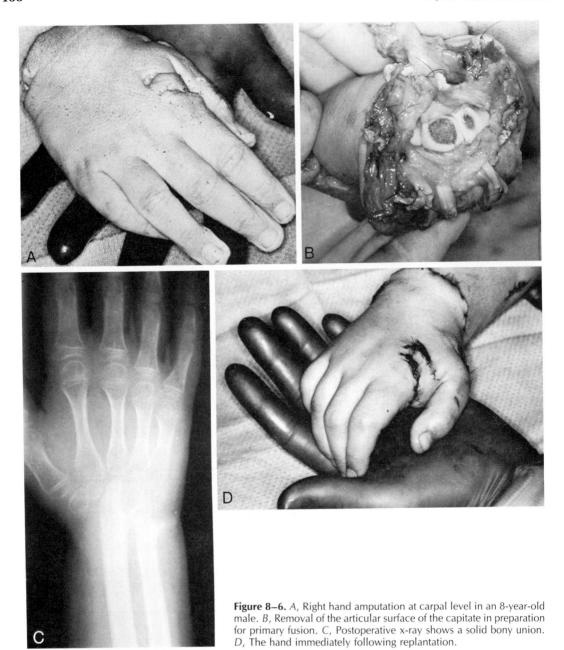

Figure 8–6. *A*, Right hand amputation at carpal level in an 8-year-old male. *B*, Removal of the articular surface of the capitate in preparation for primary fusion. *C*, Postoperative x-ray shows a solid bony union. *D*, The hand immediately following replantation.

for wrist fusion, and shortening of the ulna aids in postoperative supination and pronation. In children, the distal ulna and radial epiphysis as well as the wrist joint can occasionally be salvaged by the use of vein grafts in sharp wrist amputations.

Midpalmar amputations require the anastomosis of one major artery per finger. Repair of a single common artery can cause as many as three or four fingers to become pink initially, but vessel thrombosis is a major risk when this amputation level is treated in this way. Vessels in this region are notorious for spasm, and vein grafts are commonly required for a successful result (Fig. 8–7). If a midpalmar amputation with multiple fingers survives on a single vessel, cold intolerance is substantially greater than if one artery per finger is repaired. Hemostasis must be complete because bleeding from a superficial or deep arch produces hematomas that compromise vessel repair. Intermetacarpal

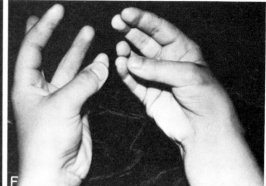

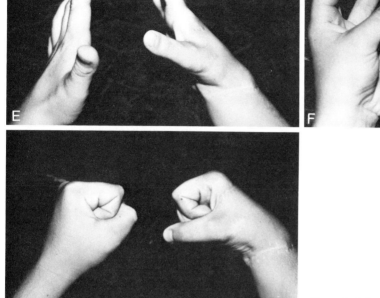

Figure 8–6. (*continued*).   Three years postoperative results: *E*, extension; *F*, opposition; *G*, flexion.

fasciotomies may help replantation survival at this level by reducing tissue pressure due to increased interstitial fluid.

Nonreplantable tissue can offer a storehouse of useful parts, including tendon grafts, skin grafts, whole joints, and articular cartilage "wafer" grafts. These parts can be utilized for primary repair of structures lost from other portions of the hand. In multiple digit amputations, a less traumatized digit may be replanted to a more important functional position. In such cases, appropriate bony shortening and tendon tension adjustments are necessary.

In certain thumb avulsions, primary repair of the flexor pollicis longus or extensor tendons may be impossible. In these cases, transfer of the index sublimis tendon to the flexor pollicis longus and/or transfer of the extensor indicius proprius to the extensor pollicis longus will aid thumb function.

Long-Term Results and Follow-Up

The objectives of pediatric replantation are to restore function and improve appearance, rather than just ensure tissue survival. The child, like the adult, frequently experiences a temporary euphoria immediately after successful replantation. This outlook is frequently replaced by a state of depression when the child realizes the replaced part will not be normal. This outcome should be discussed with the patient and family before rehabilitation is started.

In general, children adapt better and use the amputated part better than adults.[22, 44] Reinnervation is frequently excellent. Reports of digital replantations in children indicated that all had return of *at least* protective sensation.[22, 44] and in O'Brien's series, two-point discrimination averaged 4 mm.[44] In upper arm replantation, protective sensation can be anticipated if avulsion is limited and neurorrhaphy carefully done.

With current microvascular techniques, it has been reported that in adults survival rates range from 85% to 90%[39] and that in children, survival rates are between 65% and 85%, depending on the patient selections.[1, 44] Survival rates in young children with more distal injuries are lowest.

Motor function in children can also be surprisingly good but rarely normal. Cooperation in active physical therapy of

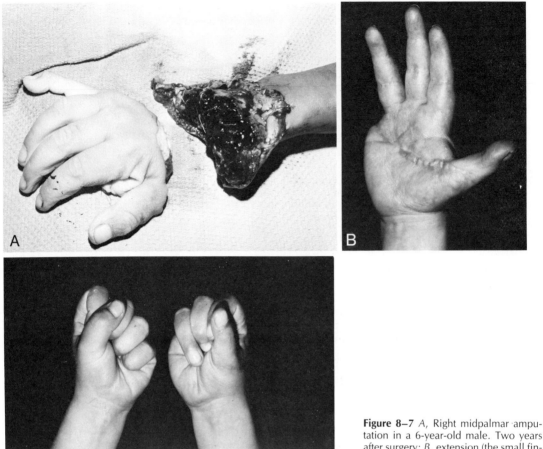

Figure 8–7 A, Right midpalmar amputation in a 6-year-old male. Two years after surgery: B, extension (the small finger was not replantable); C, flexion.

standard adult exercises is difficult in young children, so the incorporation of "play" into the usual physical therapy modalities is recommended.

The most frequent secondary procedures in children are skin revisions and tenolysis.[13, 22] The results of delayed nerve grafting in replantation children are the same as in children with other injuries. Bony nonunions are rare with current fixation techniques. Silastic arthroplasty is rarely needed but when used gives the best results at the metacarpophalangeal level.

Cold intolerance is a common complication in the replanted part and should be discussed with the children and their parents during the treatment period. As in adults, cold intolerance in children can be expected to improve with time, and gloves and appropriate protective measures should be recommended in cold weather.

In summary, replantation surgery in chil-

dren is rewarding, and the functional results justify continued replantation at all levels. Indications for such surgery should be generous, provided there are no associated life-threatening factors.

Elective Microsurgery

From an initial excitement about extremity replantation, the field of microsurgery has advanced to a point at which elective free tissue transfer is a viable alternative to traditional methods of reconstruction for congenital and traumatic defects in children.

Microvascular anastomosis of vessels less than 3 mm in diameter provides predictable patency rates, and anatomic dissections have defined vascular territories for a number of tissues. With this knowledge, the surgeon can solve a particular problem by a single stage procedure consisting of microvascular transfer of skin, muscle, bone with and without epiphyses, and composite tissue such as a myocutaneous flap or digits. Reports of toe transfer for replacement of absent thumbs and fingers, of free muscle transfer for restoration of active hand function, and of free bone transfer to bridge significant skeletal defects have appeared with increasing frequency.

TOE-TO-HAND TRANSFER

Opposable digits are a basic requirement for useful hand function. A traumatic loss or congenital absence of a thumb compromises hand function. A single-stage toe to hand transfer is one option that the surgeon can choose to replace thumb function.

Nicoladoni[69] first described a technique of transferring a toe to the hand. His technique involved a vascularized pedicle transfer, during which the hand was immobilized together with the foot. Vascularity depended on the establishment of circulation from the recipient bed, and because of the awkwardness of positioning and mediocre functional results, the method was rarely used. Buncke,[56] using microvascular technique, proved the experimental feasibility of single-stage toe to thumb transfer. The transfer was subsequently reported in China in 1966 by Cobbett[58] and later by Buncke.[55] Since then, over 500 cases of toe to hand transfer have been reported.[62, 64, 68, 72, 73] Although any thumb deficiency can be approached with this technique,[60, 66, 67, 71, 72] its use in children seems best reserved for traumatic amputations that are at or distal to the metacarpophalangeal joint or where additional amputations or congenital aplasia preclude pollicization.[61, 63] In an otherwise four-fingered hand, however, all requirements of thumb function can be met more simply and safely by traditional pollicization of either an index finger or a ring finger.[54, 57, 65]

For thumb replacement, the great toe and second toe may be selected for free transfer, but both solutions pose problems. The great toe is 1 to 1.5 cm larger than the thumb. Furthermore, loss of the great toe is disabling to the foot in that children will have weakness of push-off and pivotal motions, although they usually will not have difficulties with normal walking. Although the second toe is smaller than the thumb, its loss causes less of a functional problem for the foot. For defects at or distal to the level of the metacarpophalangeal joint, Morrison[68] has popularized the "wrap-around" technique, in which the soft tissue and the neurovascular structures from the toe are used to cover a bone graft obtained from the iliac crest. A case is represented in Figure 8–8. The young boy in this case had a traumatic amputation of his right dominant thumb at the level of the metacarpophalangeal joint. He underwent neurovascular wrap-around flap that included the nail from the big toe. The donor defect leaves the bones of the big toe intact. The plantar surface of the foot is covered with local skin flaps, and dorsally free skin grafts are used to cover the toe. Problems with the donor site include hyperkeratotic scars, particularly on the dorsum of the foot, and difficulty in durable foot coverage. It should be emphasized that skin grafts are better tolerated in the hand than in the foot and that primary closure should be performed when possible in the foot. The usefulness of this technique, however, is limited to cases in which the thumb metacarpal is present. It therefore is not indicated in congenitally deficient thumbs.

When the major portion of the metacarpal is absent, joint transfer usually provides improvement. With the great toe, this means sacrificing the metatarsophalangeal joint and the epiphyses of the toe. The differences between metatarsal joint function and metacarpal joint function must be kept in mind. The metatarsophalangeal joint is a hyperextension joint and must be converted to a flexion joint for the thumb. As has been pointed out by May,[66] this can best be accomplished by oblique osteotomy through the distal metatarsal with fixation of the transferred toe joint in extension. An analogous situation exists in the traditional pollicization procedure, in which the extensible metacarpophalangeal joint of the index finger is converted to the flexion carpometacarpal joint of the thumb.[54] Joint motion also requires transfer of both the flexor and extensor tendons, and when possible tendon repair should be done proximal to the wrist. The second toe has a problem with flexion deformities when it is used to replace a thumb or finger.

The traditional vascular anatomy of the foot has been well described by Gilbert.[59]

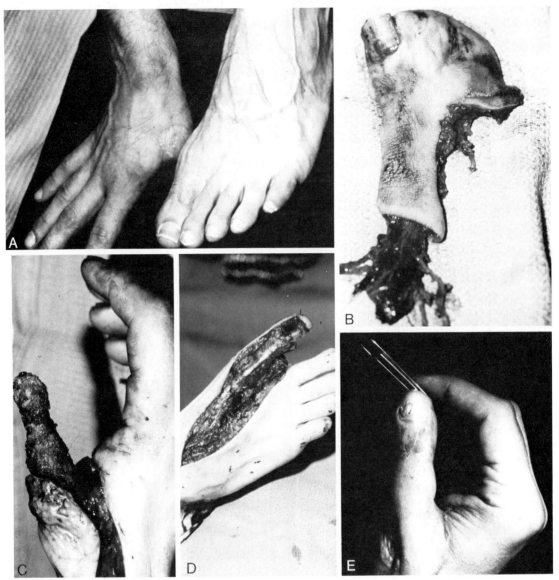

Figure 8–8. *A*, Traumatic amputation of the right dominant thumb; and the foot from which the great toe will be transferred. *B*, The skin flap, with its artery, veins, digital vessels, skin, and nail bed. *C*, The recipient site with the iliac bone graft in place. *D*, The donor defect in the foot, showing preservation of the osseous structures, which were covered with local flaps, and the plantar surface and free split-thickness skin grafts on the dorsal surface. *E*, The postoperative result at 12 months, with two-point discrimination of 8 mm.

The majority of transfers are based on the dorsalis pedis artery or its extension of the first dorsal metatarsal artery. Younger children usually require the more proximal site for a larger dorsalis pedis diameter as the level of anastomosis. The preoperative evaluation of the donor vasculature requires not only a clinical identification of a pulsing artery but also a Doppler examination. Furthermore, we feel that preoperative angiog-

raphy of both the donor sites and the recipient sites is necessary in congenital situations, in which vascular patterns are unpredictable.

Although immediate viability is determined by the arterial and venous anastomoses, the functional result depends on the outcome of the neural repair. In the traumatic amputation, neural patterns are predictable, but in congenital cases standard recipient nerves may be unavailable and some creativity is required to achieve alternate connections. For example, the dorsal ulnar sensory nerve has been made to innervate the thumb, as reported by May.[66] Children have more cortical plasticity than adults and can better integrate sensory input into functional patterns after the repair of different nerves.

In children, general anesthesia is always used, as is a stellate ganglion block for prevention of vascular spasm. A sympathetic block is not required in the lower extremity, where local methods such as 1% lidocaine (Xylocaine) control vasospasm. Two surgical teams operate simultaneously, and all dissections are done with loupe magnification. Dissection is begun proximally at the level of the dorsalis pedis and carried distally. If the first metatarsal artery is not identified, the dissection proceeds from distal to proximal. A tourniquet is used, but the limb is elevated and not exsanguinated. Once the neurovascular bundle of the toe is isolated, the tourniquet is deflated so that perfusion can be verified. In children, heparin in a bolus of 5000 units is begun at this time and repeated every hour through completion of vessel anastomosis. The transferred toe is fixed to the recipient bone with Kirschner wires. When further stabilization is indicated, it is accomplished with tendon repairs. The surgeon repairs the artery first to decrease ischemia time and sutures the vein only after adequate arterial flow is established. The tourniquet is usually used for brief periods for the venous repair. For thumb reconstruction, the recipient anastomotic vessels are on the dorsum in the area of the anatomic snuff box. The nerves are then sutured, and both donor sites and recipient sites are closed with local tissue flaps or skin grafts or both.

Postoperative care includes splinting of the foot and hand. Temperature probes are attached to the replanted digits, and, rather than upset the child by frequent poking and doctor appearances, one assesses the status of the transfer by temperature monitoring. Room temperature should be kept above 25°C. A control digital monitor helps register skin temperature. A reading 3° lower than that of an uninjured digit suggests circulatory impediment. A 5°C difference indicates severe vascular difficulties, as does a temperature reading below 26°C. One keeps the hand warm by wrapping it in a heating pad. The level of elevation is determined by whether arterial or venous problems predominate. Heparin is given by continuous infusion at a level sufficient to provide mild anticoagulation in the range of 100 to 200 units/hour. In some cases, low molecular weight dextran is used, as are aspirin and chlorpromazine (Thorazine).

Failure rates of most series range from 10% to 20%.[55, 60, 62, 64, 73] If vascular complications occur, regional blocks, changes in extremity position, boluses of heparin, and dressing changes may be helpful. If these conservative measures do not restore blood flow, reexploration is indicated.

If all is uncomplicated, hospitalization averages 1 to 2 weeks in children under 7 years of age. A long arm cast is applied for 6 weeks. The donor foot is kept in a short leg walking cast or Unna boot until skin healing is complete. Hand therapy is started in the 5- to 8-week interval, and play therapy is included.

FREE MUSCLE TRANSFER

Free muscle and free myocutaneous tissue transfers are used to treat severe soft tissue injuries that cause skin and muscle loss when tendon transfer is not an option. The most common condition in childhood that may require this technique is Volkman's contracture. Other applications include injuries that compromise wrist and finger extension and elbow flexion.

Tamai[80] in 1970 first reported free transfer of the rectus femoris of dogs with a 70% success rate. Harrii[75] reported the clinical use of a free gracilis muscle transfer in the treatment of facial palsy, and shortly thereafter Ikuta[77] reported the use of a free graft of pectoralis major to treat a severe ischemic contracture of the forearm. Manktelow[78] in his initial studies and in subsequent reports has outlined the use of gracilis for replacement of forearm finger flexion. As he noted, this muscle provides a satisfactory range of finger flexion and reasonable grip strength (50% of normal). This long muscle on the medial aspect of the thigh originates on the upper half of the pubic arch and inserts as a rounded tendon into the upper end of the tibia. Its average length is 30 to 50 cm, with two thirds being occupied by the muscle belly.[79] The nutrient artery enters the muscle in its upper third. The nerve supply is from the anterior branch of the obturator nerve, and it can be harvested with no functional deficit to the leg. The motor branch has three to four fascicles that provide good bulk for nerve suture. Skin also can be taken with the muscle. Other functioning muscles that have been used for free transfer include the pectoralis major[76] and the latissimus dorsi.

Preoperatively, mobile soft tissues are a prerequisite for all free muscle transfers. Angiography is useful in defining vascular anatomy of the donor and recipient site. A two-team approach is recommended because defining the recipient nerve is a time-consuming step. It is important that one mark the resting length of the muscle before it is detached so that this is reestablished in the recipient bed by suture to the medial epicondyle proximally and to the flexor tendon in the distal forearm. Transplanted muscle contracts with greater force from the resting length, and full digital flexion is more predictably achieved when the resting length is reestablished after transfer. The arterial anastomoses are done first so that muscle ischemia time is decreased. After transfer, nerve regeneration requires 6 to 18 months, and during this period the use of functional electrical stimulation and passive motion therapy is recommended. There are numerous reports about the success of this technique in traumatic situations,[74–78, 81] and these experiences will increase the use of this technique in children with absent muscles from birth.

FREE VASCULARIZED BONE GRAFTING

Microvascular techniques offer the surgeon another approach to skeletal reconstruction. Transfer of vascularized bone contributes more actively to the healing process than the passive scaffold, which is the contribution of the traditional bone graft. The nutrient artery supplies the endosteum and inner cortex, and the periosteal artery supplies the outer cortex and connects with the endosteal circulation (Fig. 8–9). Therefore, if a large segment of bone is to be transplanted as a living graft, it is important that the periosteal circulation be preserved. Summarizing the work of Ostrup,[92] Berggren and Weiland,[84] these points should be emphasized: (1) Complete survival of large corticocancellous grafts can be predictably obtained by microvascular anastomoses; (2) the vascularized graft participates more actively in bone heal-

ing than the conventional nonvascularized graft does; (3) reconstitution of the nutrient artery circulation is important; and (4) one should protect periosteal circulation by harvesting the graft extraperiosteally with a surrounding muscle sleeve (Fig. 8–10).

In 1975, Taylor[95] reported a successful microvascular transfer of bone. He used 22 cm of vascularized fibula to bridge a traumatic tibial defect. Union occurred at 10 months, and by 12 months the bulk of the vascularized graft was similar to the size of the contralateral uninjured tibia. Reports of other successful microvascular bone grafts followed. Use of a rib for a mandibular defect, use of osteocutaneous grafts for combined skin and bone defects, and use of vascularized grafts for en bloc tumor resection and for large nonunions[86, 87, 89–91, 93, 98, 99, 101] have been reported.

Over 60% of children with congenital pseudarthrosis failed to obtain union with conventional bone grafting. One report documents a 70% success rate of healing with vascularized bone grafting after conventional bone grafting failed. This suggests that a vascularized bone graft is, at this time, the recommended approach to congenital pseudarthrosis[82, 88, 97, 100] and should not be reserved for late treatment of this condition. One 6-year-old boy had eight unsuccessful conventional bone grafting operations for his congenital pseudarthrosis, which was then successfully treated with a vascularized fibular graft (Fig. 8–11).

Fixation of the transferred fibula is accom-

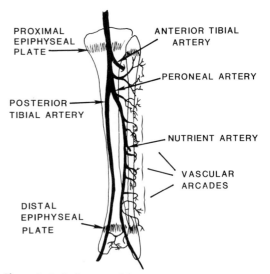

Figure 8–9. A diagram of the arterial supply to the fibula, based on the peroneal artery.

Figure 8–10. A free bone graft of the fibula with its vascular pedicle and its extraperiosteal muscular cuff.

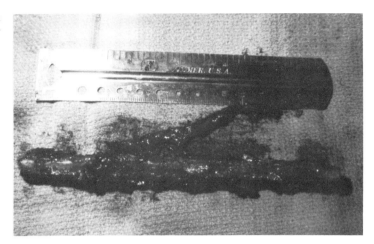

plished with small plates or intramedullary pins. After the fibula is harvested from a child, the proximal aspect of the remaining distal fibula, which includes the lateral malleolus, should be fixed to the tibia so that its upward migration and a valgus deformity at the ankle are prevented. In the future, this technique may be used to span defects created by limb-lengthening procedures[90] and to replace absent bones in congenital deformity, such as the radius in radial club hand. In the latter situation, a viable epiphysis must be included in the transfer. Sources of free bone grafts and their characteristics are shown in Table 8–1.

Postoperatively, we do not anticoagulate our patients, and have recently included a small island graft with the bone to act as a sensor for vascular viability. As shown by Berggren,[84] bone scanning is helpful in this regard if it is done within the first week. Figure 8–12 represents a bone scan of a free fibular graft used to bridge a congenital pseudarthrosis of the forearm secondary to

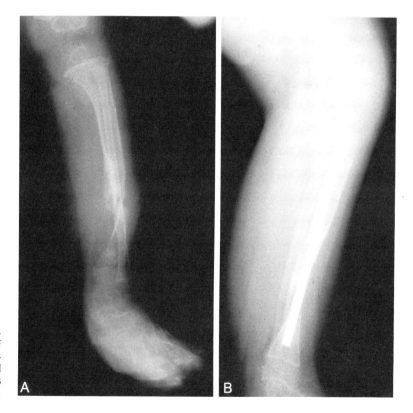

Figure 8–11. *A*, Congenital pseudarthrosis following the failure of union with conventional bone-grafting techniques. *B*, Successful union of the same pseudarthrosis following free fibular bone transfer.

Table 8–1. **Free Bone Transfers**

Characteristics	Fibula	Rib	Iliac Crest
Bone			
Length (maximum)	22–26 cm	30 cm	10 cm
Shape	Straight	Curved	Slight curve
Structure	Corticocancellous	Membranous	Corticocancellous
Vessels			
Artery	Peroneal	Posterior intercostal	Deep circumflex iliac Alternate: superficial circumflex iliac
Vein	Two venae comitantes	One intercostal	One vena comitantes
Vascular stalk	1–7 cm	3–5 cm	1–5 cm
Dissection	See ref. 91	See ref. 85	See refs. 89, 96
Options			
Articular surface	Yes	Yes	No
Epiphysis	Yes	No	No
Adjacent muscle	Yes	Yes	No (nonfunctional)
Overlying skin	Yes	Yes	Yes
Nerve	No	Yes	Yes
Complication	Minimal	Thoracotomy; venous inadequacy and thombosis	Abdominal wall hernia
Applications	Long-bone defects (extremities) Congenital pseudarthrosis	Mandibular reconstruction; composite bone-skin (extremities)	Long bone defects (extremities); composite bone-skin (extremities); mandibular reconstruction

neurofibromatosis. Note the viability of the graft as well as the epiphyseal uptake.

FREE EPIPHYSEAL AND JOINT TRANSFER

Current techniques of microsurgery have increased the feasibility of a free vascularized epiphyseal transfer. Nonvascularized methods[103, 104] are unpredictable, and although x-rays show that the epiphyseal plate stays open after transfer, there is no significant growth. Experimental work on vascularized epiphyseal plate transfers has been done by Nettlebad[106] and Tsai,[108, 109] who have shown that epiphyseal growth continues after vascular transfer in animal models. Nettlebad found an average fourfold increase in length over matched nonvascularized controls. Tsai reported the importance of achieving vascularized nutrition on both sides of the epiphyseal plate by direct suture of both the epiphyseal and nutrient arteries. Clinical cases in which free joint and free vascularized grafts were used have been reported by O'Brien,[107] Mathes,[105] and Tsai.[108, 109] It is hoped that these vascularized grafts will maintain not only an articular joint surface but also growth.

FUTURE APPLICATIONS

Clodius[110] is currently studying the treatment of chronic lymphedema by lymphovenous anastomoses. Large defects in peripheral nerves are treated with conventional autogenous nerve grafts with unpredictable results. Vascularized nerve grafting is being studied and may be superior; it would be especially helpful in the treatment of brachial plexus palsies.

Free tissue transfers are an important option in the treatment of serious upper extremity problems in children. Ohmori[112] reports that the results of using free flaps in

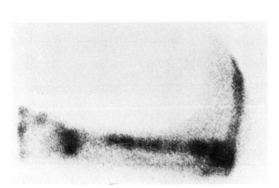

Figure 8–12. A positive bone scan of the free fibula following bone grafting for pseudarthrosis of the forearm, which resulted from nonunion of the bone due to neurofibromatosis.

children over 5 years of age are comparable to those in adults. The small caliber of the vessels in children under 5 years is associated with a high incidence of vasospasm, making elective flap transfer in this age group unwise. Within the next few years, refined microsurgical techniques will increase the number of cases of replantation and free flaps. The functional benefit of these efforts, however, must be critically evaluated so that this technique is used in appropriate situations. Conventional methods of treatment have proved effective in the past, and their place in reconstructive surgery in the child's upper extremity should not be ignored.

References

1. Berger A, Meissl G, Walzer L. Techniques and results in replantation surgery in children. Int J Microsurg 3:9, 1981.
2. Berger A, Millesi H, Mandl H, et al. Replantation and revascularization of amputated parts of extremities: a three-year report from the Viennese replantation team. Clin Orthop 133:212, 1978.
3. Branemark PI, Albrektsson B, Lindstrom J, Lundborg G. Local tissue effects of wound disinfectants. Acta Chir Scand 357:166, 1966.
4. Buncke HJ, Buncke CM, Schulz WP. Experimental digital amputation and reimplantation. Plast Reconstr Surg 36:62, 1965.
5. Buncke HJ, Buncke CM, Schulz WP. Immediate nicoladoni procedure in the rhesus monkey, or hallux-to-hand transplantation utilizing microminiature vascular anastomoses. Br J Plast Surg 19:332, 1966.
6. Buncke HJ, Daniller AI, Schulz WP, et al. The fate of autogenous whole joints transferred by microvascular anastomoses. Plast Reconstr Surg 39:333, 1967.
7. Buncke HJ, Schulz WP. Total ear reimplantation in the rabbit utilizing microminiature vascular anastomoses. Br J Plast Surg 10:15, 1966.
8. Buncke HJ, Zide BM. Colloquium: digital replantation. Ann Plast Surg 3:443, 1979.
9. Carrel A. Results of the transplantation of blood vessels, organs, and limbs. JAMA 51:1662, 1908.
10. Carrel A, Guthrie CC. Complete amputation of the thigh with replantation. Am J Med Sci 131:297, 1906.
11. Carrel A, Guthrie CC. Results of a replantation of the thigh. Science 23:393, 1906.
12. Daniel RK, Terzis JK. Replantation of upper extremity amputation. In Daniel RK, Terzis JK, eds. Reconstructive Microsurgery. Boston, Little, Brown and Co., 1977.
13. Elsahy NI. Replantation of a completely amputated distal segment of a thumb: Case report. Plast Reconstr Surg 59:579, 1977.
14. Elsahy NI. When to replant a fingertip after its complete amputation. Plast Reconstr Surg 60:14, 1977.
15. Ferreira MD, Marques EF, Azze RJ. Limb replantation. Clin Plast Surg 5:211, 1978.
16. Fujinaki A, O'Brien BM, Kureta T, Threlfall GN. Experimental micro-anastomoses of 0.4-0.5 mm vessels. Br J Plast Surg 30:269, 1977.
17. Furnas DW. Growth and development in replanted forelimbs. Plast Reconstr Surg 46:445, 1970.
18. Galway HR, Hubbard S, Mowbray M. Traumatic amputations in children. In Kostvik JP, ed. Amputation Surgery and Rehabilitation—The Toronto Experience, Edinburgh, Churchill Livingstone, 1981.
19. Harris WH, Malt RA. Late results of human limb replantation. J Trauma 14:44, 1974.
20. Hayhurst JW, O'Brien BM. An experimental study of microvascular technique, patency rates and related factors. Br J Plast Surg 28:128, 1975.
21. Hopfner E. Uber Gefassnaht, Gefasstransplantation und Reimplantation von amputierten Extremitaten. Arch Klin Chir 70:417, 1903.
22. Jaeger SH, Tasi TM, Kleinert HE. Upper extremity replantation in children. Orthop Clin North Am 12:897. 1981.
23. Kleinert HE. Techniques of axillary block. J Trauma 3:3, 1963.
24. Kleinert HE, Kasdan ML: Restoration of blood flow in upper extremity injuries. J Trauma 3:461, 1963.
25. Kleinert HE, Kasdan ML. Salvage of devascularized upper extremities including studies on small vessel anastomosis. Clin Orthop 29:29, 1963.
26. Kleinert HE, Kasden ML. Anastomosis of digital vessels. J Ky Med Assoc 63:106, 1965.
27. Kleinert HE, Kasdan ML, Romero JL. Small blood vessel anastomosis for salvage of the severely injured upper extremity. J Bone Joint Surg 45A:788, 1963.
28. Komatsu S, Tamai S. Successful replantation of a completely cut-off thumb: case report. Plast Reconstr Surg 42:374, 1968.
29. Kubo T, Ikita Y, Watari S, et al. The smallest digital replant yet? Br J Plast Surg 29:313, 1976.
30. Lee S. Microvascular surgical teaching rounds using rat organ transplantation model with twelve-year bibliography. J Res Inst Med Sci (Korea) 5:215, 1973.
31. Malt RA, Harris WH. Long-term results in replanted arm. Br J Surg 56:705, 1969.
32. Malt RA, McKhann CF. Replantation of severed arms. JAMA 189:716, 1964.
33. Malt RA, Remensnyder JP, Harris WH. Long-term utility of replanted arms. Ann Surg 176:334, 1972.
34. Marshall K, Wolfort FG, Edlich RF. Immediate insertion of silicone rods in fingers with cut flexor tendons. Plast Reconstr Surg 61:77, 1978.
35. Matsen FA, Bach AW, Wyss CR, et al. Transcutaneous PO₂:a potential monitor of the status of replanted limb part. Plast Reconstr Surg 65:732, 1980.
36. Matthews D. Microvascular free tissue transfer in children and adolescents. Presented at the 21st Annual Plastic Surgery Senior Resident's Conference, Norfolk, VA, May, 1982.
37. May JW. Digital replantation with full survival after 28 hours of cold ischemia. Plast Reconstr Surg 67:566, 1981.
38. May JW, Chait LA, O'Brien BM, et al. The no-reflow phenomenon in experimental free flaps. Plast Reconstr Surg 61:256, 1978.
39. May JW, Gallico GG. Upper extremity replantation. Curr Probl Surg 17:635, 1980.
40. May JW, Lister GD. Hand and digital replantation. In Hand Surgery, A Concise Guide to Clinical Practice. Boston, Little, Brown and Co., in press.
41. May JW, Lukash FN, Gallico GG, Stirrat CR. Re-

movable thermocouple probe microvascular patency monitor: an experimental and clinical study. Plast Reconstr Surg 72:366, 1983.

42. May JW, Toth BA, Gardner M. Digital replantation distal to the proximal interphalangeal joint. J Hand Surg 7:161, 1982.
43. O'Brien BM. Replantation surgery. Clin Plast Surg 1:405, 1974.
44. O'Brien BM, Franklin JD, Morrison WA, MacLeod AM. Replantation and revascularization surgery in children. Hand 12:12, 1980.
45. Poole MD, Bowen JE. Two unusual bleedings during anticoagulation following digital replantation. Br J Plast Surg 30:267, 1977.
46. Rosenkrantz JG, Sullivan RC, Welch K, et al. Replantation of an infant's arm. N Engl J Med. 276:609, 1967.
47. Ruby LK. Acute traumatic amputations of an extremity. Clin Orthop North Am 9:679, 1978.
48. Serafin D, Kutz JE, Kleinert HE. Replantation of a completely amputated distal thumb without venous anastomosis. Plast Reconstr Surg 52:579, 1973.
49. Snyder CC, Stevenson RM, Browne EZ. Successful replantation of a totally severed thumb. Plast Reconstr Surg 50:553, 1972.
50. Stirrat C. Temperature monitoring in digital replantation. J Hand Surg 3:342, 1978.
51. Tsai TM, Jupiter JB, Kutz JE, Kleinert HE. Vascularized autogenous whole joint transfer in the hand—A clinical study. J Hand Surg 7:335, 1982.
52. Tsui, CY, et al. Successful restoration of a completely amputated arm. Chin Med J 85:536, 1966.
53. Van Beek AL, Wavak PW, Zook EG. Microvascular surgery in children. Plast Reconstr Surg 63:457, 1979.

Toe to Hand Transfer

54. Buck-Gramcko D. Pollicization of the index finger. J Bone Joint Surg 53A:1605, 1971.
55. Buncke HJ. Free toe to hand transfer. Symposium on Microsurgery, Vol. 14. In Daniller A, Strauch B (eds.) St. Louis, CV Mosby, 1976:216–219.
56. Buncke HJ, Buncke CM, Schulz WP. Immediate Nicoledoni procedure in the rhesus monkey. Br J Plast Surg 19:332, 1966.
57. Carroll RE. Pollicization. In Green A (ed): Operative Hand Surgery. New York, Churchill Livingstone, 1982:1619.
58. Cobbett JR. Free digital transfer: report of a case of transfer of a great toe to replace an amputated thumb. J Bone Joint Surg 51B:677, 1969.
59. Gilbert A. Composite tissue transfers from the foot. Anatomic basis and surgical technique. In Daniller A, Strauch B, eds, Symposium on Microsurgery, Vol. 14. St. Louis, CV Mosby, 1976:230–242.
60. Gilbert A. Toe transfers for congenital hand deficits. J Hand Surg 7:118, 1982.
61. Holle J, Freilinger G, Mandel H, Frey M. Group reconstruction by double toe transplantation in cases of a fingerless hand and handless arm. Plast Reconstr Surg 69:962, 1982.
62. Leung PC. Second toe to hand transplantation: a clinical experience of 25 cases. Aust NZ J Surg 50:250, 1980.
63. Lichtman DM, Ahbel DE, Murphy RB, Buncke HJ Jr. Microvascular double toe transfer for opposable digits—case reports and rationale for treatment. J Hand Surg 7:279, 1982.

64. Lister GD, Kalisman M, Tsia T. Reconstruction of the hand with free microneurovascular toe to hand transfer. Experience with 54 toe transfers. Plast Reconstr Surg 71:372, 1983.
65. Littler JW. On making a thumb: one hundred years of surgical effort. J Hand Surg 1:35, 1976.
66. May JW, Smith RJ, Peimer CA. Toe to hand free tissue transfer for thumb construction with multiple digit aplasia. Plast Reconstr Surg 67:205, 1981.
67. Meals RA, Lesavoy MA. Hallux to hand transfer during ankle disarticulation for multiple limb abnormalities. JAMA 249:72, 1983.
68. Morrison WA, O'Brien B, McCleod A. Thumb reconstruction with a free neurovascular wrap around flap. J Hand Surg 5:575, 1980.
69. Nicoladoni C. Weitere Erfahrungen uber Daumenplastile. Arch Klin Shir 69:697, 1903.
70. Nygrady J, Szekeres P, Vilmos Z. Toe to thumb transfer in congenital grade III thumb hypoplasia. J Hand Surg 8:898, 1983.
71. O'Brien BM, Black MJ, Morrison WA, Maclead AM. Microvascular great toe transfer for congenital absence of the thumb. Hand 10:113, 1978.
72. Popper NK, Norris TR, Buncke HJ. Evaluation of sensibility and function with microsurgical free tissue transfer for the great toe to the hand for thumb reconstruction. J Hand Surg 8:516, 1983.
73. Wang W. Keys to successful second toe to hand transfer: a review of 30 cases. J Hand Surg 8:902, 1983.

Free Muscle Transfer

74. Harrii K. Free muscle transplantation with microneurovascular anastomoses. In Daniller A, Strauch B, eds. Symposium on Microsurgery, Vol. 14. St Louis, CV Mosby, 1976:177.
75. Harrii K, Ohmori K, Torii S. Free gracilis muscle transplantation with microneurovascular anastomosis in the treatment of facial paralysis. Plast Reconstr Surg 57:133, 1976.
76. Ikuta Y. Free muscle transfer. In Daniel RK, Terzis JK, eds. Reconstructive Microsurgery. Boston, Little, Brown and Co., 1977:270.
77. Ikuta Y, Kubo T, Tsuge K. Free muscle transplantation by microsurgical technique to treat severe Volkmann's contracture. Plast Reconst Surg 58:407, 1976.
78. Manktelow R, McKee N. Free muscle transplantation to provide active finger flexion. J Hand Surg 3:416, 1978.
79. Mathes SJ, Namai F. Classification of the vascular anatomy of muscles: Experimental and clinical correlation. Plast Reconst Surg 67:177, 1981.
80. Tamai S. Free muscle transplants in dogs with microsurgical anastomosis. Plast Reconstr Surg, 46, 219, 1970.
81. Terzis JK, Sweet RC, Dykes RW, Williams MB. Recovery of function in free muscle transplants using microneurovascular anastomosis. J Hand Surg 3:37, 1978.

Free Vascularized Bone Grafting

82. Allieu Y, Gomis R. Congenital pseudarthrosis of the forearm treated by the fibular graft. J Hand Surg 6:475, 1981.
83. Ariyan J, Finseth FJ. The anterior chest approach

for obtaining free osteocutaneous rib grafts. Plast Reconstr Surg 62:676, 1978.

84. Berggren A, Weiland AJ, Ostrup LT. Bone scintigraphy in evaluating the viability of composite bone grafts revascularized by microvascular anastomoses, conventional bone grafts, and free nonvascularized periosteal grafts. J Bone Joint Surg 64A:799, 1982.

85. Buncke HJ, Furnas DW, Gordon L, et al. Free osteocutaneous flap from a rib to a tibia. Plast Reconstr Surg 59:799, 1977.

86. Chen Z, Yan W. The study and clinical application of the osteocutaneous flap of the fibula. Microsurgery 4:11, 1983.

87. Gilbert A. Surgical techniques of vascularized transfer of the fibular shaft. Int J Microsurg 2:100, 1979.

88. Hagan KF, Buncke HJ. Treatment of congenital pseudarthrosis of the tibia with free vascularized bone graft. Clin Orthop 166:34, 1982.

89. Huong GK, Lin ZZ, Shen YI, et al. Microvascular free transfer of iliac bone based on the deep circumflex iliac vessels. J Microsurg 2:113, 1980.

90. Olerud J, Henriksson TF, Engkirst O. A free vascularized fibular graft in lengthening of the humerus with the Wagner apparatus. J Bone Joint Surg 65A:111, 1983.

91. Osterman AL, Bora FW, Jr. Free vascularized bone grafting. Orthop Clin North Am 15:131, 1984.

92. Ostrup LT, Fredrickson JM. Distant transfer of a free living bone graft by microvascular anastomoses: an experimental study. Plast Reconstr Surg 54:274, 1974.

93. Pho RWH. Malignant giant cell tumor of the distal end of the radius treated by a free vascularized fibula transplant. J Bone Joint Surg 63A:877, 1981.

94. Satom T, Tsuchiya M, Kobayaski M, et al. Experience with free composite tissue transplantation based on the deep circumflex iliac vessels. J Microsurg 3:77, 1981.

95. Taylor GI, Miller GDH, Ham FJ. The free vascularized bone graft: a clinical extension of microvascular techniques. Plast Reconstr Surg 55:533, 1975.

96. Taylor GI, Townsend P, Corlett R. Superiority of the deep circumflex iliac vessels as the supply for free groin flaps. Plast Reconstr Surg 64:745, 1979.

97. Usami F, Iketani M, et al. Treatment of congenital pseudarthrosis of the tibia by a free vascularized fibular graft. J Microsurg 3:40, 1981.

98. Weiland AJ. Current concepts review: vascularized free bone transplant. J Bone Joint Surg 63A:166, 1981.

99. Weiland AJ, Daniel RK. Microvascular bone grafts in the treatment of massive defects in bone. J Bone Joint Surg 61A:98, 1979.

100. Weiland AJ, Daniel RK. Congenital pseudarthrosis of the tibia. Treatment with vascularized autogeneous fibular groups. A preliminary report. Johns Hopkins Med J 147:89, 1980.

101. Weiland AJ, Moore JR, Daniel RK. Vascularized bone autografts. Clin Orthop 174:87, 1983.

Free Epiphyseal And Joint Transfer

102. Buncke HJ, Daniller A, Schulz WP, Chase RA. The fate of autogenous whole joints transplanted by microvascular anastomosis. Plast Reconstr Surg 39:333, 1967.

103. Freeman BA. Growth studies of transplanted epiphyses. Plast Reconstr Surg 23:84, 1959.

104. Goldberg NH, Watson HK. Composite toe (phalanx and epiphysis) transfer in the reconstruction of the aphalangic hand. J Hand Surg 9:634, 1984.

105. Mathes SJ, Buchannan R, Weeks P. Microvascular joint transplantation with epiphyseal growth. J Hand Surg 5:586, 1980.

106. Nettelblad H, Randolph M, Weiland A. Free microvascular epiphyseal plate transfer. J Bone Joint Surg 66A:142, 1984.

107. O'Brien B, Gould JS, Morrison WA, et al. Free vascularized small joint transfer to the hand. J Hand Surg 9:634, 1984.

108. Tsai TM, Jupiter JB, Kutz JE. Vascularized autogenous whole joint transfer in the hand. A clinical study. J Hand Surg 7:335, 1982.

109. Tsai TM. Free epiphyseal transfer. Presented at the fifth AOA International Symposium: Limb Reconstruction Micro or Macrosurgery. November 11, 1984.

Future Applications

110. Clodius L, Wirth W. A new experimental model for chronic lymphedema of the upper extremities. Chir Plast 2:115, 1974.

111. Daniel RK, Terzis JK. Reconstructive Microsurgery. Boston, Little, Brown and Co., 1977.

112. Ohmori K. Free flaps in children. In Daniel RK, Terzis JK, eds. Reconstructive Microsurgery. Boston, Little, Brown and Co., 1977:247.

113. Zhong-Wei C, Dong-Yhe Y, Di-Sheng C, Yu-Lin C. Microsurgery. Berlin, Springer-Verlag, 1982.

CHAPTER ○ 9 Fractures

Fractures, Ligamentous Injuries to the Hand

WILLIAM B. KLEINMAN
WILLIAM H. BOWERS

Injuries to the hand in children present unique diagnostic and therapeutic challenges. Although metacarpal and phalangeal fractures are common in this age group, most can be easily treated by closed reduction, and most heal without difficulty in 3 weeks. Those fractures near the epiphyseal plate will remodel nicely if displacement is in the plane of motion of adjacent joints; fractures near the opposite end will demonstrate little remodeling but still heal rapidly.

Regardless of the proximity of a rotational deformity to an epiphyseal plate, no degree of rotation will be remodeled. At the time of reduction of a metacarpal or phalangeal fracture, care must be taken to assure proper clinical alignment of the fingers. This is best evaluated by comparing the alignment of the fingernails of both hands following closed reduction and with the fingers in flexion.

Immobilization following either closed or open reduction is similar in children and adults. Efforts should be directed toward the "safe" position advocated by J.I.P. James,[24] maintaining the collateral ligaments of the metacarpophalangeal joints under tension for the period of immobilization. The metacarpophalangeal joints should be flexed greater than 70 degrees if swelling permits, and the interphalangeal joints flexed no more than 20 degrees (Fig. 9–1). This position is facilitated by wrist dorsiflexion of 40 degrees.

If fractures are stable and require no reduction, immobilization can be by a simple bulky compression dressing that gently controls swelling and maintains position. Low-energy fractures with minimal displacement can be splinted to an adjacent finger ("buddy taping"), which protects against angulatory forces and facilitates early active motion.

Young children have an enormous predisposition to either destroy or wiggle out of their immobilization. In the absence of internal fixation, standard casting techniques used in adults are often ineffective in children. When plaster of Paris is used to maintain a bony reduction in the hand, application of a *long* arm cast, with the elbow flexed at 90 degrees, will retard the child's ability to maneuver out of rigid immobilization.

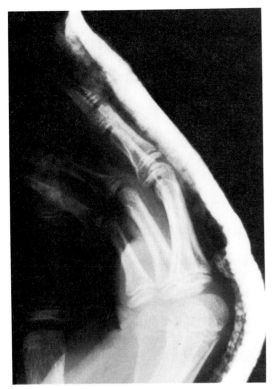

Figure 9–1. A plaster-of-Paris dorsal blocking splint can be used to maintain the "safe" position of wrist dorsiflexion and metacarpophalangeal joint flexion after fracture reduction. MCP flexion maintains the collateral ligaments under tension during the period of fracture immobilization, reducing the predisposition for extension contracture secondary to dorsal capsular tightness.

effect of either stimulation or retardation of bone growth following injury to the hand. Gentle anatomic reduction of fracture fragments will frequently accomplish this.

Neer[29] has shown that in certain types of epiphyseal plate fractures (outside the hand) angulation of up to 45 degrees and/or displacement of up to 60% can be accepted. Bony remodeling of the displaced or angulated fracture fragments will occur, and acceptable function can be restored (e.g., the proximal humerus) without manipulative reduction.

In the phalanges and metacarpals of the growing hand, some degree of angulation can be tolerated as long as it is in the plane of motion of the adjacent joints, and as long as there is growth potential left in the bone. The criteria for satisfactory reduction are much more rigid in bones adjacent to joints, which move in one plane only. In the hand, no degree of phalangeal or metacarpal rotational deformity can be accepted; if present, open or closed reduction is necessary to correct rotation (Fig. 9–2).

The indications for open reduction of phalangeal or metacarpal fractures in the child, whether or not the epiphyseal plate is involved, are similar to those in the adult. These include (1) failure to *obtain* a satisfactory reduction, (2) failure to *maintain* reduction, (3) open fractures, or (4) infected tissue.

PATHOPHYSIOLOGY OF CHILDREN'S HAND FRACTURES

Longitudinal and appositional growth are both affected by fractures of the long tubular bones of a child's hand. Inherent in the management of these injuries should be a clear understanding of the response of the cambium layer of the periosteum to injury, the susceptibility of the epiphyseal plate itself to damage, and the prognosis for each bony injury with or without alignment of fracture fragments.[21, 34, 41, 45, 52]

The effect of increased blood flow to an injured bone is to stimulate longitudinal growth. Segmuller,[42] however, reported that although half the finger fractures studied in his series had symmetric longitudinal growth after injury, retardation of growth occurred twice as commonly as increased growth. Efforts must be made to reduce the

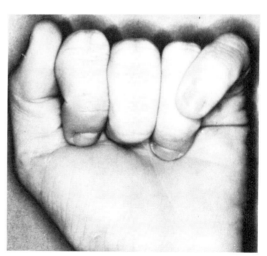

Figure 9–2. Unacceptable malunion of a metacarpal neck fracture of the little finger in a 12-year-old patient. Derotational osteotomy is indicated.

ANATOMY OF THE EPIPHYSEAL PLATE AND BIOMECHANICS OF FRACTURE

Longitudinal growth in the 19 tubular bones of the hand comes from growth plates located at the proximal ends of all phalanges and the distal ends of all metacarpals, except in the thumb metacarpal, which is located proximally (Fig. 9–3). These growth plates consist of cartilage discs located between the epiphysis and metaphysis of the tubular bone. In longitudinal sections, the epiphyseal plate consists of four distinct layers of longitudinally oriented cell columns.[41] According to Salter and Harris,[38] these four layers are (1) a resting cell zone, adjacent to the epiphyseal bone plate, consisting of metabolically inactive chondrocytes; (2) a zone of proliferating cells, with increased metabolic activity and cellular propagation; (3) a zone of cellular hypertrophy; and (4) a zone of endochondral ossification.

Siffert and Gilbert[45] refer to that section of the growth plate where randomly and sparsely dispersed germinal cells become longitudinally arranged in palisading columns as the "zone of growth" (Fig. 9–4). This

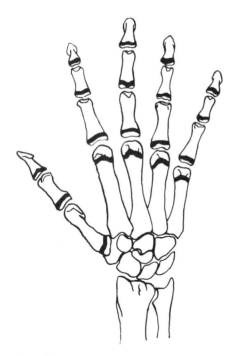

Figure 9–3. Orientation of the 19 epiphyseal plates of the hand. Each growth plate is located at the proximal end of a tubular bone, except in the metacarpals of the index, middle, ring, and little fingers; in these four bones, the plate is distally located.

cellular arrangement is a physiologic response to longitudinal bone load and joint reaction forces. The so-called zone of cartilage transformation consists of plump hypertrophying cells and a reduction in the relative amount of intercellular substance or cartilage matrix. This matrix consists of collagen fibers in an amorphous substrate containing chondroitin sulfate. The arrangement of collagen fibers is longitudinal throughout this amorphous mass, giving significant strength to the layers of the epiphyseal plate in which the concentration of matrix is high. In the zone of cartilage transformation, growth plate cells continue to hypertrophy and the relative amount of strong intercellular matrix is reduced. In this area the growth plate is quite weak to shearing and avulsion forces. Closer to the metaphysis, in this same zone, the chondroitin sulfate and collagen matrix are calcified, forming the zone of provisional calcification, with resultant increase in strength of the plate. More proximal within the plate, there is vascular ingrowth and bone formation in the final "zone of ossification."

As shear forces are applied to a growing bone, either as avulsion or in association with torque injury, bone failure occurs in the growth plate between the layers of cellular hypertrophy and provisional calcification. A consistent cleavage plane opens through the cartilage plate, separating the epiphysis from the metaphysis. It is important to note that in the hand, following cleavage and separation through this constant area, the resting and germinal cell layers remain with the epiphysis.[30, 34, 38] The epiphyses of the hand are covered by a perichondral ring and periosteum at the node of Ranvier and receive epiphyseal vessels directly (unlike the femoral epiphysis of the hip). Because of this vascular anatomy, the germinal cells remain viable and continue to grow normally following fracture reduction, unless damaged by a longitudinal crushing component to the growth plate.

The cartilaginous epiphyseal plate has been shown experimentally to be weaker than bone, but only when subjected to shearing forces.[34, 35, 38, 43, 44] The area of the plate between the hypertrophying cell layer and the "zone of provisional matrix calcification" in Siffert and Gilbert's zone of cartilage transformation (Fig. 9–4) is consistently weaker than bone, ligament, or tendon. The higher incidence of fractures through bone

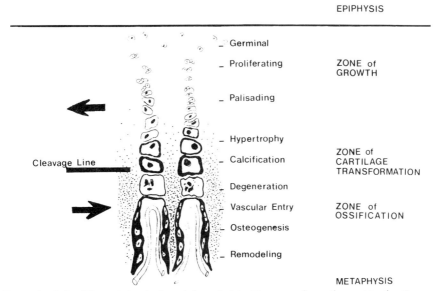

EPIPHYSIS

Germinal

Proliferating — ZONE of GROWTH

Palisading

Hypertrophy

Calcification — ZONE of CARTILAGE TRANSFORMATION

Degeneration

Vascular Entry — ZONE of OSSIFICATION

Osteogenesis

Remodeling

Cleavage Line

METAPHYSIS

Figure 9–4. Zones of cellular differentiation in the epiphyseal plate. The zone of growth consists of resting or germinal cells of low metabolic rate that undergo duplication in the proliferating area. As proliferation progresses, these cells become arranged in longitudinally oriented columns, often called the palisading area. In this area a relatively large amount of amorphous substrate is produced, and the ratio of substrate volume to cellular volume is high.

In the zone of cartilage transformation, cellular proliferation is retarded, and hypertrophic changes begin. Provisional calcification takes place in this area, and the ratio of substrate volume to cellular volume is reduced. At this point the growth plate is susceptible to forces of both shear and avulsion. As more calcification occurs in the substrate matrix, the strength of the plate again increases, into the zone of ossification. (Adapted from Siffert RS, Gilbert MD. *In* Rang M, ed. The Growth Plate and Its Disorders. Baltimore, Williams & Wilkins, 1969.)

in children, rather than injuries to the epiphyseal plate, reflects only the low incidence of pure shear as a mechanism of injury in children's hands. Bone fails preferentially to the cartilage interface between calcified and uncalcified matrix in the growth plate when the mechanism of injury involves torque, angulatory force, or compressive load. The resultant fracture anatomy depends entirely on the direction of the force of injury on the bone and on the rotational, angulatory, or shearing components associated with this force.

The epiphyseal plates of the phalanges and metacarpals of the hand are covered by periosteum, ligament, and tendon attachments. Under conditions of traumatic separation, the epiphysis, perichondral ring, and layers of germinal and palisading chondrocytes of the growth plate remain covered by soft tissue and intact epiphyseal vessels. The germinal cells are uninjured, and growth continues. Following reduction, residual separation between calcified and uncalcified cartilage is filled by avascular fibrin while germinal cells continue to proliferate.[10, 47] The growth plate widens temporarily on x-

ray, until an ingrowth of capillary buds from the metaphyseal vessels invades the proliferating cellular columns of the plate, causing resorption, narrowing, and healing. If reduction has been anatomic, healing should occur without a trace of injury (Fig. 9–5).

CLASSIFICATION OF INJURIES TO THE EPIPHYSEAL PLATE

Injuries to the epiphyseal plate occur by four mechanisms, according to Salter and Harris[38]: (1) shearing, (2) avulsion, (3) splitting, and (4) crushing. As noted earlier, the type of growth plate injury is dependent upon the components of the force causing the injury.

Although many classifications of epiphyseal injuries have been proposed,[1, 2, 30, 38] that suggested in 1963 by Salter and Harris has received the widest acceptance. Although this is not necessarily the most extensive classification,[30] the five categories of growth plate injuries using the Salter and Harris criteria provide close correlation be-

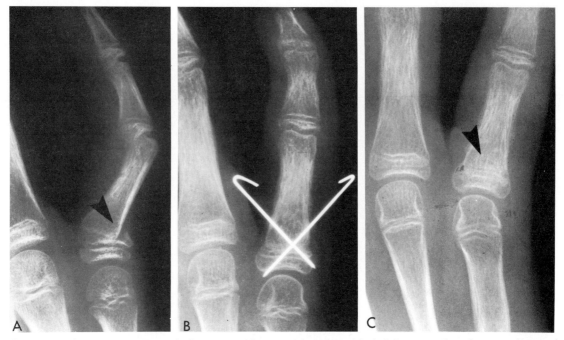

Figure 9–5. Salter-Harris type II growth plate injury to the proximal phalanx of the little finger: *A*, Shear forces are dissipated along the zone of cartilage transformation (area of provisional calcification) and through the proximal metaphyseal bone, demonstrating the Thurston-Holland sign; *B*, anatomic reduction and internal fixation with smooth percutaneous Kirschner wires; *C*, excellent bone healing with little effect on growth.

tween fracture anatomy and mechanism of injury. These authors also suggest a prognostic value for their classification, which has been clinically corroborated over the past 20 years (Fig. 9–6).

Type I. This injury results from a pure shearing or avulsion mechanism and has no bony component (Fig. 9–7). It usually occurs early in childhood, when the growth plate is thick and the hypertrophying chondrocytes are quite large. The layer along the epiphyseal side of the zone of provisional calcification is very weak (see Fig. 9–4).

These injuries are quite common in children's hands, and are often nondisplaced and misdiagnosed as sprains. Clinically, there is marked local tenderness over the growth plate. X-rays may be normal unless there is separation of the metaphyseal and epiphyseal components, which is rare (Fig.

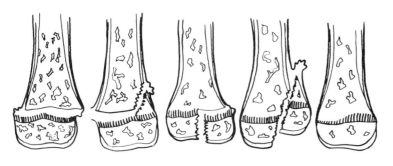

TYPE I   TYPE II   TYPE III   TYPE IV   TYPE V

Figure 9–6. The Salter-Harris classification of epiphyseal plate injuries: Type I demonstrates plate failure from shear forces dissipated through the zone of cartilage transformation (the area of provisional calcification); in type II injuries, the force dissipated through the cleavage plane of the area of provisional calcification exits through the metaphysis (the Thurston-Holland sign); those injuries classified as type III dissipate force through the provisional calcification and intraarticular zones, through the bony epiphysis, leaving an epiphyseal fragment; type IV fractures result in both metaphyseal and epiphyseal fragments remaining attached to the growth plate; in type V injuries, a portion or all of the growth potential of the plate is destroyed by insult secondary to crush, electrical or thermal burn, irradiation, frostbite, and the like, causing partial or complete growth arrest of the involved bone.

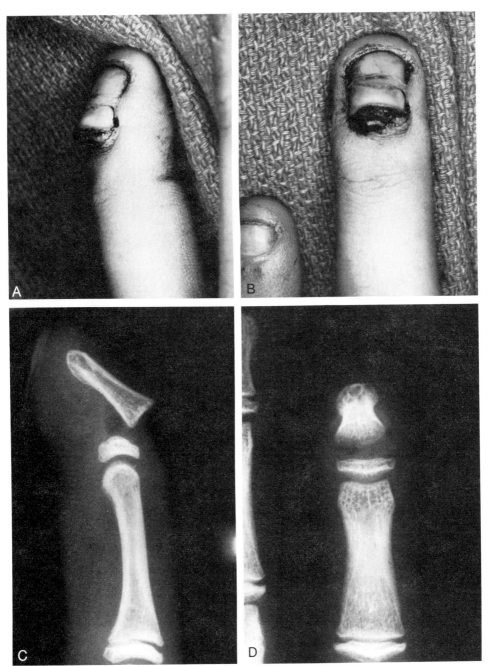

Figure 9–7. A–D, Salter-Harris type I fracture through the distal phalangeal epiphyseal plate, an unusual injury with 100% displacement of fragments.

9–7C and D). The periosteum is quite thick, usually preventing separation of the fracture fragments. Since there is no vascular compromise to the germinal layer, even if displaced, the potential for normal growth following this injury is excellent.

If nondisplaced, these injuries can be treated by immobilization for 2 to 3 weeks in a soft, plaster-reinforced, bulky dressing. If displaced, accurate reduction by open or closed means is indicated, with the understanding that gentle reduction is critical for avoiding any further damage to the plate. Immobilization following reduction should be for 3 weeks, either by cast support or by internal fixation.

Type II. These fractures are the most common of all growth plate injuries. They result from a shearing or avulsion force, with an angulatory component (Fig. 9–8). Fractures of this nature are most frequently seen after 10 years of age. They occur in conjunction with tension forces developed along the border associated with cartilage failure, and compressive forces along the opposite side, in which the metaphyseal bone fails (Fig. 9–9). As the force of injury is dissipated from the tension side to the compression side of the plate, it exits through the metaphysis, leaving a variable-sized metaphyseal fragment referred to radiographically as the Thurston-Holland sign (Fig. 9–10). The periosteum along this metaphyseal fragment remains intact and can be used to facilitate reduction, preventing overcorrection. As in type I injuries, the germinal layer of chondrocytes in type II fractures is undamaged, and the potential for normal growth is excellent. Small degrees of displacement or angulation can be accepted if occurring in the plane of motion of adjacent joints. Since the potential for remodeling is excellent, mild deformities respond to Wolff's law, leaving no permanent deformity (Fig. 9–11).

In epiphyseal plate injuries adjacent to more universal joints, such as the carpometacarpal joint of the thumb, a higher degree of displacement or angulation can be accepted because of remodeling in more than one plane of motion. This will be discussed later in this chapter.

Type III. The epiphyses of the phalanges and metacarpals of the hand are intracap-

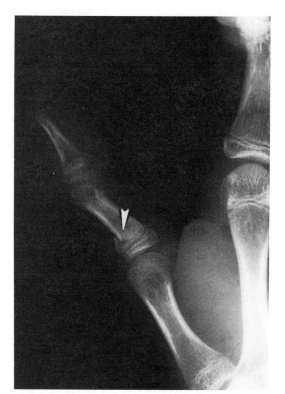

Figure 9–9. The preferential failure of the growth plate under tension and the metaphysis under compression in the Salter-Harris type II fracture.

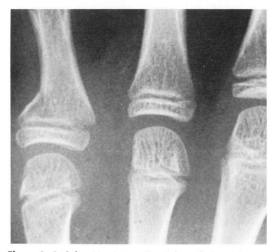

Figure 9–8. Salter-Harris type II epiphyseal plate injury to the proximal phalanx of the little finger.

sular and covered by soft tissue attachments, including the perichondral ring at the node of Ranvier, periosteum, tendons, and ligaments. The Salter-Harris type III fracture is associated with an intra-articular avulsion force, directed through these soft tissue attachments on the epiphysis and dissipated through the weak growth plate between the calcified and uncalcified layers. The type III fracture is fortunately rare. It is occasionally seen in the distal tibia (medial aspect, including the malleolus); when found in the growing hand, it is associated with avulsion injuries involving palmar plate, central tendon, or terminal tendon. For example, the flexor digitorum profundus tendon crosses the epiphysis and epiphyseal plate of the distal phalanx before inserting on the phalangeal metaphysis and mid-diaphysis. Dorsally, the terminal extensor tendon inserts predominantly on the epiphysis, with some fibers blending into the periosteal sleeve of the epiphyseal plate. The equivalent of the adult mallet finger in an adolescent is the Salter-Harris type III intra-articular growth plate injury with a variable-sized, avulsed

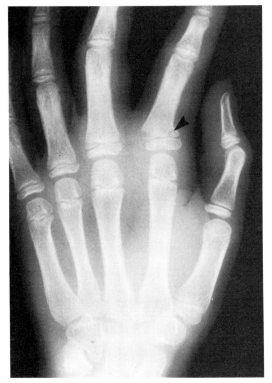

Figure 9–10. The Thurston-Holland sign (metaphyseal fragment) is associated with Salter-Harris type II epiphyseal plate injuries, displaced or nondisplaced.

bone fragment (Fig. 9–12). The mechanism of injury is avulsion of the dorsal epiphyseal fragment by the terminal tendon, as the distal phalanx is flexed by a rapidly applied axial load. The intra-articular epiphyseal component fails by tension, and the epiphyseal plate fails by shear, predictably between the uncalcified hypertrophic cell layer and the stronger area of provisional calcification.

Since the energy of the injury is dissipated from within the growth plate to within the joint through the bony epiphysis, both the germinal layer of chondrocytes *and* the congruency of the articular surface are disturbed. Unless anatomically reduced, this may lead to permanent joint irregularity and the potential for traumatic arthritis. Reconstitution of joint space congruency is essential, but there is no intact periosteal sleeve to facilitate closed reduction, as in Salter-Harris type II fractures. Therefore, open reduction with or without internal fixation is usually indicated in type III epiphyseal plate injuries. Since cleavage of the epiphyseal fragment is initiated between palisading cell columns, growth disturbance is minimal and the prognosis is good, as long as the articular surface is restored.

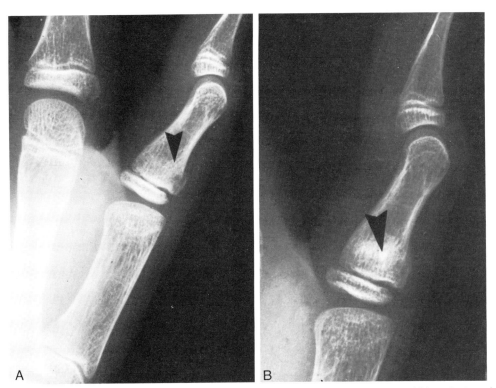

Figure 9–11. *A,* Salter-Harris type II fracture of the proximal phalanx of the thumb in a 13-year-old boy; *B,* 4 weeks after injury, the fracture is solidly healed, and early evidence of remodeling is present.

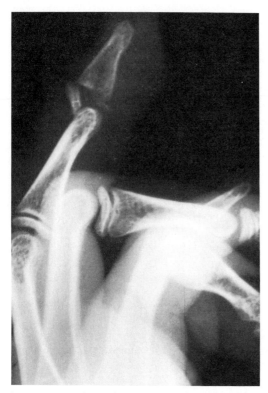

Figure 9–12. Avulsion of 60% of the distal phalangeal dorsal epiphysis, resulting in an intraarticular Salter-Harris type III fracture.

Type IV. This type of growth plate injury is fortunately quite rare in the hand. The mechanism is compressive loading of a portion of the articular surface; energy of the injury is transmitted across the epiphysis and the epiphyseal plate and is dissipated through the metaphysis. The result is an intra-articular split fracture across the growth plate, with both epiphyseal and metaphyseal components (Fig. 9–13 A and B). If displaced, these fractures should be treated by open reduction and temporary internal fixation with smooth Kirschner wires, establishing apposition of the growth plate and intra-articular fragments (Fig. 9–13 C and D). Without anatomic alignment a bony bridge may form across the plate as the fracture heals, resulting in premature closure of a portion of the epiphyseal plate and the potential for growth arrest. This injury is most commonly seen in injuries to the lateral condyle of the distal humerus and is rarely associated with injuries to the hand phalanges or metacarpals. It may also result following a rare mechanism of mallet fracture in children, as will be seen later in this chapter.

Type V. Exceedingly rare in the hand, this type of epiphyseal injury may result from a severe axial load to a portion of the epiphyseal plate. Electrical injuries, frostbite, irradiation, or thermal burns may also cause patterns of growth arrest seen in type V injuries either by a direct effect on cellular duplication or by a secondary effect on the growth plate through disruption of blood flow to this area. The result following injury by either mechanism is partial or complete growth arrest.

Trueta and Trias[51] found through their studies of injuries to rabbit epiphyseal plates that interference with growth is directly proportional to the degree of damage (amount and duration of applied force) to the epiphyseal side of the plate, i.e., the germinal cell layer.

This type of injury is usually observed in those joints that move predominantly in one plane and are subject to large loading forces, e.g., the knee. If severe abduction or adduction forces are applied to a joint that normally flexes and extends, the germinal cell layer of the plate under compressive load may be damaged, causing growth arrest in that area. The mechanism of injury should be assessed critically, as x-rays are frequently normal at the time of acute evaluation. The prognosis is poor for normal growth following this type of injury.

Conclusions. In his assessment of growth plate injuries, the surgeon should remember that although the cartilage cleavage plane between uncalcified and calcified matrix is weaker than normal bone, tendon, ligament, or joint capsule, fractures through bone are more common in children than growth plate injuries.[3, 23, 34, 38, 43, 44] Since the plate fails only when shearing and avulsion forces are applied, the mechanism of injury and the direction of applied force are responsible for this paradox. Only during the periods of rapid growth, e.g., the perinatal period and the adolescent growth spurt, do epiphyseal plate injuries seem to have a higher incidence than bone injuries in the hand.

RECOMMENDED TREATMENT FOR GROWTH PLATE INJURIES

Reduction of displaced growth plate fragments, whether achieved by closed or open means, *must* be performed gently. No additional damage should be done to the remain-

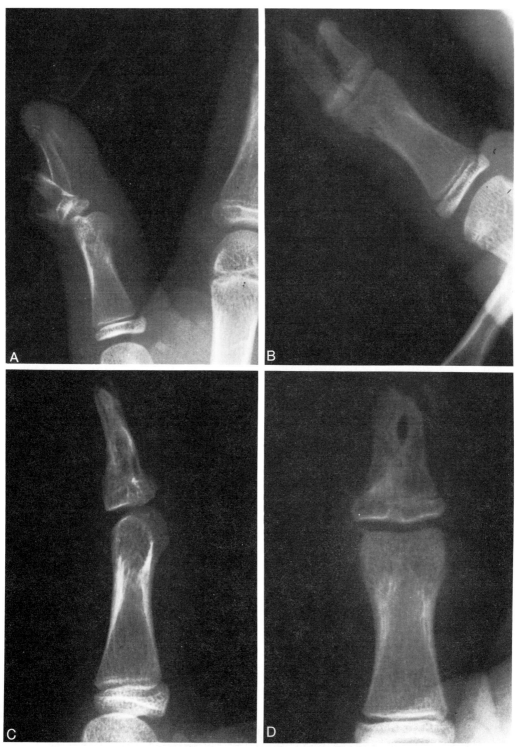

Figure 9–13. *A* and *B*, Lateral and AP x-rays of a Salter-Harris type IV injury to the thumb distal phalanx of an eight-year-old girl; *C* and *D*, lateral and AP x-rays 8 weeks following open reduction and internal fixation, demonstrating excellent reconstitution of the articular surface and good bony healing.

ing uninjured germinal cell layer of the juxtaepiphyseal area of the growth plate. Campbell, Grisolta and Zanconato[10] established that the amount of damage to the germinal layer of chondrocytes is directly proportional to the degree of growth disturbance at the epiphyseal plate. Their experimental work with immature dogs supports the better prognosis of the Salter-Harris types I and II growth plate injuries. Also established by their work is that healing of a facture line crossing both epiphysis and metaphysis (type IV) is not by cartilage but by ingrowth of undifferentiated mesenchymal tissue, which later becomes a cancellous bony bridge.[10, 47] When substantial in size, this bony bridge can cause growth arrest by anchoring the metaphysis to the epiphysis.

In type III and IV fractures, the potential disturbance to growth is minimized by open reduction and anatomic reconstitution of the articular surface and the epiphyseal plate. Campbell and coworkers[10] recommended for all displaced epiphyseal plate fractures the use of smooth thin metallic pins (e.g., Kirschner wires), inserted perpendicular to the plate from the epiphyseal fragment to the normal metaphysis (Fig. 9–14). The wire lies parallel to the longitudinally oriented palisading columns of hypertrophying chondrocytes. Use of screws or threaded pins is contraindicated, as this hardware mechanically fixes the epiphysis to the metaphysis, establishing the potential for growth arrest.

Using the principle that growth plate fractures heal in approximately one half the time required for similar bony injuries in adults, most applied internal fixation hardware can be removed within 3 weeks of reduction.

MALLET FINGERS IN CHILDREN

The childhood mallet finger deformity deserves special consideration. Its presentation is variable with respect not only to the mechanism of injury but also to the age of the patient. Unlike the adult equivalent, which is usually incurred by rapid axial loading and forced flexion of the extended distal phalanx (the basketball "jamming" injury), children incur mallet finger deformities either by forced flexion against resistive extension or by forced extension and axial loading.

In the early years of childhood, when the epiphyseal plate is thick and weak, rapid loading injuries commonly cleave the plate

between the layers of calcified and uncalcified matrix of the zone of hypertrophic cells, resulting in a displaced Salter-Harris type I fracture (see Fig. 9–7 C and D). If the same injury occurs as the adolescent epiphyseal plate is closing, the mechanism is one of terminal tendon avulsion of the dorsal bony epiphysis, the Salter-Harris type III fracture (see Fig. 9–12). The line of cleavage through the growth plate is similar to that of the type I injury; however, the dissipation of force is intra-articular. Anatomic reduction is necessary and can usually be achieved quite easily by either open or closed techniques.

If the mechanism of injury is axial loading and hyperextension of the distal interphalangeal joint, the dorsal portion of the epiphysis may fail under the compressive load. Shear forces generated perpendicular to the plate, and exiting through the dorsal metaphysis, may result in a Salter-Harris type IV fracture. As in most type IV fractures, open reduction is indicated, using percutaneous smooth Kirschner wire internal fixation.

If the terminal phalanx is axially loaded without shearing or avulsion forces to the plate, the germinal layer of the epiphyseal plate may be damaged by crushing. This Salter-Harris type V growth plate injury can result in premature growth arrest of part or all of the distal phalanx. As in all type V injuries, early radiographic examination may be normal, but the prognosis for normal growth is poor; the patient and family should be advised of the potential for either progressive angulatory deformity or significant growth retardation of the distal phalanx. If angulated, corrective osteotomy can be performed at a later date.

METACARPAL FRACTURES NOT INVOLVING THE EPIPHYSEAL PLATE

Metacarpal fractures in children are usually associated with blunt trauma or crushing injury. There may be a significant amount of damage to the periosteum and surrounding soft tissue structures (Fig. 9–15). As in most adult metacarpal fractures, loss of longitudinal stability leads to bony collapse, with palmar angulation of the distal fragment. Extrinsic wrist extensors tend to dorsiflex the proximal fragment, while the interosseous muscles palmar flex the distal fragment (Fig. 9–16A). Reduction is achieved by using the

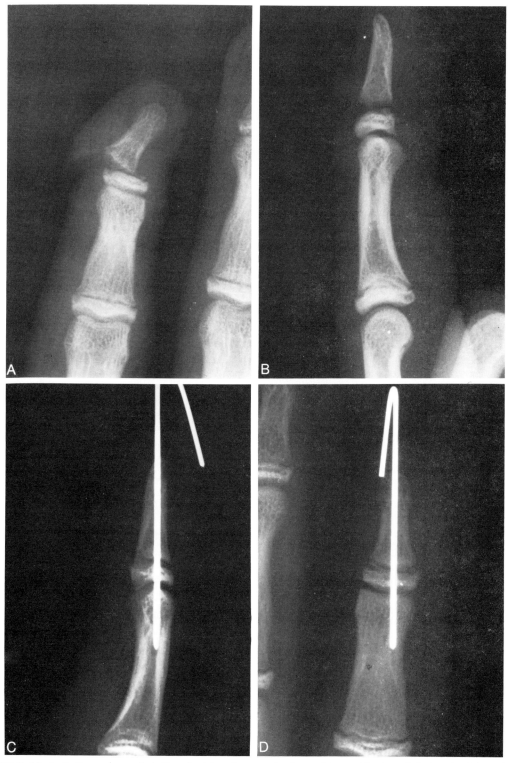

Figure 9–14. *A–D*, X-rays demonstrate the principles of open reduction and internal fixation of displaced epiphyseal plate injuries with use of smooth percutaneous Kirschner wires placed parallel to the longitudinally oriented palisading cell columns of the growth plate.

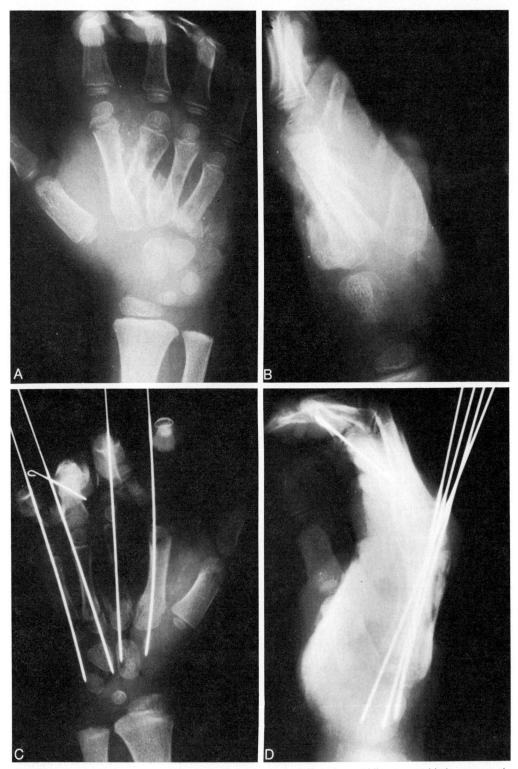

Figure 9–15. *A–D,* X-rays demonstrate severely displaced fractures of the index, middle, ring, and little metacarpals, secondary to a crushing injury, in the right hand of a 4-year-old boy. Although no fracture involved the epiphyseal plate, damage to periosteum and supporting soft tissues was extensive. Despite open reduction and Kirschner wire alignment, damage to soft tissues and loss of bone substance resulted in nonunion of the middle finger metacarpal, which was treated by bone grafting and plating.

Figure 9–16. Fractures of the metacarpals and phalanges deform and angulate in a predictable manner secondary to loss of bony support between two antagonistic forces: *A*, palmar angulation of the metacarpal neck fracture; *B*, dorsal angulation of the proximal phalangeal neck fracture; *C*, palmar angulation of the proximal fracture of the middle phalanx; *D*, dorsal angulation of the middle phalangeal neck fracture. (FDP = flexor digitorum profundus; FDS = flexor digitorum superficialis, I.O. = interossei; EDC = extensor digitorum communis; ECRL = extensor carpi radialis longus; ECRB = extensor carpi radialis brevis; ECU = extensor carpi ulnaris.)

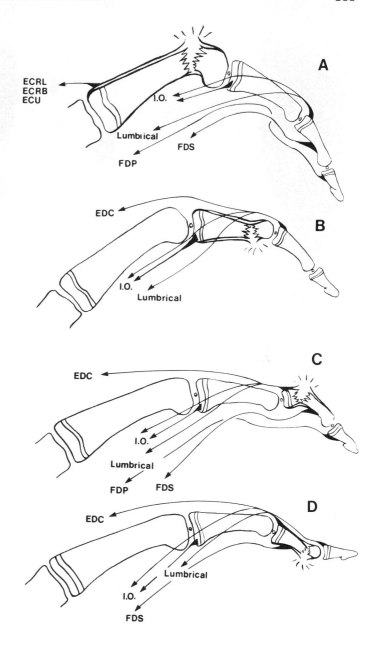

intact palmar periosteum at the metacarpal fracture site, and dorsiflexing the distal fragment with the metacarpophalangeal and proximal interphalangeal joints in flexion. The integrity of the palmar periosteum will prevent overcorrection. Following reduction, the proximal interphalangeal joint can be brought back to 10 to 20 degrees of flexion for the period of cast immobilization. No degree of malrotation should be accepted; however, some angulation in the plane of metacarpophalangeal motion may be tolerated. Factors to be considered should include the principles of fracture management in children outlined by Rang.[34] These principles may be helpful in determining the acceptability of a reduced fracture: (1) Significant remodeling will occur only if the fracture is near the growth plate and if the angular deformity is in the plane of joint motion; (2) the child must have at least 2 years of longitudinal growth remaining.

As in adults, a greater degree of angulation is acceptable in the more mobile fourth and especially fifth metacarpals. One should keep in mind that palmar angulation greater than 30 to 40 degrees may produce a tender "lump" in the palm (the metacarpal head) or

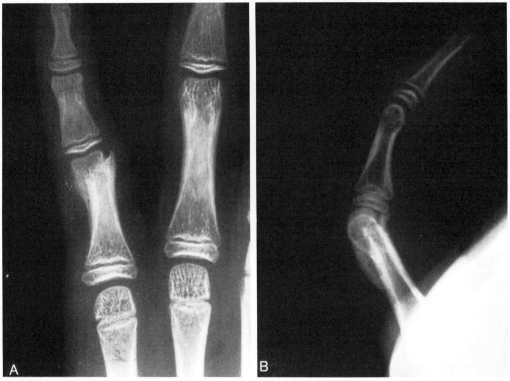

Figure 9–17. *A* and *B*, Disastrous consequences of failure to anatomically reduce a bicondylar fracture of the proximal phalanx of the little finger of an 11-year-old girl. There is marked ulnar deviation and dorsal angulation of the distal fragment associated with a bony block to flexion beyond 40°.

marked metacarpophalangeal joint hyper-extension and "claw" deformity.

The surgeon's perception of bone remodeling as a panacea can be responsible for a poor functional result. Any fracture at the end opposite the epiphyseal plate will remodel poorly (phalangeal neck or condylar fracture). Rotational deformity or angulation not in the plane of adjacent motion will not remodel (Fig. 9–17). These deformities must be reduced early and accurately by open or closed means.

PHALANGEAL FRACTURES NOT INVOLVING THE EPIPHYSEAL PLATE

The relative contributions of compression, angulatory force, and torque to the mechanism of fracture determines whether phalangeal fractures not involving the growth plate are transverse, oblique, or spiral. Dorsal angulation of the distal fragment is the usual deformity in proximal phalangeal fractures (Fig. 9–16B). The interossei pass palmar to the axis of rotation of the metacarpophalan-

geal joint and tend to displace the proximal fragment palmarly, while the central tendon and lateral bands displace the distal fragment dorsally. Manipulative reduction involves alignment of the distal and proximal fragments by gentle distraction and palmar flexion of the distal fragment. The dorsal periosteum is usually intact and prevents overcorrection. Active range of motion begins 3 weeks after reduction. Moderate displacement following reduction should be regarded critically; any "step-off" not in the plane of motion of the adjacent joints will not remodel, regardless of how near the epiphyseal plate (see Fig. 9–17). If this deformity is not corrected, joint motion will be limited by joint incongruity or tethering of extrinsic tendons by scar or bony prominences. On the palmar surface of the finger this usually is not a functional problem; the flexor digitorum superficialis tendon serves as a protective barrier to adhesions between the fracture and the glide of the flexor digitorum profundus tendon at the level of the proximal phalanx.

Similar injuries to the middle phalanx result in palmar angulation of the distal fragment if the fracture is proximal to the insertion of the flexor digitorum superficialis insertion (Fig. 9–16C). The central tendon and lateral bands pull the proximal fragment dorsally while the superficialis displaces the distal fragment palmarly.

Condylar Fractures. Distal to the insertion of the flexor digitorum superficialis are the middle phalangeal condylar fractures (Fig. 9–18A). These may be bicondylar (similar to the phalangeal neck fracture), unicondylar, or T-condylar. In bicondylar fractures, the distal fragment of the middle phalanx is angulated dorsally by the pull of the terminal tendon on the distal phalanx (Fig. 9–16D). The flexor digitorum superficialis pulls the proximal fragment palmarly.

Significant displacement of these fractures is common; frequently (especially with displaced intra-articular components), open anatomic reduction and internal fixation are indicated (Fig. 9–18B). Although there are subtle differences between middle phalangeal neck fractures and bicondylar fractures, the approach to reduction is similar (Fig. 9-

19). It is relatively easy to *obtain* reduction by gentle longitudinal traction and palmar deviation of the distal fragment, but it is difficult to *maintain* this reduction by closed means only. Condylar fractures are best immobilized for 3 to 4 weeks (depending upon the degree of displacement) following open percutaneous crossed or longitudinal K-wire fixation. Injury to the flexor and extensor tendons must be avoided (Fig. 9–20).

Intra-articular T-condylar fractures are difficult to reduce by closed techniques and should be restored anatomically using a dorsal tendon-splitting surgical approach. Fragments can be easily reduced and fixed anatomically until healed in 3 to 4 weeks.

Important in consideration of these injuries is the rapidity with which children's fractures heal. It is incumbent upon the surgeon to recognize this potential and treat the injury early. If fracture fragment displacement justifies open reduction, or if acceptable reduction can be neither *obtained* nor *maintained* by closed techniques, surgery must be performed promptly, before malunion results.

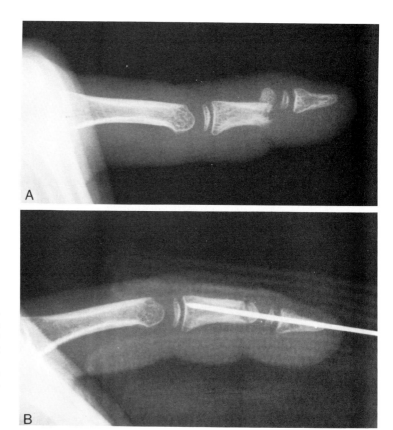

Figure 9–18. *A,* Typical dorsal angulation of the distal fragment in a middle phalangeal bicondylar fracture. Palmar displacement of the proximal fragment is by the flexor digitorum superficialis, whereas dorsal displacement of the distal fragment is by the terminal extensor tendon; *B,* open reduction and internal fixation with a single smooth, longitudinally oriented Kirschner wire.

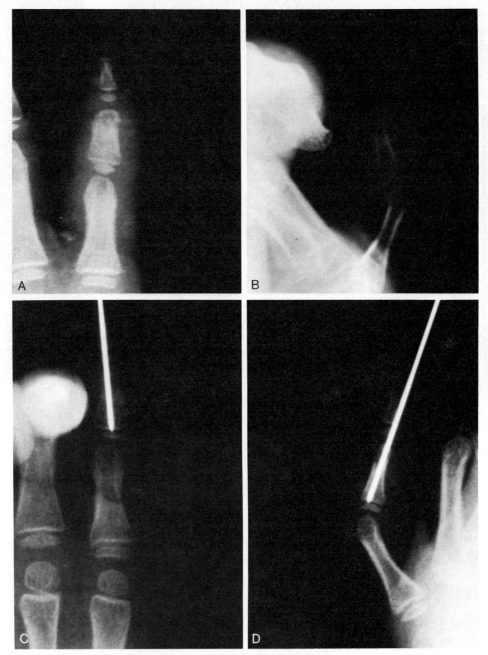

Figure 9–19. A and B, Dorsal angulation of a bicondylar fracture of the middle phalanx in a 3-year-old child; C and D, alignment with a single longitudinal Kirschner wire following open reduction. In 3 weeks the fracture should be healed well enough to remove the internal fixation and to begin active range-of-motion exercises.

METACARPAL FRACTURES AT THE BASE OF THE THUMB

Fractures at the base of the thumb in adults have been classified by Green and O'Brien[20] into three basic types (Fig. 9–21): (1) the intra-articular Bennett fracture, (2) the Y-shaped intra-articular Rolando fracture, and (3) the extra-articular proximal metaphyseal fracture. The mechanism of injury is forced lateral or palmar abduction with axial loading of the carpometacarpal joint.

As in adults, children's injuries in this area are associated with avulsion forces generated

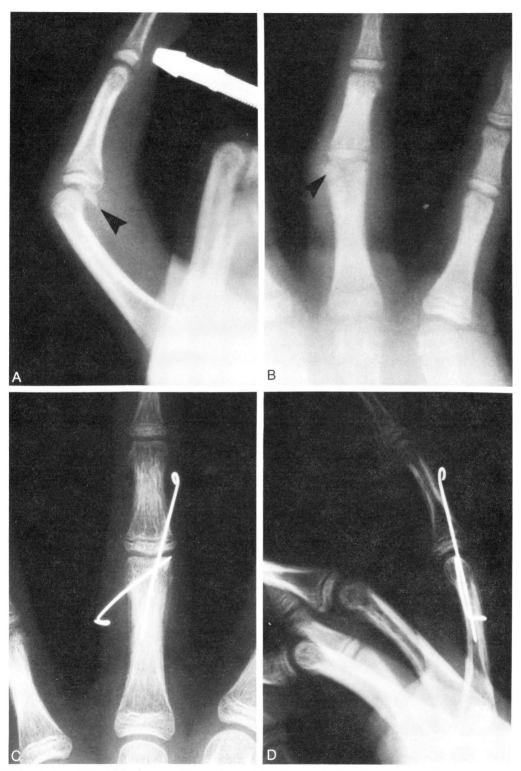

Figure 9–20. *A–D*, Unicondylar fracture of the radial condyle of the proximal phalanx of the ring finger in a 14-year-old boy, treated by open reduction of the condyle and internal fixation with percutaneous Kirschner wires.

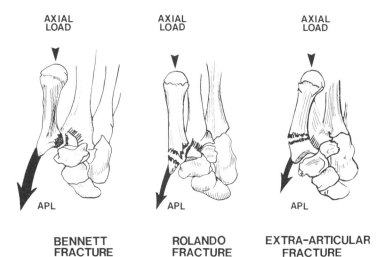

AXIAL
LOAD

APL

AXIAL
LOAD

APL

AXIAL
LOAD

APL

BENNETT
FRACTURE

ROLANDO
FRACTURE

EXTRA-ARTICULAR
FRACTURE

Figure 9–21. Classification of fractures involving the base of the thumb metacarpal. (Adapted from Green DP, O'Brien ET. South Med J 65:807–814, 1972.)

by the abductor pollicis longus. The distinct difference in children, however, is that the deforming force is manifest by shear across the epiphyseal plate, dissipated through the medial metacarpal metaphysis (Salter-Harris type II fracture). The strong interosseous ligament complex anchoring the first and second metacarpal bases supports the medial metaphysis of the thumb metacarpal, and predisposes to type II rather than type I injury. In children this medial ligament complex is responsible for the metaphyseal fragment radiographically seen in the type II injury (the Thurston-Holland sign) (Fig. 9–22A).

Since the carpometacarpal joint of the

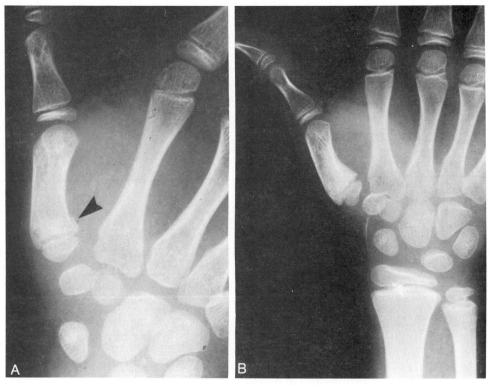

Figure 9–22. *A,* Acute Salter-Harris type II fracture of the base of the thumb metacarpal in a 10-year-old boy. The arrow indicates the Thurston-Holland radiographic sign indicating the metaphyseal fragment; *B,* 10 weeks following injury, considerable remodeling has occurred without reduction, and range of motion is complete.

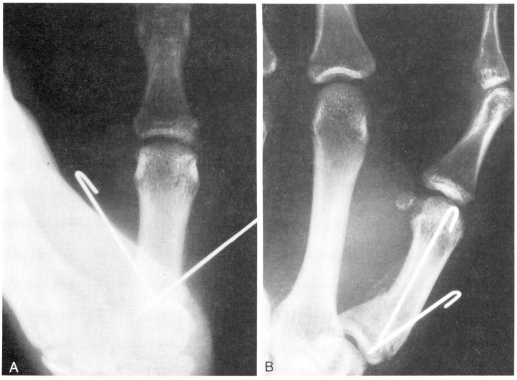

Figure 9–23. A and B, Open reduction and internal fixation by crossed percutaneous Kirschner wires of a basilar thumb metacarpal fracture in a 21-year-old woman with closed epiphyseal plates.

thumb is the most mobile joint of the hand, and since motion at this joint is universal and not in one plane, significant remodeling of moderately displaced fractures can be expected at this site (Fig. 9–22B). Closed injuries in this area with fracture displacement of 40% or less, or angulatory deformity of 40 degrees or less, can be expected to do quite nicely if the child has greater than 2 years of growth left from this epiphyseal plate. Open injuries, or those with greater displacement and angulation, should be reduced openly and fixed with smooth percutaneous Kirschner wires. The technique is similar to that used in adults (Fig. 9–23). These wires can be removed and active motion begun in 3 to 4 weeks.

Small Joint Injuries in Children

Injuries to ligaments cause pain on joint motion, and the resulting ligamentous instability can lead to subluxation or dislocation. More force is required to rupture a ligament or its attachment to bone than to fracture the hypertrophic zone of the epiphyseal plate, and for this reason epiphyseal injuries are more frequent than ligamentous injuries in children.[7]

The ligamentous injuries described here can be divided into grade I sprains with fiber disruption but no joint instability, grade II sprains with fiber disruption resulting in ligamentous laxity, and grade III sprains with fiber disruption and joint dislocation on stress testing. In all these injuries, however, joint congruity is maintained after the injury and after stress testing.

Grade I sprains have minimal fiber disruption and hemorrhage and can be treated with buddy taping for 3 weeks. Grade II sprains have moderate fiber disruption. On clinical examination, they elicit capsule laxity and should be treated with immobilization for 2 weeks and then buddy taping for 2 weeks. When the joint has a full range of painless motion, normal activities can be resumed. Grade III sprains have a complete rupture of one of the ligaments stabilizing the joint and require immobilization for at least 3 weeks. In most patients with grade III injuries, x-ray shows a small fracture that represents the avulsion of the ligament from the bone. If this is protected for 3 weeks, the cells in the injured area will reattach the ligament to the bone and prevent joint instability. No dynamic splinting is recommended in children until stability is determined by stress testing (6 to 8 weeks); however, in children, dynamic splinting is usually not necessary. On rare occasions, grade III injuries develop articular incongruity; in those instances, open repair of the ligament is recommended. The decision to repair a ligament is made if joint incongruity is seen in the true AP and lateral x-rays. If the ligament cannot be sutured directly and the main injury is between the ligament and bone, a drill hole is made in the bone distal to the epiphyseal plate and the ligamentous attachment is placed within the medullary cavity so that a teno-osseous repair will occur. This necessitates making a drill hole in the bone on the side of the injury large enough for the suture holding the ligament to pull the ligament into the medullary cavity of the bone. The drill hole on the contralateral side is smaller, as only the suture need pass and be tied over a button (Fig. 9–24).

Collateral ligament stability of the thumb MP joint varies considerably in the general population; if one suspects an injury, it is best to compare it with the uninjured opposite side. The collateral ligaments are tightest in flexion, and when a small (10 degree) lateral discrepancy exists in maximum

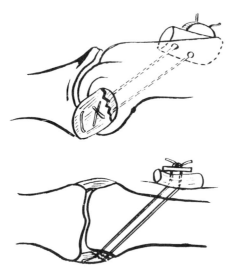

Figure 9–24. The pull-out suture method of repair for a ligament injury. The suture should be a synthetic monofilament strong enough to allow extraction.

flexion, a collateral ligament injury can be assumed.[64] If the joint is in any other position, however, a diagnosis of ligament instability is valid only if lateral deviation exceeds 30 degrees. An ulnar collateral ligament injury weakens pinch; arthrography of the MP joint may demonstrate a capsular tear and help with the diagnosis.[60] In some cases the ligament is in the joint (Stener's lesion[65]); in this injury and those of complete rupture, suture of the ligament is indicated. Afterwards, repair of the ligament should be protected for 5 weeks.

VOLAR PLATE INJURIES AND JOINT DISLOCATIONS

Volar plate injuries including dorsal subluxation, may end in dorsal dislocation.[57–59] As volar stress increases, tension develops within the volar plate and accessory collateral ligaments. If stress is applied slowly, the proximal attachments of the ligaments attenuate and ultimately fail. The joint may sublux or dislocate dorsally, pulling the intact volar plate and accessory collateral ligament over the condyles. The slow application of tension is a clinical rarity. The usual force is rapid, avulsing a piece of the volar metaphysis from the middle phalanx, but just as often the thick central volar plate corresponding to the meniscoid portion of the volar plate will rupture without a bony fragment. (Fig. 9–25). This first-degree volar capsular injury is painful but not destabilizing. If the stress continues, the distal lateral attachments of the volar plate fail and the tear extends proximally between the accessory collateral and proper collateral ligament. The middle phalanx is ultimately forced dorsally, hinging on the proper collateral ligament origins, and the joint may be completely dislocated without disruption of the proper collateral ligaments. Reduction of the joint is by closed hyperextension followed by flexion of the middle phalanx over the proximal, positioning the joint in flexion. One should not apply traction to pull the joint into flexion, as this may result in entrapment of tissues within the joint and prevent reduction. After reduction, the collateral ligaments are tested for stability. First-degree volar plate injury requires buddy taping for about 2 weeks and invariably heals without problems.

Both the patient with a "chip" fracture and

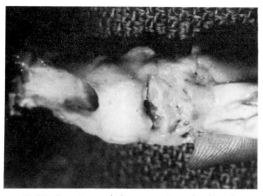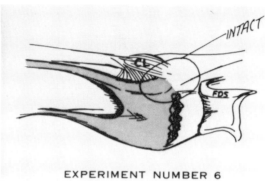

EXPERIMENT NUMBER 6

Figure 9–25. Experimental demonstration of a first degree volar plate injury. The injury is painful but *not* destabilizing, because the critical corners are intact. No bony fragment is attached to the volar plate rupture.

the patient with a negative x-ray film may demonstrate complete loss of volar stability with hyperextension stress. If the volar instability is present and recognized, a dorsal blocking splint, preventing full extension but allowing flexion, is recommended for 3 weeks. If the injury is unrecognized and not treated, the condyles will eventually buttonhole through the volar plate and a chronic hyperextension deformity—a swan-neck deformity—will develop at the proximal interphalangeal joint level (Fig. 9–26). If this defect is a functional problem, suture or reattachment of the ruptured volar plate is indicated.

Volar PIP dislocations are rare and involve injury to the central slip and one or both collateral ligaments. A straight volar dislocation ruptures the central slip, whereas a volar and lateral dislocation ruptures the central slip and one or both collateral ligaments. These injuries are usually reducible by closed methods, after which the PIP joint should be held in extension by a static splint for 1 month. The DIP joint should be free, so that lateral band gliding is possible in its usual position dorsal to the axis of PIP joint motion. Irreducible volar dislocations (Fig. 9–27) with soft tissue interposition require open reduction and splinting in extension for 1 month, with the terminal joint free to move so that the lateral bands will not become adherent at the PIP joint level. Old volar dislocations of the PIP joint require open reduction and soft tissue replacement of the structures that were involved in the injury.

The "pseudoboutonniere" deformity of a digit is similar in appearance to the true boutonniere except that the central slip is intact

and flexion of the PIP joint is caused by an increase in fluid within the joint from an acute injury or scarring of volar joint structures from an old injury. In these injuries, the course of the lateral bands is increased because of swelling or scarring which causes an extension contracture of the DIP joint. This injury is common in adolescents. The collateral ligaments, the volar plate proximal attachment and the oblique retinacular ligaments may be involved. X-rays may show calcification along the lateral cortex of the proximal phalanx, a finding usually seen on oblique views (Fig. 9–28). The injury causes a PIP joint flexion contracture and distal interphalangeal joint extension and represents an old injury. Treatment is usually nonsurgical with static or dynamic splinting of the PIP joint into extension and the DIP joint into flexion. If a fixed flexion deformity of the PIP joint does not respond to conservative measures, release of the proximal volar plate contracture may be required.

Dorsal MP joint dislocations are rare and usually occur in the thumb, index finger, and little fingers. The volar capsule of the metacarpophalangeal joint has a strong distal attachment to the proximal phalanx, while the weaker proximal attachments are to the flexion tendon sheaths and not to bone. MP joint dorsal dislocations frequently have volar plate interposition, which prevents closed reduction. The diagnosis of this injury is made by observing dimpling of the volar skin, a sign that is more obvious in thumb than in finger dislocation because the latter occurs at the level of the distal palmar crease. This crease has a normal skin fascia dimple, which obscures the dimpling from the dislocation. Displacement and angulation as

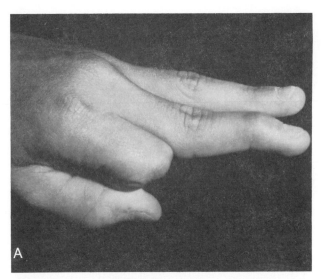

Figure 9–26. *A*, Hyperextension deformity at the PIP joint is shown. *B*, the condyles are seen buttonholed through the chronic volar plate disruption (VP).

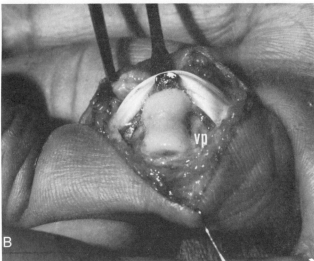

well as widening of the joint are seen on x-ray. Occasionally, sesamoid bones are seen in the joint, and open reduction of this dislocation is required. A volar incision exposes the volar plate, which can be removed from the joint to make reduction possible. The joint is placed in flexion for 4 weeks, at which time joint motion is started. Volar dislocation of the MP joint has been reported but is a rare injury.

INTRA-ARTICULAR FRACTURES

Some intra-articular fractures are marginal capsular disruptions and should be treated accordingly. These are the middle phalangeal volar chip fractures associated with hy-

perextension injury at the interphalangeal joints or the dorsal chip fracture of the middle phalanx at the central slip insertion. Most of these are tension injuries and usually involve only small amounts of the articular cartilage surface. The prognosis for return of motion after 3 weeks of splinting is good.

Fractures associated with compressive forces produce cartilage damage, bone impaction, and articular surface incongruity. These are unstable and usually associated with unicondylar or bicondylar fractures. Fracture-dislocations result from greater compressive forces to the interphalangeal joints and result in significant intra-articular surface disruptions. They are associated with significant morbidity *even with good treatment*. Typical examples are the dorsal sur-

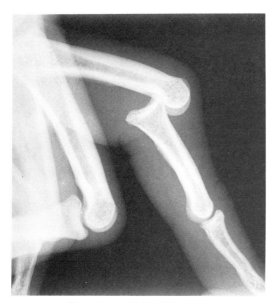

Figure 9–27. Volar dislocation.

face fractures associated with the relatively rare volar dislocation and the volar surface fractures associated with the relatively common dorsal dislocation. In these cases, a closed reduction should be attempted and if congruity of the remaining intact articular surfaces is obtained, splinting is applied as recommended by McElfresh.[63] The results of this treatment are satisfactory. If a satisfactory reduction is not obtained or is lost during treatment (a diagnosis made by follow-up x-rays), bone and ligament reconstruction is indicated. Usually the impacted surface is fragmented, and its excision with volar plate advancement is carried out. Occasionally, a single large fragment is present; in such cases, cartilage congruity is restored by fragment fixation using interosseous wiring or pins. In my experience, the unseen damage to the opposing joint surfaces in this injury precludes a good result with any technique. In such cases, Eaton[61] recommends a trans-articular pin, which is removed at 3 weeks, followed by active flexion with a dorsal blocking splint. If a pull-out wire is used, it should be removed at 4 weeks. After immobilization is discontinued, Eaton recommends a dynamic splint if full extension is not obtained by 5 weeks in a child. Static splints may be used at night to maintain correction obtained by exercises and dynamic splinting. However, in the author's experience, dynamic splinting is not usually necessary since flexion contractures rarely persist for more than 3 to 4 months.

Fractures of the metacarpal and phalangeal condyles are best seen in the original anterioposterior x-ray, but the diagnosis is more difficult to confirm in young children. These injuries are unstable, and if the condyle is depressed or rotated, it cannot be treated by closed reduction. Open reduction and internal fixation with Kirschner wires or interosseous wires are required for proper bone realignment. The internal fixation should remain in place for 3 weeks and rehabilitation, although somewhat prolonged, is usually satisfactory. After removal of the internal fixation device, protective splinting for 2 to 3 weeks is recommended.

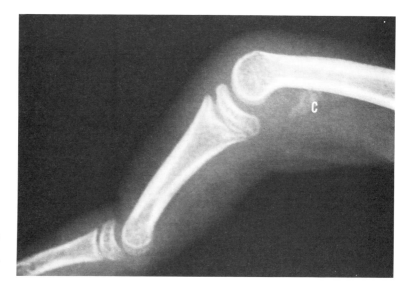

Figure 9–28. Pseudoboutonnière deformity. Note the calcification in the area of the proximal volar plate (C).

DISLOCATION OF THE THUMB, RING, AND LITTLE CARPOMETACARPAL JOINTS

These injuries are rare in children but are usually reducible, and immobilization in a cast for 3 weeks gives a satisfactory result. If the dislocation recurs, reduction and fixation with percutaneous Kirschner wires for 1 month is recommended. In such cases, external splinting is required.

Fracture-dislocations of the thumb and fourth and fifth carpometacarpal joints are injuries that are suspected by clinical examination and confirmed by appropriate x-rays. In the case of the fourth and fifth carpometacarpal joints, a 30 degree supinated oblique view is recommended to confirm the injury. Comminuted fractures may dislocate with external splinting, and in these cases, Kirschner wires and cast immobilization are required.[56] Large fragments in older children and old injuries may require open reduction and compression screw fixation.

References

Fractures

1. Aitken AP. Fractures of the epiphyses. Clin Orthop. 41:19–23, 1965.
2. Aitken, AP. Fractures of the epiphyses of the upper extremity. *In* Flynn JE (ed). Hand Surgery. Baltimore, Williams & Wilkins, 1966:161–183.
3. Barton NJ. Fractures of the phalanges of the hand in children. Hand 11:134–143, 1979.
4. Barton N. Fractures of the phalanges of the hand. Hand 9:1–10, 1979.
5. Blair WF, Marcus NA. Extrusion of the proximal interphalangeal joint: a case report. J Hand Surg 6:146–147, 1981.
6. Bolton H. Fractures of the hand in children. *In* Stack HG, Bolton H (eds). Proceedings of the Second Hand Club. London, British Society for Surgery of the Hand, 1966:388–390.
7. Bora FW Jr, Ignatius P, Nissenbaum M. The treatment of epiphyseal fractures in the hand. J Bone Joint Surg (Am) 58:286, 1976.
8. Bora FW Jr, Nissenbaum M, Ignatius P. The treatment of epiphyseal fractures in the hand. Orthop Digest 4:11–13, 1976.
9. Brown JE. Epiphyseal growth arrest in a fractured metacarpal. J Bone Joint Surg (Am) 41:494–496, 1959.
10. Campbell CJ, Grisolia A, Zanconato G. The effects produced in the cartilaginous epiphyseal plate of immature dogs by experimental traumata. J Bone Joint Surg 41:1221–1242, 1959.
11. Ceilley RI, Sebben JE. Nail deformity with nonunion of distal phalanx. Arch Dermatol 114:1717, 1978.
12. Cowen NJ, Kranik AD. An irreducible juxta-epiphyseal fracture of the proximal phalanx: report of a case. Clin Orthop 110:42–44, 1975.
13. Dixon GL, Moon NF. Rotational supracondylar fractures of the proximal phalanx in children. Clin Orthop 83:151–156, 1972.
14. Dobyns JH, Beckenbaugh RD, Bryan RS, et al. Fractures of the hand and wrist. *In* Flynn JE (ed). Hand Surgery, 3rd ed. Baltimore, Williams & Wilkins, 1982:111–180.
15. Eaton RB, Burton RI. Fractures of the hand. *In* Kilgore ES, Grantham WP (eds). The Hand: Surgical and Non-Surgical Management. Philadelphia, Lea & Febiger, 1977:121–142.
16. Engber WD, Clancy WG. Traumatic avulsion of the fingernail associated with injury to the phalangeal epiphyseal plate. J Bone Joint Surg (Am) 60:713–714, 1978.
17. Frackelton WH. Injuries of the hand. *In* Blount WP (ed). Fractures in Children. Baltimore, Williams & Wilkins, 1955:112–128.
18. Green DP. Hand injuries in children. Pediatr Clin North Am 24:903–918, 1977.
19. Green DP, Andersen JR. Closed reduction and percutaneous pin fixation of fractured phalanges. J Bone Joint Surg (Am) 55:1651–1654, 1973.
20. Green DP, O'Brien ET. Fractures of the thumb metacarpal. South Med J 65:807–814, 1972.
21. Green DP, Rowland SA. Fractures and dislocations in the hand. *In* Rockwood, CA Green, DP (eds). Fractures, Vol I. Philadelphia, JB Lippincott, 1975:265–327.
22. Hager DL. Hand injuries in children. Contemp Orthop 4:631–655, 1982.
23. Hanlon CR, Estes WL Jr. Fractures in childhood: a statistical analysis. Am J Surg 87:312–323, 1954.
24. James JIP. Common simple errors in the management of hand injuries. Proc R Soc Med 63:69–71, 1970.
25. Leonard MH, Breck LW, Ellis OH, et al: Finger fractures in children: 263 consecutive cases. J Bone Joint Surg (Am) 49:1242–1243, 1967.
26. Leonard MH, Dubravik P. Management of fractured fingers in the child. J Bone Joint Surg (Am), 51:812–813, 1969.
27. Leonard MH. Open reduction of fractures of the neck of the proximal phalanx in a child. Clin Orthop 116:176–179, 1976.
28. Michelinakis E, Vourexaki H. Displaced epiphyseal plate of the terminal phalanx in a child. Hand 12:51–53, 1979.
29. Neer CS II, Horwitz BS. Fractures of the proximal humeral epiphyseal plate. Clin Orthop 41:24–31, 1965.
30. Ogden JA. Skeletal Injury in the Child. Philadelphia, Lea & Febiger, 1982.
31. Pratt DR. Exposing fractures of the proximal phalanx of the finger longitudinally through the dorsal extensor apparatus. Clin Orthop 15:22–26, 1959.
32. Pulvertaft R. Injuries of the fingers and metacarpal bones and joints. *In* Pulvertaft RG (ed). Clinical Surgery, Vol 7. Philadelphia, JB Lippincott, 1966.
33. Quigley TB, Banks HH, Leach RE, et al. Advances in the management of fractures and dislocations in the past decade. Orthop Clin North Am 3:793–825, 1972.
34. Rang M. Children's Fractures. Philadelphia, JB Lippincott, 1974.
35. Rank BK, Wakefield AR, Hueston JT. Surgery of Repair as Applied to Hand Injuries, 3rd ed. Baltimore, Williams & Wilkins, 1968:126–154.
36. Reed MH. Fractures and dislocations of the extremities in children. J Trauma 17:351–354, 1977.

37. Rockwood CA, Green DP. Fractures. Philadelphia, JB Lippincott, 1975.
38. Salter RB, Harris WR. Injuries involving the epiphyseal plate. J Bone Joint Surg (Am) 45:587–622, 1963.
39. Samuel AW. Epiphyseal plate injuries in the hand. Injury 12:503–505, 1981.
40. Saypal GH, Slattery LR. Observations on displaced fractures of the hand. Surg Gynecol Obstet 79:522–525, 1944.
41. Schenk R. Basic histomorphology and physiology of skeletal growth. *In* Weber BG, Brunner C, Freuler F (eds). Treatment of Fractures in Children and Adolescents. New York, Springer-Verlag, 1980:3–19.
42. Segmuller G, Schonenberger F. Fractures of the hand. *In* Weber B, Brunner C, Freuler F (eds). Treatment of Fractures in Children and Adolescents. New York, Springer-Verlag, 1980:218–225.
43. Seymour N. Juxta-epiphyseal fracture of the terminal phalanx of the finger. J Bone Joint Surg (Br) 42:347–349, 1966.
44. Sharrard WJW. Orthopaedics and Fractures, Vol II, 2nd ed., Oxford, Blackwell Scientific Publications, 1979:1484–1553,
45. Siffert RS, Gilbert MD, Anatomy and physiology of the growth plate. *In* Rang M (ed). The Growth Plate and Its Disorders. Baltimore, Williams & Wilkins, 1969.
46. Sokolay MP, Berg E. X-ray principals and pitfalls in skeletal trauma. Curr. Concepts Trauma 5:4–8, 1982.
47. Stein F. Skeletal injuries of the hand in children. Clin Plast Surg 8:65–81, 1981.
48. Strickland JW. Bone, nerve and tendon injuries of the hand in children. Pediatr Clin North Am 22:451–462, 1975.
49. Swanson AB. Fractures involving the digits of the hand. Orthop Clin North Am 1:261–274, 1970.
50. Tachdjian MO. Fractures and dislocations. *In* Tachdjian MO (ed). Pediatric Orthopedics, Vol II. Philadelphia, WB Saunders, 1972:1532–1545.
51. Trueta J, Trias A. The vascular contribution to osteogenesis. The effect of pressure upon the epiphyseal cartilage of the rabbit. J Bone Joint Surg (Br) 43:800–813, 1961.
52. Von Raffler W. Irreducible juxta-epiphyseal fracture of a finger. J Bone Joint Surg (Br) 46:229, 1964.
53. Weber BG. Fracture healing in the growing bone and in the mature skeleton. *In* Weber BG, Brunner C, Freuler F (eds). Treatment of Fractures in Children and Adolescents. New York, Springer-Verlag 1980:20–57.
54. Weckesser EC. Rotational osteotomy of the metacarpal for overlapping fingers. J Bone Joint Surg (Am) 47:751–756, 1965.
55. Wood VE. Fractures of the hand in children. Orthop Clin North Am 7:527–542, 1976.

Ligamentous Injuries

56. Bora FW Jr, Didzian NH: The treatment of injuries to the carpometacarpal joint of the little finger. J Bone Joint Surg (Am) 56 (7):1459–1463, 1974.
57. Bowers WH. Capsular injuries of the proximal interphalangeal joint. *In* Cowan NJ (ed). Practical Hand Surgery. Chicago, Year Book Medical Publishers, 1980:305–314.
58. Bowers WH. The proximal interphalangeal joint volar plate. II. A clinical study of hyperextension injury. J Hand Surg 6:77–81, 1981.
59. Bowers WH, Wolf JW Jr, Nehil JL, et al. The proximal interphalangeal joint volar plate. I. An anatomical and biochemical Study. J Hand Surg 5:79–88, 1980.
60. Bowers WH, Hurst LC. Gamekeepers thumb. Evaluation by arthrography and stress roentgenography. J Bone Joint Surg (Am) 59 (4):519–524, 1977.
61. Eaton RG, Mallerich MM. Volar plate arthroplasty for the proximal interphalangeal joint—a ten year review. J Hand Surg 5:260, 1980.
62. McCue FC, Honner R, Gieck JH, et al. A pseudo-boutonniere deformity. Hand 1:166–170, 1975.
63. McElfresh EC, Dobyns JH, O'Brian ET. Management of fracture-dislocation of the proximal interphalangeal joint by extension-block splinting. J Bone Joint Surgery (Am) 54,1705, 1972.
64. Palmer AK, Louis DS. Assessing ulnar instability of the metacarpophalangeal joint of the thumb. J Hand Surg 3 (6):542–546, 1978.
65. Sterner B. Displacement of the ruptured ulnar collateral ligament of the metacarpophalangeal joint of the thumb. J Bone Joint Surg (Br) 44:869–879, 1962.
66. Thompson JS, Eaton RG. Volar dislocation of the proximal interphalangeal joint. J Hand Surg 2:232, 1977.

Injuries to and Developmental Deformities of the Wrist and Carpus

BARRY P. SIMMONS

DEVELOPMENT OF THE WRIST AND CARPUS

The wrist and carpus form embryologically as separate cartilaginous units. Subsequent joint development proceeds from chondrification of the mesoderm, to cavitation, and then to development of a synovial lining.[70] Failure of differentiation of the individual carpal bones or the radiocarpal or radioulnar joints results in congenital fusions.[54] Congenital fusion of all these joints has been reported but is more common across the intercarpal joints than across the other two.[60] Proximal congenital radioulnar synostosis may occur with synostosis of almost the full length of radius and ulna,[69] but isolated distal radioulnar synostosis is extremely rare.[42]

Ossification of the carpus and distal radial and ulnar epiphyses occurs in a predictable pattern.[34] The normal neonate rarely shows ossification of any of these structures; the ossification center appears first in the capitate at 3 months, followed closely by the hamate. Thereafter, there is generally ossification of the triquetrum (2 to 3 years), lunate (3 to 3½ years), trapezium (3½ to 4 years), and trapezoid and scaphoid (4½ to 6 years). The ossific nucleus tends to appear earlier in females than in males. Another difference related to sex is that the scaphoid may appear slightly before the trapezium in males; however, in both sexes the centers of the trapezium, trapezoid, and scaphoid appear within 1 to 3 months of each other. The distal radius ossific nucleus appears at approximately 1 year of age, and the distal ulna appears at 6 years.

Carpal Coalition

As already noted, the carpus is entirely cartilaginous at birth.[14, 58, 59] Failure of differentiation of the individual carpal bones results in congenital fusions, or coalitions. These may occur as part of an isolated event or as part of a syndrome of congenital malformations. Coalitions associated with syndromes tend to involve more than two bones and/or bridge the proximal and distal row.[65] These conditions can also bridge the radiocarpal joint.[11] Syndromes in which carpal fusions are commonly seen include arthrogryposis, diastrophic dwarfism, dyschondrosteosis, Ellis-van Creveld syndrome, hand-foot-uterus syndrome, otopalatodigital syndrome, Holt-Oram syndrome, synphalangism, and Turner's syndrome.[44]

Other carpal anomalies may be seen in some of these syndromes, including extra or absent carpal bones, accessory bones (see further on), irregular carpal margins or carpal slopes, and decreased or increased carpal angles. These latter abnormalities can be seen in other syndromes, including epiphyseal dysplasia, Fanconi's anemia, and homocystinuria.

Isolated coalitions tend to occur in the same row and involve only two bones. Virtually every combination of coalitions has been described.[16, 27, 40, 44, 55, 59, 60] Undoubtedly, the most common is lunate-triquetral coalition, followed by, in order of decreasing frequency, capitate-hamate, pisiform-triquetral, and trapezium-trapezoid coalitions. Other coalitions tend to occur as part of a syndrome rather than as an isolated event.

Lunate-triquetral coalition was first described in a cadaver by Sandifort in 1779,[68] but the first clinical case was reported by Carson in 1908.[17, 18] The incidence in the general population is estimated to be between 0.08% and 0.13%, but can be nearly 100 times higher in blacks (9.5%).[27, 40, 59] Numerous series have documented the relatively high incidence in people of African descent. The ratio of affected females to affected males is as high as 2:1, and there is a strong familial tendency. It is not classically sex-linked but multifactorial in nature. It is often bilateral, especially in blacks; in one study, a 61.5% bilateral incidence in Nigerians was reported.[14, 55]

Lunate-triquetral coalitions are not always radiologically complete. Minaar divides the coalitions into four categories: (1) incomplete fusion resembling a pseudarthrosis, (2) fusion with a notch of varying depth, (3) complete fusion, and (4) complete fusion associated with other anomalies (Fig. 10–1).[55]

Of the other reported carpal coalitions not associated with multiple additional anomalies, capitate-hamate is the next most common.[14] Cockshott also reports a pisiform-triquetral coalition.[14] Both these coalitions occur most frequently in blacks.

Can carpal coalitions be symptomatic? Fractures of carpal coalitions have been reported, but carpal coalitions, unlike tarsal coalitions, are generally considered asymptomatic.[21, 44] This author has seen a single patient with Minaar type I associated with

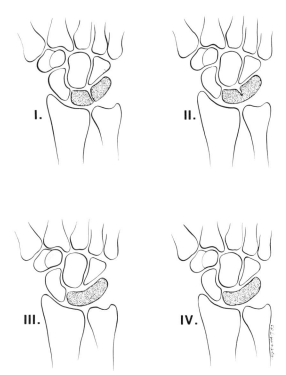

Figure 10–1. Lunate-triquetral coalitions can be classified according to the degree of fusion and the associated anomalies.

pain that did respond to surgical completion of the lunate-triquetral coalition (Figure 10–2). Furthermore, three other cases have been seen in which Minaar type I lunate-triquetral coalition was associated with triquetral-hamate medial column instablility (Fig. 10–3). Completion of the coalition plus triquetral-hamate fusion resulted in a painless wrist.

Bipartite Carpal Bones

Bisection of the carpal bones has been reported in the trapezium, triquetrum, hamate, lunate, and scaphoid.[58, 61] The scaphoid is the most common, however, and the most significant because of its clinical implications.

As the carpus develops, a single ossific nucleus in each carpal bone is usually seen; the most common exception is the scaphoid, which may have separate proximal and distal centers of ossification.[34] Bipartition therefore could occur and in fact has been reported by various authors.[10, 24, 32, 35, 58, 59, 63, 64, 85] Despite this, its existence as an entity is still in doubt. Pfitzner and Gruber's conclusions were based on anatomic dissections done prior to the advent of radiography. Because of the absence of clinical history, their conclusions can be questioned.

The criteria for diagnosis of a bipartite scaphoid cannot clearly be separated from traumatic bipartition (i.e., a fracture). The following factors are considered to be supportive of congenital bipartite scaphoid:[12, 58] (1) absence of history of trauma, (2) the presence of bilateral scaphoid bipartition, (3) equal size and density of both ossicles, (4) absence of degenerative changes in the radioscaphoid articulation, and (5) a clear space between fragments with smooth edges at the joint surfaces. However, all the criteria can be seen in fractures. Louis and associates, reviewing a large series of x-rays and fetal dissections, concluded that bipartite scaphoid is of traumatic, not congenital, origin and should be treated as such.[49] The problem is discussed in greater detail in the section on carpal fractures, further on in this chapter.

Accessoria

As many as 25 accessory bones have been reported to occur about the wrist and carpus.[58, 61] They can be located anywhere in the carpus. Generally, they fuse to their adjacent bones at puberty and are rarely symptomatic. Among the most common accessory carpal bones are the os centrale, os triangulare, and os styloideum.

The os centrale is a dorsal ossicle that forms between the scaphoid, capitate, and trapezoid and usually is seen separate from them only in the embryo. The ossicle fuses with the dorsal, distal, ulnar side of the scaphoid before birth. The os triangulare also is seen only in the embryo, and its location varies somewhat from the ulnar side of the radius, to the ulnar styloid, to the lunate and triquetrum. Most often, it is located close to the ulnar styloid.

The only potentially symptomatic ossicle is the os styloideum. It is located dorsally between the trapezoid, capitate, and second and third metacarpals. It may fuse to the third metacarpal styloid process and become symptomatic because of its prominence. This "carpal boss" is seen more commonly in young women and, if symptomatic, will usually respond to immobilization or anti-inflammatory medications or both. Those that do not may require excision.[19]

ABNORMALITIES OF THE WRIST

Carpal Osteolysis

Carpal osteolysis is an extremely rare syndrome associated with tarsal osteolysis and generally occurs during early childhood.[6]

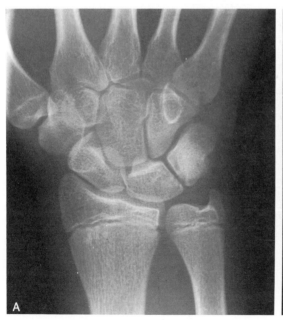 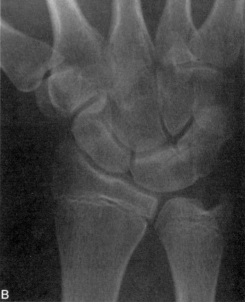

Figure 10–2. *A,* Symptomatic Minaar type 1 carpal coalition. *B,* Surgical fusion of the incomplete coalition.

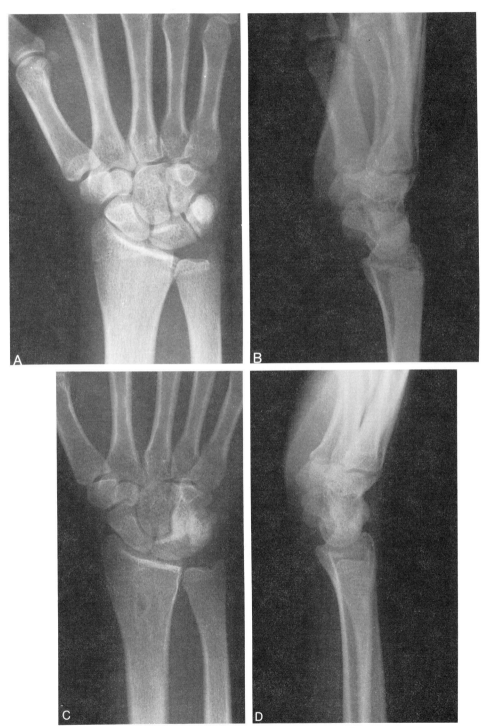

Figure 10–3. *A*, 16-year-old female with Minaar type 1 lunate-triquetral carpal coalition associated with triquetral-hamate (medial column) instability. *B*, Note the palmar flexion of the lunate and scaphoid on the lateral view. *C*, Completion of the coalition and triquetral-hamate fusion produced a painless wrist. *D*, Palmar flexion is corrected on postoperative x-ray.

Since Gorham first described the syndrome of massive osteolysis (disappearing-bone disease) in 1955,[33] there have been multiple case reports of more selective peripheral osteolysis that involves primarily the carpal and tarsal bones.[2, 6, 18, 33, 57] The case reports identify patients presenting from 1 to 12 years of age, with spontaneous onset of painful swelling that usually occurs first in the feet and then in the hands. Laboratory evaluation may show an elevated erythrocyte sedimentation rate, but other tests for juvenile rheumatoid arthritis are negative. Despite this, several patients were given a course of steroids that failed to relieve the symptoms.

Radiologically, there is a spectrum of changes ranging from irregularly shrunken or crenated carpal bones to complete absence of the carpus. The appearance of these is characteristically different from that in rheumatoid arthritis.

Clinically, the course seems to be progressive and unremitting. Often, patients will show evidence of problems of the proximal joints including the forearms, elbows, ankles, and knees. Spine involvement with scoliosis can occur. Furthermore, patients may develop proteinuria as a first sign of nephropathy. Reviewing the literature, Beals[6] identified nine of 14 patients with renal involvement, a few of whom subsequently died of renal failure. There is no definitive treatment for the musculoskeletal problem. The paucity of cases makes classification difficult. Beals has suggested the following:

1. Farber's disease—Onset in infancy, abnormal fibroblast mucopolysaccharide metabolism, progressive bone destruction, and joint contracture diffusely.

2. Carpal and tarsal osteolysis—Onset at 1 to 5 years of age, recessive: (a) increased acid mucopolysaccharides in cell culture and progressive joint destruction, primarily of wrist, feet, and elbows;[88] (b) mucopolysaccharide studies not performed, principally destruction of carpus and tarsus;[80] (c) mucolipidosis III (pseudo-Hurler polydystrophy), progressive destruction of carpus and tarsus, multiple contractures, Hurler-like facies, short stature, normal intelligence and longevity, absent mucopolysaccariduria, and abnormal polysaccharide storage in skin fibroblasts.

3. Carpal and tarsal osteolysis—Onset at 1 to 5 years of age, dominant; mostly affects carpus, tarsus, and elbows; occasionally associated with osteoporosis, abnormally

shaped skull, and minimal reduction of adult height; high percentage of cases involve severe nephropathy.

4. Neurogenic acro-osteolysis—Onset in childhood, mainly phalangeal osteolysis, recessive and dominant, associated with sensory neuropathy.

5. Acro-osteolysis of Joseph: Onset in childhood, autosomal recessive inheritance, only distal phalangeal osteolysis in otherwise normal boys.[41]

6. Acro-osteolysis of Shinz—Onset in second decade, autosomal dominant, phalangeal osteolysis in hands and feet associated with ulcerations without neurologic abnormalities.[45]

7. Arthrodento-osteodysplasia (Hadju-Cheney syndrome)—Onset in second decade, autosomal dominant, osteolysis in distal phalanges, generalized bone dysplasia including multiple fractures, early loss of teeth, hypoplastic mandible, prominent occiput, failure of tubulation of long bones, and generalized osteoporosis.[39]

8. Lipodermatoarthritis—Onset at 30 years of age, inheritance unknown, inflammatory process producing severe joint destruction associated with papular and nodular skin lesions.[5]

9. Massive osteolysis of Gorham—Onset at 20 years of age, inheritance unknown, unifocal lesion of proximal skeleton, painless, due to hemangiomas.[33]

Madelung's Deformity

In 1878, Madelung described a painful deformity of the wrist that usually presents during adolescence.[50] Although this description has been attributed to Madelung, he pointed out that it had previously been described by several other authors, including Dupuytren (1834), Malgaigne (1855), Weber (1859), and Nelaton (1847).[50] Clinically, the most striking feature is prominence of the distal ulna and a foreshortened forearm (Fig. 10–4). Further examination discloses a volar and ulnar tilt to the distal radius and limited supination in the forearm.

Radiological evaluation discloses abnormalities of the radius, ulna, and carpus (Fig. 10–5).[22, 25] Abnormalities in the radius include (1) prolonged curvature, dorsal and ulnar, (2) shortening, (3) triangularization of the distal radial epiphysis, (4) premature fusion of the medial half of the radial epi-

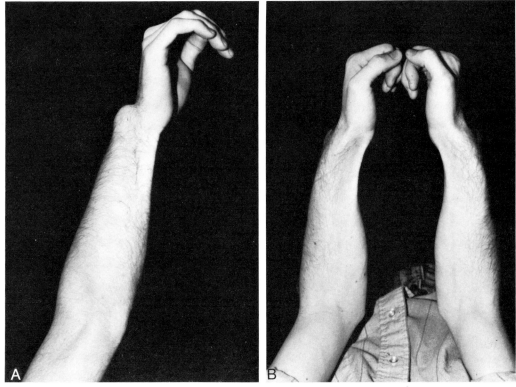

Figure 10–4. *A*, Prominence of the distal ulna is the most apparent deformity in Madelung's deformity. *B*, Bowed, fore-shortened forearms are also present. This also demonstrates the marked limitation of supination.

physis, (5) a localized area of lucency along the ulnar border of the radius, (6) osteophyte formation along the inferior ulnar part of the radius, and (7) ulnar and volar angulation of the distal radial articular surface.

Ulnar abnormalities include (1) dorsal subluxation, (2) enlargement and distortion of the ulnar head, and (3) decreased length. Abnormalities seen in the carpus include (1) wedging of the central portion of the carpus between the deformed radius and protruding ulna, (2) a triangular configuration with the lunate at the apex, and (3) arched curvature in a lateral projection as a direct continuation of the arc of the posterior bowing of the radial epiphysis.

Anton and colleagues[3] reported on the most extensive series, which consisted of 171 cases. Of these, one third were thought to be inherited, and transmission was believed to follow an autosomal dominant pattern. The ratio of affected females to affected males is 4:1, and the deformity is bilateral twice as often as it is unilateral. In six of the 171 cases reported by Anton's group, the radius had a reverse deformity. In these cases, the bowing of the radius was volar and ulnar, and the distal articular surface faced dorsally. The accentuated ulnar inclination persists in a "reverse Madelung's," however. The resultant ulnar protuberance is thus volar rather than dorsal.

The etiology of true Madelung's deformity is unknown except for the inheritance patterns already mentioned. Other disorders may mimic Madelung's but are uncommon. These include trauma, dyschondrosteosis, Turner's syndrome, multiple enchondromatosis, and Morquio's syndrome.[1, 7, 28, 38]

The clinical picture is variable, depending on the severity of the deformity. The initial abnormality may be present as early as 7 or 8 years of age, but it usually does not become apparent until the pubertal growth spurt. That is also the age at which patients are likely to become symptomatic. The major complaint is pain over the distal radioulnar joint, accentuated by supination. Examination discloses the deformity previously described, limitation of supination, accentuation of ulnar deviation, and, on occasion, limitation of dorsiflexion.

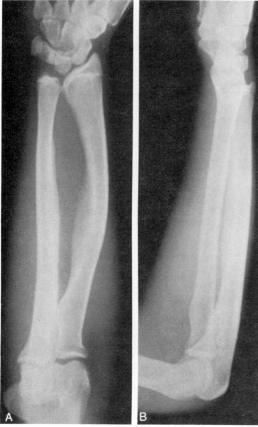

Figure 10–5. *A,* Radiologic evaluation of Madelung's deformity in the AP plane discloses the marked bowing and ulnar tilt of the distal radius and triangulation of the carpus. *B,* On the lateral view, the dorsally displaced ulna is noted.

good maintenance of correction, variable improvement in forearm rotation, elimination of pain, and increase in grip strength. Seven patients with deformity not considered "severe" underwent only excision of the distal ulna. This produced good relief of pain and increased motion, but follow-up x-rays indicated an increasing ulnar translocation of the carpus, suggesting future problems. To avoid this in one patient, this author performed resection of the articulating surface of the ulna. Although initially there was increased supination as well as relief of pain, eventually some of the limitation of motion returned; the patient did remain free of pain, however. Nevertheless this may be the preferred approach because the amount of motion regained after distal ulnar resection is unpredictable and subsequent ulnar translocation of the carpus may occur.

Another alternative is arthrodesis of the distal radioulnar joint with resection of 1 or 2 cm of the ulna proximal to the fusion (Lauenstein's procedure). This obviously must be delayed until the physes have closed. Although not a new procedure, it has not been applied to Madelung's deformity and should be used with caution.

INJURIES OF THE RADIOCARPAL JOINT

Intraarticular fractures of the radiocarpal joint are unusual, especially in the younger age group, because of the cartilaginous makeup of the radial epiphysis and carpus. At the time of puberty, as elsewhere in the skeleton, the physes are more at risk. Intraarticular fractures at the radiocarpal joint are thus usually problems in adults.

Intraarticular fractures, when they occur, need the same meticulous restoration of a joint surface as elsewhere in the skeleton. A review of a large series of children's digital fractures[36] disclosed a significant deterioration in functional results of anatomic reduction if restoration of significant intraarticular fractures was not achieved. Children may remodel fractures, but they do not remodel displaced joint surfaces (Fig. 10–6). The eventual result of allowing a displaced intraarticular fracture to heal is likely to be a painful, arthritic joint requiring arthroplasty or arthrodesis. Open physes is not a contraindication to open reduction if a

Treatment

Treatment of the disorder is indicated only if a patient is having pain.[56] Because many patients become symptomatic during the most progressive stage—at the time of growth spurt—splinting may suffice to tide them over that period. If splinting fails, surgical treatment is undertaken, consisting of resection of the distal ulna (Darrach procedure) with or without a radial osteotomy. Ranawat and associates examined the long-term (average 8 years) follow-up of surgical treatment.[66] Patients were considered to have a severe deformity if the angle between the distal radial articular surface and radial axis was less than 60°, the forearm to third metacarpal angle was more than 15°, and the lunate was more than 50% ulnarly translocated from the lunate facet on the distal radius. These patients (five in all) underwent osteotomy and distal ulnar resection with

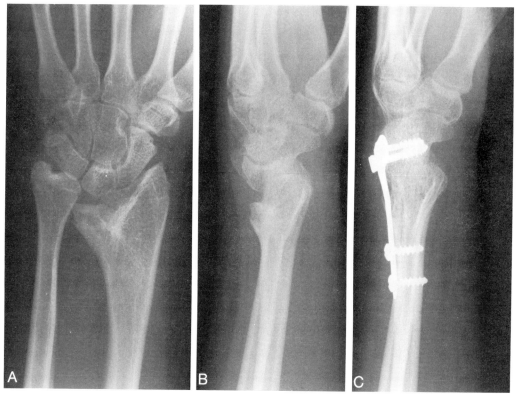

Figure 10–6. This intraarticular fracture occurred at age 8 and was left unreduced (*A* and *B*). Because of increasing pain, the patient required radiocarpal fusion after her physes closed (*C*).

closed reduction fails to give satisfactory alignment of the joint surfaces.

FRACTURES OF THE CARPUS

Although uncommon, fractures of the carpal bones occur far more frequently than those at the radiocarpal joint. Although fractures can involve virtually any carpal bone, the scaphoid is the one most commonly involved in both children and adults.[9, 20, 81] Scaphoid fractures are most common in the 15- to 30-year-old age group, but, in a 14-year period, Vahvanen and Westerlund found 108 scaphoid fractures in the 10- to 14-year-old group.[23, 53] Usually, the mechanism of injury was, as in the adults, a fall on an outstretched hand, and in 4.6% there was another fracture in the same extremity, most commonly in the radius.

Analysis of scaphoid fractures in children discloses a different pattern than that seen in adults. Whereas in adults approximately 70% of these fractures are at the waist in the middle third of the scaphoid, only 12% are at that level in children.[81] The vast majority

of fractures, 87%, occur in the distal third, and of these 44% are avulsion fractures, especially of the tubercle. Only one fracture in Vahvanen's study involved the proximal pole. Most striking, however, is that the fractures in all 108 patients in Vahvanen's series healed, usually in 4 to 8 weeks, with only below-elbow immobilization used.

It should be noted, however, that nonunions of the scaphoid in this age group can occur.[71] All the nonunions were in the middle third fractures, and all healed after a bone graft through a volar approach.

Is the bipartite scaphoid a real entity? As mentioned earlier, it is unlikely.[49] Even if it does exist, the discussion may be academic, in light of more recent understanding of the important role of the scaphoid in the biomechanics of wrist motion. A more appropriate question would be: Does a bipartite scaphoid, whether of congenital or traumatic origin, lead to degenerative arthritis of the wrist? The answer would have to be *yes* in a large percentage of cases. Even Pfitzner, while acknowledging the congenital bipartite scaphoid, mentioned traumatic arthritis in one of his cases.[63] Thus, "bipartite" scaphoids in children should be considered to be of traumatic origin and treated accordingly.

Treatment

Cast Immobilization

Cast immobilization of acute, uncomplicated fractures of the scaphoid should be the first step in all cases, regardless of the fracture's location within the scaphoid. Scaphoid tubercle fractures can be treated in short arm thumb spica casts. In waist or proximal pole fractures, however, despite Vahvanen's findings, a long arm cast is preferable for the first 6 weeks.

In established nonunions that have never been immobilized, cast immobilization is a reasonable first step, as long as there is no carpal collapse (see further on). This may be the place for electrical stimulation. If there is no evidence of healing after 3 months in a cast, or if there is a definite nonunion after 6 months in a cast, the patient should undergo a bone graft. This can be done through a volar (Russe) or dorsal (Matti) approach.[15, 51, 67] Use of an intraosseous compression screw will also lessen the postoperative period of immobilization.[37] Regardless of technique, over 80% of nonunions will heal after a bone graft.

Should asymptomatic nonunions be treated? The vast majority of scaphoid nonunions will develop radiologic evidence of degenerative arthritis of the radioscaphoid and/or scaphocapitate joint in time. Although it cannot be predicted which of these will be symptomatic, a high percentage of them are. Thus, every attempt should be made to correct scaphoid nonunions, especially in children who obviously have a long anticipated life span.

Surgical Technique

The scaphoid can be approached through either a palmar[67] or a dorsal[51] incision with equally good results.[15] The palmar approach is as described by Russe. A 4- to 5-cm incision is planned between the flexor carpi radialis and radial artery from a point over the scaphoid tubercle distally. Bone graft can be obtained from the distal metaphyseal portion of the distal radius, and the incision should be brought proximally enough to allow this exposure. This can be felt as a "down slope" proximal to the wrist joint. It is useful to

mark the incision prior to inflating the tourniquet, as one can then palpate the radial artery and make sure of its location. If there is any question, the dissection can be brought down through the flexor carpi radialis sheath directly. Under tourniquet control, the antebrachial fascia is divided, exposing the wrist joint beneath it. The joint is often more proximal than one anticipates—being at the level of, or slightly proximal to, the proximal wrist crease. Once the joint is identified, the capsule is incised longitudinally in the direction of the incision, and the capsular insertion is elevated sharply, both radial and ulnar, from the radius proximally and scaphoid distally. Incision of the capsule in the longitudinal direction allows it to be repaired subsequently in a snug fashion and avoids the potential problems for carpal instability that could occur if a transverse incision were made through the volar radiocarpal ligaments. If one has trouble identifying the site of nonunion, radial deviation of the wrist will help, as will distal traction on the thumb. If there is still any question, intraoperative x-rays should be obtained so that the location can be confirmed. Once the nonunion is identified, the nonarticular portion of the scaphoid, from where the capsule has been removed, is the ideal site for placement of a corticocancellous or cancellous strut of bone. The nonunion site is entered, and a trough is then fashioned. This can be done with a small curette and/ or rongeur, and all of the bony work should be done with nonpower instruments. Most of the avascular bone should be removed; if the proximal pole is markedly avascular, aggressive removal of this bone is necessary. All of the sclerotic margin of the nonunion should be curetted back to bleeding bone.

Occasionally, the scaphoid appears healed. This may be due to a firm fibrous union. Rather than sacrificing the stability this gives or trying to "confirm" the nonunion with more aggressive dissection (which will create a less stable situation), the surgeon should leave a portion of this fibrous union intact and graft the remainder. Subsequent union, if achieved, will progress along the entire fracture line.

Attention is then turned proximally to obtain the graft. The pronator quadratus can be identified easily on the palmar aspect of the radius at the site of the distal metaphysis. The dissection should be carried sufficiently far radially so that the tendon of the pronator quadratus can be identified. This tendon is then incised along both the radial and the distal edges in an L-shaped fashion. Subperiosteal dissection is then possible. Using small osteotomes, the surgeon can remove the corticocancellous strut of appropriate size. The natural curve of the distal radial metaphysis closely approximates that of the ulnar edge of the scaphoid, allowing for a good fit. Once the corticocancellous strut is removed, multiple curetting of cancellous bone from the distal radius is possible. The pronator quadratus can then be brought back over the window in the distal radius and repaired with a resorbable suture. This helps with hemostasis.

Attention is then turned back to the scaphoid, and the depth of the scaphoid is packed liberally with cancellous bone. The corticocancellous or cancellous strut can be placed in the previously fashioned trough. This should give stability. If it does not, one or two parallel 0.035- or 0.045-inch wires can be placed to hold the alignment.

One of the advantages of the palmar approach is that in long-standing nonunions, there may be loss of bone along the volar aspect with collapse through the scaphoid and, obviously, collapse through the rest of the carpus as well. This can be corrected through the palmar approach. One should carefully analyze the patient's x-rays preoperatively; if there is evidence of carpal collapse, the volar approach is preferable to the dorsal.

Once the graft is in place, the capsule can be closed with a nonabsorbable suture, and the tourniquet can be released. After irrigation and hemostasis, the skin edges can be closed. The immediate postoperative dressing is a radial gutter splint, which is removed after 7 to 10 days and replaced with a long arm thumb spica cast. The cast is removed at 6 weeks, and, after new x-rays are obtained, a short arm thumb spica cast is applied until union is complete. Wires, if used, should be removed at 6 weeks, regardless of the appearance of the fracture. They may serve to distract the fracture fragments and actually delay healing rather than enhancing it.

If the dorsal approach is preferred, one can go between the first and second dorsal compartments in a dorsoradial approach or through the second compartment. The latter approach is somewhat easier in that it decreases the threat to the superficial radial nerve and the dorsal branch of the radial ar-

tery and allows access to the second dorsal compartment, where excellent bone graft can be obtained. With this approach, a 4- to 5-cm incision is planned over the second dorsal compartment. The dorsal retinaculum is incised, and the wrist joint can be entered. Again, the graft should be placed on the nonarticular surface of the scaphoid. Bone graft can be obtained from the second dorsal compartment, as mentioned. The remainder of the technique and postoperative care are as mentioned previously.

LIGAMENTOUS INJURIES OF THE WRIST AND CARPUS

Significant ligamentous injuries of the wrist occur far less commonly in children than in adults. Injuries to the wrist are usually bony and proximal to the carpus. This is especially true in younger children; significant ligamentous injury is rare before adolescence. As children enter adolescence, their injuries more closely resemble those of adults. At this stage, with an ossified carpus but open distal radius and ulna physes, ligamentous injuries start to occur more commonly and are the same as those in adults.

Although rotary subluxation of the scaphoid has been recognized for a long time, the more recent work of Taleisnik, Linscheid, and Dobyns has clarified the ligamentous anatomy and mechanics of the carpus.[48, 76–78]

LIGAMENTOUS ANATOMY OF THE WRIST

Normal mechanics of the carpal motion depend on an intact ligamentous apparatus (Fig. 10–7). Taleisnik has helped devise a classification of wrist joint ligaments that clarifies the most important structures.[77] The extrinsic ligaments are best divided into proximal, or radiocarpal, and distal, or carpometacarpal ligaments (Table 10–1).

For analysis of wrist instability, the proximal extrinsic ligaments are the important ones. They can be subdivided into superficial and deep ligaments. The superficial fibers of the extrinsic ligaments, when visualized from the palmar surface of the wrist joint, appear to be somewhat random; however, generally they assume a V-shaped pat-

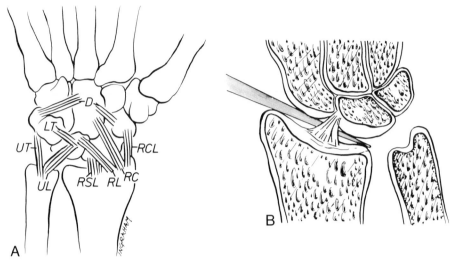

Figure 10–7. *A,* The schema of the palmar aspect of the right wrist identifies the important ligaments. The extrinsic, deep, proximal, radiocarpal complex of the radiocapite (RC), radiolunate (RL), and radioscapholunate (RSL) prevents scapholunate dissociation. RCL = radial collateral ligament; UL = ulnolunate ligament; UT = ulnotriquetral ligament; LT = lunate-triquetral ligament; D = deltoid or volar intercarpal ligament. *B,* The radioscapholunate ligament can be seen to be intrarticular, and by blending with the dorsal intermediate intrinsic interosseous scapholunate ligament, this articulation is partially surrounded (180°) by a strong ligamentous complex.

tern with the apex at the capitate and lunate and the two arms spreading laterally to the radius and ulna.[43]

The deep, proximal, extrinsic radiocarpal ligaments consist of the radiocapite (RC), radiolunate (RL), and radioscapholunate (RSL) ligaments. Fibers of the RSL course from the volar portion of the radius distally and dorsally to insert on the adjacent artic-

Table 10–1. **Wrist (Carpus) Ligaments**

I. Extrinsic
  A. Proximal
    1. Superficial
    2. Deep
      a. Volar radiocarpal
        (1) Radiocapite
        (2) Radiolunate
        (3) Radioscapholunate
      b. Triangular fibrocartilage complex
        (1) Radioulnar
        (2) Articular disk
        (3) Meniscal hemologue
        (4) Ulnar collateral
        (5) Extensor carpi ulnaris sheath
      c. Radial collateral
      d. Dorsal radiocarpal
  B. Distal
II. Intrinsic
  A. Short
  B. Intermediate
    1. Scaphotrapezium
    2. Scapholunate
    3. Lunate-triquetral
  C. Long
    1. Volar intercarpal
    2. Dorsal intercarpal

ular surfaces of the scaphoid and lunate, where they join the fibers of the dorsal intermediate intrinsic interosseous ligament (see further on). Thus, the scapholunate articulation is encompassed circumferentially by a ligamentous network; rupture of some or all of these fibers results in partial or complete diastasis of these two carpal bones.

Further ulnar is the origin of the ulnocarpal complex, or triangular fibrocartilage mplex (TFCC), as defined by Palmer.[62] The TFCC consists of the radioulnar ligament, articular disk, meniscal homologue, ulnar collateral ligament, and sheath of the extensor carpi ulnaris (Fig. 10–8).

The radioulnar ligament (RUL) of the TFCC consists of two thick bundles, one dorsal and the other volar, which diverge from the ulnar edge of the radius adjacent to the lunate fossa to insert on the caput ulnae and ulnar styloid; between these bundles, which form a triangular pattern, sits the articular disk. On the ulnar edge sits the somewhat thin ulnar collateral ligament and more substantial meniscal homologue, which are joined by fibers from the RUL and originate on the ulnar styloid and caput ulnae to insert in the triquetrum, hamate, and base of the fifth metacarpal. The sheath of the extensor carpi ulnaris is dorsal and, with the remainder of the TFCC, constitutes the ligamentous support for the distal radioulnar joint. Thus, one sees that the ulnocarpal articulation seen in lower primates has been replaced by a lig-

Figure 10–8. The triangular fibrocartilage complex including the sheath of the extensor carpi ulnaris provides ligamentous support for the distal radioulnar joint.

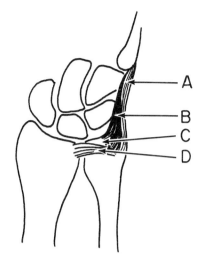

A Ulnar collateral ligament
B Meniscal homologue
C Articular Disc
D Radioulnar ligaments

} Triangular Fibrocartilage Complex

amentous sling that rests on the ulna and supports the ulnar side of the carpus.[43]

The remaining deep extrinsic radiocarpal ligaments consist of the laterally placed radial collateral ligament, running from the radius to the tubercle of the scaphoid, and the dorsal radiocarpal ligament (Fig. 10–9). This latter structure courses from the radius to the dorsum of the proximal carpus and is relatively weak when compared with the stout volar structures.

Less important are the intrinsic ligaments running between the carpal bones. The volar ligaments are thicker and stronger than the

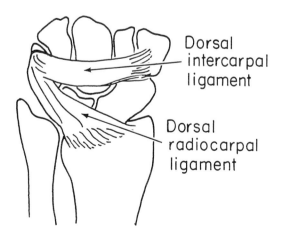

Dorsal intercarpal ligament

Dorsal radiocarpal ligament

Figure 10–9. Diagram depicting dorsal carpal ligaments, which include the extrinsic dorsal radiocarpal ligament and the intrinsic dorsal intercarpal ligament.

dorsal. Taleisnik separates these into short, intermediate, and long. The short intrinsic ligaments are stout and traverse the distal carpal row, binding these four bones into a single functional unit. The three intermediate intrinsic ligaments are the scaphotrapezium, scapholunate, and lunate-triquetrum. The scaphotrapezium allows a considerable amount of motion as the scaphoid flexes and rotates during flexion/extension and radial/ulnar deviation. The scapholunate, as mentioned, has volar and dorsal portions that, in conjunction with the radioscapholunate ligament, surround this articulation. There is room for motion, however, as the scaphoid normally rotates about 30° more than the lunate, especially with wrist flexion and radial deviation. The lunate-triquetral ligament is a stouter volar structure that binds the lunate and triquetrum tightly.

The two long, intrinsic ligaments are divided into volar and dorsal, and, as in most of the other ligamentous structures, the volar is strongest and most important. It stabilizes the capitate, from which it originates, with two arms coursing proximally in a V-shaped pattern to the scaphoid laterally and to the triquetrum medially (Fig. 10–7). This does leave a potential hiatus of weakness over the lunate, through which it can dislocate (space of Poirier). The dorsal ligament is thinner and runs from the triquetrum to the scaphoid and trapezium (Fig. 10–9).

MECHANICS OF WRIST MOTION

The carpus is a complex mechanical structure allowing motion in multiple planes. The distal carpal row, because of its tight ligaments, follows the metacarpals, with which it articulates. Thus, all the motion comes in the radiocarpal joint and the intercarpal joints both between the proximal and distal carpal row and between the bones within the proximal carpal row themselves. Furthermore, because the carpus has no direct tendinous attachments, it is an intercalated ligament (i.e., a segment whose position depends on forces acting distal to it). Thus, the position of the carpals depends on how their ligamentous attachments and geometric configurations allow them to respond to these distal-to-proximal forces. As Fisk noted in his Hunterian Lecture in 1968, there is a resultant "concertina effect," with the tendency towards collapse into a zigzag pattern being countered by the integrity of the ligaments and the scaphoid.[26]

To clarify the mechanics of wrist motion, Taleisnik has conveniently adapted the so-called columnar concept of wrist motion first proposed by Navarro.[76, 77] Taleisnik's modifications divide the carpus into three vertical columns: (1) the central column (entire distal carpal row plus lunate), (2) the lateral column (scaphoid), and (3) the medial column (triquetrum). The pisiform does not participate in these movements and is excluded. Thus, the scaphoid, lunate and capitate unit, and triquetrum are the keys to carpal mechanics; not coincidentally, they are the site of the concentration of ligamentous structures previously noted.

The central column, or flexion-extension column, is the major weight-bearing column of the wrist. As forces are transmitted down the capitate, the lunate, because of its shape and ligaments, responds in a reciprocal manner. The connecting rod, or linkage bar, in this link is the scaphoid or lateral column. Navarro also called this the mobile column.

Another approach to understanding this complex link is to observe the movements of the normal carpus in radial and ulnar deviation. In either motion, the respective lateral or medial column has to "get out of the way" as the height of the carpus lessens (i.e., descent of the carpus). In radial deviation, the scaphoid diminishes by rotating and flexing, and the lunate, because of its tight ligamentous attachments, follows. Thus, a lateral x-ray of the wrist in radial deviation shows a palmar flexed scaphoid and palmar flexed lunate (Fig. 10–10). There is room for some motion between the scaphoid and the lunate, and the lunate flexes only approximately half the distance of the scaphoid.

This finding can also be noted on an anteroposterior x-ray (Fig. 10–10). In a normal wrist in neutral, the lunate is not tipped and the scaphoid is midway between its flexed and extended position. On a radial deviation view, because the scaphoid has to flex and rotate to allow the carpus to descend and the lunate follows the scaphoid, the scaphoid is foreshortened with a cortical circle sign and the lunate can be noted to be tipped. On a maximum ulnar deviation view, the scaphoid dorsiflexes as it is pulled out to its maximum length so that the cortical circle sign disappears. Again, the lunate is noted to be tipped, although a lateral view is required to show that it is dorsiflexed, not palmar flexed as in radial deviation.

Navarro also called the triquetrum, or medial column, the rotational column. This column is more fixed as the central column rotates on it. This is due to the helicoid nature of the triquetral-hamate articulation. In a normal wrist, on ulnar deviation the medial column "diminishes" by a rotational or "screw home" effect on the central column. Thus, a lateral x-ray in maximum ulnar deviation shows dorsiflexion of the triquetrum and similarly, now released by the scaphoid, dorsiflexion of the lunate (Fig. 10–10). Thus, it is clear that the lunate's position depends on the ligamentous integrity to its adjacent proximal carpal bones.

WRIST INSTABILITY AND CARPAL BONE INJURIES

Although the concept of wrist instability was first mentioned in the literature by Gilford in 1943,[31] the classification of patterns of instability was proposed by Linscheid and Dobyns in 1972.[48] By analysis of clinical cases and cadaver dissections, they proposed the widely used classification of dorsal intercalated segmental instability (DISI) patterns and volar intercalated segmental instability (VISI) patterns (the latter also known as palmar intercalated segmental instability [PISI]). The key in this classification is the lunate. If, on a true lateral x-ray with the wrist in neutral flexion/extension and radial/ulnar deviation, the distal articulating surface of the lunate faces dorsally, there is a

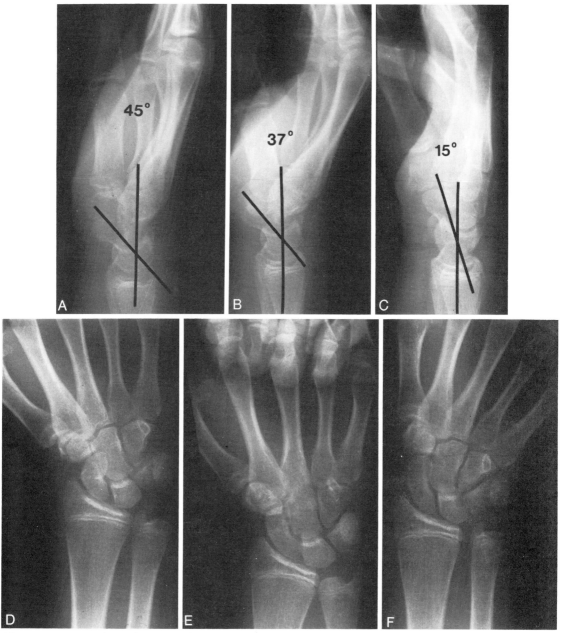

Figure 10–10. Normal carpal motion is demonstrated on these lateral x-rays in radial deviation (A), neutral (B), and ulnar deviation (C). The angle described is between the radius and the scaphoid. On radial deviation the scaphoid must flex to allow descent of the carpus, and the lunate follows, to a lesser degree. On ulnar deviation the scaphoid extends to full length, and the triquetrum dorsiflexes to allow descent of the ulnar aspect of the carpus. In this case, the lunate follows the triquetrum into dorsiflexion. Disruption of the radiocarpal ligaments (scapholunate dissociation) leaves the scaphoid palmar-flexed and the lunate-triquetrum dorsiflexed in maximum ulnar deviation (dorsal intercalated segmental instability [DISI] pattern). However, lunate-triquetral dissociation leaves the lunate "free" to follow the scaphoid, producing a palmar (or volar) intercalated segmental instability (PISI) pattern. An anteroposterior (AP) x-ray demonstrates the same findings as does the lateral view. On radial deviation (D), the scaphoid is flexed or foreshortened, also producing a cortical circle sign. The lunate follows into flexion acquiring a slightly triangular shape. The triquetrum also follows, so that it rides "high" on the hamate. In addition, there is a smooth arc in the intercarpal joints or "Shenton's line" of the wrist. On a compression view in neutral (E), the lunate is more trapezoid, and the scapholunate gap is still less than 2 mm (negative "Terry Thomas" sign). On ulnar deviation (F), the scaphoid extends to length with disappearance of the cortical circle sign; the scapholunate gap is less than 2 mm (negative "Terry Thomas" sign); the triquetrum rides "low" on the hamate; and the lunate again appears slightly triangular, this time because it follows the triquetrum into dorsiflexion. Again, there is a smooth "Shenton's line" of the wrist.

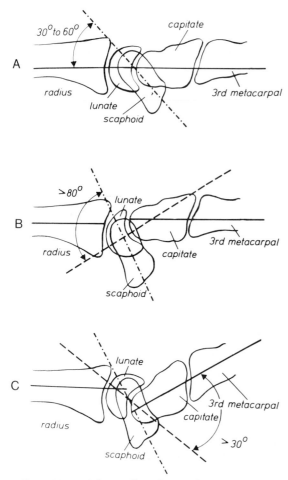

Figure 10–11. Schema of lateral x-rays demonstrate the normal 30° to 60° scapholunate angle (*A*) and an intact radiolunate-capitate colinear line. *B*, Scapholunate disruption results in scaphoid palmar flexion and lunate dorsiflexion, producing a scapholunate angle greater than 80° and disruption of the colinear line, a dorsal intercalated segmental instability (DISI) pattern, because the lunate faces dorsally. *C*, Other forms of instability (proximal carpal row, lunate-triquetral, and triquetral-hamate may allow the lunate and scaphoid to palmar flex together, producing a palmar intercalated segmental instability pattern (PISI). Note the abnormal angle between the lunate and the capitate as well.

DISI pattern; if the lunate faces volarly, there is a VISI pattern (Fig. 10–11). Other roentgenographic abnormalities can exist that will be mentioned subsequently.

Utilization of the columnar concept helps clarify wrist instability; these classifications will be used here in conjunction with DISI and PISI patterns when applicable.

Lateral column instability can occur at three articulations; the scaphotrapeziotrapezoid (STT), the scaphocapitate, and the scapholunate. The first two are extremely rare, but, interestingly, the only acute STT dissociations mentioned in the literature and

seen in this author's personal experience were in children.[75] Both were the result of thumb abduction injuries and responded to reduction and immobilization. Scaphocapitate dissociation has not, to this point, been reported in children.

Scapholunate dissociation, or rotary subluxation of the scaphoid, is the most common dissociation in the carpus. Although the mechanism of injury is often difficult to determine, most injuries to the wrist occur in dorsiflexion. There usually is a rotary component as well. Mayfield and associates have demonstrated that loading of a cadaveric wrist in dorsiflexion, ulnar deviation, and intercarpal supination puts the greatest stress on the volar, extrinsic radiocarpal ligaments.[52] As these sequentially rupture, four stages of progressive perilunar instability occur. Stages 1 and 2 signify initial and then greater tears of the scapholunate ligaments, resulting in scapholunate dissociation. Additional force tears the lunate-triquetral ligamentous supports, resulting in perilunate dislocations (stage 3), and then the dorsal ligament as well, resulting in lunate dislocations (stage 4). It is interesting to recall that the helicoid nature of the distal articulating surface of the triquetrum provides for supination normally during ulnar deviation and that injury occurs when there is a force exerted that ruptures the ligamentous apparatus.

Thus, scapholunate dissociation results in a scaphoid that is independent of the adjacent carpus. In this situation, the scaphoid palmar flexes, but the lunate, which remains attached to the triquetrum, dorsiflexes. Thus, on a true lateral x-ray, the scaphoid is excessively flexed, but the lunate is now dorsiflexed rather than neutral (Fig. 10–11). In a normal wrist, the scapholunate angle is 30° to 60°; in scapholunate dissociation, it is greater than 80°. Furthermore, because the intercalated segment (i.e., proximal carpal row) has dorsiflexed, the distal carpal row must flex, creating a zigzag deformity. This disrupts the colinear line of the radius and capitate. This is a DISI pattern of instability. One may be able to elucidate the abnormal findings with lateral x-rays in maximum ulnar and radial deviation.

On an anteroposterior view, the carpus may look normal. However, instability can be accentuated by stress views: AP in maximum radial deviation, maximum ulnar deviation, and neutral with the patient making a tight fist (compression view) (Fig. 10–12).

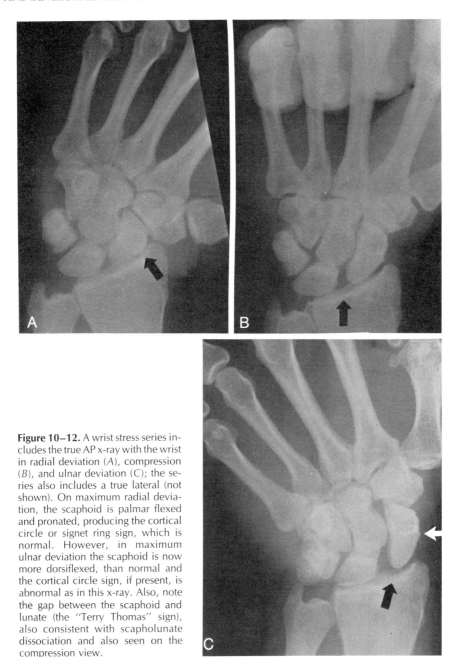

Figure 10–12. A wrist stress series includes the true AP x-ray with the wrist in radial deviation (*A*), compression (*B*), and ulnar deviation (*C*); the series also includes a true lateral (not shown). On maximum radial deviation, the scaphoid is palmar flexed and pronated, producing the cortical circle or signet ring sign, which is normal. However, in maximum ulnar deviation the scaphoid is now more dorsiflexed, than normal and the cortical circle sign, if present, is abnormal as in this x-ray. Also, note the gap between the scaphoid and lunate (the "Terry Thomas" sign), also consistent with scapholunate dissociation and also seen on the compression view.

In radial deviation, one expects to see the scaphoid foreshortened with a positive cortical circle sign because that is the normal mechanical position.[86, 87] However, when the wrist comes over into ulnar deviation, the scaphoid does not follow because of disruption of the scapholunate ligament complex (Fig. 10–12). As a result, the scaphoid remains foreshortened with a positive cortical circle sign, and there is a gap between the scaphoid and the lunate, informally referred to as the "Terry Thomas" sign. In this case, the lunate follows the triquetrum. On a comparison view, the capitate can be seen descending between the scaphoid and the lunate as the ligamentous tear allows these two carpal bones to spread. Also, this capitate descent disrupts Shenton's line of the wrist, which is a smooth arc that one normally sees between the two carpal rows.

There may be a normal stress series, and the patient still has lateral column instability in the scapholunate area. This is the hall-mark of dynamic instability and distinguishes this pattern from static instability. Like patients with static instability, patients with dynamic instability present either with or without a history of trauma, complaining of intermittent episodes of pain that is poorly localized in the wrist but generally experienced in the dorsoradial area. They will mention that the wrist "catches" as the scaphoid obviously snaps from subluxation to a reduced position. This is painful. If radioscaphoid arthritis has already developed, a highly unusual situation in children, this pain may be more persistent. In these cases, there may be synovitis, significant limitation of motion, and decreased grip strength. However, in many cases, if the scaphoid is reduced, there will be a normal range of motion and grip strength.

In dynamic cases, one will see the positive findings of DISI pattern only if the patient can hold the scaphoid in the subluxed position. Often, this is best ascertained on physical examination. While palpating the tubercle of the scaphoid on the palmar side of the wrist, one can feel it make its normal smooth transition from flexion, when the wrist is in radial deviation, to extension, when the wrist is in ulnar deviation. If this is disrupted or the scaphoid can be made to "click," the physician should be highly suspicious of a dynamic instability pattern. A wrist arthrogram may help in that situation. Dye introduced into the radioscaphoid joint should traverse the radiocarpal joint and fill the bursa at the distal end of the ulnar side of the medial aspect of the wrist. However, there should be no communication between the radiocarpal and the intercarpal joint. If the dye now is noted to flow down the radioscaphoid joint and up between the scaphoid and the lunate to surround the scaphoid, the existence of a scapholunate dissociation is certain. The physician should perform the arthrogram and watch the dye flow. Obviously, dynamic instability is stage 2 ligamentous injury as classified by Mayfield.[52]

Medial column instability is far less common than lateral column instability, especially in the pediatric age group. Again, as the carpus matures, carpal instability can occur in the face of an open distal radial epiphysis. These are "adult" injuries. Medial column instability has not been selectively reported in the literature in the adolescent age group. This author has seen one case that, interestingly, occurred in association with a Minaar type I carpal coalition, which has already been mentioned (see Fig. 10–3). Medial column instability is far more commonly a dynamic instability pattern than a static one. The x-ray may appear normal except for the type I Minaar carpal coalition. Patients may complain of a "click" that may be reproduced by attempting pronation and supination through the carpus with the wrist over in maximum ulnar deviation while axial compression forces are being applied.[47]

The other types of carpal instability are even rarer, and, except for ulnar translocation occurring in patients with juvenile rheumatoid arthritis, there are no reports of such instability in the literature.

Can carpal instability occur in the true pediatric group—that is, patients with an immature carpus? There is a report of one case in the literature, and this author also has seen a single patient with the same problem.[30] Interestingly, both patients showed the same picture of precocious ossification of the carpus with narrowing of the joint spaces in the intercarpal and radiocarpal areas (Fig. 10–12).

Treatment of Carpal Instability

Acute carpal instability is usually recognized only when it involves the scapholunate area, resulting in acute scapholunate dissociation. Aggressive treatment is required in these cases. Reduction can be attempted with longitudinal traction and, it is hoped, held with a long arm cast that also immobilizes the index and middle metacarpophalangeal joints and the thumb with the forearm in pronation. Frequent x-rays are necessary to ensure that the reduction is held. It is probably best to reduce the disruption under adequate anesthesia and then hold it with percutaneous K-wires across the carpus. If a reduction cannot be achieved with longitudinal traction, the patient should undergo an operative repair of the volar radiocarpal extrinsic ligaments and the dorsal interosseous ligament through a combined volar approach through the carpal canal and dorsal approach through the fourth dorsal compartment. Although in adults one can consider using wires across the radiocarpal joint to hold the reduction, this technique should be avoided in children because of their open physes. Every attempt should be made to hold the reduction with wires only in the carpus. These should remain in place for 8 weeks, and the initial rehabilitation should proceed slowly. Patients should be aware that some stiffness may result.

Chronic instability presents a greater problem. In lateral column instability at the scapholunate joint in the adolescent age group, intercarpal fusion is preferred. Ligamentous reconstruction has been unsatisfactory when approached from the dorsum.[48] There has been some greater success with a volar approach, but intercarpal fusion gives a more predictable result.[78] Theoretically, this could be accomplished between any bone adjacent to the scaphoid, but the largest series with the longest follow-up involves fusion of the scaphotrapeziotrapezoid joint.[83, 84] This approach has the additional advantage of allowing the most motion in comparison to fusion at the other two sites. Another reason to avoid ligamentous reconstruction in the adolescent age group is the persistence of an open distal radial epiphysis.

Treatment of lateral column instability at the scapholunate area that involves the patient with an immature carpus is extremely rare and represents a much greater problem. The case cited earlier involved a 3-year-old girl who underwent open reduction and internal fixation for her acute injury but still developed a painful, stiff wrist (Fig. 10–13). If this instability is recognized acutely, it needs to be treated vigorously, as mentioned previously. However, despite this management, the patient may reacquire the instability, as in the one case known to this author. In the other case cited, the patient presented with chronic instability at age 7 years. Although ligamentous reconstruction did eliminate her pain, it left her with a total range of motion of 40°.[30] Furthermore, the extremity was somewhat atrophic, and the x-rays disclosed joint space narrowing and precocious ossification suggestive of juvenile rheumatoid arthritis (which was ruled out). At present, there appears to be no good surgical solution for the chronic cases.

As for medial column instability, this has

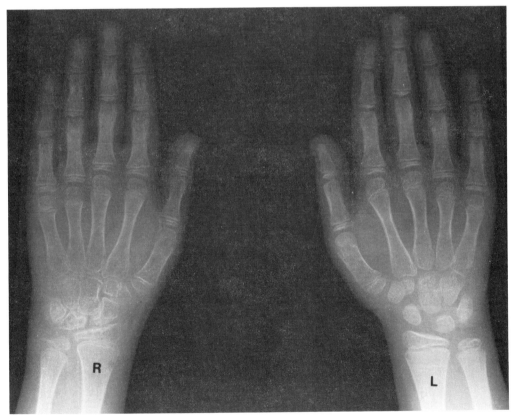

Figure 10–13. This 5-year-old female sustained a ligamentous injury to her right wrist 2 years earlier. Despite open reduction and K-wire fixation, she developed a stiff, painful wrist. X-rays show the diffuse degenerative arthritis as well as precocious ossification.

been recognized only in the adolescent age group and not in younger children. In the single patient mentioned, completion of the lunate-triquetral coalition plus hamate-triquetral fusion resulted in relief of symptoms (see Fig. 10–3).

Surgical Technique

The surgical approach to intercarpal fusion obviously depends on the bones to be fused; it also depends on the necessity for visualization of the radiocarpal joint itself. If scaphotrapeziotrapezoid fusion is planned and there is no degenerative arthritis in the radioscaphoid joint, a transverse incision is preferable.[84] This is virtually always the case in children. By palpation, one can identify the area of the scaphotrapeziotrapezoid joint on the dorsoradial aspect of the hand. The common tendency is to place the incision too far ulnar. Once the area is identified, a 3- to 4 cm transverse incision is made. Several small filaments of the superficial radial nerve will often be encountered subcutaneously and can be preserved. Postoperative dysesthesias have not been a problem. The extensor pollicis longus is mobilized and can be retracted either radially or ulnarward, whichever is easiest. This brings one directly over the joint, which is incised transversely. The scaphoid has an extremely broad surface, and it should be fully identified. The articular surface and a very small portion of subchondral bone can then be removed with the use of a curette, rongeur, or power burr. This should be done on the scaphoid, trapezium and trapezoid, not only at the junction of the last two with the scaphoid but also with each other.

Bone graft can then be obtained from the second dorsal compartment. If a longitudinal incision has been used, this should be placed over the second dorsal compartment. If a transverse incision is used distally, a separate transverse incision can be made over the second dorsal compartment proximally. A 2- to 3-cm incision is used, and the dorsal retinaculum incised, longitudinally rather than transversely because the wrist extensors can be mobilized more easily in this fashion. The flat surface of the distal radius is identified, and the periosteum is elevated. A rectangular portion of corticocancellous bone can be removed to be placed over the anticipated graft area. Multiple curettings of cancellous bone are then available. Care must be

taken to avoid the physis. The physis is easily identified by two factors: (1) an abundance of small epiphyseal vessels, and (2) a change in the periosteum to perichondrium, as the latter is considerably more difficult to elevate. The tendons are then allowed to lie back in their bed in the second dorsal compartment, and the dorsal retinaculum is closed with a resorbable suture.

An alternative method to entering the second dorsal compartment is to gain access to the distal radius entirely subperiosteally. This can be done by incising the periosteum longitudinally directly over Lister's tubercle between the second and third dorsal compartments. A subperiosteal dissection radially brings one beneath the second dorsal compartment. This has the advantage of decreasing postoperative discomfort somewhat. If more than three intercarpal joints are to be fused, it is best to obtain graft from the iliac crest.

Once the graft has been obtained, placement of double-pointed 0.045- or 0.054-inch wires is undertaken. One wire is individually placed retrograde in the trapezium and then in the trapezoid for subsequent insertion into the scaphoid. However, these should not be driven antegrade until cancellous bone graft is placed deep in the fusion site. After accomplishing this, one can drill the wires across the fusion site, thus providing the necessary stability. More bone graft can then be packed around the area. Another wire is also passed from the trapezium across into the trapezoid. The wires are left buried just beneath the skin.

The surgeon should note that the removal of the normal articular surfaces and the subchondral bone will leave a gap. This gap should not be compressed in an attempt to obtain bony apposition between the carpal bones themselves, but should be filled with cancellous bone. Attempted bony apposition by compression may ultimately produce malalignment.

If the patient has dynamic instability, alignment of the scaphoid should be easy to accomplish. However, if there is static instability, the scaphoid will have to be reduced. One should take care to avoid dramatic dorsiflexion of the scaphoid because this may produce problems with the radiocarpal joint.

The capsule can then be closed with a resorbable suture, and the skin with nylon. A long arm splint incorporating the thumb is initially applied; in 7 to 10 days this is removed and a long arm thumb spica cast applied. Some authors do suggest incorporating the index and the middle fingers, but if the wires are firmly placed, this may not be necessary. The cast is removed at 6 weeks, and x-rays are obtained. Often, plaster immobilization is necessary for another 4 to 6 weeks; this can be accomplished with a short arm cast.

If patients have medial column instability, the fusion will be between the triquetral-lunate or triquetral-lunate-hamate-capitate joints. These joints can also be approached by a transverse incision if the diagnosis is clear and no inspection of the radiocarpal joint is necessary. Otherwise, they should be approached through an incision through the fourth dorsal compartment. The mechanics of the fusion are as noted for a scaphotrapeziotrapezoid fusion.

PERILUNATE AND LUNATE DISLOCATION

Perilunate and lunate dislocations are the end stage of disruption of the volar radiocarpal ligamentous complex. As noted by Mayfield, a dorsiflexion and ulnar deviation force combined with intercarpal supination result in tearing of the volar radiocarpal ligaments.[52] Initially, one produces two stages of scapholunate dissociation. As all of the ligaments tear on the palmar side, the carpus is allowed to sublux dorsally, producing a perilunate dislocation (Fig. 10–14). In the final, stage 4, there is also disruption of the remaining dorsal ligaments, resulting in a palmar lunate dislocation.

Treatment

Treatment of perilunate and lunate dislocations demands attention to the points previously made in discussing wrist instability because these are the logical extension of that injury. Longitudinal traction often reduces the perilunate dislocation. In the lunate dislocation, one may need palmar flexion with direct pressure on the lunate to produce a reduction. Should closed traction fail to result in reduction, then open reduction is necessary and in these cases the force is so great that it is best to combine the palmar and dorsal approach so that after the reduction is achieved the ligamentous injury can be repaired in hopes of preventing subsequent carpal instability.

If reduction is achieved closed, one has to be critical of post-reduction views, not only as to whether the dislocated carpus is reduced, but also as to whether there is any

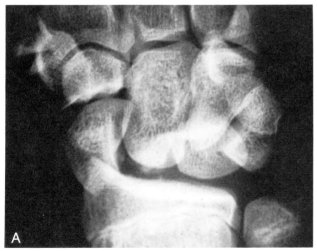
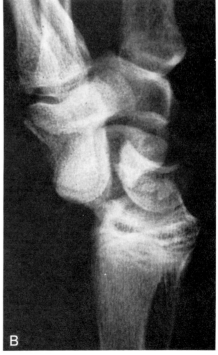

Figure 10–14. Perilunate dislocation as a result of a fall on an outstretched hand. *A*, Note the triangular appearance of the triquetrum on the AP view. *B*, Lateral views show the carpus dorsal to a palmar flexed lunate.

subsequent instability pattern. If such is noted, one needs multiple K-wires to hold a satisfactory reduction, and if this cannot be achieved closed, then again open reduction is indicated. The wrist should be held immobilized for 8 weeks after the reduction.

As in lateral column carpal instability, lunate and perilunate dislocations can occur in the adolescent age group and should be treated as an adult injury. The author is unaware of their occurrence in the patient with an immature carpus.

OTHER CARPAL BONE INJURIES

Virtually all combinations of fractures and fracture dislocations of the carpus have been reported. Again, if dislocation occurs in children, it is in the adolescent age group. Description of all these combinations is beyond the scope of this chapter; however, the principles of carpal dissociations (i.e., accurate reduction of the carpus) apply to these other dislocations. For example, transscaphoid perilunate dislocations are generally quite easily reduced with longitudinal traction. However, accurate alignment of the scaphoid must be achieved. A displaced scaphoid has not only a lesser chance of uniting but also an increased chance of causing pain because of the associated carpal instability that persists.[86, 87] Thus, failure to obtain accurate reduction of the scaphoid fracture is an indication for open reduction. In these cases, internal fixation with a compression screw, as suggested by Herbert, may be advisable.[37] Although use of a Herbert screw is associated with no higher incidence of union than that reported for conventional techniques, it has the distinct advantage of allowing mobilization at 8 weeks with less resultant stiffness.

If closed reduction is successful, the wrist should be immobilized in slight flexion and slight radial deviation with the forearm in pronation in a long arm cast including the thumb. From what has been presented on carpal mechanics, one knows that this position is the one most likely to bring the scaphoid fragments into apposition and reduce the tensile forces on the torn ligaments. However, because radial deviation may also cause flexion through the scaphoid fracture site, critical evaluation of postreduction x-rays is essential. Failure to achieve satisfactory reduction with good apposition between the scaphoid fracture fragments is an indication

for open reduction. Again, the intraosseous compression screw may be indicated in these cases. The carpus should be approached both dorsally through the fourth compartment and palmarly through the carpal canal so that the torn ligaments can be repaired.

AVASCULAR NECROSIS OF THE LUNATE

Avascular necrosis of the lunate, or Kienböck's disease, is generally a disorder that affects young people in the 15- to 35-year-old age group and occurs three times more frequently in males than in females. Although its etiology is still open to some debate, this disorder is probably of traumatic origin.[8] As elsewhere in the skeleton, the initial trauma produces a fracture, and as part of the healing process there may be fragmentation and collapse of the lunate. Like other traumatic injuries of the wrist previously mentioned, Kienböck's disease can be seen in the adolescent age group in patients with open physes (Fig. 10–15A, B). It is not a disorder of the immature carpus.

Adolescents with avascular necrosis of the lunate may have symptoms before the x-ray findings become apparent on plain films. Patients will present with complaints of diffuse wrist pain that is somewhat worse dorsally and often exacerbated by activity. The findings on examination may often be variable, depending on the stage of the disease. However, often there is tenderness over the lunate, mild synovitis, a mild limitation of motion, and decreased grip strength. Even if the x-rays are considered normal for such a patient, the physician should have a high level of suspicion. In cases of persistent wrist pain that does not respond permanently to plaster immobilization for 4 to 6 weeks, repeat x-rays should be obtained. If these are normal and the patient remains symptomatic, tomograms or a bone scan or both may help confirm the diagnosis.

Should patients with avascular necrosis of the lunate undergo treatment? Is the natural history of the disease such that they will become symptomatic? In most cases, they will become symptomatic. Although not all patients progress to severe pain, a large number will eventually develop symptoms of an arthritic wrist, with both limitation of motion and pain. The options then are less good than

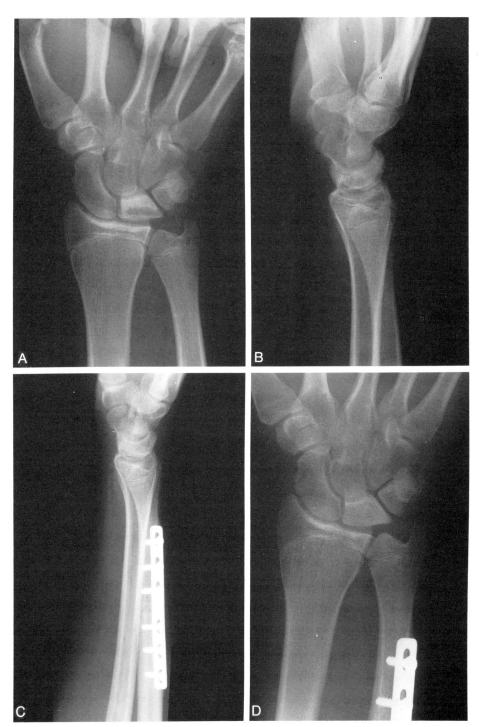

Figure 10–15. A 17-year-old male with early Kienböck's disease. Preoperative AP (*A*) and lateral (*B*) x-rays show sclerosis, cystic changes, and very slight collapse at the usual site (i.e., the ulnar edge of the radius). Postoperative x-rays 7 months later show the site of the ulnar lengthening (*C*) and healing of the once avascular lunate with no further collapse (*D*). Note the change in ulnar variance.

if progression can be prevented. In the vast majority of cases, with or without plaster immobilization, there will be progressive collapse of the lunate and subsequent carpal collapse.

Considerable controversy continues to exist about the best treatment for Kienböck's disease. However, the best rationale for treatment should be postulated on biological and biomechanical grounds. As already noted, revascularization of necrotic bone allows for a period of weakening of the bone and subsequent collapse. Once the lunate is collapsed, regardless of whether it maintains a good radiolunate and lunate-capitate joint surface (which is not usually the case), the patient is left with a "collapsed carpus" that is due to the loss of height of the lunate. Carpal collapse then results in biomechanical abnormality, which will often be symptomatic.

Lichtman and colleagues have classified Kienböck's disease in four stages[46]: (1) pain with no radiological evidence of Kienböck's, (2) pain with radiological evidence of Kienböck's, (3) pain with lunate collapse but without arthritis, and (4) pain with lunate collapse and arthritis. It is wise to add another element when analyzing radiographs of patients with Kienböck's disease— namely, carpal collapse (Table 10–2). This offers a rationale for treatment.

Reviewing a large series of radiographs, authors have noted that a statistically significant number of wrists with Kienböck's disease also have a "short" ulna.[29] This has been described as ulnar variance. A line through the flattest portion of the articulating surface of the distal radius will go through the distal portion of the ulna in a patient with "zero ulnar variance." When the distal ulna protrudes longer than the neutral position, the patient has a "positive ulnar variance"; when it extends shorter than this line, there is a "negative ulnar variance." Positive ulnar

variance may correlate with problems with the triangular fibrocartilage complex or the "lunate impaction syndrome" or both, but these disorders are beyond the scope of this chapter and will not be described further.

Biomechanically, most forces across the wrist are transmitted down the central column through the capitate, lunate, and lunate fossa of the radius. Because it is well known that avascular bone will subsequently collapse if submitted to the normal forces, it is an attractive conjecture that "unloading the lunate" will allow for healing without deformity. Based on the observation that a large number of patients with Kienböck's disease have had a negative ulnar variance, either ulnar lengthening or radial shortening is proposed. By doing such, one could transmit the forces either medially or laterally in the carpus so that the lunate would be unweighted. Reports of a large series of ulnar lengthenings suggest that this rationale may indeed be true.[4, 79] In fact, patients with Kienböck's disease with no or only a moderate amount of lunate collapse are candidates for either procedure (Fig. 10–15C, D).

Of the two alternatives, ulnar lengthening is used in the largest series, but radial shortening is somewhat simpler and does not require the use of an iliac crest bone graft. The degree of shortening or lengthening depends on the amount of ulnar variance, but generally this is in the range of 3 to 5 mm. If there is no evidence of carpal collapse, in the author's opinion, lengthening or shortening also may be advisable in a neutral ulnar variance to unload the lunate. Obviously, one would not choose to add or shorten more than 3 mm. Thus, in stage 1, 2, or 3, an extraarticular unloading procedure is advised.

If a patient has progressed to stage 4, there is collapse of the lunate and collapse of the carpus but no arthritis. Arthritis is unlikely to occur in adolescents; it is more commonly seen in young adults with a closed radial

Table 10–2. **Classification of Kienböck's Disease***

Stage	Pain	Plain Radiographs	Lunate Collapse	Carpal Collapse	Arthritis
1	+	−	−	−	−
2	+	+	−	−	−
3	+	+	Mild	−	−
4	+	+	Severe	+	−
5	+	+	+	+	+

* Kienböck's disease can be classified according to radiographic findings. Stage 1 or 2 is most likely in the adolescent age group.

physis. Clearly, in these cases, an extraarticular procedure may unload the lunate but will not restore the biomechanical integrity of the carpus; thus, the wrist may go on to degenerative arthritis despite healing of the lunate. In this case it is best to go into the carpus. One can unload the lunate by diverting the forces to either the medial or the lateral column. In the former case, a capitate-hamate fusion accomplishes this,[13] but this approach might invite further problems with medial column instability, especially between the lunate-triquetral joints. Follow-up is not long enough to confirm this. However, it appears that it is wisest to transmit the forces to the lateral column, the scaphoid. This can be done with a fusion of either the scaphotrapeziotrapezoid joints or the scaphocapitate joint. Considerable experience with scaphotrapeziotrapezoid fusions has been gained in the treatment of lateral column carpal instability. These fusions result in better motion than scaphocapitate fusions do, and they seem preferable in cases in which there is not severe collapse.[82, 84] In cases of severe collapse, scaphocapitate fusion is advisable.

How does one handle the lunate in patients with severe collapse? There is no great experience, but conjecturally, if there is only a moderate amount of collapse and no evidence of degenerative arthritis, intercarpal fusion alone seems to suffice. If, however, there is evidence of severe fragmentation of the lunate and arthritis, replacement arthroplasty is advisable. This can be accomplished with the lunate Silastic spacer described by Swanson,[72, 73] although a rolled-up piece of tendon may suffice. Swanson's lunate prosthesis and other types of implants (many hand-carved) have been performed successfully since the late 1960s. However, certain long-term problems, although rare, have been noted. The most dramatic one has been symptomatic silastic synovitis, with or without fragmentation of the prosthesis. Cineradiographic studies of the wrist with a lunate Silastic prosthesis have shown that, without diversion of forces from the central column, there is elastic deformation of the prosthesis. Thus, if implantation of a lunate prosthesis is considered, it is best done in conjunction with intercarpal fusion, which will divert the forces from the central column. Certainly, in adolescents and young adults, because of the anticipated longevity of these patients, it would be best to avoid using a prosthesis.

Vascularized Bone Grafts

The concept of using vascularized bone grafts for the treatment of avascular necrosis of the lunate is appealing. One can use either a piece of pisiform rotated on two branches from the ulnar artery or bone from the volar aspect of the radius based on a pronator quadratus muscle flap. However, the idea overlooks the fact that revascularization, although an important step in bone healing, leaves bone in its weakest state and therefore vulnerable to collapse. Perhaps vascularized bone graft can be used in conjunction with "unloading" by utilization of an external fixator. At this time, however, the use of vascularized bone graft for the treatment of Kienböck's disease should be considered experimental.

Surgical Technique

Ulnar lengthening is performed as suggested by Armistead.[4] The procedure is performed with the patient under general anesthesia because an iliac bone graft is necessary. A longitudinal incision is made slightly dorsal to the ulnar border of the ulna over its distal third. The area between the extensor carpi ulnaris and the flexor carpi ulnaris is identified, and the periosteum is incised and stripped both dorsal and palmar so that one has access to the ulna. The plate can be placed either dorsal or volar, wherever it fits best. Generally, this is on the dorsal side. One must take care to keep the plate proximal to the ulnar physis. A slotted plate with four or more holes is preferred. The site for plate placement is identified, and the area between the central two holes is marked. An osteotomy is then made three fourths of the way through the ulnar portion of the ulna. The plate is then applied to the ulna with the standard technique, but the screws are not tightened. The remaining portion of the ulna is then divided.

A piece of corticocancellous bone is then obtained from the iliac crest. The brim of the crest should be used because this has a shape that approximates the site of the graft placement. In measuring the graft to be taken, one must remember that the width of the saw removes up to 1 mm of bone. Therefore, it is wise to mark the width of the graft to be used and cut to the outside of each mark. One should take care not to overlengthen the ulna because this can cause problems with the distal radioulnar joint and limitation in forearm rotation. As a general rule, a 3- to 5-mm graft is correct. If there is a negative ulnar variance, it should be corrected with up to a maximum of 5 mm of lengthening.

After obtaining the graft, the surgeon can lengthen the ulna by distracting the osteotomy site with a lamina spreader. Once the graft is in place, the site of the osteotomy should be allowed to compress on both sides of the graft, and the screws should then be tightened. A long arm splint is initially applied and replaced with a long arm cast at 7 to 10 days. The long arm cast is removed at 6 weeks, and a short arm cast is applied if the site is not united. Generally, another 6 weeks of immobilization will be necessary.

If a radial osteotomy is preferred, it should be done through a longitudinal incision over the dorsum of the wrist extensors. The oblique muscles of the extensor pollicis longus and extensor pollicis brevis will have to be retracted. If the surgeon prefers to use a plate, a standard compression plate can be used. Generally, a T-plate is not necessary. Again, one must take care not to impose on the physis. Because this also requires removal at a later time, one may prefer using several 0.062-inch wires. In such cases, the osteotomy should be performed further distally in the metaphysis because there will be more bone for apposition and healing in this area. Postoperative care is the same as that used with ulnar lengthening.

References

1. Aegerter E, Kirkpatrick JA. Orthopedic Diseases, 3rd ed. Philadelphia, WB Saunders, 1968:205.
2. Amer OE, Mossman DL. Bone agenesis. A case involving the carpus and tarsus. J Bone Joint Surg 40A:917, 1958.
3. Anton JI, Reitz GB, Spiegel MB. Madelung's deformity. Am Surg 108:411, 1938.
4. Armistead RB, Linscheid RL, Dobyns JH, Beckenbaugh RD. Ulnar lengthening in the treatment of Kienböck's disease. J Bone Joint Surg 64A:170, 1982.
5. Bartz AI, Merville V. Lipoid dermato-arthritis and arthritis mutilans. Am J Med 30:51, 1961.
6. Beals RK, Bird CB. Carpal and tarsal osteolysis: a case report and review of the literature. J Bone Joint Surg 57:681, 1975.
7. Beals RK, Lourien EW. Dyschondrosteosis and Madelung's deformity. Report of three kindreds and review of the literature. Clin Orthop Rel Res 116:24, 1976.
8. Beckenbaugh RD, Shives TC, Dobyns JH, Linscheid RL, Kienböck's disease: The natural history of Kienböck's disease and consideration of lunate fractures. Clin Orthop Rel Res 149:98, 1980.
9. Blount WP. Fractures in Children. Baltimore, Williams & Wilkins, 1955:94.
10. Boyd GI. Bipartite carpal navicular bone. Br J Surg 20:455, 1933.
11. Boyes JH. Bunnell's Surgery of the Hand, 5th ed. Philadelphia, JB Lippincott, 1970:82.
12. Boyes JH. Bunnell's Surgery of the Hand, 5th ed. Philadelphia, JB Lippincott, 1970:592.
13. Chuinard RG. Personal communications.
14. Cockshott WP. Carpal fusion. Am J Roentgenol 89:1260, 1963.
15. Cooney WP, Dobyns JH, Linscheid RL. Non-union of the scaphoid. Analysis of the results from bone grafting. J Hand Surg 5:343, 1980.
16. Cope JR, Carpal coalition. Clin Radiol 25:261, 1974.
17. Corson ER. Fusion of the semilunar and cuneiform bones (os lunatum and os triquetrum) in both wrists of an adult male negro—shown by the x-ray. Anat Rec 2:143, 1908.
18. Counahan R, Simmons MJ, Charlwood GJ. Multifocal osteolysis with nephropathy. Arch Dis Child 51:717, 1976.
19. Cuono CB, Watson HK. The carpal boss: surgical treatment and etiological considerations. Plast Reconstr Surg 63:88, 1979.
20. Croundy M. Fractures of the carpal scaphoid in children. Br J Surg 56:523, 1969.
21. Curr JR. Congenital fusion of lunate and triquetrum. J Bone Joint Surg 34:99, 1946.
22. Dannenburg M, Anton JA, Spiegel MB. Madelung's deformity. Consideration of its roentgenological diagnostic criteria. Am J Roentgenol 42:671, 1939.
23. Dunn AW. Fractures and dislocations of the carpus. Surg Clin North Am 52:1513, 1972.
24. Faulker DM. Bipartite carpal scaphoid. J Bone Joint Surg 101:284, 1928.
25. Felman AH, Kirkpatrick JA Jr. Madelung's deformity: observations in 17 patients. Radiology 93:1037, 1969.
26. Fisk GF. Carpal instability and the fractured scaphoid. Ann Roy Coll Surg Eng 46:63, 1970.
27. Garn SM, Frisancko AR, Poznanski AK, et al. Analysis of triquetral-lunate fusion. Am J Phys Anthrop 34:431, 1971.
28. Gelberman RH, Bauman T. Madelung's deformity and dyschondrosteosis. J Hand Surg 5:338, 1980.
29. Gelberman RH, Salamon PB, Jewist JM, Posch JL. Ulnar variance in Kienböck's disease. J Bone Joint Surg 57A:675, 1975.
30. Gerard FM. Post-traumatic carpal instability in a young child. J Bone Joint Surg 62:131, 1980.
31. Gilford WW, Bolton RH, Lambrinudi C. The mechanism of the wrist joint with special reference to fractures of the scaphoid. Guy Hosp Rep 92:52, 1943.
32. Gollasch W. Congenital bipartite carpal scaphoid bones. Arch Orthop Unfallchir 40:269, 1939.
33. Gorham LW, Stant AP. Massive osteolysis (acute spontaneous absorption of bone, phantom bone, disappearing bone). Its relationship to hemangiomatosis. J Bone Joint Surg 37A:985, 1955.
34. Greulich WW, Pyle SJ. Radiographic Atlas of Skeletal Development of the Hand and Wrist, 2nd ed. London, Oxford University Press, 1959.
35. Gruber, W. Os naviculare carpi bipartitum. Arch f Pathol Anat 69:391, 1877.
36. Hastings HH II, Simmons BP. Hand fractures in children: a statistical analysis. Clin Orthop Rel Res 188:120, 1984.
37. Herbert TJ, Fisher WE. Management of the fractured scaphoid using a new bone screw. J Bone Joint Surg 66B:114, 1984.
38. Herdman RD, Langer LO, Good RA. Dyschondrosteosis: the most common cause of Madelung's deformity. J Pediatr 88:432, 1966.

39. Hermann J, Zugibe FT, Gilbert EF, Opitz JM. Arthro-dento-osteo dysplasia (Hadju-Cheney syndrome). Review of a genetic "acroosteolysis syndrome." Z Kinderheik 114:93, 1973.
40. Hughes PCR, Tanner JM. The development of carpal bone fusion as seen in serial radiographs. Br J Radiol 39:943, 1966.
41. Joseph R, Nezelof C, Guerard L, Job JC. Acro-osteo-lyse idiopathique familiale. Sem Hop Paris 35:622, 1959.
42. Kanavel AB. Congenital malformations of the hands. Arch Surg 25:11, 1932.
43. Kaplan EB. Functional and Surgical Anatomy of the Hand, 2nd ed. Philadelphia, JB Lippincott, 1965:125.
44. Kelikian H. Congenital Deformities of the Hand and Forearm. Philadelphia, WB Saunders, 1974.
45. Lamy M, Manteaux P. Acro-osteolyse dominante. Arch Fr Pediatr 18:693, 1961.
46. Lichtman DM, Mack GR, MacDonald RI, et al. Kien-böck's disease: the role of silicone replacement ar-throplasty. J Bone Joint Surg 59A:899, 1977.
47. Lichtman DM, Schneider JR, Swafford AR, Mach GR. Venar midcarpal instability—clinical and lab-oratory analysis. J Hand Surg 6:515, 1981.
48. Linscheid RL, Dobyns JH, Beaubout JW, Bryan RS. Traumatic instability of the wrist: diagnosis, clas-sification and pathomechanics. J Bone Joint Surg 54:1612, 1972.
49. Louis DS, Calhoun TP, Gan SM, et al. Congenital bipartite scaphoid—fact or fiction? J Bone Joint Surg 58A:1108, 1976.
50. Madelung U. Die spontane Subluxation der Hand nach Vome. Verh Dtsch Ges Chir 7:259, 1878.
51. Matti H. Technik und Resultate meiner Pseudoar-throsenoperation. Z Chir 63:1442, 1936.
52. Mayfield JK, Johnson RP, Kilcoyne RK. Carpal dis-locations: pathomechanics and progressive perilu-nar instability. J Hand Surg 5:226, 1980.
52a. Mayfield JK, Johnson RP, Kilcoyne RK. Mechanism of carpal injuries. Clin Orthop Rel Res 149:43, 1980.
53. Mazet R Jr, Hohl M. Fractures of the carpal navi-cular. J Bone Joint Surg 45A:82, 1963.
54. McCredie J. Congenital fusion of bones: radiology, embryology and pathogenesis. Clin Radiol 26:47, 1975.
55. Minaar AB deV. Congenital fusion of the lunate and triquetral bones in the South African Bantu. J Bone Joint Surg 34B:45, 1952.
56. Nielsen JB. Madelung's deformity. A follow-up of 26 cases and a review of the literature. Acta Orthop Scand 48:379, 1977.
57. Normad ICS, Dent MP, Smellie JM. Disappearing carpal bones. Proc Roy Soc Med 55:978, 1962.
58. O'Rahilly R. A survey of carpal and tarsal anomalies. J Bone Joint Surg 35A:626, 1953.
59. O'Rahilly R. Developmental deviations in carpus and tarsus. Clin Orthop Rel Res 10:9, 1957.
60. O'Rahilly R. A survey of carpal and tarsal anomalies. J Bone Joint Surg 35:261, 1974.
61. Pallardy R, Chevrot A, Galmicke JM, Galmiche B. In Tubiana R, ed. The Hand. Philadelphia, WB Saun-ders, 1981:665.
62. Palmer AK, Weiner FW. The triangular fibrocarti-lage complex of the wrist—anatomy and function. J Hand Surg 6:153, 1981.
63. Pfitzner W. Beitrage zur Kenntniss des men-schlichen Extremitatenskelets VI. Die Variationen in Aufbau der Handskelets. Morphol Arbeit von Schwalbe, Zeitschr Morphol 4:347, 1895.
64. Pfitzner W. Beitrage zur Kenntniss des men-schlichen Extremitatenskelets. VIII. Die morpho-gischen Elemente des menschlichen Handskelets Zeitschr Morphol 2:77, 365, 1900.
65. Poznanski AK, Hoh JF. The carpals in congenital malformation syndromes. Am J Roentgenol 112:443, 1971.
66. Ranawat CS, Defiore J, Straub LR. Madelung's de-formity. An end-result study of surgical treatment. J Bone Joint Surg 57A:772, 1975.
67. Russe O. Fracture of the carpal navicular: diagnosis, non-operative treatment, and operative treatment. J Bone Joint Surg (Am) 42:759, 1960.
68. Sandifort E. Observations anatomics pathologicae. Liber 3:136, 1779.
69. Simmons BP, Southmayd WW, Riseborough EJ. Congenital radioulnar synostosis. J Hand Surg 8:829, 1983.
70. Sledge CB. Developmental anatomy of joints. In Res-nick D, Niwayama G, eds. Diagnosis of Bone and Joint Disorders. Philadelphia, WB Saunders, 1981.
71. Southcott R, Rossman MA. Non-union of carpal sca-phoid fractures in children. J Bone Joint Surg 59B:20, 1977.
72. Swanson AB. Silicone rubber implants for the re-placement of the carpal scaphoid and lunate bones. Orthop Clin North Am 1:299, 1970.
73. Swanson AB. Flexible Resection Implant Arthro-plasty in the Hand and Extremities. St. Louis, CV Mosby, 1973:240.
74. Szaboky GT, Muller J, Melnick J, Tamburie R. Anomalous fusion between lunate and triquetrum. J Bone Joint Surg 51:1001, 1969.
75. Tachahara SS. A case of trapezio-scaphoid sublux-ation. Br J Clin Pract 31:162, 1977.
76. Taleisnik J. The ligaments of the wrist. J Hand Surg 1:110, 1976.
77. Taleisnik J. Wrist: Anatomy, Function and Injury. AAOS Instr. Course Lecture XXVII. St. Louis, CV Mosby, 1978:61.
78. Taleisnik J. Post-traumatic carpal instability. Clin Orthop Rel Res 149:73, 1980.
79. Tiberg B. Kienböck's disease treated with osteotomy to lengthen the ulna. Acta Orthop Scand 39:359, 1968.
80. Torg JS, DiGeorge AM, Kirkpatrick JA, Trujillo MM. Hereditary multicentric osteolysis with recessive transmission. A new syndrome. J Pediatr 75:243, 1969.
81. Vahvanen V, Westerlund M. Fracture of the sca-phoid in children. Acta Orthop Scand 51:909, 1980.
82. Watson HK. Limited wrist arthrodesis. Clin Orthop Rel Res 149:126, 1980.
83. Watson HK, Goodman ML, Johnson TR. Limited wrist arthrodesis. Part II. Intercarpal and radiocar-pal combinations. J Hand Surg 6:223, 1981.
84. Watson HK, Hempton RF. Limited wrist arthrodesis. Part I: Triscaphoid joint. J Hand Surg 5:320, 1980.
85. Waugh RL, Sullivan RI. Anomalies of the carpus with particular reference to the bipartite scaphoid. J Bone Joint Surg 32A:682, 1950.
86. Weber ER. Biomechanical implications of scaphoid waist fractures. Clin Orthop Rel Res 149:83, 1980.
87. Weber ER, Chao EY. An experimental approach to the mechanism of scaphoid wrist fractures. J Hand Surg 3:142, 1978.
88. Winchester P, Crossman H, Lim WN, Domes BS. A new acid mucopolysaccharidosis with skeletal de-formities simulating rheumatoid arthritis. Am J Roentgenol 106:121, 1969.

Injuries to the Forearm

PAUL P. GRIFFIN

RESPONSE TO INJURY

Presence of the growth plate and bone remodeling are characteristics that make the treatment and complications of children's fractures different from those of adults.

In the child the periosteum is thicker than it is in the adult, and it usually remains intact after a fracture. This periosteal sleeve, if properly used, can assist in and add stability to the reduction of the fracture. In the periosteum of the child great osteogenic activity occurs, producing a large callus that accelerates fracture healing. Also, a child's cortex is more porous than an adult's, which makes it possible for a long bone to bend or to fracture as a greenstick. A further difference between the mature and immature skeleton is the epiphyseal plate or physis. A healthy physis responds to the stimulus of malalignment by differential growth on the concave and convex side of a deformity in order to realign the two ends of a long bone. Injury to the physis may result in premature closure that results in the bone being short or angulated or both. Unless the physis is injured, it responds to a fracture by growing more rapidly for some months afterward.

Anatomy of the Forearm

The radius, the ulna, and the distal radioulnar joint are designed to allow the radius to rotate around the ulna.[1] The interosseous membrane between the ulna and the radius helps to maintain this relationship between the two bones. If the interosseous space is allowed to become narrow after a fracture, rotation of the forearm will be limited.

The distal radius and ulna are held together by the triangular fibrocartilage in the radioulnar joint and by the joint capsule. Disruption of this joint may tear these ligaments, disrupting the relationship of the distal radius and ulna, a deformity that limits forearm rotation and may become a cause of chronic pain.[3]

Proximally the circumferential articular surface of the head of the radius rests in the radial notch of the ulna. The annular ligament attaches to the distal edge of the notch and stabilizes the head in the notch.

Principles of Rotational Force

Except for a fracture secondary to a direct blow to the forearm, there is a rotational force in effect for all forearm fractures. Evans pointed out that all fractures of the forearm resulting from a fall on the outstretched hand have a rotational force that determines the direction of the deformity.[1] Depending upon the direction of motion of the body in relation to the position of the hand on the ground, the distal fragment may pronate or supinate on the proximal fragment. When the fracture of the radius is a greenstick fracture, there is a rotational deformity that persists and should be corrected. If the fracture of the radius is complete, the rotated position of the proximal fragment is produced by muscle forces acting on it. Reduction of a complete fracture is obtained by rotating the distal fragment into proper alignment with the proximal fragment.

FRACTURES OF THE RADIUS

Fracture of the Distal Epiphysis

Fracture of the distal epiphysis of the radius is the most common epiphyseal injury. A dorsal displacement with volar angulation is the typical injury but, on occasion, the displacement of the distal fragment is volar with a dorsal angulation.* Reduction is usually easy to achieve by manipulation to increase the angulation of the distal fragment so as to appose the cortex of the two fragments then straighten the distal fragment by appropriate flexion or extension. The fracture is stable after reduction and should be immobilized in a well-molded cast for 4 weeks. Severe flexion is not necessary for immobilization, because in a properly molded cast both the flexion and extension reductions can be maintained with the wrist at neutral.

Incomplete Fractures of the Radius

The torus (buckle) fracture of the radius is a stable incomplete fracture in which the cortex is compressed, usually asymmetrically.

---

* The direction of the apex of the fracture site is used to describe the angulation (e.g., if the apex is volar, the fracture is said to be angulated volarly).

Significant deformity is rare, and immobilization by volar and dorsal splints for 3 to 4 weeks is sufficient treatment.

The cortex on the concave side of the fracture is compressed, and correction of the rotation usually aligns the radius adequately. If the radius is markedly angulated after the rotation has been corrected, pressure at the apex of the deformity will further correct the angular deformity, but in my experience, this latter maneuver is seldom necessary.

The most common fracture of the diaphysis in children is a greenstick fracture of the radius.[3] Only 6% of fractures of the radius in young children are complete. Greenstick fractures of the radius are caused by a combination of compressive and rotational forces that occur when the child falls with outstretched hand (wrist extended) against a stationary object, usually the ground. The fracture is caused by the compression force, but the direction of angulation is caused by rotation of the distal fragment. There are two types of greenstick fractures of the radius, volar and dorsal angulated. Volar angulation, which is the most common deformity,[6] results from supination of the distal fragment in relation to the proximal fragment (Fig. 11–1). The dorsal angulated type has pronation

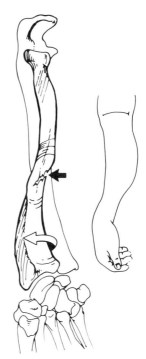

Figure 11–1. A schematic drawing illustrating the deformity of a greenstick supination fracture.

of the distal fragment relative to the proximal fragment (Fig. 11–2).

The deformity can be corrected by reversing the rotation. If the distal fragment is supinated on the proximal fragment (a volar angulation fracture), pronation of the forearm will simultaneously restore the rotatory alignment and correct the angulation (Fig. 11–3). This principle is true regardless of the location of the fracture. Occasionally, a severe fracture may not be completely corrected by the rotation maneuver, and in these cases direct pressure at the apex of the fracture will further realign the fragments. With this technique there is no need to complete the greenstick fracture of the radius or ulna.

If the distal fragment pronates on the proximal fragment, the apex of the deformity will be dorsal, and the distal fragment will be angulated volarly. This deformity can be reduced by supinating the forearm (Fig. 11–4).

A rule of thumb for correction of a greenstick fracture of the radius is to rotate the forearm so that the thumb turns toward the apex of the deformity. If the apex of the deformity is volar, pronate the forearm; if the

apex is dorsal, supinate the forearm. When uncertain as to whether a fracture is a greenstick, realign the radius by direct pressure over the apex; make certain to complete the fracture; then follow the principles for its treatment (see Complete Fractures of the Radius, below). If a complete fracture is treated by the greenstick principles, the result usually is not satisfactory.

There is controversy concerning the final position in which to immobilize the arm after reduction. Evans[1] casted the reduced fracture in pronation for volar-angulated greenstick fractures and supination for dorsal-angulated fractures. Pollen,[7] however, believes that all greenstick fractures should be immobilized in supination to relieve the deforming force of the brachioradialis. I recommend the greenstick fracture be held in a long arm cast for 6 weeks in the position that reduces the fracture.

The Bowed Forearm

The forces that cause a greenstick fracture of the radius may bend the radius rather than break it, and the ulna may also bend with the radius from the compression. When the radius is bowed, the rotational force causes the deformity, and the treatment is to correct the rotation as if it were a greenstick fracture. (Fig. 11–5). Pronate the forearm if the apex is volar; supinate it if the apex is dorsal. Direct pressure over the apex may be needed to completely correct the alignment of the ulna. The rotation applied to the forearm corrects the deformity, and completely fracturing the radius is not necessary.

A long arm cast with the elbow flexed to 90 degrees and the forearm in the rotation position required to reduce the fracture (supination or pronation) will maintain the reduction. Six weeks immobilization is sufficient for union of either a bowed radius or a greenstick fracture.

Complete Fractures of the Radius

The immediate relationship of the proximal and distal fragments of the radius after complete fracture is determined by the forces acting on the forearm and the resistance of the surface against the outstretched hand. The direction of the rotational force directs the angulation, and the pull of muscles and soft tissue determines the position of the proximal fragment. If distal radial fragment ov-

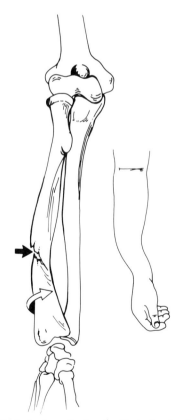

Figure 11–2. A schematic drawing illustrating the deformity of a greenstick pronation fracture.

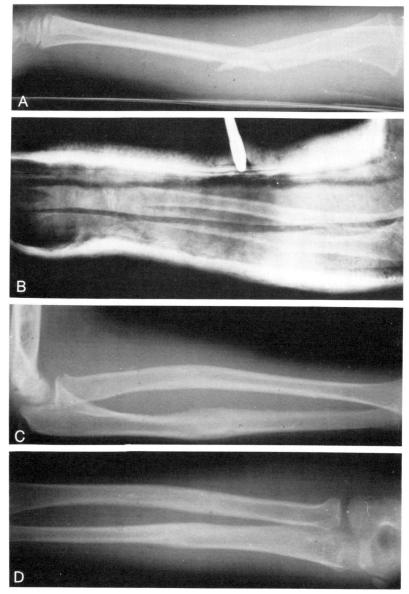

Figure 11–3. *A*, A greenstick supination fracture. There is volar angulation. *B*, By pronating the forearm, the deformity is corrected. *C*, AP view of forearm after healing. *D*, Lateral view of forearm after healing. A slight bow remains, but the forearm appearance and rotatory motion is normal.

errides the proximal fragment, a fracture of the ulna, a bend of the ulna (incomplete fracture), or a disruption of the radioulnar joint occurs.

Three observations are helpful in determining the rotation of the proximal fragment: the contour of the forearm proximal to the fracture, the x-rays of the fracture fragments, and the position of the bicipital tubercle as shown by x-ray. By palpating the uninjured forearm, one can determine the width the interosseous space should be after reduction. Evans[1] reported that the position of the bi-

cipital tubercle of the radius is a guide to forearm rotation. Anterior-posterior (AP) x-rays of the bicipital tubercle of the normal radius in zero degrees, 30 degrees, and 60 degrees of supination are compared to the anterior-posterior (AP) x-ray of the injured forearm, which helps determine the position of rotation of the fragments on the fractured side. The width of the interosseous space on the x-ray also helps to determine the position of the fragments. If the space is either abruptly wider or abruptly narrower, malrotation is present. Angular deformity of the ulna

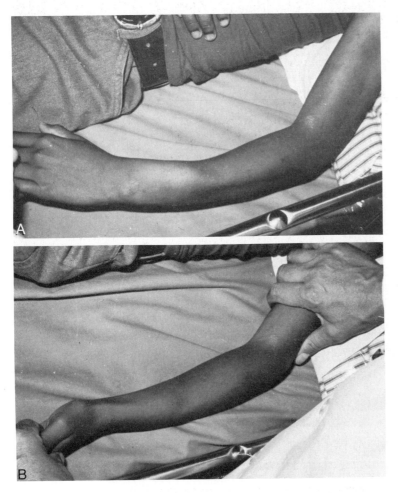

Figure 11–4. *A,* Appearance of a greenstick pronation fracture. There is dorsal angulation of the fracture. *B,* Supination is limited. Correction of the alignment was obtained by completely supinating the forearm.

must be corrected, or it will limit rotation of the radius by blocking its rotational movement and will limit distal radioulnar joint motion as well.

A common complete fracture of the distal radius occurs 1.5 inches from its distal end; the distal fragment is displaced dorsally with a dorsal periosteal hinge. Reduction is achieved by increasing the deformity and by rotating the distal fragment to align the proximal fragment. The distal fragment is then translocated so that the width of the radius on the injured side is equal to the width on the contralateral side (Fig. 11–6A, B).

Most fractures of the distal radius require the distal fragment to be rotated in pronation, but a few may require supination. The latter injuries generally have medial displacement of the distal fragment and subluxation of the radioulnar joint. In adults the Galleazzi fracture, a fracture of the distal third of the radius, with disruption of the radioulnar joint, requires open reduction and internal fixation. In children closed reduction of this injury is adequate, because the radioulnar joint does well if both the fracture and the joint are reduced. When pronation of the distal fragment is needed to correct the rotational deformity, supination of the forearm may be required to reduce the distal radioulnar joint. Pronation reduces the fracture and supination reduces the radioulnar joint after the fracture is reduced. Extremity immobilization in a long arm cast with the elbow flexed 90° for 6 weeks is required for bone and joint healing.

FRACTURES OF BOTH RADIUS AND ULNA

Simultaneous fractures of the two bones in the distal third of the forearm require correction in both rotation and angulation

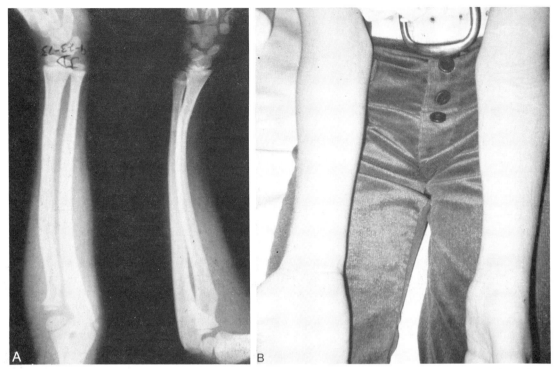

Figure 11–5. AP and lateral views of a bowed radius and ulna. The distal radius is pronated, causing the dorsal angulation. B, The deformed arm will not supinate as shown in A. Correction of the alignment was obtained by completely supinating the forearm.

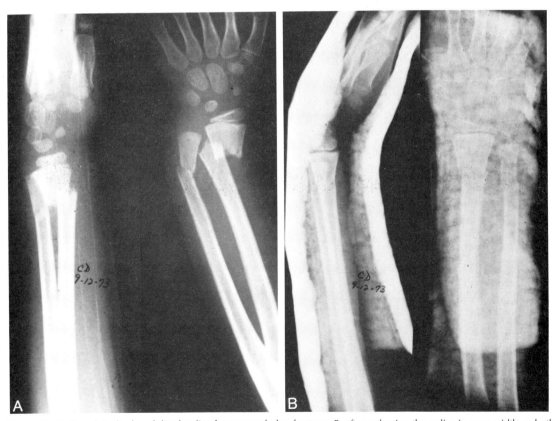

Figure 11–6. Complete displaced distal radius fracture and ulna fracture; B, after reduction the radius is same width on both sides of the fracture. The forearm is immobilized in neutral rotation for 6 to 8 weeks.

planes for a satisfactory result. To have end-to-end apposition is desirable, but not essential. One bone cannot override if the other is reduced, end to end. Rang[6] warns against immobilizing fractures of the distal radius and ulna in full pronation or supination because one fragment will be angulated anteriorly while the other is posteriorly angulated. A neutral position is recommended for the forearm, and to maintain reduction, the cast distal and proximal to the fracture should be molded.

Fractures of the mid- and proximal thirds of the diaphysis of both bones are difficult to reduce and to maintain in the reduced position. I recommend that the patient be supine, with the fingers in a finger trap. Countertraction is then applied to the arm, with the elbow at a right angle. The tendons and muscles have a tendency to improve the angulation and rotation with this longitudinal traction force. The first step in reduction, correction of the rotation deformity, is accomplished by rotating the distal radial fragment so that it is in proper alignment with the proximal fragment. The next step is to oppose the ulna fragments and then to straighten them in order to correct the angulation. Finally, to lever the radial fragments into position, use the ulna as a fulcrum. Check the position of the fragments with x-rays, and if satisfactory, with the elbow flexed 90 degrees, apply a long, circular arm cast from the palm to the axilla. The cast should be molded to fit the contour of the arm and should be flat on the ulnar side. Attach a sling through a loop at the level of fracture to prevent sagging of the cast, which could allow sagging of the fracture after swelling subsides. It is important to follow these patients with x-rays on a weekly basis for 2 weeks or longer if it is suspected that the fracture may lose position. A long arm cast for 6 to 8 weeks is required for bone healing.

MALUNION

The degree of malunion acceptable in a child's forearm has never precisely been determined. There are many variables that influence how much the remodeling process during growth will correct a deformity. These include: age, rotation of the fracture and the direction of the malunion. Children under 8 years who have had forearm fractures rarely have significant angulation at maturity.[2] Fractures at the distal ends of the radius and the ulna remodel more than proximal fractures of these bones, and when there is angulation in the plane of the adjacent joints, the joints compensate for the malunion; the result is more satisfactory in comparison with similar malunions in other planes. Very little remodeling occurs when angulation is at right angles to the motion of the adjacent joints. It appears that remodeling is quicker and more complete when the apex of angulation is on the flexor, rather than the extensor, side. No more than 15 degrees of angulation should be accepted in any direction in patients over age 10. Most fractures are satisfactorily aligned at the time of the initial reduction but lose position because of a poorly made cast, an inappropriate sling position or the lack of one, or failure to correct the rotation. The loss of position frequently occurs after the swelling subsides and during the first 2 weeks of treatment.

The most common disability resulting from malunion of forearm fractures is limited rotation, caused by rotation malunion, disruption of the distal radioulnar joint, or angulation of the radius that blocks its rotation around the ulna. Fuller[2] reported that children under age 8 with early malunion had no residual limitation of rotation in follow-up examination. He concluded that a rotation deformity in young children corrected itself with growth. My experience leads me to agree with other authors that rotational malunion does not correct itself with growth. In children over 10 years old, remodeling of angulation in the middle and proximal thirds of the radius is limited, and in teenage patients open reduction should be considered if closed manipulation fails to align the fragment in a normal position.

The major correction of malunion in a growing bone is by asymmetrical growth at the epiphyseal plate and by remodeling at the fracture site. Growth at the epiphysis realigns that end of the bone with the linear axis of the bone. Remodeling at the fracture site reduces the sharp edge on the convex surface. The concave side fills in by new bone deposition. The major change from local remodeling at the fracture site is a change in the contour of the bone, rather than a change in the alignment of the fragments.

MONTEGGIA FRACTURE

In 1841 Monteggia described the fracture of the ulnar shaft associated with dislocation of the head of the radius. The radial head may be displaced anteriorly, posteriorly, or laterally, and in some instances the ulna is bowed rather than fractured (Fig. 11–7). For diagnosis of an isolated fracture of the ulna x-rays should always include the elbow, to determine the position of the radial head (Fig. 11–8). A line along the center of the radius must intersect the capitellum in all views with the elbow flexed, and if this relationship is not present, the head is dislocated. The usual mechanism of injury is forced pronation.

Closed reduction of the radial head and the ulnar shaft is almost always successful. With the child supine, the elbow is flexed, and pressure is exerted over the radial head as the forearm is supinated. Reduction should be checked by a lateral x-ray. A line drawn through the center of the diaphysis of the radius and the center of the radial head should intersect the capitellum of the humerus. Unlike the Monteggia fracture in the adult, in the child the annular ligament does not pull free from the ulna and will function satisfactorily if the fracture-dislocation is reduced. In rare instances open reduction of an acute ulnar fracture is necessary, and in those cases the bone is fixed with an intramedullary pin or a plate. In cases treated sev-

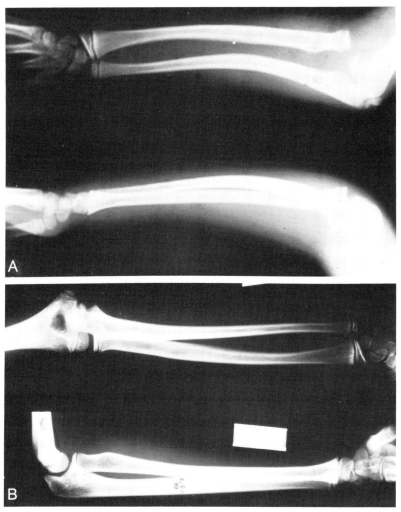

Figure 11–7. *A,* Monteggia injury with ulna bowed, rather than fractured; *B,* after healing the ulna had to be osteotomized and straightened before the radial head could be reduced.

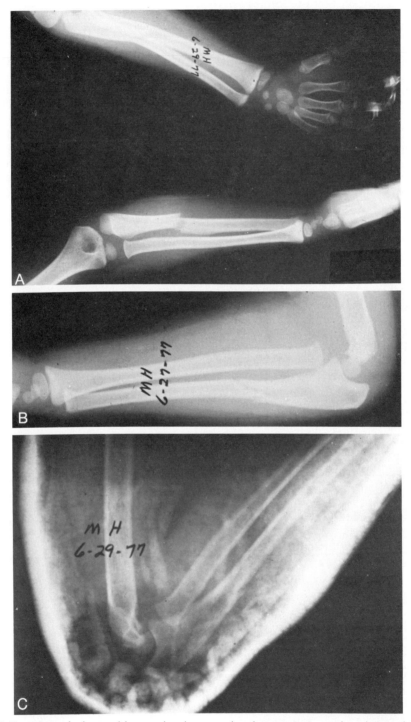

Figure 11–8. *A*, Two views of a fractured forearm that shows an ulnar fracture. *B*, Correct lateral view of the same fracture shows the radial head dislocated. *C*, Lateral view after reduction. Note the degree of flexion necessary for reduction.

eral months later it may still be possible to relocate the radial head by open reduction, but in these cases osteotomy of the ulna with internal fixation (plate or pin) is usually required to correct ulnar malunion.

FRACTURE OF THE NECK OF THE RADIUS

Fractures of the proximal radius usually occur in the neck, and rarely in the head. Other injuries that frequently occur at the same time include fractures of the olecranon or the medial epicondyle, and dislocation of the elbow or the proximal radioulnar joint. A fall on the outstretched hand produces a valgus stress that angulates the head from the radius (see Fig. 11–10A); the fracture is usually a type I or type II Salter-Harris but may extend entirely through the metaphysis. There is disagreement as to the degree of angulation that is acceptable, but I believe that an angle of as much as 30 degrees remodels sufficiently to give acceptable forearm rotation. Others report that no more than 15 degrees of angulation is acceptable.[4] If reduction is required, after the child is anesthetized, I apply pressure with my thumb directly over the radial head while the fore-

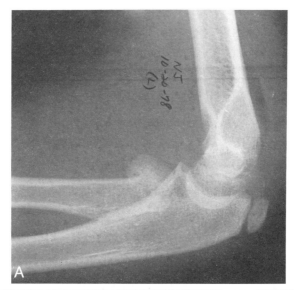

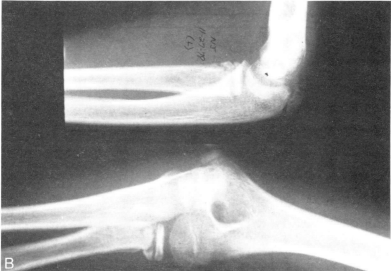

Figure 11–9. *A,* Lateral view of elbow shows anterior angulation of radial neck fracture; *B,* AP and lateral views after manipulation under anesthesia.

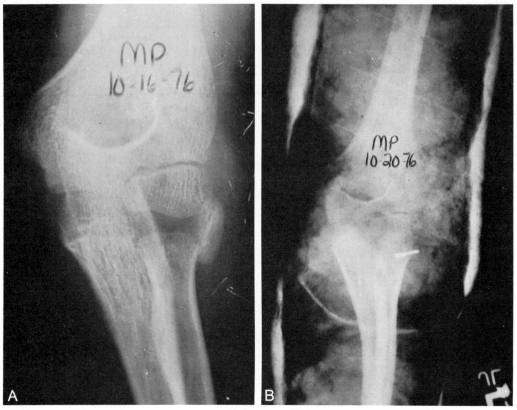

Figure 11–10. A, Complete separation of radial head; B, after reduction, fixation is with K-wire placed tangentially to maintain reduction.

arm is pronated and supinated. If full supination and pronation are present under anesthesia, pressure will reduce the angled radial head (Fig. 11–9). If this method fails, a K-wire is introduced percutaneously and can be used to lever the head into alignment under observation by x-ray.

Closed reduction is not adequate for the completely displaced radial head and open reduction is required (Fig. 11–10). The head should be reduced without disturbing its soft tissue attachments, and if the head is not stable after reduction, a Kirschner wire should be placed obliquely across the corner of the head into the metaphysis of the radius for fracture fixation. The pin should be removed at 3 weeks, and at that time exercises should begin. The author does not recommend placing a pin through the capitellum to hold the radial head in position, because he has observed pin fracture within the joint. A completely displaced radial head should not be removed, but replaced by open reduction and internal fixation. Removal of the radial head is not indicated in young chil-

dren because it inhibits growth and causes a proximal shift of the radial shaft, a complication that impairs distal radio-ulnar joint motion with growth. A devascularized radial head will slowly revascularize and, although causing deformity and limited motion, have a better result than removal.

References

1. Evans EH. Fractures of the radius and ulna. J. Bone Joint Surg 33B:548–561, 1951.
2. Fuller DJ, McCullough CJ. Malunited fractures of the forearm in children. J Bone Joint Surg 64B:364–367, 1982.
3. Gaudhi RK, Wilson P, Mason-Brown JJ, et al. Spontaneous correction of deformity following fractures of the forearm in children. Br J Surg 50:5, 1962.
4. Jones ERL, Esah M. Displaced fractures of the neck of the radius in children. J Bone Joint Surg 53B:429–439, 1977.
5. Patrick J. A study of supination and pronation with special reference to the treatment of forearm fractures. J Bone Joint Surg 28:737, 1946.
6. Rang M. Children's fractures. Philadelphia, JB Lippincott, 1983:211.
7. Pollen AG Fractures and Dislocation in Children. Baltimore, Williams & Wilkins, 1973.

CHAPTER ○ 1 2

Injuries to and Developmental Deformities of the Elbow in Children

KURT M. W. NIEMANN
JOHN S. GOULD
BARRY SIMMONS
F. WILLIAM BORA, JR.

DEVELOPMENT AND GROWTH OF THE ELBOW JOINT [1, 2, 5]

The elbow joint, whose development has been studied by Gray and Gardner[1] and by Wadsworth,[2] begins as mesenchyme at 34 days of fetal life. By day 37, the humerus, radius, and ulna are apparent by cell aggragates of mesoderm; the radius begins to chondrify at 41 days and the ulna at 44 days. As chondrification of the humerus, radius, and ulna progresses, an interzone is formed at the junction between their articular ends. Gradually, this interzone loosens and cavitation occurs, which develops into a joint space at day 57. Ossification occurs in the chondrified radius and ulna at 8 weeks, and the ligaments of the elbow joint develop at the same time.

At birth, the articular surfaces are covered with cartilage, the only difference from the adult being that the trochlear groove is shallower. With subsequent growth and development the secondary epiphyseal ossification centers appear in regular sequence: the capitellum at 5 months in the male and 4 months in the female. The radial head appears at 5 years in the male and 4 years in the female, followed by the medial epicondyle at 7 years and 5 years, respectively. The trochlea is present at 9 years in the male and 8 years in the female, the olecranon process at 10 years, and finally, the lateral epicondyle at 12 years in the male, and 11 years in the female (Fig. 12–1). With continuing skeletal maturation, the capitellum, trochlea, and lateral epicondyle fuse at puberty; this mass fuses to the lower humeral shaft at age 17 years in the male and 14 years in the female. The apophysis of the medial epicondyle fuses to the humeral shaft at 18 years in the male and 15 years in the female. The olecranon fuses to the ulnar shaft in the male at 15 to 17 years and in the female at 14 to 15 years. The radial head fuses to the radial shaft at 15 to 17 years in the male and 14 to 15 years in the female. The order of appearance of the ossification centers is consistent in the same extremity, but it should be noted that there may be considerable variation from the left to the right side in the same individual. If there is variation in appearance, ordinarily the right side will precede the left. The reasons may be that advanced skeletal maturation has been observed with

213

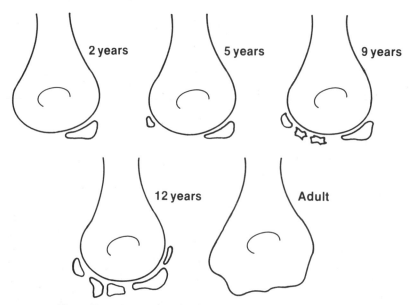

Figure 12–1. Stages of ossification of the distal humeral epiphysis.

use and that most children are right-handed.[5]

ANATOMY OF THE ELBOW JOINTS [3, 4, 6]

The elbow functions as a ginglymus or hinge joint and is made up of three joints— the ulnohumeral joint, the radiohumeral joint, and the proximal radioulnar joint. The joint between the proximal radius and ulna is a trochoid joint, with rotation the only motion. The radial head, whose contour fits that of the capitellum, slides on flexion-extension of the elbow joint. The trochlea of the humerus fits accurately into the trochlear notch of the ulna. When the elbow is fully extended, the medial and lateral epicondyles and the olecranon form a straight line. With the elbow in 90 degrees of flexion, these three prominences line up as an equilateral triangle. This point is important in recognition of traumatic deformities of the elbow. The trochlea has a central groove, and the ulna has an elevated ridge with concave medial and lateral surfaces that correspond to the convex surface of the trochlea. The distal end of the humerus is formed by the trochlea and capitellum which are anterior to the humeral shaft, at an angle of 45 degrees.

Active flexion of the elbow (150 degrees) is limited by the muscle bulk of the forearm and upper arm muscles. Passive flexion is limited by compaction of the radial head against the radial fossa, by the coronoid process against the coronoid fossa, and by the posterior capsule and the triceps. Extension is limited by bone impaction of the olecranon process into the olecranon fossa and by tension in the anterior capsule and the biceps and brachialis muscle-tendon units. The extension-flexion range of elbow motion is 0 to 150 degrees, respectively. Pronation and supination are measured from a neutral forearm position with the elbow at 90 degrees of flexion and are each 80 degrees.

The ligaments of the elbow joint are formed as thickenings of the capsular membrane. The anterior and posterior capsular ligaments are quite thin but with growth are supported by strong muscle-tendon units (brachialis and biceps anteriorly and triceps-olecranon unit posteriorly.) The lateral elbow ligament attaches proximally to the lateral epicondyle and distally to the annular ligament and to the radial notch of the ulna. The medial ligament[6] is composed of three distinct bands that are continuous with each other. The anterior band originates from the anterior aspect of the medial epicondyle and attaches to the medial edge of the coronoid process. The thin middle section arises from the inferior surface of the medial epicondyle and attaches to the medial edge of the coronoid process and to an oblique band that extends between the distal ends of the anterior and posterior bands. The posterior band originates from the posterior aspect of the medial epicondyle and attaches to the medial edge of the olecranon process. The middle section of the ligament has a grooved surface that is in contact with the ulnar nerve. The annular ligament forms approximately four fifths of a circle. The remaining fifth consists of the radial notch in the ulna that articulates with the radial head. The notch and ligament form a cup-shaped socket that is narrower distally, thereby preventing distal migration on the head.

The articulation of the forearm bones with the distal humerus, the shape of the distal humerus, and the length of the forearm bones all influence the angular relationship between the forearm and humerus. This is the carrying angle, and with the elbow in full extension, the relation of the ulna to the humerus is 15 degrees of valgus. The carrying angle has been reported to increase with age.[4] The carrying angle will be influenced by a wide variety of conditions, both congenital and traumatic.[3] Chromosome anomalies that decrease vertical height tend to increase the carrying angle, and conversely, anomalies that increase vertical height tend to decrease or reverse the carrying angle. In childhood, injury to the distal growth plate of the humerus may change the normal carrying angle.

CONGENITAL SYNOSTOSIS OF THE RADIUS AND ULNA [7–25]

Congenital synostosis of the proximal radius and ulna is a rare malformation of the upper limb. The first anatomic description of this entity was given by Sandifort in 1793. One hundred years later, Morrison described a clinical case and reported the classic physical findings.[17]

During the embryonic period of fetal development, the upper limb bud arises from the unsegmented body wall at between 25 and 28 days. Growth and differentiation continue until 48 to 50 days, when all external characteristics of the adult limb are present.[21] The elbow is first discernible at 34 days. At this stage, three connected cartilaginous anlagen are present, which are destined to become the humerus, the radius, and the ulna. Soon thereafter, longitudinal segmentation produces a separation of the distal radius and ulna, but for a time the proximal ends are united and share a common perichondrium.[16] Abnormal genetic or teratogenic factors operating at this time, therefore, would interrupt subsequent proximal radioulnar joint morphogenesis.

If an event does occur to prevent cavitation of the cartilage and subsequent joint formation, the stage is set for enchondral ossification of the proximal cartilaginous tissue, which will lead to a bony synostosis. If some joint development occurs before a period of arrest, one would anticipate seeing a less severe degree of coalition and a more normal elbow joint, such as a radial head.

During this period of intrauterine development, the forearm is in a position midway between neutral and full pronation.[24] Thus, failure of proximal radioulnar joint differentiation leaves the forearm forever in its fetal position. With one exception,[13] in all previous clinical cases the forearm has been fixed in varying degrees of pronation.[24]

Although the etiology is unknown, there appears to be a genetic basis for some cases of congenital radioulnar synostosis. Positive family histories have been reported,[8–10, 14] and the condition is seen in disorders such as acropolysyndactyly (Carpenter's syndrome), acrocephalosyndactyly (Apert's syndrome), arthrogryposis, and mandibulofacial dysostosis.[25] It is also seen in nondysfunctional sex chromosomal abnormalities, especially Klinefelter's syndrome and its variants.[11, 15, 18, 24]

Clinical Presentation

Patients with congenital radioulnar synostosis may present either unilaterally or bilaterally and may have associated anomalies.[36] There is a 3:2 male predominance, and it is usual for children to be brought to medical attention before the age of 3 years.

Functional complaints are variable and include (1) difficulty in holding or using small objects such as a spoon or pencil, (2) inability to dress owing to poor manipulation of belt buckles or buttons, (3) backhanded positioning in holding objects such as bottles or toys (Fig. 12–2), and (4) difficulty competing in sports requiring upper extremity dexterity. Feeding and accepting objects with an open palm are difficult functions in patients with bilateral involvement and in those with more severe degrees of fixed pronation, whether it is bilateral or unilateral (Fig. 12–3).

Associated anomalies may involve the musculoskeletal, cardiovascular, thoracic,

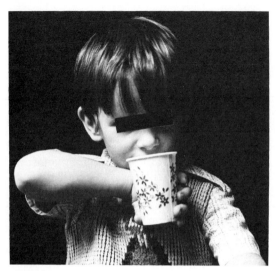

Figure 12–2. In bilateral cases in which there is hyperpronation, patients may have difficulty getting objects to their mouths, resulting in "backhanded" positioning.

gastrointestinal, renal, and central nervous systems. In the hand, thumb aplasia or hypoplasia, polydactyly, syndactyly, and congenital constriction ring syndrome occur. In the wrist, various degrees of carpal coalition have been observed. Cardiac anomalies include tetralogy of Fallot and ventricular septal defects; thoracic anomalies include hy-poplasia of the first and second ribs and the pectoral musculature. In the central nervous system, associated problems include microcephaly, hydrocephalus, encephalocele, mental retardation, delay in attaining developmental milestones, and hemiplegia. One case of unilateral hypoplasia of the kidney and umbilical hernia has also been reported.

On physical examination, the elbow often has loss of its normal carrying angle and has a flexion deformity. Noticeable shortening of the forearm is present, which is more apparent in unilateral cases.

Rotational hypermobility of the wrist with an arc of motion of 45 degrees through the radiocarpal and intercarpal joints appears to be an adaptive phenomenon from rotational stress on the wrist in the absence of forearm rotation. There is usually no hypermobility in the other planes of wrist motion. Retrospective studies evaluating adults with this condition indicate that despite this ligamentous laxity, patients do not appear to develop symptoms of carpal instability.[20]

As mentioned, all patients save one reported in the literature present in pronation.[10, 12, 13, 20, 24] Approximately 40% of patients presented in fixed pronation of less than 30 degrees, 40% with more than 60 degrees, and the remaining 20% fixed between 30 and 60 degrees.

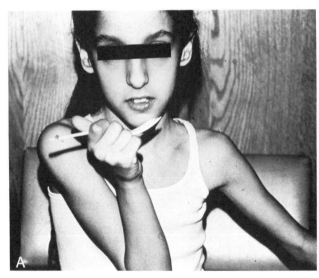

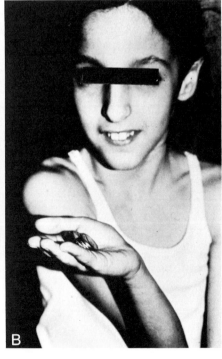

Figure 12–3. Fixed pronation makes it awkward for patients to feed themselves (*A*), or accept objects in an open palm (*B*).

Radiographic analysis of patients with congenital radioulnar synostosis shows anatomic variations from minor radial head deformities, in patients with a 45 degree arc of forearm rotation, to a full synostosis across the whole length of the radius and ulna, with no rotation. More extensive synostoses are usually fixed in more pronation. X-rays are most helpful in defining the clinical picture (Fig. 12–4).

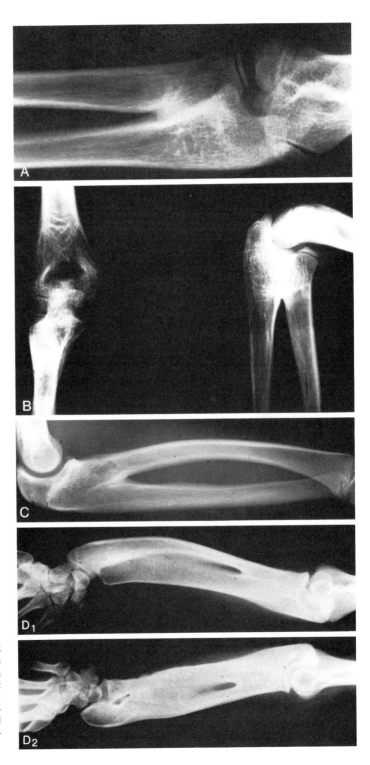

Figure 12–4. A wide spectrum of anomalous findings may be present radiologically from a small synostotic segment proximally with a dislocated radial head (A), a small synostotic segment with a subluxed radial head, (B), larger proximal synostotic segment with absent radial head (note accentuated radial bowing) (C), to a virtually complete synostosis (D).

Treatment

The ideal treatment would be to restore forearm rotation, but surgical attempts to do so have failed. Reported procedures include simple division of the bony bridge,[24] resection of the synostotic proximal radius saving the bicipital tuberosity with [7, 15, 17, 19, 25] and without[22] muscle interposition and with division of the interosseous membrane.[14] An ingenious idea of placing a metallic swivel in the intramedullary canal of the radius between the supinator and pronator teres, with resection of the distal ulna and transfer of the flexor carpi ulnaris to the dorsum of the hand to help restore supination, has been reported to work in post-traumatic proximal radioulnar synostosis.[15] One instance of using this procedure in congenital radioulnar synostosis, however, gave disappointing results.[23]

Patients with less than 30 degrees of fixed pronation, unilateral or bilateral, generally do not need surgery. Their restrictions include accepting objects in an open palm, performing very specific athletic activities such as pull-ups, and difficulty in eating if the affected extremity is the dominant one. Furthermore, changing the position of the forearm will not improve performance in these activities. A report of a large series of children with less than 60 degrees of pronation concluded that surgery would not be beneficial.[9]

If the child's function is limited and surgery is thought advisable, the goal is to place the forearm, hand, and wrist unit in a more functional position. This can be accomplished by derotational osteotomy and is best done before the child reaches school age. Although the derotational osteotomy can be done anywhere along the forearm, it is technically easier if done through the proximal radioulnar synostosis. Under tourniquet control, a skin incision is made along the subcutaneous border of the ulna, which allows the fascia along the anconeus and the extensor carpi ulnaris to be opened longitudinally. The osteotomy can be performed subperiosteally within the synostotic mass distal to the radial head, if present. A smooth Steinmann pin is placed in the medullary canal, fixing the bone fragments longitudinally but permitting a change in fragment rotation along the longitudinal axis. Although a variety of transfixing devices can be used, including another pin or staple, it is best to avoid placing a device internally, so that the rotation position can be changed if vascular complications occur. A single transcutaneous Steinmann pin distal to the osteotomy site will control rotation of the distal fragment, and the pin can be easily removed so that the fragment positions can be reversed if there are vascular complications (Fig 12–5). Once proper rotation of the fragments is obtained, the pin can be incorporated in a long-arm cast. The external K-wire is removed at 6 weeks and the long-arm cast at 6 to 12 weeks, depending on the bone healing. The intramedullary K-wire can be easily removed after bony union if it is left subcutaneously at the tip of the olecranon.

Derotation of up to 45 degrees can be accomplished in a single stage, but if more is required, it is best done in two stages. This is because the change in fragment rotation can cause vascular compromise, a complication that must be watched for carefully in the early postoperative period. Although compartment pressures may be helpful, clinical signs are the most reliable indicators. Reversal of the rotated segment usually improves the vascular situation, and in such cases, fasciotomies are rarely necessary. Sub-

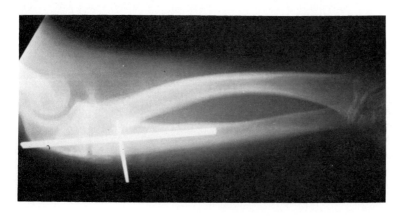

Figure 12–5. The osteotomy is technically easiest within the synostosis. An intramedullary device controls alignment, and the transcutaneous wire controls rotation.

sequent correction can be restored by manipulation with parenteral analgesics without another trip to the operating room.

If there is unilateral involvement, the optimum final position should be 20 degrees of pronation. If there is bilateral involvement, the dominant extremity should be rotated to 20 degrees of pronation and the nondominant extremity individualized for each patient. Some authors [12, 13] believe that the nondominant extremity is best casted in 20 degrees of supination; however, long-term follow-up on some of these patients has shown that supination does not allow the child to receive objects in an open palm without placing the elbow in an awkward position. If 20 degrees of supination is selected, the child must abduct his shoulder for eating or for any two-handed task that involves bilateral forearm pronation, such as typing. This is an awkward and fatiguing position (Fig. 12–6). If bilateral surgery is performed, it is probably best to place the dominant forearm in 20 degrees of pronation and the nondominant forearm in neutral, hoping that hypermobility of the wrist will allow for good function. If the child is older and has chosen a career, the position of correction should be suited for the tasks involved in the job (Table 12–1).

CONGENITAL RADIAL HEAD DISLOCATION [26–28]

This condition has a lateral prominence and an elbow flexion deformity. Dislocation of the radial head is anterior in 50%, posterior in 40%, and lateral in 10% of the cases. Pronation and supination are nearly normal in young children, but supination becomes restricted later. If the radial head fails to develop, it becomes dome-shaped rather than the normal trumpet shape.

Radial head dislocation occurs in conditions that affect the relative growth of the radius and ulna. Nail-patella syndrome,[28] Ollier's disease, and multiple hereditary osteocartilaginous exostoses have a short ulna and cause dislocation of the radial head. Attempts to reduce the radial head and replace the orbicular ligament have been reported to have limited success in young children. If limited motion, pain, and a cosmetic deformity occur, resection of the radial head at the end of the growth period is indicated (Fig. 12–7). Congenital dislocation must be differentiated from a traumatic injury; the former is always bilateral and the latter, unilateral (Table 12–1).

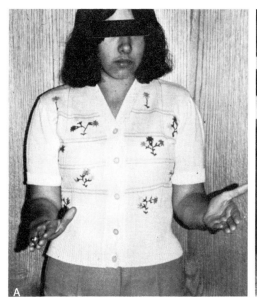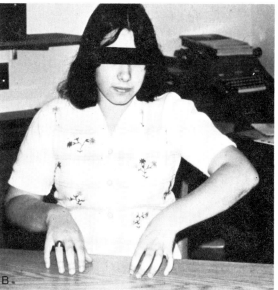

Figure 12–6. *A*, Bilateral congenital radioulnar synostosis with the dominant arm in pronation and the other in supination. *B*, Fixation in supination is cosmetically and functionally undesirable. This position requires shoulder abduction, which is both fatiguing and awkward for daily activities.

Table 12–1. A Comparison of Congenital Forearm Deformities

	Etiology	Involvement	Symptoms	Signs	X-Ray	Treatment	Comments
Congenital Dislocation of the Radial Head	Genetic defect Family history (+)	Bilateral (100%)		Elbow and forearm: Limitation of supination mild flexion-extension block Cubitus valgus Radial head bump	Anterior (50%) Posterior (40%) Lateral (10%) Dome radial head Reversal posterior ulnar border	Resect radial head after maturity Early relocation with orbicular ligament replacement	Difficulty with activities requiring supination Adults have minimal functional problems
Traumatic Dislocation of the Radial Head	History of trauma	Unilateral			Normal trumpet-shaped radial head Normal posterior ulnar border		
Congenital Radioulnar Synostosis	Genetic	Bilateral (60%)		Elbow and forearm: Fixed pronation Extension also limited with radial head dislocation	*Type I*—proximal fusion radius-ulna *Type II*—proximal fusion radius-ulna + dislocation of radial head	Osteotomy through area of synostosis Resection synostosis with material interposition Bilateral cases: dominant hand 20 degrees pronation, subdominant hand neutral to 20 degrees supination	Patients can adjust to 40 degrees of pronation or less More severe deformities helped by osteotomy Osteotomy recommended at 6 years of age
Madelung's Deformity	Traumatic Bone dysplasia Chromosomal (Turner's syndrome) Idiopathic	Bilateral (66%)	Wrist pain	Forearm and wrist: Flexion—increased; extension—decreased; pronation—blocked; supination—full Short forearm Ulna-styloid bump	Premature fusion of the medial half of the distal growth plate of the radius Dorsal subluxation of the distal ulna	Darrach—mild Biplanar osteotomy and Darrach Fusion distal radioulnar joint and nonunion ulna more proximal (Lauenstein procedure) Wrist fusion	

220

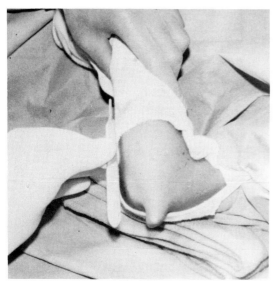

Figure 12–7. Congenital dislocation of the radial head.

CONGENITAL FUSION OF THE ELBOW [35, 36, 39, 43]

Congenital fusion of the elbow is a rare anomaly that may involve the humerus, ulna, and radius or the humeroradial[35, 36, 39,] and/or humeroulnar articulation (Fig. 12–8). Associated anomalies[43] frequently occur in the forearm and hand, such as variations in the numbers of digits, but hand function is usually satisfactory. Prosthetic treatment is

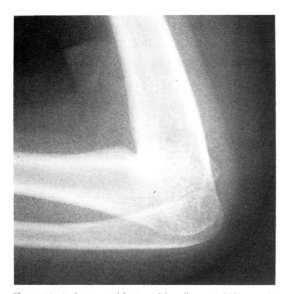

Figure 12–8. Congenital fusion of the elbow (radiohumeral).

rarely necessary because hand function enables children to compensate for fused elbow position. Resection of the fusion has had limited success because of recurrence and deficient elbow motors. A recent case, however, was reported in which a congenital radiohumeral synostosis was resected and useful elbow motion was obtained.[35] This suggests that resection may be rewarding, with the use of advanced management techniques such as the continuous passive motion machine.

DISLOCATION OF THE ELBOW [29–34, 37, 38, 40–42, 44]

Elbow dislocations in children are not very common (Fig. 12–9), but when they do occur, a hyperextension force is the usual cause. In these cases, the anterior capsule and brachialis muscle attachment are injured. Elbow dislocation can be distinguished from supracondylar fracture of the humerus by determining the relationship of the medial and lateral epicondyles and the olecranon with the elbow extended. They remain in a straight line in the supracondylar fracture, but this line is disrupted in the elbow dislocation. Elbow dislocations may compress the brachial artery and the median and ulnar nerves. Since separation of the medial epicondyle is a frequent concurrent injury, determining its position may be helpful in establishing the diagnosis.

Reduction of the elbow dislocation is accomplished by straight traction on the forearm and countertraction on the upper arm. Muscle relaxation by general anesthesia is usually necessary. After a successful reduction, full elbow motion should be present. The force causing the dislocation may fracture the medial epicondyle, placing it in the joint. In such cases a valgus stress and tension on the flexor-pronator muscle mass, or redislocation of the elbow, may be necessary to extract the medial epicondyle from the joint. If the medial epicondyle remains separated for a significant distance, reduction and fixation by percutaneous wire or by an open procedure may be necessary. Recurrent dislocation is rare (Fig. 12–10). Limited elbow motion is common after dislocation; hence, following reduction, limited exercises are started 10 days after casting.

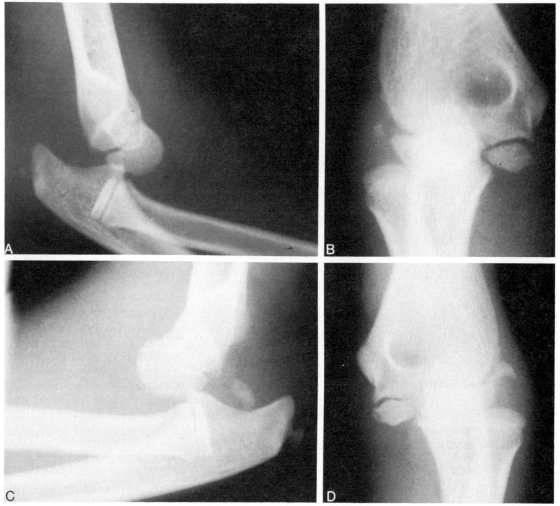

Figure 12–9. *A,* Traumatic dislocation of the elbow (lateral view). Note the shallow ulnar notch. *B,* Traumatic dislocation of the elbow (AP view). *C,* Recurrent traumatic dislocation of the elbow associated with lateral epicondylar avulsion fracture (lateral view). *D,* Recurrent traumatic dislocation of the elbow with lateral epicondylar fracture (AP view).

SUBLUXATION OF THE RADIAL HEAD (NURSEMAID'S ELBOW AND PULLED ELBOW) [45–49]

Subluxation of the radial head is an injury sustained in toddlers. Dissections performed in young children (aged 2 to 5 years) show that the radial head is very similar to that in the adult, even though x-rays project the head as round rather than flared, as seen in the adult. It is unlikely, therefore, that the annular ligament flips over the radial head with this injury, as has been reported. These dissections also show that in young children the annular ligament has an elasticity that permits the radial head to sublux on the capitellum when the arm is pulled, causing ef-fusion and hemorrhage (unpublished data). This increase in fluid within the joint causes pain because the capsule is distended. The mechanism of injury is a sudden pull on the extended arm with the forearm in pronation as the child is held by a helping hand to restrain a fall. Immediately after the episode the child will refuse to use the arm, and it hangs at his side. The elbow is held in slight flexion and the forearm in midpronation. Attempts to rotate the forearm and extend the elbow beyond a small range are resisted, and the child cries with the pain. The diagnosis is clinical, as x-rays are normal.

Reduction is accomplished by applying pressure over the radial head as the forearm is progressively supinated as the elbow is extended from 90 degrees of flexion. A palpable

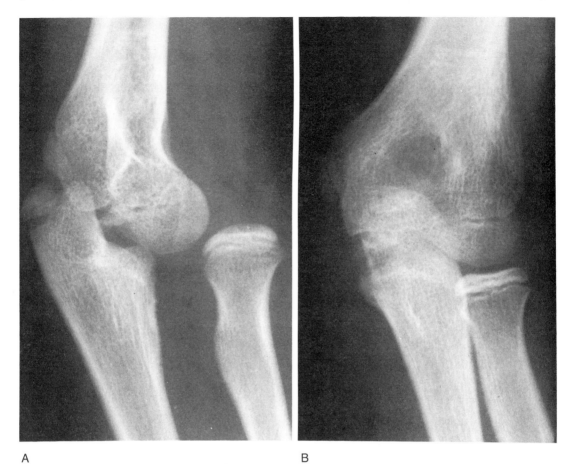

A   B

Figure 12–10. *A*, Recurrent dislocation of the elbow after trauma; *B*, postreduction (both AP views).

click is usually felt, and the symptoms disappear quickly. Late injuries (7 days) respond to the same maneuver, but symptoms take longer to resolve. Protection in a sling for a few days is all that is necessary. Although uncommon, the radial head subluxation on the capitellum may be repeated in the same child. Sling immobilization is recommended for several weeks in these repeated injuries, and after this treatment additional symptoms are rare.

SUPRACONDYLAR FRACTURE [50-71]

The most common elbow fracture in children is the supracondylar, which represents 60% of elbow fractures and usually occurs between the ages of 3 to 10 years. The most frequent mechanism of injury is a fall on the outstretched hand, forcing the hand into hyperextension and driving the distal fragment posteriorly. If the force continues, the distal end of the proximal fragment rides anteriorly

and the distal fragment posteriorly in either a medial or a lateral position. The displacement may be extreme and may resemble an elbow dislocation. Occasionally, the fracture is incomplete, showing prominence of the anterior and posterior fat pads on x-ray (Figs. 12–11 and 12–12). This injury should be treated with a long-arm cast for 1 month, with the elbow at 90 degrees and the forearm in neutral. A fall on the elbow in flexion causes rotation and anterior displacement of the distal condyles. The displacement of the fragments is less in the flexion type than in the extension supracondylar fracture (Fig. 12–13).

Treatment

The more common closed posterior supracondylar fracture can be reduced by traction and anterior translocation of the distal fragment, if treated soon after the injury. If an anteroposterior x-ray shows a gap between

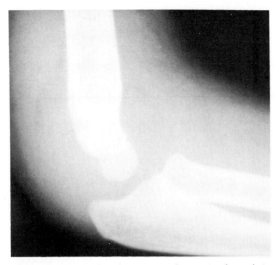

Figure 12–11. Displaced anterior and posterior fat pads in an undisplaced supracondylar fracture.

the lateral edges of the fracture fragments, the gap can be closed with forearm pronation provided that the fracture fragments are aligned in other planes. If the fracture fragments are not aligned, pronation of the fore-

arm will produce a valgus tilt of the distal fragment. The use of supination to reduce a supracondylar fracture may destabilize the distal fragment, causing a varus deformity. This will produce a gunstock deformity, a complication to be avoided (see Fig. 12–17). A delay permits swelling to occur, making closed reduction difficult. Reduction is maintained by placing the elbow in a long-arm cast, with the elbow flexed to 90 degrees, for 1 month. If acute flexion is required to maintain reduction, vascular compromise to the forearm and hand muscles may occur; in such cases the elbow position must be changed to accommodate the vascular situation. Alternative methods of treatment include skin traction (Dunlop's) or skeletal traction (utilizing a transolecranon pin holding the arm at the child's side or overhead in 90-90 traction). The method we have found best to reduce edema and maintain reduction without complications is the olecranon winged traction screw, which is inserted opposite the coronoid process of the ulna and distal to the physis and which has a series of holes that allow one to adjust to the tilt of

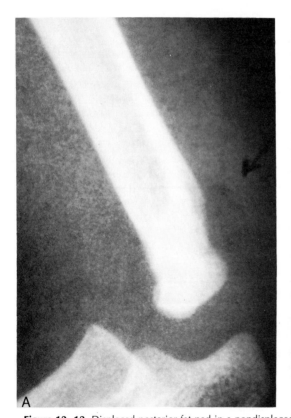

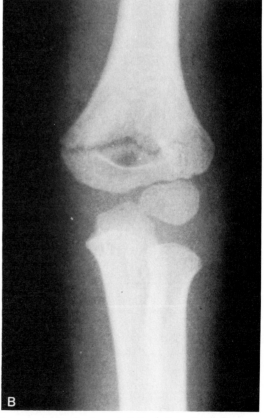

Figure 12–12. Displaced posterior fat pad in a nondisplaced supracondylar fracture. A, Lateral view; B, AP view.

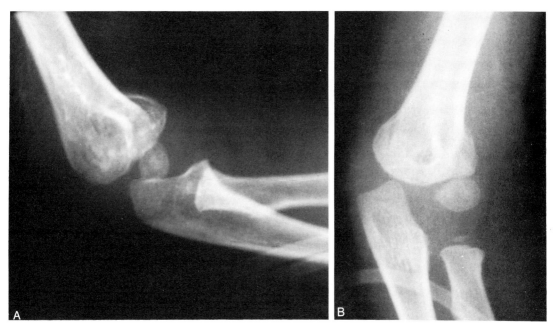

Figure 12–13. Anterior (flexion type) supracondylar fracture. *A,* Lateral view. *B,* AP view.

the distal fragment (Fig. 12–14). The screw is inserted under local anesthesia in the emergency room and traction is begun immediately, eliminating the usual delays in getting the patient to the operating room. The arm is placed in overhead 90-90 traction, a position that reduces swelling quickly and allows monitoring of the neurovascular status as well as fracture reduction. After 2 weeks, the bone is healed enough so that the child can be placed in a long-arm cast suspended from his neck with a sling through a plaster ring. The cast is worn for 3 weeks. The availability of image intensification in the operating room has popularized another treatment option, the percutaneous pinning of fragments with Kirschner wires. After closed reduction is checked by x-ray, Kirschner wires are introduced into the epicondyles and run across the fracture site at an angle of 40 degrees to the long axis of the humeral shaft. This method is more useful in older children, in whom it is easier to visualize the distal fragment by x-ray, enabling passage of the wire through bone in the distal fragment. After pinning, the elbow is placed in a splint at 90 degrees of flexion, or in whatever position is most satisfactory to accomplish fracture reduction. This technique has the advantage of accomplishing quick fracture stabilization, and it avoids a longer period of hospitalization, which is required by the skeletal traction techniques. The splint

is worn for 3 weeks, and then elbow motion is gradually started. If vascular complications occur, the K-wire fixation techniques permit soft tissue decompression without loss of the fracture reduction.

The presence of a supracondylar fracture should alert the clinician to the possibility of vascular compromise—either arterial or venous. Insufficient arterial inflow is the result of direct injury to the brachial artery by fracture fragments (Fig. 12–15) or brachial artery spasm. Venous obstruction is caused by swelling from the injury and pressure from a tight cast. The placement of the elbow in acute flexion to maintain fracture reduction may also impair circulation. If there is a vascular complication, circumferential dressings should be removed and the elbow positioned in less flexion. If the vascular situation improves, the extremity should be immobilized in a nonconstrictive dressing, iced, and elevated. The vascular situation should be followed closely by evaluating capillary filling and taking digital pressure recordings and temperature. Frequent clinical examinations and direct compartmental pressure measurements are helpful in assessment. If there is no improvement in circulation, the brachial vessels should be explored (Fig. 12–16). Spasm should be treated by topical lidocaine and arterial injury by excision and arterial reanastomosis or interposition vein graft. If the problem is venous,

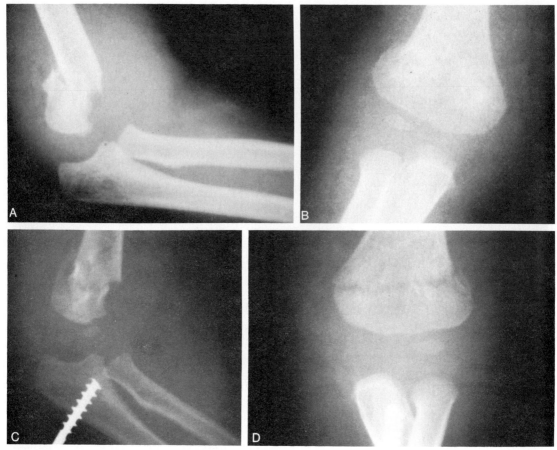

Figure 12–14. Posterior (extension type) supracondylar fracture. *A*, Lateral view. *B*, AP view. *C*, Lateral view postreduction with winged traction screw. *D*, AP postreduction view.

release of the facia and epimysium of individual muscles is necessary.

The complication of vascular insufficiency resulting from supracondylar fracture is Volkmann's ischemic contracture. Ischemic necrosis of the flexor muscles causes contracture of the flexors of the wrist, fingers, and thumb; this, combined with intrinsic paralysis due to nerve impairment, causes the "claw hand" position, hyperextension of the metacarpophalangeal joints, flexion of the interphalangeal joints, contracture of the thumb web, and flexion of the wrist. Six to 12 months of physical therapy, including dynamic splinting is recommended to prevent additional deformities. When serial clinical examinations and electrical studies show no improvement, removal of the scarred muscle to improve joint positioning and joint motion is necessary. If most of the involved muscles have been replaced by scar tissue, tendon transfer or a vascularized free muscle transfer is needed to provide power after the scar tissue has been removed. Impaired function

from nerve compression may be helped by neurolysis or nerve grafting in severe cases.

If malunion occurs, its alignment is altered with growth. This remodeling process has the greatest capacity for improving function if the deformity is in the axis of elbow motion (flexion-extension). Shoulder motion compensates for fractures that heal in positions of moderate malrotation. The common causes of poor results are fractures that heal in excessive medial or lateral tilts of the distal fragment. The gunstock deformity (cubitus varus) after a supracondylar fracture is the most disabling to upper extremity function and is a complication that should be avoided (Fig. 12–17).

FRACTURE OF THE LATERAL CONDYLE [72–78]

Fractures of the lateral condyle of the humerus are common and account for 20% of elbow fractures in children. The mechanism

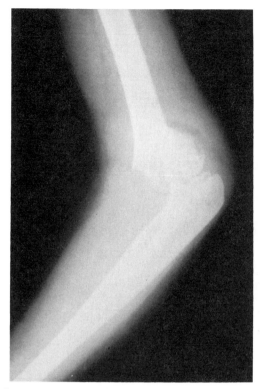

Figure 12–15. Anterior bone spike from proximal fragment injuring brachial artery.

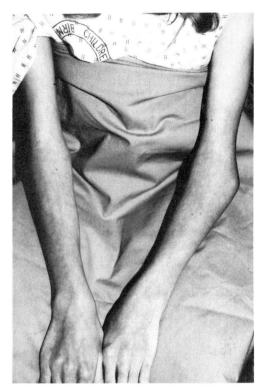

Figure 12–17. Gunstock deformity of the elbow (cubitus varus) after old supracondylar fracture.

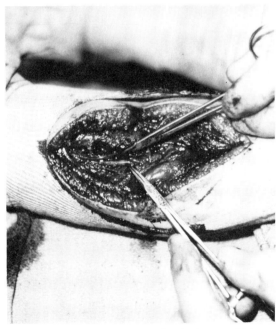

Figure 12–16. Hemostat points to brachial artery which was explored following injury from supracondylar fracture.

of injury is a fall on the outstretched hand with the force directed laterally. As the radial head impacts on the capitellum, the forearm goes into extension and the capitellum is fractured (Fig. 12–18A). If the injury is severe and the force continues, the elbow may dislocate. The fracture line begins in the trochlea and passes obliquely upward into the metaphysis above the capitellum and then out to the lateral epicondyle. Wadsworth[78] described four types of lateral condyle fractures: type 1, a metaphyseal fracture without displacement of the trochlea cartilage, which is stable and is treated with a cast; type 2, a fracture of the metaphysis and the trochlea cartilage with displacement, which is best seen in the lateral view and can be treated with closed reduction and casting; type 3, a displaced fracture of the lateral condyle, which is rotated 90 degrees and in which the articular surface opposes the bony metaphysis, requiring open reduction (Fig. 12–18C); and type 4, an injury resulting from repeated stresses rather than acute fracture and appearing as a form of osteochondritis dissecans on x-ray. This injury should be immobilized with a posterior splint or a cast with a collar and cuff until bone remodeling is seen on x-ray (6 to 8 weeks).

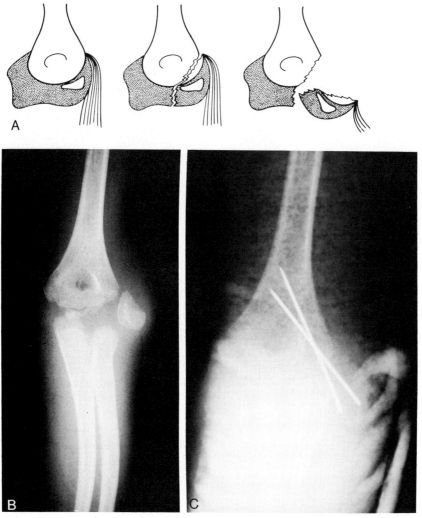

Figure 12–18. *A,* Illustration of the mechanism of lateral condylar fracture; *B,* lateral condylar fracture, displaced and rotated 90°; *C,* postreduction with crossed Kirschner wires.

All patients with displaced lateral condyle fractures are taken to the operating room, and a closed reduction is attempted under x-ray control. If the reduction is satisfactory, two smooth Kirschner wires are percutaneously passed across the fracture. It does not seem to make any difference if the wires are parallel or crossed. In some instances, the lateral condyle fracture is small; in such cases a Kirschner wire may have to be passed into the capitellum and across into the opposite cortex of the humerus for fixation. Small metaphyseal fragments may be difficult to visualize under image intensification; if there is any question about the position, open reduction and internal fixation are recommended. In such cases, the fragment is fixed with wires that are left long, so that after the skin is closed and swelling subsides, the wires can be removed through small stab wounds in the skin. The extremity is immobilized in a long-arm cast for 4 weeks, at which time the cast and pins are removed and exercises started. We have not observed growth plate disturbances from this pin-fixation technique.

Nonunion is a complication of this injury (Fig. 12–19). In such cases, the medial side of the distal humerus continues to grow and the lateral side lags behind, causing a progressive angular deformity. In some cases, the ulnar humeral articulation migrates laterally, increasing the carrying angle. Elbow extension is limited, but flexion is usually

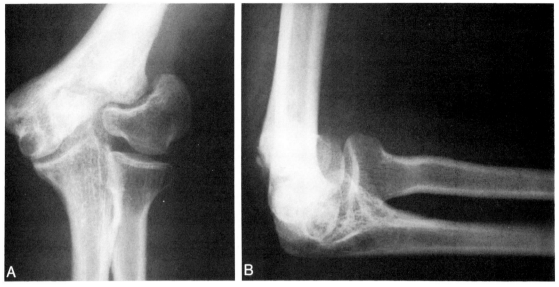

Figure 12–19. Nonunion of the old lateral condylar fracture with displacement and cubitus valgus: *A*, AP view; *B*, lateral view.

normal. Tardy ulnar palsy may result from stretching of the ulnar nerve many years (15 to 20) after the injury. Tardy ulnar palsy may require transposition of the ulnar nerve at a later date.

Jeffrey,[75] in 1958, recommended drilling the nonunion area and packing it with cancellous bone; Tajima[77] recommended taking down the nonunion, inserting an iliac bone graft, and osteotomizing the distal humerus to re-establish a normal carrying angle. Both these operations are difficult and have unpredictable results. Osteotomy of the distal humerus to restore a normal carrying angle may be indicated, but at a later time and in selected children. In the child, the nonunited fragment should not be excised.

Malunion of the lateral epicondyle is usually the result either of failure to recognize the displacement or of inadequate fixation after reduction. The fragment usually unites in a lateral position, and subsequent growth produces a V-shaped notch in the distal humerus, which has been described by Wadsworth[78] as a fishtail deformity. If the displacement is recognized early, it is possible to refracture the lateral condyle and obtain healing in a more satisfactory position. Lateral condyle fractures may stimulate overgrowth of the capitellum. In such cases, the normal carrying angle may be changed to neutral, but the overgrowth is usually not enough to alter normal elbow motion.

MEDIAL CONDYLE FRACTURES [79–82]

Fractures to the medial condyle or trochlear epiphysis are rare but may cause ulnar and/or median nerve palsy. A significant amount of soft tissue injury is seen with medial condyle fractures. If closed reduction of the fracture is unsatisfactory, open reduction and internal fixation with K-wires are recommended. Secure fixation usually results in prompt union and satisfactory elbow function.

INJURIES TO THE MEDIAL EPICONDYLE [83–87]

Blount[83] reported that fractures of the medial epicondyle account for 8% of elbow injuries in children. This injury is usually an avulsion fracture caused by a fall on the outstretched hand and extended elbow (Fig. 12–20). Elbow dislocation may result from a maximum force causing this injury. If a dislocation has not occurred and displacement of the medial epicondyle is only 1 or 2 mm, immobilization of the elbow in 90 degrees of flexion for 1 month is satisfactory treatment. The fragment will usually heal by bony union, but occasionally a fibrous union may result. If fragment displacement is 10 mm or more, reduction and fixation by percutaneous pinning or open fixation are neces-

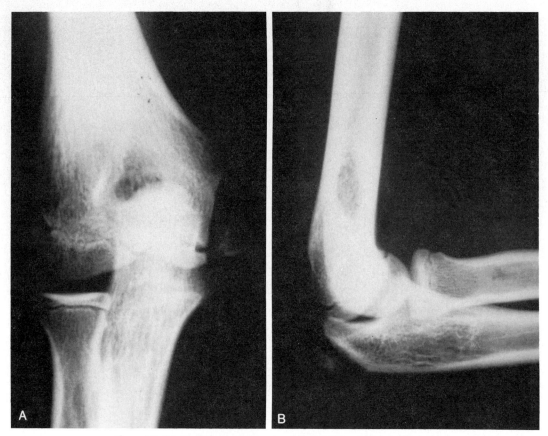

Figure 12–20. Medial epicondylar fracture, AP (*A*) and lateral (*B*) views.

sary. If the medial epicondyle is displaced in the elbow, its removal, reduction, and internal fixation are required. We have not observed any growth disturbance from this treatment. These fractures occasionally have ulnar nerve symptoms requiring release and transposition.

BICONDYLAR OR T-FRACTURES [80–90]

Bicondylar or T-fractures are quite common in the adult but rare in the child. These fractures are the result of severe trauma, and the clinical deformity is similar to that seen in the supracondylar fracture. One must reduce this fracture early to prevent neurovascular injuries. Reduction of the condylar fragments by skeletal traction is more important than the relationship of the fragments to the humeral shaft. A winged traction screw in the ulna or transverse ulnar pin with overhead 90-90 traction may be used. If traction fails to align the condyles, open reduction and internal fixation are required.

SEPARATION OF THE LOWER HUMERAL EPIPHYSIS [91–97]

Separation of the lower humeral epiphysis is an unusual injury and usually occurs in the infant. It is caused by a fall and may be a sequela of the battered child syndrome. The child presents with a markedly swollen elbow, and the displacement of the epiphysis is best recognized by comparative x-rays of the opposite elbow. Comparative elbow x-rays will also differentiate this injury from dislocation of the elbow and fractures of the lateral condyle. Since, in infants, elbow sepsis has a similar clinical presentation, if blood studies and systemic signs (temperature and pulse rate) suggest infection, joint aspiration is recommended. X-rays usually make the diagnosis, and if the injury is seen early, closed reduction is easily accomplished. As often occurs, the injury may be seen late, with significant callus and periosteal new bone. In these cases, a conservative program of splinting, exercise, and observation is recommended. Satisfactory remod-

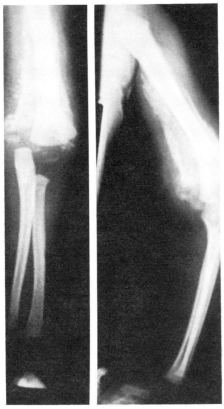

Figure 12–21. Healing Salter type I fracture of the lower humeral epiphysis with persistent displacement (in a battered child). Note the alignment of the callus and, therefore, of the epiphysis, with the proximal ulna. Remodeling from growth satisfactorily realigned the distal humerus.

eling of the bone after fracture usually occurs, and surgery is rarely required (Fig. 12–21).

INJURIES TO THE OLECRANON [98–101]

Injuries to the olecranon are uncommon in childhood. The mechanism is usually a fall on the bent elbow, by direct trauma to the olecranon. In most instances, displacement is not severe, and immobilization in a long-arm cast with the elbow at 90 degrees is all that is necessary (Fig. 12–22). Motion is started at 1 month. In the older child, the fracture may be angulated, with separation of the bone at the subcutaneous border of the ulna. In these cases, open reduction and fixation with smooth Kirschner wires or small Rush pins are recommended. We have not observed a growth disturbance of the olecranon epiphysis with this treatment.

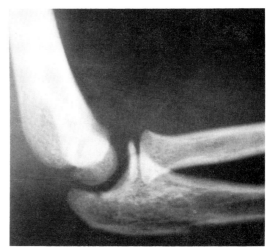

Figure 12–22. Undisplaced fracture of the olecranon.

References

Fetal Development of the Elbow

1. Gray DJ, Gardner E. Prenatal development of the human elbow joint. Am J Anat 88:429, 1951.
2. Wadsworth TG. The Elbow. New York, Churchill Livingstone, 1982.

Postnatal Development

3. Baugham FA Jr, Higgins JV, Wadsworth TG, et al. The carrying angle in sex chromosome anomalies. JAMA 230(5):718, 1974.
4. Beals RK. The normal carrying angle of the elbow. A radiographic study of 422 patients. Clin Orthop 119:194, 1976.
5. McCarthy SM, Ogden JA. Radiology of postnatal skeletal development. VI. Elbow joint, proximal radius and ulna. Skeletal Radiol 9(1):17, 1982.
6. Schwab GH, Bennett JB, Woods GW, et al. Biomechanics of elbow instability: the role of the medial collateral ligament. Clin Orthop 146:42, 1980.

Congenital Radioulnar Synostosis

7. Cross AR. Congenital bilateral radioulnar synostosis. Am J Dis Child 58:1259, 1939.
8. Davenport CB, Taylor HL, Nelson LS. Radio-ulnar synostosis. Arch Surg 8:705, 1924.
9. Dawson HGW. A congenital deformity of the forearm and its operative treatment. Br Med J 2:833, 1912.
10. Fahlstrom S. Radio-ulnar synostosis. J Bone Joint Surg 14:395, 1932.
11. Fergeson-Smith EA, Johnston AW, Handmaker SD. Primary amentia and micro-orchidism associated with an XXYY sex chromosome constitution. Lancet 2:184, 1960.
12. Green WT, Mital M. Congenital radio-ulnar synostosis: Its surgical treatment. J Bone Joint Surg (Am) 51:1042, 1969.
13. Green WT, Mital M. Congenital radio-ulnar synostosis: Surgical treatment. J Bone Joint Surg (Am) 61:738, 1979.

14. Henson HO, Andersen ON. Congenital radio-ulnar synostosis. Acta Orthop Scand 41:255, 1970.
15. Kelekian H, Doumanian A. Swivel for proximal radio-ulnar synostosis. J Bone Joint Surg (Am) 39:945, 1957.
16. Lewis WH. The development of the arm in man. Am J Anat 1:169, 1901.
17. Morrison J. Congenital radio-ulnar synostosis. Br J Med 2:1337, 1892.
18. Robinson GC, Miller JR, Dill FJ, et al. Klinefelter's syndrome with the XXYY sex chromosome complex. J Pediatr 65:266, 1964.
19. Roth PB. Case of congenital radio-ulnar synostosis after operation in a boy aged 10. Proc R Soc Med (Surg) 15:4, 1921–1922.
20. Simmons BP, Southmayd WW, Riseborough EJ. Congenital radioulnar synostosis. J Hand Surg 8:829, 1983.
21. Sledge CB. Some morphologic and experimental aspects of limb development. Clin Orthop 44:241, 1966.
22. Stretton JL. Congenital synostosis of radio-ulnar articulations. Br Med J 2:1519, 1905.
23. Tachdjian MO. Pediatric Orthopedics. Philadelphia, WB Saunders, 1972:105.
24. Wilkie DPD. Congenital radio-ulnar synostosis. Br J Surg 1:366, 1914.
25. Wynn-Davies R. Heritable Disorders in Orthopedic Practice. Oxford, Blackwell Scientific Publications, 1973:175.

Congenital Radial Head Dislocation

26. Danielisz L. Congenital dislocation of the head of the radius and elbow injury. Arch Chir Neerl 23:163, 1971.
27. Exarhou EI Antoniou NK. Congenital dislocation of the head of the radius. Acta Orthop Scand 41:551, 1970.
28. Fidalgo-Valdueza A. The nail-patella syndrome. A report of three families. J Bone Joint Surg (Br) 55:145, 1973.

Congenital Fusion of the Elbow; Dislocation of the Elbow

29. Bucknill TM. Anterior dislocation of the radial head in children. Proc R Soc Med 70(9):620, 1977.
30. Danielsson LG, Theander G. Traumatic dislocation of the radial head at birth. Acta Radiol (Diagn) (Stockh) 22(3b):379, 1981.
31. DeLee JC. Transverse divergent dislocation of the elbow in a child. Case report. J Bone Joint Surg (Am) 63(2):322, 1981.
32. Fowles JV, Rizkallah R. Intra-articular injuries of the elbow: pitfalls of diagnosis and treatment. Can Med Assoc J 114(2):125, 1976.
33. Green NE. Entrapment of the median nerve following elbow dislocation. J Pediatr Orthop 3(3):384, 1983.
34. Hallet J. Entrapment of the median nerve after dislocation of the elbow. A case report. J Bone Joint Surg (Br) 653(3):408, 1981.
35. K'iery L, Wouters HW. Congenital ankylosis of joints. Arch Chir Neerl 2(2):173, 1971.
36. Leisti J, Lachman RS, Rimoin DL. Humeroradial ankylosis associated with other congenital defects (the boomerang arm sign). Birth Defects 11(5):306, 1975.
37. Lloyd-Roberts GC, Bucknill TM. Anterior dislocation of the radial head in children: etiology, natural history and management. J Bone Joint Surg (Br) 59(4):402, 1977.
38. MacSween WA. Transposition of radius and ulna associated with dislocation of the elbow in a child. Injury 10(4):314, 1976.
39. Murphy HS, Hanson CG. Congenital humeroradial synostosis. J Bone Joint Surg 27:712, 1945.
40. Naidoo KS. Unreduced posterior dislocations of the elbow. J Bone Joint Surg (Br) 64(6):603, 1982.
41. Strauss RH, Lanese RR. Injuries among wrestlers in school and college tournaments. JAMA 248(16):2016, 1982.
42. Tayob AA, Shiveley RA. Bilateral elbow dislocations with intra-articular displacement of the medial epicondyles. J Trauma 20(4):332, 1980.
43. Williams, PF. The elbow in arthrogryposis. J Bone Joint Surg (Br) 55(4):834, 1973.
44. Zeier FG. Recurrent traumatic elbow dislocation. Clin Orthop (169):211, 1982.

Nursemaid's Elbow

45. Dimon JH III. Pulled elbow or babysitter's elbow. ONAJ 6(2):72, 1979.
46. Hardy RH. Pulled elbow. J R Coll Gen Pract 28(189):224, 1978.
47. Illingsworth CM. Pulled elbow: A study of 100 patients. Br Med J 2(5972):672, 1975.
48. Miller TO, Insall J. Radial head subluxation in adolescence. NY State J Med 75(1):80, 1975.
49. Salter RB, Zaltz C. Anatomic investigations of the mechanism of injury and pathologic anatomy of "pulled elbow" in young children. Clin Orthop 77:134, 1971.

Supracondylar Fracture

50. Aino VL, Lluch EE, Ramierz AM, et al. Percutaneous fixation of supracondylar fractures of the humerus in children. J Bone Joint Surg (Am) 59(7):914, 1977.
51. Arnold JA, Nasca RJ, Nelson CL. Supracondylar fractures of the humerus. The role of dynamic factors in prevention of deformity. J Bone Joint Surg 59(Am):386, 1977.
52. Bhuller GS, Hardy AE. Ipsilateral elbow and forearm injuries in children. Aust NZ J Surg 51(1):65, 1981.
53. Bongers KJ, Ponsen RJ. Use of Kirschner wires for percutaneous stabilization of supracondylar fractures of the humerus in children. Arch Chir Neerl 31(4):203, 1979.
54. Carcassone M, Bergoin M, Hornung H. Results of operative treatment of severe supracondylar fractures of the elbow in children. J Pediatr Surg 7(6):676, 1972.
55. Childress HM. Transarticular pin fixation in supracondylar fractures at the elbow in children. A case report. J Bone Joint Surg (Am) 54(7):1548, 1972.
56. Crawford AH, Oestreich AE. Danger of loss of reduction of supracondylar elbow fracture during radiography. J Pediatr Orthop 3(4):523, 1983.
57. D'Ambrosia RD. Supracondylar fractures of the humerus—prevention of cubitus varus. J Bone Joint Surg 54(Am):60, 1972.

58. D'Ambrosia RD, Zink W. Fractures of the elbow in children. Pediatr Annu 11(6):541, 550,1982.
59. Dodge HS. Displaced supracondylar fracture of the humerus in children—treatment by Dunlop's traction. J Bone Joint Surg 54(Am):1408, 1972.
60. Dowd GS, Hopcroft PW. Varus deformity in supracondylar fractures of the humerus in children. Injury 10(4):297, 1979.
61. Dunlop J. Transcondylar fractures of the humerus in childhood. J Bone Joint Surg 21:59, 1939.
62. Flynn JC, Matthews JG, Benoit RL. Blind pinning of displaced supracondylar fractures of the humerus in children. Sixteen years' experience with long-term follow-up. J Bone Joint Surg (Am) 56(2):263, 1974.
63. Fowles JV, Kassab MT. Displaced supracondylar fractures of the elbow in children. A report on the fixation of extension and flexion fractures by two lateral percutaneous pins. J Bone Joint Surg (Br) 56(3):490, 1974.
64. Kirk AA, Herndon W. Supracondylar fractures. VA Med Mthly 103(9):637, 1976.
65. Micheli LJ, Skolnick MD, Hall JE. Supracondylar fractures of the humerus in children. Am Fam Physician 19(3):100, 1979.
66. Morris PK. Supracondylar fracture of the humerus involving the elbow joint. Proc Mine Med Off Assoc 50(408):33, 1970.
67. Palmer EE, Niemann KMW, Veseley D, et al. Supracondylar fracture of the humerus in children. J Bone Joint Surg. 60(Am):653, 1978.
68. Rogers LF, Malave S Jr, White H, et al. Plastic bowing, torus and greenstick supracondylar fractures of the humerus: radiographic clues to obscure fractures of the elbow in children. Radiology 128(1):145, 1978.
69. Smith DN, Lee JR. The radiological diagnosis of post-traumatic effusion of the elbow joint and its clinical significance: the "displaced fat pad" sign. Injury 10(2):115, 1978.
70. Wieland AJ, Meyer S, Tolo VT, et al. Surgical treatment of displaced supracondylar fractures of the humerus in children. J Bone Joint Surg 60(Am):657, 1978.
71. Yousefzadeh DK, Jackson JH. Lipohemarthrosis of the elbow joint. Radiology 128(3):643, 1978.

Fractures of the Lateral Condyle

72. Flynn JC, Richards JF Jr. Non-union of minimally displaced fractures of the lateral condyle in the humerus in children. J Bone Joint Surg (Am) 52(6):1096, 1971.
73. Hardacre JA, Nahigian SH, Froimson AI, et al. Fractures of the lateral condyle of the humerus in children. J Bone Joint Surg (Am) 53(6):1083, 1971.
74. Holmes JC, Hall JE. Tardy ulnar nerve palsy in children. Clin Orthop (135):128, 1978.
75. Jeffrey CC. Non-union of the epiphysis of the lateral condyle of the humerus. J Bone Joint Surg 40(Br):396, 1958.
76. Micheli LJ, Santore R, Stanitski CL. Epiphyseal fractures of the elbow in children. Am Fam Physician 22(5):107, 1980.
77. Tajima T. Treatment of un-united fractures of the lateral humeral condyle. Personal communication, 1980.
78. Wadsworth TG. Injuries of the capitular (lateral humeral condyle) epiphysis. Clin Orthop 85:127, 1972.

Medial Condyle Fractures

79. Chacha PB. Fracture of the medial condyle of the humerus with rotational displacement. Report of two cases. J Bone Joint Surg (Am) 52(7):1433, 1970.
80. Fahey JJ, O'Brien ET. Fracture-separation of the medial humeral condyle in a child confused with fracture of the medial epicondyle. J Bone Joint Surg 53(6):1102, 1971.
81. Ho KC, Marmor L. Entrapment of the ulnar nerve at the elbow. Am J Surg 121(3):355, 1971.
82. Varma BP, Srivastava TP. Fracture of the medial condyle of the humerus in children: A report of 4 cases including the late sequelae. Injury 4(2):171, 1972.

Injuries to the Medial Epicondyle

83. Blount WP. Injuries about the elbow. *In* Blount WP (ed). Fractures in Children. Baltimore, Williams & Wilkins, 1954: 26–75.
84. Chessare JW, Rogers LF, White H, et al. Injuries of the medial epicondylar ossification center of the humerus. AJR 129(1):49, 1977.
85. Haw DW. Avulsion fracture of the medial epicondyle of the elbow in a young javelin thrower. Br J Sports Med 15(1):47, 1981.
86. Papavasiliou VA. Fracture-separation of the medial epicondylar epiphysis of the elbow joint. Clin Orthop (171):172, 1982.
87. Silberstein MJ, Brodeur AE, Graviss ER, et al. Some vagaries of the medial epicondyle. J Bone Joint Surg (Am) 63(4):524, 1981.

Bicondylar or T-Fractures

88. Bryan RS, Bickel WH. "T" condylar fractures of distal humerus. J Trauma 11(10):830, 1971.
89. Dangles C, Tylkowski C, Pankovich AM. Epicondylotrochlear fracture of the humerus before appearance of an ossification center. A case report. Clin Orthop (171):161, 1982.
90. Johansson H, Olerud S. Operative treatment of intercondylar fractures of the humerus. J Trauma 11(10):836, 1971.

Separation of the Lower Humeral Epiphysis

91. Dameron TB Jr. Transverse fractures of the distal humerus in children. AAOS Instructional Course Lectures 30:224, 1981.
92. Kaplan SS, Reckling FW. Fracture separation of the lower humeral epiphysis with medial displacement. Review of the literature and report of a case. J Bone Joint Surg (Am) 53(6):1105, 1971.
93. Laud NS, Babulkar SS. Rare epiphyseal injuries. A study of 6 cases with review of literature. J Postgrad Med 16(2):92, 1970.
94. Mizuno K, Hirohata K, Kashiwagi D. Fracture-separation of the distal humeral epiphysis in young children. J Bone Joint Surg (Am) 61:570, 1979.
95. Peiro A, Mut T, Aracil J, et al. Fracture-separation of the lower humeral epiphysis in young children. Acta Orthop Scand 52(3):295, 1981.
96. Rogers LF, Rockwood CA Jr. Separation of the entire distal humeral epiphysis. Radiology 106(2):393, 1973.
97. Specht EE. Epiphyseal injuries in childhood. Am Fam Physician 10(4):101, 1974.

Injuries to the Olecranon

98. Grandham SA, Kiernan HA Jr. Displaced olecranon fracture in children. J Trauma 15(3):197, 1975.

99. Torg JS, Moyer RA. Non-union of a stress fracture through the olecranon epiphyseal plate observed in an adolescent baseball pitcher. J Bone Joint Surg (Am) 59(2):264, 1977.

100. van der Horst CM, Keeman JN. Treatment of olecranon fractures. Neth J Surg 35(1):27, 1983.

101. Wilpulla E, Bakalim G. Fractures of the olecranon. Fractures complicated by forward dislocation of the forearm. Ann Chir Gynaecol Fenn 60(2):105, 1971.

CHAPTER ○ 13

Injuries to and Developmental Deformities of the Shoulder

ROBERT J. NEVIASER

Disorders of the shoulder in the pediatric population can be divided into congenital and traumatic types. Fortunately, the first type is rare, and the second uncommon. In order to appreciate the developmental, or congenital, anomalies better, a brief review of the intrauterine development of the shoulder girdle is appropriate.[3, 18]

ANATOMIC DEVELOPMENT OF THE SHOULDER

The development of the shoulder girdle occurs in the first 8 weeks following fertilization. Therefore, anomalies that may result in complete or partial absence or in duplication of parts occur during this time. The migration of the scapula or scapulohumeral complex from a position in the cervical region to the thoracic region begins at approximately the fifth week, and the migration is complete by the eighth week. The lower pole of the scapula moves from the level of the fifth cervical vertebra to a position opposite the fifth thoracic vertebra.

The upper end of the humerus evolves from three centers of ossification. The center for the humeral head appears between the fourth and sixth months after birth, uniting with those of the greater and lesser tuberosities between the seventh and fourteenth years. The ossification center for the greater tuberosity initially appears in the second or third year of life and the center for the lesser tuberosity appears in the fifth year. The tuberosities fuse together at this time as well. The complete fusion of the head of the humerus with the shaft occurs by the nineteenth year.

The scapula has several ossification centers. The one for the body is present at birth. The coracoid process develops from two centers, one near the middle appearing in the first year, and another at its base in the tenth year. The latter center also contributes to glenoid development. These ossification centers unite with the body of the scapula by age 15. A small ossification center at the tip of the coracoid appears at puberty and occasionally does not unite. The acromion process arises from two centers that appear at puberty and unite by age 22. Failure of union also occurs in the acromial ossification centers. The superior portion of the glenoid develops from the ossification center that appears at the base of the coracoid at age 10 and fuses by age 15. A lower center, horseshoe in shape, appears at puberty. If it does not appear, glenoid dysplasia results. Finally, two centers, one for the vertebral border and one for the inferior angle of the scapula, appear at puberty and unite at about 21 years.

The clavicle arises from two cartilaginous centers present at birth—the medial for the inner two thirds and the lateral for the outer third. Their failure to unite can lead to cleidocranial dysostosis or congenital pseudarthrosis of the clavicle.

Phylogeny

The evolution of the human shoulder demonstrates several important changes from mammalian shoulders. These changes are directly related to the functional demands of the human shoulder.[5] The deltoid tubercle has migrated distally, and the acromion has increased in size. Coupled with the marked increase in mass in the deltoid muscle, these changes emphasize the progressive importance of the deltoid in the human as opposed to other mammals. Additionally, the infraspinatus fossa is relatively larger in man, whereas the supraspinatus fossa is relatively smaller. These differences represent the importance of the deltoid-infraspinatus complex,[10] as opposed to the biceps-supraspinatus complex, in elevating the shoulder.

There also are evolutionary changes in the biceps mechanism. The bicipital groove migrates medially in association with the rotational development of the humerus. As a result, the biceps takes a less direct course over the humeral head to the scapula. The caudal migration of the scapula also shortens the distance between the center of rotation of the humeral head and the origin of the long head of the biceps. As a result, the biceps has no role in shoulder abduction or elevation in the human, whereas in lower forms it acts as a strong abductor and external rotator. The depth of the bicipital groove also varies considerably, and with flattening of the groove, attritional changes can occur that result in subluxation or dislocation of the long head of the biceps. These changes, in turn, can also be associated with tendinitis of the long head of the biceps.

CONGENITAL ANOMALIES

The congenital or developmental anomalies of the shoulder can be categorized according to the bone involved: the body of the scapula, the glenoid, the clavicle, and the upper end of the humerus.

Anomalies of the Scapula

Sprengel's Deformity. This congenital anomaly consists of a high, small malrotated scapula. Although it had been described earlier, in 1891 Sprengel stated that he believed this anomaly was a failure of descent of the scapula. Since that time the anomaly has borne his name. Nearly two thirds of affected youngsters have associated anomalies, including scoliosis; hemivertebra; abnormalities of the rib or vertebral segmentation; an omovertebral bone; spina bifida; clavicular malformation; renal anomalies; or hypoplasia of various muscles, including the pectoralis major, the trapezius, the rhomboid, the serratus anterior, and the latissimus dorsi.

The etiology is unclear. As mentioned, the scapula on the affected side is higher than normal, smaller, and malrotated (Fig. 13–1). In as many as 50% of the patients, there is an associated fibrous, cartilaginous, or osseous bar known as the omovertebral bone that extends from the vertebral border of the superior medial aspect of the scapula to the posterior elements of one of the fourth through seventh cervical vertebrae. The scapula is usually malrotated so that its inferior angle is situated dorsally and laterally, and the superior angle is located ventrally and medially. The clavicle on the affected side is usually straight. Scapulothoracic motion is usually limited, but glenohumeral motion should be normal. The amount of motion is often affected by the presence or absence of the omovertebral bone. Because of the straight configuration of the clavicle, there may be compression of the brachial plexus and the vessels between the scapula and the first rib, creating a thoracic outlet syndrome. This development must also be considered when surgical correction of the overall condition is contemplated.

The treatment of Sprengel's deformity depends on the degree of disability and loss of motion, the presence or absence of an omovertebral bone, the age of the child, associated

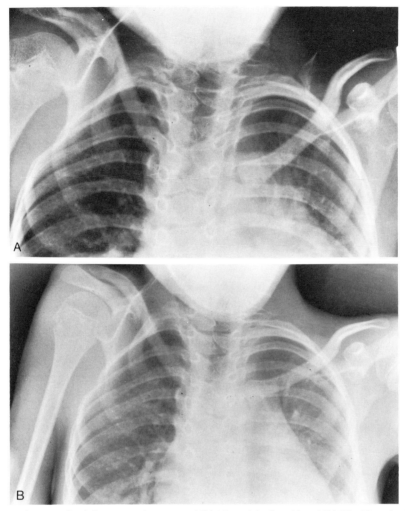

Figure 13–1. Typical Sprengel's deformity in the young child (A) and in the older child (B). (Note the high-riding small scapula on the right in both instances.)

abnormalities, and the skill and experience of the physicians involved. Generally, surgery is not indicated before a child is 3 to 4 years of age. An active exercise program to encourage shoulder motion is advisable but does not alter the basic underlying process or its functional limitations.

Between the ages of 3 and 7 one may consider operative correction of the deformity in a youngster who is significantly handicapped. In those who have minimal or only slight functional impairment, surgical correction should be undertaken only in the most unusual circumstances. There are a number of operative procedures which have been described to relocate the scapula at a lower position.[2, 6] Putti, Schrock, Ober, Green, and Woodward have described pro-

cedures that release the scapular attachments of the scapular muscles, resect the omovertebral bone, and lower the scapula. Subperiosteal dissection of the scapula has been advocated by Schrock and Ober, whereas resection of the supraspinous portion of the scapula has been utilized by Woodward, Green, and Schrock. The scapula is relocated to a more normal position in all procedures, and this position is maintained on a temporary basis by using either a traction wire, as described by Green, or heavy sutures to the ribs. An important adjunct to consider in those patients with a significantly straight clavicle is subperiosteal excision of the mid three-quarters of the clavicle with morcellation of the bone fragments and their replacement into the periosteal sleeve, which is subsequently sutured. This procedure avoids problems of thoracic outlet compression and allows the bone to remodel to accomodate the new position of the clavicle. Muscles that have been detached are then resutured to the scapula in its new position. Postoperative care includes immobilization in a Velpeau for 3 to 4 weeks, followed by an active rehabilitation program.

In those patients with a milder deformity, simple excision of the superior angle of the scapula and the omovertebral bone or band, if present, may give functional and esthetic improvement. This operation can be done in patients over age 8, whereas the more extensive scapular repositioning should not be done after that age.

Congenital Absence of the Scapula. Fortunately, this anomaly is quite rare and is almost invariably associated with amelia of the upper extremity on the affected side. Use of an upper limb prosthesis may improve bimanual function.

Nonunion of Ossification Centers of the Scapula. The three most common sites of failure of union are the tip of the coracoid, the acromion, and the lower epiphysis of the glenoid. The first two are far more common than the latter. Occasionally, the acromial nonunion site is misinterpreted as a fracture, especially when there is a history of injury. However, there is usually no evidence of ecchymosis or local tenderness, but x-ray examination reveals a regular, smooth line, which is usually bilateral. These anomalies do not require treatment.

Congenital Dysplasia or Hypoplasia of the Glenoid

This uncommon condition is due to failure of formation of either the upper or lower glenoid epiphysis, more commonly the lower one. The glenoid is flattened. Occasionally, it may be associated with various congenital anomalies such as Holt-Oram, Hurler's, Apert's, and other syndromes. Usually, however, the condition is an isolated anomaly, often bilateral. It is frequently asymptomatic, often being discovered on a routine x-ray (Fig. 13–2).

Occasionally, when the affected youngster reaches the mid-teens, glenohumeral instability may appear. Depending on the severity of symptoms and functional impairment, management varies from exercises to osteot-

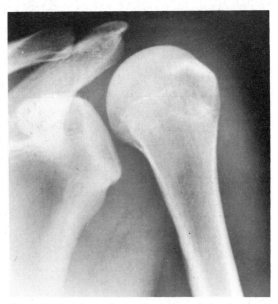

Figure 13–2. A hypoplastic glenoid in a skeletally mature individual. This condition noted on routine shoulder x-rays for other problems. This patient had no instability.

omy of the neck of the scapula, with an interpositional bone graft to improve the glenoid contour and reduce the symptoms of instability.

Anomalies of the Clavicle

Cleidocranial Dysostosis. This anomaly is an autosomal dominant condition that involves intramembranous bone formation. It results in bilateral absence of the clavicles, although on occasion portions of the clavicle may be ossified (Fig. 13–3). A dramatic clinical finding is the ability of the shoulders to touch in the mid-line when absence is bilateral. There is no treatment for this condition, although when small segments have been ossified and are hypermobile, these can be removed if necessary.

Congenital Pseudarthrosis of the Clavicle. This rare condition has been reported to be transmitted as an autosomal dominant trait, although many of the cases seem to be nonfamilial. Virtually all reports have involved the right clavicle. This condition should not be confused with the nonunion of a clavicular fracture occurring at birth: it is thought to arise from a failure of union between the medial and lateral ossification centers of the clavicle. In congenital pseudarthrosis of the clavicle, a painless, nontender, bony prominence is often noted immediately following

Figure 13–3. Cleidocranial dysostosis with small remnant of clavicle, medially.

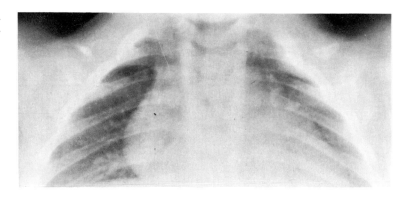

birth. The deformity increases with advancing age (Fig. 13–4, A and B). Fractures occurring at birth are associated with pseudoparalysis, pain on passive motion, and progressive callous formation noted on x-rays. Congenital pseudarthrosis, however, shows no reactive bone, and the ends of the fragments usually are well rounded. The typical "sucked candy" appearance seen in congenital pseudarthrosis of the tibia or other pseudarthroses associated with neurofibromatosis is not seen in congenital pseudarthrosis of the clavicle (Fig. 13–4, C, D, and E). As the child grows older, asymmetry of the shoulder girdle, winging of the scapula, and abnormal mobility of the fragments can be noted.

Indications for surgery include significant functional impairment or, in females, an appearance that is esthetically unacceptable.[7] To date, the most successful method of obtaining union is cancellous bone grafting with secure internal fixation (Fig. 13–4, F and G).[9] The recent popularity of electrical stimulation may eventually secure a place in the treatment of this entity but cannot be recommended now. External electrical stimulus is not useful because of the difficulty in proper positioning of the electrodes. Internal stimulus has been reported to achieve union, but the rate of complication from pin breakage and pin tract infection is significant.

Coracoclavicular Bar. This anomaly consists of a fibrous, a cartilaginous, or a bony bridge between the undersurface of the clavicle and the coracoid process. When present, the bridge restricts clavicular rotation and may limit shoulder motion. In the incomplete form, which is more common, the function may not be significantly impaired. The long-term outcome of the complete bar may be premature degenerative changes in the acromioclavicular joint, although these changes are also common in the general population. On a rare occasion, excision of a complete bar may be justified in order to improve shoulder motion.

Anomalies of the Humerus

Congenital or Developmental Humerus Varus. This affliction is rare. The developmental form is more common than the congenital, and it may be associated with fracture or epiphyseal injury to the proximal humerus during birth.[1] The condition may also be associated with osteochondrodystrophy and with metabolic disorders such as renal osteodystrophy and hypothyroidism.

The normal neck-shaft angle of the upper humerus is approximately 50 degrees. In humerus varus this angle may increase to as much as 90 degrees. In those patients in whom the epiphyseal plate is also in a varus position, the resulting shortening is severe, because 80% of the longitudinal growth of the humerus occurs at the proximal end. In those instances in which the growth plate is more normally oriented, the functional impairment is mild. It is rarely necessary to perform corrective osteotomies for this condition, because the functional limitation is rarely significant. When indicated, humeral osteotomy is generally successful and should be associated with an anterior-inferior acromioplasty and coracoacromial ligament resection.

Abnormalities of the Bicipital Groove. Flattening of the bicipital groove is a common anomaly (Fig. 13–5, A). When the medial wall is significantly flat and the groove is sufficiently wide, the long head of the biceps moves abnormally from side to side. This subluxation (Fig. 13–5, B) can result in

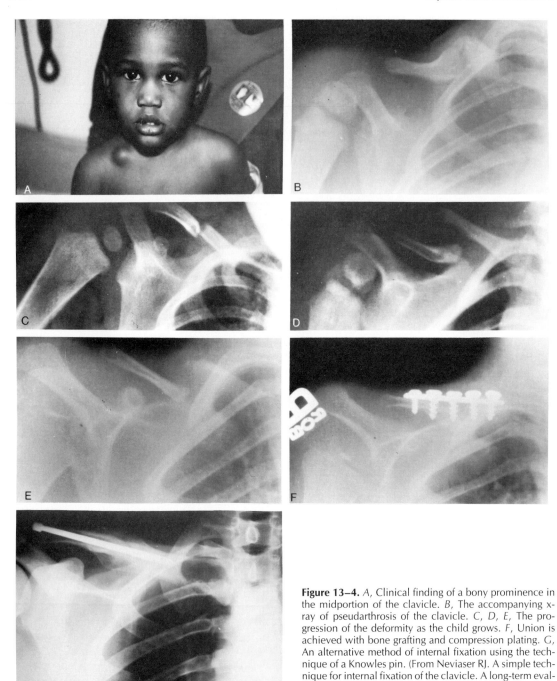

Figure 13–4. *A*, Clinical finding of a bony prominence in the midportion of the clavicle. *B*, The accompanying x-ray of pseudarthrosis of the clavicle. *C, D, E,* The progression of the deformity as the child grows. *F,* Union is achieved with bone grafting and compression plating. *G,* An alternative method of internal fixation using the technique of a Knowles pin. (From Neviaser RJ. A simple technique for internal fixation of the clavicle. A long-term evaluation. Clin Orthop Rel Res 109:103–107, 1975, by permission.)

an associated biceps tenosynovitis. Dislocation of the biceps tendon can only occur with an associated tear of the insertion of the subscapularis.[12, 13] Biceps tenosynovitis is usually part of a painful shoulder syndrome. It rarely becomes symptomatic before full maturity.

Treatment initially includes local or systemic antiinflammatory drugs, heat application prior to vigorous use, ice application after use, gentle stretching exercises, and a temporary avoidance of the offending activity. In those unusual instances in which nonoperative means are not successful in alle-

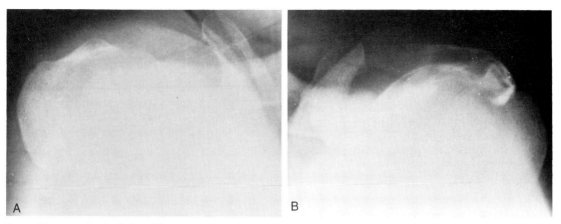

Figure 13–5. *A,* Flattened, broad bicipital groove. *B,* Subluxation of the biceps tendon medially associated with the hypoplastic bicipital groove. (This is an arthrographic demonstration.)

viating the pain and the problem sufficiently hampers the patients' normal lifestyle, a subacromial decompression, including a coracoacromial ligament resection, an anterior-inferior oblique acromioplasty, and an acromioclavicular arthroplasty, should be combined with tenodesis of the biceps in the groove to the transverse humeral ligament, with resection of the intraarticular portion.[11, 14, 15]

Muscle Anomalies About the Shoulder

Congenital or developmental absence of muscles about the shoulder is seen with some frequency. The most common abnormality is absence of the pectoralis major that involves either the sternal head, the clavicular head, or the entire muscle. These conditions are often associated with anomalies of the ipsilateral extremity, especially in the hand.

The presence of fibrotic bands involving the middle portion of the deltoid may be either congenital or iatrogenic. Repeated injections, especially of tetracyclines, into this muscle in children have been reported to lead to fibrotic bands in the middle portion of the deltoid. Whether congenital or iatrogenic, these bands create an abduction contracture of the shoulder and a peculiar posture. Treatment includes excision of the fibrotic portion of the deltoid, and a satisfactory result can be anticipated.

TRAUMATIC AFFLICTIONS OF THE SHOULDER

Trauma to the shoulder can be divided into fractures, epiphyseal injuries, and problems of instability.

Fractures of the Clavicle

The most frequently fractured bone in childhood is the clavicle. It is especially common in the newborn as a result of difficult deliveries. The displacement of the fragments is similar to that seen in adults from the pull of the sternocleidomastoid on the medial fragment.

The clinical picture often appears as a pseudoparalysis; the infant lies with the arm immobile at the side and cries on any attempt to move the extremity. The neurologic examination, including a check of reflexes and distal motor function, should be evaluated and found to be normal. This injury must be differentiated from brachial plexus injuries with true paralysis, in which the arm lies limply at the side but is not painful on attempts at motion. Treatment in the infant involves simply supporting the arm inside the nightshirt until it is healed. The deformity will mold and disappear with growth. In young children, a soft figure-of-eight dressing may be used. In teenagers, treatment is the same as for an adult, with a figure-of-eight dressing. The patient's raising of the arm above 30 degrees of abduction or forward flexion should be limited and its use should be restricted to below waist level.

Fractures of the Proximal Humeral Epiphysis

Although injury to the proximal humeral epiphysis is most common between the ages of 11 and 15, it can also be seen as a result of traumatic delivery. The injury is far more common in males than in females. In the infant a type of pseudoparalysis can be found. In the older child, the usual findings of fracture, including local swelling and tenderness with ecchymosis, are present. The arm may appear shortened with some prominence at the anterior axillary fold. Diagnosis should be confirmed by x-rays in the anterior-posterior (AP) and axillary dimensions, and comparison with the opposite side should be made. In infancy the diagnosis may be difficult because of the immaturity of the proximal humeral ossification centers.

Most fractures that are angulated more than 15 degrees are candidates for reduction. This decision, of course, depends on the age and remodeling potential of the child. The younger the child, the greater the remodeling potential. Incomplete remodeling is more common over age 11. Inability to achieve a closed reduction is rare, but when necessary, an open reduction can be justified. Internal fixation may or may not be needed but if required should be minimal. A technique using smooth Kirschner wires combined with a tension band is often sufficient. Threaded wires or other threaded devices, such as screws, across the epiphyseal plate should not be used.

Problems of Instability

Acromioclavicular Separation

Acromioclavicular dislocation in the young child is uncommon but does exist (Fig. 13–6, A). In the late teens, it is more common especially in athletic individuals (Fig. 13–6, B). The mechanism of injury is usually a blow on the anterior lateral aspect of the acromion that drives the scapulohumeral complex inferiorly. This action ruptures the acromioclavicular and coracoclavicular ligaments. These injuries have been classified into types I, II, and III, or sprains, subluxations, and dislocations, respectively. In type I, or sprain, the acromioclavicular ligaments are merely stretched. In type II, or subluxation, the acromioclavicular liga-

ments are disrupted, and the coracoclavicular ligaments are sprained but not completely ruptured. In type III all the supporting ligaments about the acromioclavicular joint are disrupted.

Physical examination usually demonstrates tenderness about a prominent distal clavicle. Upward pressure on the arm and downward pressure on the clavicle can reduce this obvious prominence. X-rays will show varying degrees of superior displacement of the clavicle in relation to the acromion. This deformity is produced by the weight of the arm pulling the scapula inferiorly, rather than by a force pulling the clavicle superiorly. Standing x-rays of both shoulders are helpful for comparison of both acromioclavicular joints, because occasionally one sees a normal acromioclavicular joint with apparent subluxation. Adding weights to the arms is not indicated, because it distorts the basic injury and gives a false interpretation to the degree of separation.

Treatment in types I and II is usually symptomatic. Support of the arm for a short time, while the acute reaction subsides, followed by progressive rehabilitation usually results in a functional shoulder. Type III, the complete separation, can also be treated symptomatically. Over a long period of time, with scarring in the region, the degree of separation will reduce. The functional result is often satisfactory, despite the prominence of the outer clavicle. Some authors advocate open reduction and pin fixation.[4] In the young child, care must be taken to use only a small, smooth pin that will not disrupt the epiphyseal plate. For those patients with chronic separations who are symptomatic, reduction with transfer of the coracoacromial ligament by detaching it from the coracoid and turning it superiorly to form a new superior acromioclavicular ligament has proved successful. In the patient with closed epiphyses, resection of the outer centimeter of the clavicle should also be part of the procedure.

Anterior Glenohumeral Instability

Anterior glenohumeral instability is seen in two forms: recurrent subluxation and recurrent dislocation. Both are far more common in the older teenager than in the younger child. Recurrent anterior subluxation has received greater attention in the recent literature than previously.[16] The group of patients

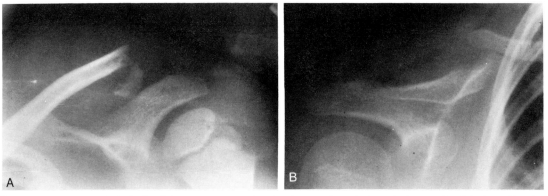

Figure 13–6. *A,* Acromioclavicular dislocation associated with a fracture through the articular margin of the lateral border of the clavicle. *B,* Acromioclavicular dislocation in a young child.

with this problem includes those who have had no overt dislocation, but who develop a "dead" feeling in the arm when it is in abduction, extension, and external rotation. Occasionally, they note a sense of the joint popping in and out of the socket. Those patients with recurrent anterior subluxation have been further classified into the involuntary and voluntary groups. The involuntary group includes those who cannot control the subluxation at all times. Although these patients can intentionally sublux their shoulders, they cannot prevent subluxation at other times, for example, during overhead motions such as serving in tennis. Those individuals in the voluntary group, on the other hand, have complete control over the mechanism, often performing this maneuver as a party trick or to gain sympathy from family and peers. These patients have no episodes of involuntary subluxation. It is important to differentiate these two groups because those in the latter group are rarely, if ever, candidates for surgery, and indeed may require psychiatric help. Such patients occasionally demonstrate hyperlaxity of all joints, the so-called Ehlers-Danlos syndrome. Patients in the involuntary group, however, usually have no precipitating emotional problems but may be significantly handicapped by the tendency of the shoulder to subluxate during athletic or other activities involving the abducted, externally rotated, extended position of the shoulder.

Physical examination of patients in the voluntary group demonstrates that they are able to subluxate their shoulder on command. Increased glenohumeral laxity can also be reproduced readily by the examiner and does not cause a sense of apprehension

or resistence on the part of the patient. Members of the involuntary group are able to subluxate the joint on command, but they are fearful to do so. The examiner can produce an apprehension sign by placing a thumb behind the humeral head and pressing it forward while the arm is held in 90 degrees of abduction, external rotation, and extension. The patient may resist placement of the arm in this position or performance of the maneuver, but the joint can occasionally be subluxated by the examiner causing the patient's arm to go "dead" or the patient's knees to buckle.

The pathologic anatomy of the involuntary subluxator is usually a Bankart lesion consisting of tear of the anterior-inferior portion of the glenoid labrum and the inferior glenohumeral ligaments. The voluntary type usually has only capsular redundancy.

Treatment of the voluntary type should be an exercise program and, when indicated, counseling for emotional problems. Treatment for the involuntary type should consist of exercises designed to strengthen the abductors and internal rotators first. Once these are strengthened, a program to strengthen external rotators should be undertaken. Before considering any surgical reconstruction, an adequate trial of 3 months of exercises is indicated. If the exercise program has been followed faithfully and is unsuccessful, surgical repair should be considered. Although many procedures have been described, the one that provides the most consistent success in alleviating the subluxation and in allowing the maximum postoperative motion is the Bankart procedure. When no overt Bankart lesion is present the modified Bankart procedure can be used.

Those patients with recurrent dislocation have long received the attention of the orthopedic community. When the initial dislocation occurs under the age of 20, the incidence of recurrent dislocation is extremely high.[17] Immobilization after the first episode of dislocation with the arm at the side and in internal rotation for a period of 3 weeks can reduce the recurrence rate by 10 to 15 percent. This still, however, leaves a rate of recurrence of approximately 75 to 80 percent. Immobilization following subsequent episodes of dislocation has no effect on altering the rate of recurrence.

The mechanism of injury is usually a forceful displacement of the involved arm into external rotation, abduction, and extension. The physical findings include a loss of the normal contour of the deltoid and the underlying humeral head, compared with the opposite side; the presence of the humeral head anteriorly; and the loss of prominence of the coracoid. X-rays should be taken in the routine AP plane and the axillary plane and will demonstrate an anterior displacement of the humeral head in relation to the glenoid. The pathologic anatomy of the dislocation is the Bankart lesion, consisting of detachment of the anterior-inferior glenoid labrum, which is an extension of the inferior glenohumeral ligaments.

When an acute dislocation is first seen by a physician, examination for a neurologic deficit should be undertaken prior to attempting the reduction. This examination specifically includes the axillary nerve, which has a variable sensibility pattern over the outer aspect of the skin of the shoulder overlying the deltoid muscle. Other neurologic lesions are uncommon, although branches of the brachial plexus are occasionally injured in severe associated trauma. Reduction can be affected by any one of a number of maneuvers. A frequently successful technique is to place the patient prone on a table with the involved shoulder and arm dangling over the side. After an intravenous dosage of analgesic, downward traction on the arm with one hand while placing the other in the axilla and directing the humeral head toward the glenoid can succeed in reducing a dislocation. Postreduction x-rays should be obtained in the anterior-posterior and the axillary plane. As long as the arm is kept anterior to the plane of the body and the hand in front of the head, dislocation will not recur when obtaining the axillary view.

After reduction, the arm should be maintained at the side and in internal rotation in a Velpeau' bandage. As indicated previously, if the dislocation is the first one, immobilization in this position for 3 weeks reduces the rate of recurrence slightly. If the dislocation is not the first, immobilization should be continued only for a few days for comfort; progressive use of the arm then should be allowed.

Once the second dislocation has occurred, discussion with the patient and the family concerning surgical reconstruction should ensue. The decision is, of course, an elective one, but the chance of redislocation is extremely high, and appropriate counseling and advice should be given so that the family can make an informed decision regarding surgical reconstruction. When the decision to proceed with surgery has been made, any number of procedures are available. The one most closely related to normal anatomy is the Bankart procedure, which restores the inferior glenohumeral ligaments to their natural attachment at the anterior-inferior glenoid labrum. When done properly, this procedure not only has an extremely high rate of success in preventing further dislocations but also provides more motion than any other procedure. If untreated, multiple dislocations can produce a posttraumatic arthropathy over a period of many years. In the older patient, an associated rotator cuff tear can accompany a violent anterior dislocation, but this complication is extremely rare in the young patient. Axillary nerve injuries do occur in varying degrees of severity, but rarely is the entire axillary nerve permanently damaged. When axillary nerve injury does occur, a baseline electrical study should be obtained at 3 weeks and shoulder function should be evaluated at subsequent office visits. Usually, within 6 months satisfactory function of the deltoid returns. In the interim, exercises to prevent stiffness of the shoulder should be undertaken.

Multidirectional Instability

This disorder is related to the problem of recurrent anterior subluxation. Those patients with multidirectional instability, however, have posterior and inferior instability as well. Many patterns of combined instability can be seen with this disorder: e.g., anterior and posterior, anterior and inferior, posterior and inferior (Fig. 13–7), or anterior, poste-

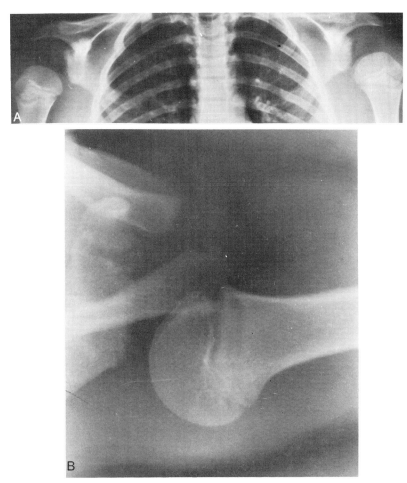

Figure 13–7. A, Anterior-posterior x-ray of a 10-year-old child with bilateral multidirectional instability. The shoulders subluxate inferiorly on this view. B, Axillary view of the same child demonstrating the posterior subluxation on one side.

rior, and inferior.[8] Many of these patients have hypermobility in other joints of their bodies. The pathologic defect of this lesion is capsular laxity. There is rarely a definitive history of injury, and an associated Bankart lesion is usually not present.

The diagnosis is sometimes difficult. The patient must be evaluated thoroughly to determine in which direction the shoulder is unstable. Occasionally, one can mistake the maneuver by which an anterior subluxation is reduced for posterior instability. Accordingly, unless the diagnosis is absolutely certain, examination under anesthesia and with the assistance of fluoroscopy may be necessary to establish the correct direction of the instability so that the appropriate therapy may be undertaken.

Therapy should consist of a program of strengthening exercises, specifically to strengthen the abductors of the shoulder and the appropriate muscles that control rotation. This means that if the instability is posterior and inferior, the exercises to strengthen the deltoid and external rotators should be given initially, whereas if the instability is anterior and inferior, exercises to strengthen external rotation and abduction should be given. Later, exercises for the rotators in the opposite direction should also be prescribed. Generally, a period of 6 to 12 weeks is necessary to evaluate whether or not the program will be successful. As a general rule, the exercise program can be very helpful in controlling the problem. If it is unsuccessful, surgical reconstruction is available but, fortunately, is rarely indicated. If the instability is anterior and inferior, a Bankart repair combined with an anterior-inferior capsular tightening is indicated. If the instability is posterior, a posterior Bankart procedure should be performed together with a posterior-inferior capsular tightening.

References

1. Bollini G, Rigault P. Humerus varus. Chir Pediatr 21:369–376, 1980.
2. Carson WG, Lovell WW, Whitesides TE Jr. Congenital elevation of the scapula. Surgical correction by the Woodward procedure. J Bone Joint Surg 63A:1199–1207, 1981.
3. Chung SMK, Nissenbaum MM. Congenital and developmental defects of the shoulder. Orthop Clin North Am 6:381–392, 1975.
4. Eidman DK, Siff SJ, Tullos HS. Acromioclavicular lesions in children. Am J Sports Med 9:150–154, 1981.
5. Inman VT, Saunder JB, Dec M, et al. Observations on the function of the shoulder joint. J Bone Joint Surg 26:1–30, 1944.
6. Klisick P, Filipovic M, Uzelac O, et al. Relocation of congenitally elevated scapula. J Pediatr Orthop 1:43–45, 1981.
7. Kohler R, Chappuis JP, Daudet M. Congenital pseudarthrosis of the clavicle, report of seven cases. Chir Pediatr 21:201–207, 1980.
8. Neer CS, Foster CR. Inferior capsular shift for involuntary inferior and multi-directional instability of the shoulder: a preliminary report. J Bone Joint Surg 62A:897–908, 1980.
9. Neviaser RJ, Neviaser JS, Neviaser TJ, et al. A simple technique for internal fixation of the clavicle. A long-term evaluation. Clin Orthop Rel Res 109:103–107, 1975.
10. Neviaser RJ. Anatomic considerations and examination of the shoulder. Orthop Clin North Am 11:187–195, 1980.
11. Neviaser, RJ. Lesions of the biceps and tendinitis of the shoulder. Orthop Clin North Am 11:343–348, 1980.
12. Neviaser RJ. Tears of the rotator cuff. Orthop Clin North Am 11:295–306, 1980.
13. Neviaser RJ, Neviaser TJ. Lesions of the musculotendinous cuff of the shoulder: diagnosis and management. Part A: Tears of the rotator cuff. AAOS Instructional Course Lectures vol 30. St. Louis, CV Mosby, 1981:239–250.
14. Neviaser TJ, Neviaser RJ. Lesions of the musculotendinous cuff of the shoulder: diagnosis and management. Part B: Lesions of the long head of the biceps tendon. AAOS Instructional Course Lectures, vol 30. St. Louis, CV Mosby, 1981:250–257.
15. Neviaser TJ, Neviaser RJ, Neviaser JS, et al. Four-in-one arthroplasty for the painful arc syndrome. Clin Orthop Rel Res 163:107–112, 1982.
16. Rowe CR, Zarins B. Recurrent transient subluxation of the shoulder. Bone Joint Surg 63A:863–872, 1981.
17. Rowe CR. Acute and recurrent anterior dislocations of the shoulder. Orthop Clin North Am 11:253–270, 1980.

CHAPTER ○ 1 4

Injuries to the Brachial Plexus

A. O. NARAKAS

The frequency of obstetrical palsy varies from 0.3 per 1000 births in developed countries to 8 per 1000 in underdeveloped regions. Adler and Patterson[1] reported the incidence of brachial palsy in the Hospital for Special Surgery in New York between 1928 and 1939 to be 1.56 per 1000, and in the period between 1939 and 1962 to be 0.38 per 1000; they attributed the decrease to improved delivery techniques. Sever[36-40] reported no difference in occurrence between boys and girls but found that the right upper limb was more frequently affected than the left because the former is usually delivered first (64%).

HISTORICAL REVIEW OF ETIOLOGY AND PATHOLOGY

Brachial plexus palsies of the newborn are probably as old as mankind but were not reported in the medical literature until the eighteenth century. Smillie,[41] in his book on midwifery, mentions a bilateral upper limb palsy at birth, after a forceps delivery. The condition he reported impressed his contemporaries and healed in a few days. Doherty[8] reported a palsy of the upper arm of a newborn, and Jacquemier[17] an isolated axillary nerve palsy that healed in 20 days. Danyau[6] was the first to do an autopsy on a baby who died 8 days after a forceps delivery; in this case, the brachial plexus was found infiltrated with blood and was in continuity with the spinal cord. DePaul[7] published observations of the extremity deformity without localizing the site of injury. Duchenne[9] was the first to report the clinical features of upper trunk lesions. Drawings from Duchenne's book show proximal and distal extremity deformities from obstetrical palsy (Fig. 14–1).

Erb[10] used electrical diagnostic techniques (in adults and in one child) to pinpoint the lesion to the upper trunk of the brachial plexus. This area has since been called Erb's point and the C5–C6 palsy was labeled an Erb-Duchenne palsy. Flaubert[13]* described a

* Flaubert described an iatrogenic lesion. An attempt was made to reduce a dislocated shoulder of 2 months' duration by violent traction on the upper limb. An avulsion of the plexus from the spinal cord resulted, with rupture of the subclavian artery. The patient died. The famous French writer, Gustave Flaubert, was the son of this surgeon of the Hôtel Dieu of Rouen.

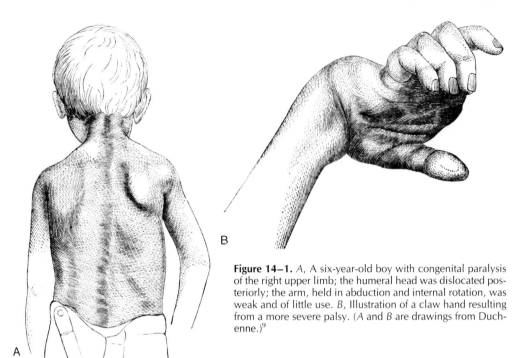

Figure 14–1. *A,* A six-year-old boy with congenital paralysis of the right upper limb; the humeral head was dislocated posteriorly; the arm, held in abduction and internal rotation, was weak and of little use. *B,* Illustration of a claw hand resulting from a more severe palsy. (*A* and *B* are drawings from Duchenne.)[9]

more severe type of iatrogenic palsy affecting the entire upper limb and associated with a Horner syndrome, which was thoroughly studied by Klumpke.[19]† Trombetta's analysis[48] of the forces acting on the plexus during delivery popularized the subject during that period, and a thesis by Cibert[5] reported a symposium on obstetrical palsy held in Paris. A summary from that meeting concluded that while traction or crush lesions between the clavicle and the first rib would heal if they were in continuity, ruptures of the nerves or avulsion from the spinal cord would not heal and would leave deformities.

Other historical papers on the causes of obstetrical palsy were by Weil,[51] Erlacher,[11] Rupilius,[31] Buda,[4] and Laurence,[22] who reported that the palsy occurred during fetal life by compression of the umbilical cord, abnormal position of the fetus, and shoulder dislocation. Van Neck[50] reported on two patients with aplasia of the brachial plexus, an observation made at surgery. Weil[51] and

Schubert[32] reported that genetic factors were responsible for obstetrical palsy, and Valentin[49] and Ombredanne[30] recorded obstetrical palsy in association with other deformities, including limb paralysis, underdevelopment of the scapula and clavicle, torticollis, scoliosis, spina bifida, and clubfoot.

Metaizeau et al.,[24] using stillborn infants, reported that continued traction on the head will progressively increase plexus damage. When the shoulder is forcibly depressed during a cephalic delivery, injury to the upper trunk (C5–C6) produces paralysis of the shoulder muscles with normal hand and wrist function. If the shoulder further impinges on the pelvic brim while being delivered, the C7 root may be stretched or avulsed from the spinal cord, resulting in a more complete palsy. Severe shoulder depression may injure or avulse C8 and T1 and cause a complete brachial plexus palsy with a Horner sign. Their observations were in agreement with those of Wickstrom.[52]

In the newborn, anterior flexion of the head produces an elongation of 25% of the upper trunk. If, at the same time, the shoulder is depressed and the head deviated and rotated to the opposite side, as in the cephalic delivery, the limits of elasticity of the upper trunk may be reached. Additional

---

† Augusta Klumpke was one of the four brilliant daughters of an American businessman. She studied medicine in Lausanne, Switzerland and went to Paris for residency. Her plans were barred by the famous neurologist, Dejerine, who opposed women who wanted to be doctors. Nevertheless, she married him seven years later.

force will stretch the trunk like dominoes— C5, C6, and the lower roots in numerical succession. This mechanism explains why C5–C6 lesions are more common in the cephalic delivery.

In breech delivery, the same mechanism is responsible if the upper extremity is delivered first and the shoulders are pressed by the obstetrician's finger while the head is not yet free. Also, traction on the lower roots when the arm is held above the head may result in a brachial palsy. Initially the lower roots would be involved, but with sufficient force the entire plexus may suffer. Bilateral upper extremity involvement is reported to be more frequent in breech deliveries. The distribution of lesions in 54 patients reported by Wickstrom[52] revealed a much higher percentage of upper plexus lesions (60%) when compared with the lower plexus (7%), with the remainder involving the entire plexus. These workers found lesions of the upper plexus to be functionally less severe than those occurring elsewhere. From these reports and more recent experiences, observers agree that most brachial plexus palsies are

due to an injury during delivery and are caused by stretch.

My classification of obstetrical palsy (Table 14–1) is based on the clinical course of children during the first 8 weeks after birth. These observations are correlated with nerve injuries (Fig. 14–2), classified in three types by Seddon and in five degrees by Sunderland (Table 14–2),[43, 44] and include a time frame recovery of specific muscle groups. Mild cases of upper trunk involvement (C5–C6) (type 1) have temporary shoulder and arm muscle palsy that heals in a few weeks. In more severe cases (Type 2), C5–C6 ruptures and C7 may be partially involved (neurapraxia-axonotmesis), producing shoulder and elbow paralysis and weak wrist and digit extension. The prognosis is unpredictable during the early weeks of life. Active shoulder motion rarely recovers, but elbow function is usually satisfactory. In such patients, the shoulder joint becomes limited in external rotation, and the child tries to compensate for shoulder motion with scapulothoracic motion. If the trapezius is not involved, the scapula is elevated. Over a

Table 14–1. **Classification and Prognosis in Obstetrical Palsy**

	Clinical Picture	Pathology Grades (Sunderland's degrees)	Recovery
Type I	C5–C6	1 & 2	Complete or almost in 1–8 weeks
Type II	C5–C6	Mixed 2 & 3	Elbow flexion: 1–4 wks Elbow extension: 1–8 wks
	C7	Mixed 1 & 2	Limited shoulder: 6–30 wks
Type III	C5–C6	4 or 5	Poor shoulder: 10–40 wks Elbow flexion: 16–40 wks
	C7	2 or 3	Elbow extension: 16–20 wks Wrist: 40–60 wks
	C8–T1 (no Horner sign)	1	Hand complete: 1–3 wks
Type IV	C5–C7	4 and/or 5	Poor shoulder: 10–40 wks Elbow flexion: 16–40 wks
	C8	Mixed 2–3	Elbow extension incomplete, poor: 20–60 wks or nil
	T1 (temporary Horner sign)	1 and 2	Wrist: 40–60 wks Hand complete: 20–60 wks
Type V	C5–C7 C7	5 or avulsed	Shoulder and elbow as above
	C8	3 or avulsed	Wrist poor or only extension; poor flexion or none
	T1	2 and 3	
	C8–T1 (Horner sign usually present)	Avulsed	Very poor hand with no or weak flexors and extensors; no intrinsics

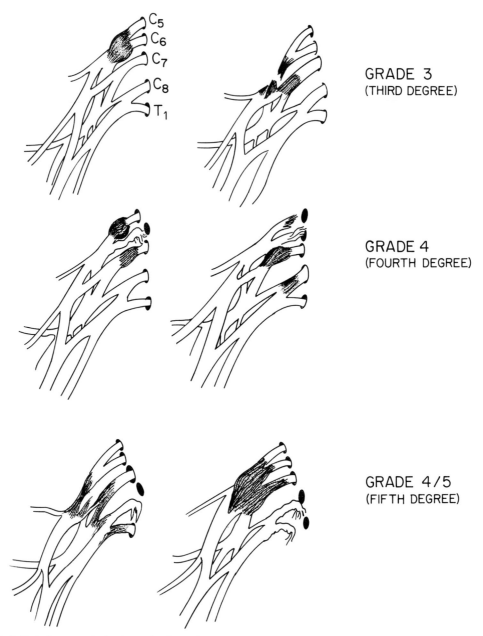

GRADE 3
(THIRD DEGREE)

GRADE 4
(FOURTH DEGREE)

GRADE 4/5
(FIFTH DEGREE)

Figure 14–2. Pathology seen in the types of palsy outlined in Table 14–1. No macroscopic alterations are seen in grades 1 and 2, which are not illustrated here. (Narakas; compare with Sunderland, Table 14–2).

period of time, the scapula, clavicle, and humerus become significantly smaller than on the contralateral univolved side. A few of the children in this group may not recover active wrist and digit extension, and tendon transfers to replace these functions are indicated.

More severe cases (Type 3) involve the upper trunk, with avulsion of C7 and stretch of C8–T1 roots. In such cases the palsy may be complete at birth with a temporary Horner sign, but hand and wrist function usually is

present in a few weeks. Flexor carpi ulnaris function returns early and, unopposed, pulls the wrist into ulnar deviation and volar flexion (Fig. 14–3).

A greater force avulses C8 and T1 (Type 4) and usually causes a persisting Horner sign (Fig. 14–4). I observed that a significant part of C_5 and C_6 function returned in 93 children who had complete paralysis when first examined. Severe injury involving all the nerve roots (Type 5) usually causes a permanent

Table 14–2. **Correlation of Seddon and Sunderland Classification of Nerve Injuries.**

		Sunderland					
		First	Second	Third	Fourth	Fifth	(Degree)
Seddon	Neurapraxia	▨					
	Axonotmesis		▨	▨			
	Neurotmesis				▨	▨	

Shaded areas indicate equivalent terms.

From Omer G Jr, Spinner M, eds. Management of Peripheral Nerve Problems, Philadelphia, WB Saunders, 1980, by permission.

Horner syndrome. The presence of a Horner sign and paralysis of the rhomboids, levator scapulae, and serratus anterior are ominous, for they indicate root damage and probable avulsion.

In evaluation of sympathetic function (e.g., Horner) it must be remembered that all roots of the plexus carry postganglionic sympathetic fibers to the periphery. The relative percentage contribution of sympathetic fibers to each individual root of the plexus varies. There are more postganglionic fibers in the eighth cervical root (25 to 45%) than in any other, and fewer postganglionic fibers in the fifth cervical root (1 to 5%). The sixth and seventh are intermediate (in cross-sectional density of postganglionic fibers). Therefore, 40 to 70% of the postganglionic fibers in the brachial plexus are contained in the lower trunk. This anatomic arrangement explains why lesions of the lower roots have greater sympathetic impairment than do upper root lesions. Forni and Giordani[14] observed that plexus lesions may also have peripheral nerve lesions; in the 164 cases they studied, 10% had radial nerve lesions at various levels.

At 1 year, most children with untreated brachial plexus palsy present with the shoulder in internal rotation, the elbow flexed, the wrist in extension, the metacarpophalangeal joints straight, and the interphalangeal joints flexed. The web between the thumb and index finger may be contracted, and in some cases active finger flexion is present. If T1 is spared, or if there is a contribution from T2 to the medial cord (as is seen in 2% of my operated cases), intrinsic activity may be fair, increasing hand function. Narakas[28, 29] and Alnot and Huten[2] reported that T1 may give a fiber contribution to the median nerve, explaining why some infants with C8 avulsion recover finger flexion. Flexion is enhanced by the phenomenon of the quadrigia effect of tendinous crossover between the flexor digitorum profundus tendons.

The deformity from obstetrical palsy becomes more obvious between the second and eighth months. Dislocation of the shoulder may occur, and in some cases the humeral head becomes oval and appears to articulate

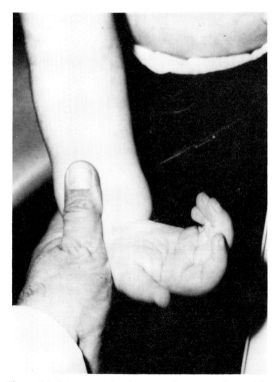

Figure 14–3. In type 3 involvement, there is paralysis of the wrist at birth, but after a few weeks flexor carpi ulnaris function returns, placing the wrist in flexion and ulnar deviation as seen in this patient.

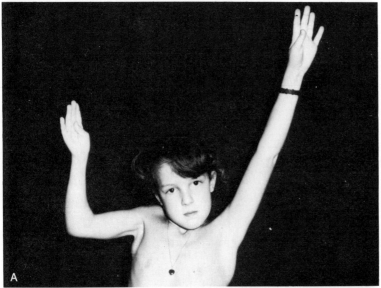

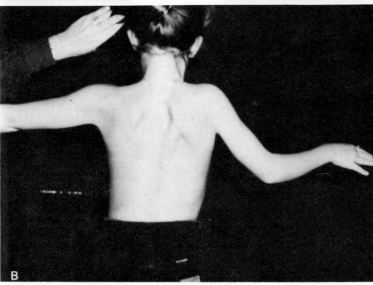

Figure 14–4. Type 4 lesions show early recovery of hand function and poor recovery of the muscles innervated by the upper three roots of the brachial plexus. Abduction "external rotation" is severely limited, and shoulder elevation is accomplished by scapulothoracic motion (*A* and *B*).

with both the acromion and the glenoid. Dislocation of the elbow has been reported in one third of the patients. Forearm and wrist deformities also appear, the former usually in supination and the latter in ulnar deviation. It is interesting that children rarely complain of pain with brachial plexus palsies—a problem that occurs frequently and is difficult to treat in adults. Sensory abnormalities are present in children with obstetrical palsy and depend upon the severity and extent of the lesion. Hyperesthesia appears when nerve regeneration occurs, and in severe cases sensation gradually changes from anesthesia to protective sensation after 2 years.

EARLY HISTORY OF THE TREATMENT OF OBSTETRICAL PALSY

The British surgeon Kennedy[18] reported operating on three patients with obstetrical palsy in 1902, including one, aged 2 months, who was observed to have scarring in the upper trunk (C5–C6). The scar was excised and direct nerve suture with chromic catgut was done. Active shoulder abduction to 90 degrees and good elbow flexion occurred 9 months later. Subsequently, various surgeons (Lange,[20] Fairbank,[12] Spitzy,[42] Thornburn,[47] and Wyeth and Sharpe[53]) have reported their results using direct suture, nerve grafting, nerve tubes, and nerve transfers (neurotization).

The classic reports of Sever[36–40] showed that many obstetrical palsies improved spontaneously and suggested that the satisfactory results of surgery in previous reports might have occurred without the surgery. Further reports by numerous authors (Bentzon,[3] Ombredanne,[30] Thomas,[46] Seddon,[33–35] Merle D'Aubigné,[23] and Guilleminet[16]) indicated that although spectacular results occasionally occurred with surgery, many traumatic injuries fared as well with conservative management.

Until the late 1960s, the standard of care consisted of immobilizing the involved extremity across the chest to prevent additional stretch on the plexus. Every time the baby was changed, the shoulder was passively abducted, externally rotated, and elevated (as were all joints distal to the shoulder) to prevent contractures. At 3 weeks, physiotherapy and intermittent splinting were recommended for short periods each day. In the late 1960s the advances in diagnostic technology—the EMG and the myelogram—made it possible to determine which injuries were unlikely to improve spontaneously. Armed with these methods and the new advances of surgical technology (magnification, fine instruments, and atraumatic sutures) physicians started treating selected cases of obstetrical plexus injury with surgery and obtained encouraging results.

THE SURGICAL TREATMENT OF OBSTETRICAL PALSY

Millesi[25, 26] in 1964 and Narakas[28,29] in 1965 started using microsurgical techniques in the treatment of brachial plexus injuries. When these cases were evaluated in the early seventies, the results were more satisfactory than those of earlier surgical treatment. Lascombes[21] reported on 12 operative cases of brachial plexus injuries in children in Nancy, and Tassin[45] reported on 230 cases seen in Paris. The latter report included 114 children who were operated on by Gilbert.[15] Gilbert's results were more satisfactory than those in all previous reports.

Three surgical maneuvers—neurolysis, autogenous nerve grafting, and neurotization—have been reported to improve func-

tion in selected cases of obstetrical palsy. Neurolysis is helpful in patients in whom there has been no improvement after a series of repeated clinical examinations and in whom, at surgery, perineural scar and scar in the epineurium were found and removed. Sometimes, it is not possible to remove the scar tissue, thus in some patients, after neurolysis, the improvement of muscle power is of no functional significance. In other patients, neurolysis has improved the power of the antagonist muscle and detracted from overall function of the limb. In my series, neurolysis has been helpful in only a few cases. Stretch lesions causing nerve gaps can be bridged by autogenous nerve tissues, which are satisfactory conduits of axon regeneration. Autogenous nerve grafting cannot be used in avulsion injuries, but it is especially helpful when the graft can be attached to a specific nerve, such as the musculocutaneous, for elbow flexion. Muscle paralysis from root avulsions may have function improved by nerve transfers, a procedure referred to as neurotization. Nerve-to-nerve transfer, using the intercostal to a peripheral nerve, yields favorable results in youngsters and adults, who can be taught to perform a new muscle function by the transplanted nerve. It is difficult to tell a 6-month-old baby to breathe deeply to contract his biceps, the objective of the intercostal to musculocutaneous neurotization procedure. In my experience, intercostal nerve transfers have had unsatisfactory results in young children. In a few cases in which I have observed improved function after nerve transfer, the muscle innervated by the transfer acts as an isolated entity and not in synchrony with other working muscles. In rare instances, exploration of the plexus has shown nerve lesions that could be repaired directly; in these cases the surgeons should seize the opportunity and do a direct suture.

Indications and Surgical Technique

I have treated 93 children for obstetrical palsy and have observed that if the biceps has not become active at 3 months, the baby will have minimal shoulder control. If the biceps has not recovered by 10 months, shoulder function will be very poor. In my clinic a child with a brachial palsy has a muscle test in the first week, at 1 month, and at 2 months. If shoulder and elbow muscle groups are paralyzed at 3 months, surgical exploration of the upper plexus is performed.

The operation should be performed by a surgeon trained in microsurgery and in brachial plexus surgery. A transverse incision across the subclavian groove or a combination of a transverse and an oblique incision on the neck, along the posterior border of the sternocleidomastoid muscle, exposes the scalene outlet and the upper three spinal nerves. In a complete palsy the incision is extended in front of the shoulder, and the clavicle and subclavius muscle are divided to expose the lower plexus. If neuromas are observed on the trunks and intraoperative electrical tests show no conduction, they are excised and the gap filled with sural nerves harvested from the legs. If nerve roots are avulsed, they are identified and the operation abandoned. Wound closure includes fixing the clavicle with a suture or pin and the routine closure of soft tissue layers. The extremity is immobilized across the chest, and the baby is put in a previously made splint, which holds his head, neck, and shoulders, for 3 weeks. If at 8 months there is limitation of external rotation, a subscapularis muscle release from the scapula is performed, avoiding the shoulder joint. Other reconstructive procedures may be required at a later time (2 to 3 years).

Older Children

The results of surgery for obstetrical plexus lesions in older children are less rewarding. When surgery is undertaken, the parents must be informed that some recovered function (elbow flexion) may be lost temporarily while nerve regeneration is occurring.

Results of Operative Treatment

Gilbert[15] (Paris) has operated on 160 children and has followed over 100 patients for two years. He reported an improvement in 65%, results being better in types 3 and 4 compared with type 5 (Table 14–1). Fifty percent of those in type 3 (involvement of C5–C6 with mild damage to C7) (Table 14–1) improved showing abduction and elevation of the shoulder above 150 degrees with satisfactory external rotation and normal elbow

and forearm function (Figs. 14–5 to 14–7). In 25% of the patients, abduction and elevation of the shoulder ranged from 120 to 140 degrees, with external rotation to neutral. Elbow flexion in these cases was good. The

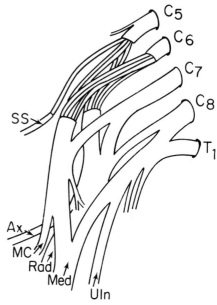

Figure 14–5. A drawing of the surgical procedure performed at 7 months in a grade 3 lesion, in which a neuroma was removed from C-5 and C-6, and the gap is treated with autologous grafting. C-7 had a stretch injury that did not require surgery.

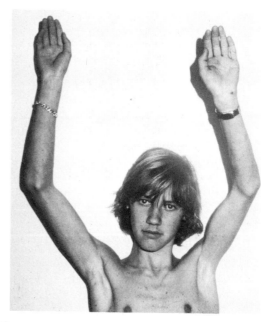

Figure 14–6. Twelve years after the surgery depicted in Figure 5, the youth is left with a short left upper extremity but with satisfactory function.

Figure 14–7. The same youth, who has limited external rotation of the shoulder but good flexion of the elbow and good hand and wrist function.

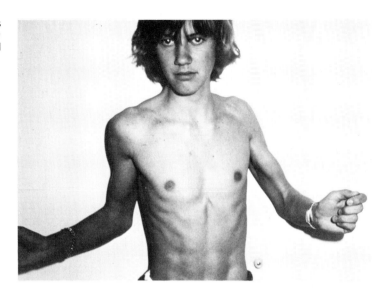

remaining 25% obtained limited shoulder motion to 90 to 100 degrees (abduction, elevation) with external rotation of the shoulder to neutral (Fig. 14–8). In the older child the extremity is several centimeters (4 to 8 cm) shorter than the contralateral univolved side (Fig. 14–9). These type 3 patients may require additional reconstructive surgery around the shoulder at a later date (2 to 3 years). Twenty-five percent of patients in type 4 can be improved to type 2 (Table 14–1), with the remaining 75% having poorer re-

sults. Half will reach type 2 shoulder function but will have limited function of the elbow and difficulties in pronation and supination. Their hand will be awkward and smaller and their extremity 4 cm shorter

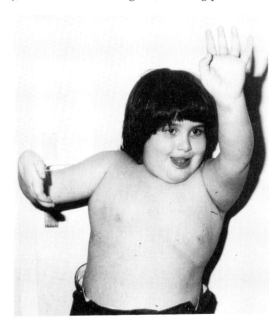

Figure 14–8. A child with a severe type 3 lesion has recovery of abduction to 90 degrees with recovery of external rotation to neutral.

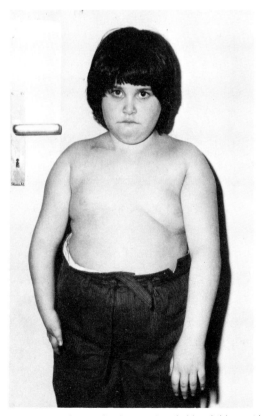

Figure 14–9. The involved extremity of older children with unilateral brachial plexus palsy is 4 to 8 cm shorter than the contralateral, uninvolved side.

when compared with the contralateral uninvolved side at age 3 years. Twenty-five percent of the children operated on were type 5 patients (Table 14–1); 25% of these type 5 patients obtained acceptable prehension and limited elbow motion, with a marked supination deformity and an extremity 6 cm shorter than the contralateral univolved side at age 5 years. Their Horner sign persists for life. Another 25% of group 5 was improved to type 4 (Table 14–1), and the remaining 50% of type 5 who had surgery were not improved. Morelli[27] operated on 28 cases and reached similar results.

BRACHIAL PLEXUS INJURIES FROM OTHER CAUSES

Over the past 20 years, 1100 brachial plexus injuries have been referred to the author for evaluation. In this series, 31 children (under 15 years) were seen; of these injuries, 17 resulted from motor vehicle accidents, two from skiing, and one from playing a game. Four patients had lacerations—two from gunshot wounds, one from electrical current, and one from iatrogenic causes after a cervical node excision. Seven other patients had brachial plexus impairment—three from vaccinations, two from tumors, and two from congenital malformations (partial plexus aplasia). Eleven of the 17 children with brachial plexus injuries from motor vehicle accidents had surgery, 8 of whom had supraclavicular lesions with avulsion of the upper roots (C5–C7) from the spinal cord. The other three patients had rupture of C5 with traction lesions of the remaining roots.

Clinical evaluation, electrical diagnostic studies, myelography, and computerized tomography were used to define the lesion before surgery. In one case, computerized tomography showed that C5–C6 roots were avulsed and that C7 was stretched, a diagnosis that once could not have been made before surgery.

The exposure for traumatic brachial plexus lesions in children is the same as has been previously described for obstetrical palsy. Avulsion injuries have been reported to be treated with intercostal nerve transfers (neurotization), a procedure that has not produced any useful muscle reinnervation in my series. Small children have difficulty in making the central transition to voluntarily initiate muscle action in a nerve that was intended for an entirely different function.

After surgery the extremity is immobilized across the chest for 3 weeks, and, after wound healing, all paralyzed joints are carried through a full range of passive motion until muscle innervation appears. In some cases, low-frequency electrotherapy is used as a means of muscle stimulation. It is important that rehabilitation modalities not interfere with school education.

I have operated on 11 children with traction injuries, and although this is not enough to allow any statistical evaluation, it is my impression that they do better than adults (350 operated). These children with traumatic palsy do not do as well as the children with obstetrical palsy after surgery. The violence of trauma may effect the regeneration potential of the nerve cells. These children also frequently have serious injuries affecting other parts of their body, which makes rehabilitation more difficult.

Children with avulsions of the lower roots (C7–C8 and T1) have the greatest problems with sensory dysfunction because their hand is insensate. Even if these children recover muscle control of the shoulder and elbow, the extremity is repeatedly injured and is placed in an awkward and extreme posture, such as leaning on the dorsum of the wrist when crawling. Children with this injury frequently suck their thumbs, and I have observed one child who destroyed the thumb to the level of the metacarpophalangeal joint by causing repeated infections and ulcerations. Chronic infection of the fingertips is a frequent complication in these cases.

Pain problems do exist in children with traction injuries, although they are not the major problem that they are in adults. The surgical removal of the extremity for pain is not indicated because the central interpretation of the pain persists (phantom limb) and the clinical situation is not improved. Sensory tests in our clinic show protective sensation to return 2 years after surgery.

Self-portraits by children with traumatic brachial plexus injuries show an altered body image (Fig. 14–10). It is interesting that these children seem to draw a projected image rather than a mirror image of themselves. One child in my series sustained a traumatic injury to the levels of C5–T1 at age 2 1/2 years and had this injury surgically treated with nerve grafting. Electrical diagnostic studies showed fair to good reinner-

Figure 14–10. *A*, Self-portrait of a child after an extremity implantation at the shoulder (the arm was insensate) shows an altered body image. The head is asymmetric and tilted, and the involved extremity is absent or articulating with the body at an abnormal location (the head or neck). *B*, The same child drew this self-portrait 6 years and 2 months after implantation. The limb, though deformed, has regained sensation.

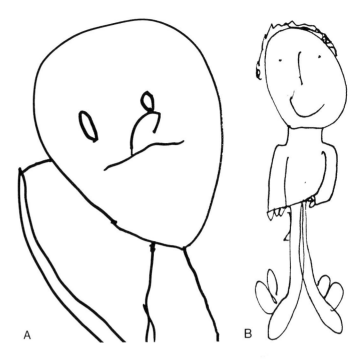

A   B

vation 2 years after the surgery, but the child did not use the extremity for activities. At age 13 years, the child became more conscious of his body and his external world and started using the extremity; at age 14 years, he developed satisfactory active motion of the shoulder, elbow, wrist, and fingers.

Three children sustained lacerations of the brachial plexus that were repaired within a few weeks, with very satisfactory results. Direct suture and nerve grafts were used in each case. No difference was noted in the results of injury at similar levels that were treated by direct suture and nerve grafting. Shoulder, elbow and wrist motion, and strength were satisfactory in these cases, and median and ulnar intrinsic function returned to 50% of normal at 5 years.

Extremity function with a fixed internal rotation contracture may be improved by lengthening the subscapularis tendon. However, if the deltoid and external rotators are weak, this procedure is not helpful because a tight shoulder joint stabilizes the humerus to the glenoid so that the extremity can be moved by the muscles that control the scapula.

Other reconstructive procedures that improve shoulder function include tendon transfers and humeral shaft osteotomy. Tendon transfer using the pectoralis major, latissimus dorsi, or sternocleidomastoid has been reported to improve elbow flexion.

Hand function may be improved by capsulotomies to improve motion of stiff joint deformities and by tendon transfers to provide active joint motion. After nerve surgery on the brachial plexus these procedures should be delayed for 2 to 3 years to be sure nerve regeneration is maximal.

The author wishes to express his thanks to Professor M. Bettex, Head of the Paediatric Surgery Department, University Hospital of Berne, and Professor N. Genton, Head of the Paediatric Surgery Clinic, University of Lausanne, for the operative facilities given him to treat patients in their respective departments.

References

1. Adler J. Erb's palsy: Long term results of treatment in 88 cases. J Bone Joint Surg 49A:1052–1064, 1967.
2. Alnot JY, Huten B. La systematisation du plexus brachial. Rev Chir Orthop 63:27–34, 1977.
3. Bentzon PGK. De obstetriske lammelser af plexus brachialis. Disputats Levin of Munksgaard, Kobenhavn, 1922.
4. Buda R. Isolierte Phrenikuslahmung bei einem Saügling mit Schwieglig entartetem Musculus Sternocleidomastoideus. Ost Z Kinderf 1:98–102, 1947.
5. Cibert M. Thèse: Paralysies radiculaires obstetricales, No. 130, Lyon, 1897.
6. Danyau M. communication d'un cas de paralysie du membre supérieur. Bull Soc Chir 2:48–51, 1851.
7. Depaul. Gaz Hôpitaux 90, 1867.
8. Doherty. Nervous affections in young infants. Dublin J Med Sci 25:82, 1844.
9. Duchenne. De l'électrisation localisée et de son ap-

plication à la pathologie et à la thérapeutique. 3:357–362. Paris, Baillière, 1872.

9a. Duval et Guillain. Pathogénie des accidents nerveux consécutifs aux luxations et traumatismes de l'épaule. Arch Gén Med 2:143, 1898.

10. Erb WH. Uber eine eigenthümliche Localisation von Lähmungen im Plexus Brachialis. Verhandl D. Naturnist Ver Heidelberg 2:130–137, 1874.

11. Erlacher P. Zur Entstehung de angeborenen Plexus oder Schulterlahmung. Arch Orthop Unfallchir 21:28–42, 1923.

12. Fairbank H. Subluxation of the shoulder joint in infants and young children. Lancet 1:1217–1223, 1913.

13. Flaubert M. Mémoire sur plusieurs cas de luxation. Rep Gén Anat Phys Pathol 3:55–69, 1827.

14. Forni L, Giordani C. Le paralysie ostetrichi tronculari dell arto superiore. Chir Org Mov 40:120–139, 1954.

15. Gilbert A. Personal communication, 1983.

16. Guilleminet M. Les paralysies obstetricales du membre supérieur à la période initiale. Ann Chir Infant 3:6–31, 1962.

17. Jacquemier. Manuel des accouchements 2:785, 1846.

18. Kennedy R. Further notes on the treatment of birth paralysis of the upper extremity by suture of the 5th and 6th cervical nerves. Br Med J 2:1065–1068, 1904.

19. Klumpke A. Contribution à l'étude des paralysies radiculaires du plexus branchial. Rev Med 5:591–790, 1885.

20. Lange W. Schultergelenkdistorsion und Entbindugslähmung. Verh Deutsch Gesell Orthop 11:348, 1912.

21. Lascombes P. Thèse: les paralysies obstricales du plexus brachial chez le nourrisson. Resultats du traitement précoce par micro-chirurgie plexulaire (A propos de 12 observations), 1982.

22. Laurence. Cited by C Fritsch, Thèse: Etude clinique des paralysies brachiales obstetricales, 1983.

23. Merle d'Aubigné R. Chirurgie orthopédique des paralysies. 122–139, 1956.

24. Metaizeau J, Gayet C, Plenat F. Les lésions obstetricales du plexus brachial. Chir Paediatr 20:159–163, 1979.

25. Millesi H. Résultats tardifs de la greffe nerveuse interfasciculaire. Chirurgie réparatrice des lésions du plexus brachial. Rev Med Suisse Romande, 511–519, 1973.

26. Millesi H. Surgical management of brachial plexus injuries. J Hand Surg 2:367–379, 1977.

27. Morelli E, Raimondi PL, Saporiti E. Le paralisi ostetriche. Il loro trattamento precoce. In Pipino F (ed). Le Paralisi Ostetriche. Bologna, Aulo Gaggi, 1984:57–76.

28. Narakas A, Verdan C. Les greffes nerveuses.

29. Narakas A. Plexo braquial. Terapeutica quirurgica directa. Tecnica. Indicacion operatoria. Resultados. In cirurgia de los nervios perifericos. Rev Orthop Trauma 16 Ib:860–925, 1972.

30. Ombredanne S. Des paralysies obstetricales qui ne sont pas du tout obstetricales. Gaz Méd France 630, 15 mai 1932.

31. Rupilius K. Ein Betrag zur gemeinsamen Genese der angeborenen Zwerchfellslähmung der Plexusläh-mung des Schiefhalses. Arch Orthop Unfallchir 34:628–633, 1934.

32. Schubert A. Die Átiologie der Geburtslahmung. Zbl Chir 49:363–365, 1922.

33. Seddon HJ. Three types of nerve injury. Brain 66:237, 1943.

34. Seddon HJ. Brachial plexus injuries. J Bone Joint Surg 31B, 1:3–4, 1949.

35. Seddon H. Nerve grafting J Bone Joint Surg 45B:447–461, 1963.

36. Sever J. Obstetrical paralysis, its etiology, pathology. Clinical aspects and treatment. Am J Dis Child 12:541–561, 1916.

37. Sever J. A research on obstetrical paralysis: its causation and anatomy. Boston Med Surg J 174:327, 1916.

38. Sever J. Obstetric paralysis: report of eleven hundred cases. JAMA 85:1862–1865, 1925.

39. Sever J. Obstetric paralysis. Surg Gynecol Obstet 44:547–549, 1927.

40. Sever J. Obstetric paralysis. Pub Health Nursing 32:187–196, 1940.

41. Smillie. Collection of preternatural cases and observations in midwifery compleating the design of illustrating his first volume on that subject. 3:504–505, London, 1764.

42. Spitzy Lange. Chirurgie und Orthopaedics und Fractures. Oxford, Blackwell Scientific Publications, 1971.

43. Sunderland S. A classification of peripheral nerve injuries producing loss of function. Brain 74:491–516, 1951.

44. Sunderland S. Nerve and nerve injuries, 2nd ed. New York, Churchill Livingstone, 1978: 1046.

45. Tassin. Personal communication, 1983.

46. Thomas A. Les paralysies obstetricales du membre supérieur. Gynecol Obstet 2:76, 3:175, 1946.

47. Thornburn W. Obstetrical paralysis. Lancet 640, 1920.

48. Trombetta. Sullo Stiramento dei Nervi, 1880.

49. Valentin, B. Pathologisch Anatomisch Beiträge zur Kenntnis der Geburtslähmung. Z Orthop Chir 15:337–353, 1924.

50. Van Neck M. Lésions congénitales ou obstetricales de l'épaule et du plexus brachial. J Méd Bruxelles 133–142, 12 mars 1914.

51. Weil S. Die Atiologie de Plexuslähmung der Neugeborenen. Arch Orthop Unfallchir 10:222–231, 1921.

52. Wickstrom J. Birth injuries of the brachial plexus: Treatment of defects in the shoulder. Clin Orthop 23:187–196, 1962.

53. Wyeth J, Sharpe W. The field of neurological surgery in a general hospital. Surg Gynecol Obstet 24:29, 1917.

PART III

Upper Extremity in Systemic Disease

CHAPTER ○ 15

Rheumatoid Diseases

BALU H. ATHREYA
F. WILLIAM BORA, JR.
RICHARD P. DUSHUTTLE

JUVENILE RHEUMATOID ARTHRITIS (JRA)

Juvenile rheumatoid arthritis (known in Europe as juvenile chronic arthritis or juvenile arthritis) is a syndrome with chronic synovitis as the basic pathologic feature.[10,13,26,42] It is a chronic disease in which involvement of the joints of the upper extremity is common. The number of children in the United States with this disease is estimated to be between 12,700 and 63,700.

Clinical Features

There are three major types of JRA (Table 15–1). Classification is based on the characteristics of the disease during the first 6 months of illness.[10]

The systemic type of JRA is most common in early childhood, although recently this clinical picture has been recognized in adults also. The course is characterized by high spiking fever (reaching up to 41°C), an evanescent maculopapular rash, lymphadenopathy, hepatosplenomegaly, pericarditis, and pleurisy. Earlier in the course, arthralgia is prominent, but true arthritis may not be present. Diagnosis may be particularly difficult because clinical features of leukemia, neuroblastoma, and various infectious diseases may resemble the signs and symptoms of JRA. Therefore, careful cultures and bone marrow examination should be done to rule out these other diseases before the diagnosis of JRA is considered. Once arthritis develops, it is relatively easy to make the diagnosis. In the usual course of systemic JRA, fever subsides over a period of 6 months to 2 years, and polyarticular arthritis persists. The common laboratory features of children in this group include anemia, leukocytosis (up to 30,000 mm³), elevated platelet count, and elevated erythrocyte sedimentation rate (ESR). Sera of these patients do not show rheumatoid factor (RF) or antinuclear factor (ANF). However, HLA-B35 has been shown to be associated with this systemic type of JRA.

The pauciarticular type of JRA is characterized by involvement of four joints or fewer. There are three subtypes. Pauciarticular type I predominantly affects young girls, a majority of whom carry ANF in their serum and are at high risk of developing

Table 15–1. **Classification of Juvenile Rheumatoid Arthritis**

Mode of Onset	Percentage of all JRA Cases	Incidence Age	Sex	Clinical Findings	Laboratory Findings	Prognosis
Systemic	30	<10	1.5:1 (F:M)	Fever, rash, polyarticular arthritis; heart, liver, spleen, and lymph nodes involved; iridocyclitis seen occasionally	Anemia; leukocytosis; Elevated ESR; ANA rarely +; RF −	All disease mortality in this group (1% to 2% of all JRA patients); 40% evidence of joint destruction
Pauciarticular (<5 joints)	45	<10	6:1 (F:M)	Lower extremity arthritis	ANA +, ESR	Continuous: 25%; arthritis rarely erosive; eventual remission 60%
Subtype 1 (iritis)		<10	Almost all females	Iritis	ANA +; HLA-DRw5 +	10%: functional blindness; 55%: acute; 45%; chronic
Subtype 2 (HLA-B27 +)		>10	1:9 (F:M)	Heel pain, tendinitis, SI and lumbar spine arthritis later. No iritis or HLA-B27 +	HLA-B27 +	Juvenile ankylosing spondylitis later
Polyarticular (>4 joints)	25			Acute or insidious onset symmetric arthritis in upper and lower extremities	HLA-DTMo ESR	Best outlook for recovery Mortality: 0; duration longer, more crippling; 25% remission
Subtype 1 (RF +)		>10	Mostly female	Resembles adult RA	RF +	
Subtype 2 (RF −)					RF −	Less crippling than RF +

(Reproduced from Brewer EJ, et al, eds. Juvenile Rheumatoid Arthritis. Philadelphia, WB Saunders, 1982, by permission.)

chronic iridocyclitis. HLA-DRW5 has been shown to be associated with this subtype.

In contrast, pauciarticular type II predominantly affects boys in late childhood or adolescence and is not associated with the presence of ANF in serum. A majority of these children carry HLA-B27, and acute iridocyclitis may occur in a small percentage, as opposed to the chronic iridocyclitis of pauciarticular type I disease.

Another subtype of pauciarticular arthritis has been recognized. Children in this group have no iritis, do not carry HLA-B27, carry a new HLA antigen called T_{mo} (related to DW7 and 8), and have a good chance for recovery.

Polyarticular arthritis in childhood resembles adult type rheumatoid arthritis (RA), with insidious onset, low-grade fever, morning stiffness, and symmetric polyarticular arthritis of small and large joints. This group is divided into seropositive and seronegative subgroups, depending on the presence or absence of rheumatoid factor (RF) in the serum. Approximately 10% of all children with JRA have RF in the serum (compared with 80% of adults with RA). Children with seropositive JRA tend to be older, develop nodules more often, and develop severe hip disease more often than do children with seronegative JRA. The usual laboratory abnormalities in this group include mild anemia, elevated ESR, elevated levels of C3 and immunoglobulins in the serum, and negative ANF. In seropositive JRA, C3 may be low, particularly in association with systemic features. Seropositive JRA resembles adult seropositive RA with respect to symptoms as well as HLA type (HLA-DR4).

Diagnosis

JRA is a clinical diagnosis and a diagnosis of exclusion. There is no one laboratory abnormality that is characteristic of JRA. Testing for RF in the serum and synovial biopsy does not help because RF may be present in the sera of children with other diseases and synovial biopsy usually shows nonspecific chronic inflammatory changes.

In the presence of systemic features such as fever, rash, and lymphadenopathy, every effort must be made to exclude infectious diseases, leukemia, and neuroblastoma. When a child presents with pauciarticular arthritis, arthritis caused by infectious agents

and spondyloarthropathies have to be ruled out. Mechanical derangements and local lesions, such as pigmented villonodular synovitis, must be excluded in the presence of arthritis of single joints. Symmetric polyarticular arthritis of large and small joints can occur in any of the rheumatic diseases, such as systemic lupus erythematosus (SLE) and progressive systemic sclerosis (PSS).

Radiologic features of JRA include soft tissue swelling, juxta-articular osteoporosis, and periosteal elevation in the early stages. These abnormalities are particularly evident in x-rays of the hand. Later, loss of cartilage space, erosions, deformities, and ankyloses are seen.

Medical Management

Although there is no specific cure for JRA, the disease can be controlled. The overall prognosis for recovery is good for JRA, although there are variations within subgroups (Table 15–1). Physicians treating children with JRA must take into account the many organ systems involved as well as the growth and development of the child. Finally, diagnosis and management require the expertise of many disciplines. One physician, preferably a pediatrician, should coordinate the input from this multidisciplinary team.

Absolute bed rest is not indicated except during acute illness or in the presence of pericarditis. The child should be encouraged to partake in activities to tolerance, except in the presence of acutely inflamed joints, which should be rested with splints. However, these splints should be removed twice daily, and the child should be encouraged to move the joint actively.

Good nutrition is necessary for any child with chronic illness, but there is no scientific basis for many special diets promoted as cures for arthritis. Many children are anemic. Oral iron may be tried, although response to therapy is not consistent.

The pharmacologic management of JRA includes four groups of drugs: (1) aspirin and/or one of the nonsteroidal anti-inflammatory drugs (NSAIDs) (Table 15–2); (2) disease-modifying (DMD) or slow-acting antirheumatic drugs (SAARDs) (Table 15–3); (3) steroids and immunosuppressives; and (4) newer experimental drugs.

It is best to start treatment with aspirin or one of the NSAIDs and to increase the dose

Table 15–2. **Rheumatic Disease Medications: Nonsteroidal Anti-Inflammatory Drugs (NSAID)**

A. Salicylates*—60 to 80 mg/kg/day in four doses
B. Indomethacin group
  1. Tolmetin (Tolectin)*—15 to 45 mg/kg/day in four doses
  2. Indomethacin (Indocin)—1.5 to 2.5 mg/kg/day in four doses
  3. Sulindac (Clinoril); no pediatric studies—two divided doses
C. Propionic acid group
  1. Fenoprofen (Nalfon)—900 to 1800 mg/m^2/day in four doses
  2. Ibuprofen (Motrin)—1200 to 1600 mg/m^2/day in four doses
  3. Naproxen (Naprosyn)—10 mg/kg/day in two doses
  4. Pirprofen (Rengasil)†—20 mg/kg/day with maximum of 600 mg/day in four doses
  5. Ketoprofen (Orudis)†—100 to 200 mg/m^2/day in three to four doses
D. Other
  1. Sodium meclofenamate (Meclomen)—4 to 7.5 mg/kg/day in three to four doses
  2. Phenylbutazone (Butazolidin or Tandearil)—3 to 6 mg/kg/day in two to four doses
  3. Proquazone (Biarsan)†—400 to 800 mg/m^2/day in three to four doses
  4. Acetaminophen (Tylenol, Tempra, and many other preparations); not usually considered anti-inflammatory—60 to 80 mg/kg/day in four doses

* Approved for use in children by the Food and Drug Administration.
† Not released for market in United States at time of publication.
(Modified from Brewer EJ, et al, eds. Juvenile Rheumatoid Arthritis. Philadelphia, WB Saunders, 1982 by permission.)

gradually until there is clinical response or evidence of toxicity. The dosage and toxicity of these drugs are listed in Table 15–2. Response to therapy with this group of drugs usually is seen in 2 to 6 weeks. If there is no response or if there is an undesirable side effect with one of the drugs (from the list of

Table 15–3. **Rheumatic Disease Medications: Slower-Acting Antirheumatic Drugs (SAARD)**

A. Gold salts
  1. Gold sodium thiomalate (Myochrysine)*—after test dose, 1 mg/kg/wk IM × 20 wks, then every other wk
  2. Aurothioglucose (Solganol)*—after test dose, 1 mg/kg/wk IM × 20 wks, then every other wk
  3. Auranofin (Ridaura)—in process of study
B. Hydroxychloroquine (Plaquenil)—6 to 7 mg/kg/day once daily
C. D-Penicillamine (Cuprimine, Depen)—10 mg/kg/day once daily

* Approved for use in children by the Food and Drug Administration.
(Modified from Brewer EJ, et al, eds. Juvenile Rheumatoid Arthritis. Philadelphia, WB Saunders, 1982 by permission.)

NSAIDs), it is reasonable to try another NSAID. The majority of children with pauciarticular and RF-negative polyarticular disease, and some with systemic and RF-positive disease, will respond to an NSAID and go into remission within 3 to 6 months.

If there is no response or only partial response to these drugs, one drug from the SAARD group should be added (Table 15–3). For mild disease, one can try hydroxychloroquine. However, our own preference is for gold in injectable form. Oral gold is currently available only on experimental protocol. D-Penicillamine is associated with more serious and less reversible toxic effects. Its use should be limited to cases in which other drugs in this group are not effective; however, the patient's liver and kidney function should be carefully monitored for possible side effects.

For severe systemic disease associated with high fever (not responsive to aspirin or NSAID) and pericarditis, oral steroid is the drug of choice.

In contrast with systemic steroids, intra-articular steroids are used during the acute phase of more localized diseases. They are used for (1) strictly localized disease in one or two joints not being controlled by an NSAID, and (2) polyarticular disease under reasonable control with antirheumatic drugs, but with persistent activity in one or two joints only. Local steroids are also used for the treatment of iridocyclitis.

All children with JRA should have their eyes examined for iridocyclitis at the time of diagnosis and periodically thereafter. The frequency of re-examination during the active phase of disease should be every 3 months for chidren with pauciarticular arthritis and positive ANF and every 6 months for those with other types of arthritis. Even after the disease goes into remission, eye examinations should be continued once a year for 5 years or whenever there are symptoms referable to the eye.

Frequency of Involvement of the Joints of the Upper Extremity in JRA

The frequency with which various joints are affected in *adults* with RA is summarized in Table 15–4. For comparison, see Table 15–5 for the frequency of involvement of joints of

Table 15–4. **Frequency of Involvement of the Joints of the Upper Extremity in Adult RA**

	Percentage Initially Involved			Percentage Ultimately Involved
	Right	*Left*	*Bilateral*	
MCP	65	58	52	87
Wrist	60	57	48	82
PIP	63	53	45	63
Shoulder	37	42	30	47
Elbow	20	15	14	21

(Modified from Harris ED Jr. Rheumatoid arthritis: the clinical spectrum. *In* Kelley WN, et al, eds. Textbook of Rheumatology. Philadelphia, WB Saunders, 1981: 932 by permission.)

Table 15–5. **Joints of the Upper Extremity Involved in Juvenile Rheumatoid Arthritis**

	Percentage of Involved Joints (Within 1 Year)		Percentage of Involved Joints (Within 5 Years)	
	Right	*Left*	*Right*	*Left*
MCP	16	15	7	5
Wrist	55	54	37	37
PIP	19	18	8	6
Shoulder	7.6	7.8	10	10
Elbow	28	26	22	21

(Reproduced from Arden GP, Ansell BM. Surgical Management of Juvenile Chronic Polyarthritis. London, Academic Press, 1978 by permission.)

the upper extremity in JRA. Metacarpophalangeal (MCP), proximal interphalangeal (PIP), and shoulder joints are involved less frequently in JRA than in adult RA. Initially, the wrists are involved at about the same frequency. On follow-up, it appears that wrists are not involved as commonly in children as in adults—37% versus 82%.[2, 11, 41] However, Nalebuff and his associates reported severe wrist disease in 80% of patients with JRA followed 20 years or more after onset.[38]

A review of published studies suggests that the wrist is the most commonly involved joint of the upper extremity. Ansell and Arden[2] noted the wrist to be the most commonly affected joint of the upper extremity and the second most commonly affected joint in the body during the first year of disease when all JRA is considered as a single group. If, however, pauciarticular and polyarticular varieties were considered separately, the elbow was most commonly affected in pauciarticular disease, and the wrist was af-

fected most commonly in polyarticular disease. Small joints of the hand (MCP and PIP joints) were involved in 15% to 19% of cases and the shoulder in 7.6% to 7.8% of the cases.

In another large series from Finland,[14] wrist joints were found to be the most commonly affected joints (56% of all cases). Flexion deformities of the MCP, PIP, and distal interphalangeal (DIP) joints were seen in 32% of cases in the 0- to 4-year age group, in 20% of the 5- to 12-year group, and in only 4% of the 13- to 15-year group.

In a series from Houston,[16] involvement of the wrist with loss of extension was the most common clinical observation (about 50%). Approximately 20% to 25% of children had decreased flexion of MCP and PIP joints. In a review of clinical and radiological features of JRA in 200 patients, the same authors noted involvement of the wrist in 24.5% of these patients. MCP and PIP joints were involved in almost 50% of the patients, and DIP joints were involved in 19% of patients.

In our clinic, with an unselected group of patients with JRA, the wrist was found to be the most commonly affected joint of the upper extremity (35.6%). Fingers were involved in 27.4% of cases.

When the thumb is considered separately, approximately 25% of children have thumb involvement, with subluxation the most common abnormality.[3]

Flexor tendon sheath involvement is reported in 61% to 64% of adults with RA[41] but in only 7% of children with JRA.[16]

Patterns of Involvement of the Joints of the Upper Extremity in JRA

Shoulder. As mentioned earlier, this joint is less commonly affected in JRA than in adult RA. Even when the shoulder is involved, symptoms are mild and overshadowed by problems in the weight-bearing joints and in the wrists. The common manifestations of involvement of the shoulder joint are pain and limitation of range of movement resulting in functional limitations in dressing and grooming. Swelling is not easily detectable unless there is swelling of the subacromial bursa. Children with JRA tend to keep the shoulders in a position characterized by drooping and forward movement of the scapula. Limitations of abduction and external rotation are common findings. Limitation of internal rotation is seen later in the course of the disease.[18] Superior subluxation of the humeral head and rupture of biceps tendon are less common in JRA than in adult RA.

Another relatively uncommon finding is a synovial cyst, arising out of the shoulder joint and descending along the biceps. On clinical exam a mass is usually noted along the anterior aspect of the upper arm. The mass may be firm in the early stages but later becomes fluctuant. This complication is seen most often in children with systemic JRA.[5, 15]

X-ray findings include osteoporosis, subcortical erosions, and loss of cartilage space.[18] Subchondral cysts lead to erosions (Fig. 15–1). Further progression of disease results in flattening of the head of the humerus, proximal subluxation of the humeral head, and erosions of the glenoid. Rarely, resorption of the distal portion of the clavicle may be seen as evidence of involvement of the acromioclavicular joint.[34]

Elbow Joints. Involvement of the elbow is often manifested by limitation of extension even before evidence of synovitis is present. Even with elbow flexion contractures of up to 30°, these children remain functional; in contrast, loss of flexion is more disabling because it prevents the child from activities of daily living such as putting his hand to his mouth. Swelling of the elbow is common, but pain is not. On physical examination, obliteration of the normal dimples of the extended elbow on either side of the olecranon

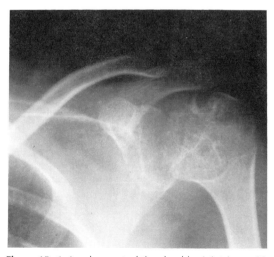

Figure 15–1. Involvement of the shoulder joint in an 11-year-old girl with JRA. Note destruction of the humeral head, erosions, and cystic changes.

process suggests effusion or synovitis or both. The elbow may be warm to touch. Soft synovium with a velvety feeling is easily palpated laterally between the olecranon process and the head of the radius. In addition to demonstrating the aforementioned features, the elbows are common sites for the presence of rheumatoid nodules.

X-rays of the elbow often show effusion and demineralization. Erosions, subchondral cysts, and bony ankylosis are late findings. Extensive erosions of the articular surfaces with widening of the joint space and subluxation are seen in end-stage disease.[23]

Wrist and Hand. Involvement of the wrist is more common in systemic and polyarticular JRA than in the pauciarticular variety. Swelling and limitation of motion are the most frequent findings. Involvement of the PIP joints produces swelling, which leads to a spindle-shaped digit. In seronegative polyarticular JRA, involvement of both the radiocarpal and intercarpal joints commonly results in diffuse swelling of the entire wrist. Swelling of radioulnar joints is more common in the seropositive variety.

On physical examination, limited extension is the most common and earliest feature of involvement of the wrist joint. This finding is associated with muscle weakness and poor grip. Later, flexion and lateral movements also are affected. Tendency to early ankylosis is a particularly disturbing feature of juvenile onset arthritis.[38]

During the early stages, in the presence of acute inflammation, there is often spasm of flexor muscles, and the wrist tends to stay in flexed posture. This should be corrected with suitable night splinting and with measures that will reduce the muscle spasm. Later in the course of the disease, there is volar subluxation (Fig. 15–2) and ankylosis.

Dorsal prominence of the ulnar head due to stretching of the ulnar collateral ligament by infiltrating synovium and instability of the distal radioulnar joint is seen in JRA as often as in adult RA. Carpal tunnel syndrome, however, is extremely unusual in JRA.

Both ulnar deviation and radial deviation of the wrist can occur. Chaplin and colleagues reported that deviations of the wrist are more common in children than in adults.[14] Specifically, ulnar deviation was more common in children (34%) than in adults (26%) (Table 15–6 and Fig. 15–3). In our series, we noted ulnar deviation in nine

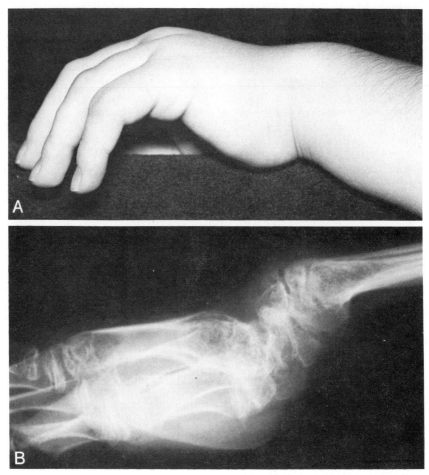

Figure 15–2. *A*, Volar subluxation of the wrist in a 10-year-old girl with seronegative polyarticular JRA. *B*, X-rays of the hand from the same child.

children and radial deviation in seven.[3] Cranberry and Mangum measured wrist deviation as the angle between the shaft of the radius and the axis of the second metacarpal bone and showed that ulnar deviation is more common than radial deviation.[16] In contrast, radial deviation of the wrist with ulnar deviation of the fingers at the metacarpophalangeal is a more common abnormality in adult RA.[50]

X-ray changes in early stages include periarticular swelling, particularly near the ulnar styloid, and periostitis of the metacarpals or phalanges. In addition, accelerated appearance of ossification centers of carpal bones is a feature typically seen in JRA, although it can occur with any chronic inflammation (Fig. 15–4). Later in the course, there is uniform loss of cartilage between the bones, and the appearance of bony erosions.[28] These

Table 15–6. **Hand Deviation in Juvenile Rheumatoid Arthritis**

	Total Number of Wrists	Percentage Deviated to Ulnar Side	Percentage Deviated to Radial Side	Percentage With No Deviation
Juvenile cases with wrist involved	487	34	23	43
Juvenile cases with wrist not involved	341	22	9	69
Adult cases with wrist involved	400	26	25	49

(From Chaplin D et al. Wrist and finger deformities in juvenile rheumatoid arthritis. Acta Rheum Scand 15:206–223, 1969 by permission.)

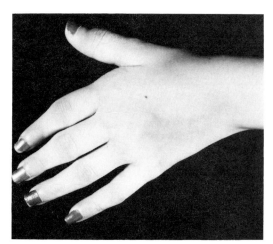

Figure 15–3. Ulnar deviation of the wrist in a 10-year-old girl with seropositive polyarticular JRA.

Wrists are probably the most commonly ankylosed peripheral joints in JRA, with carpometacarpal joints of the second and third fingers affected most commonly. Intercarpal ankylosis is less common, and radiocarpal ankylosis is rare. The longer the disease remains active, the greater is the tendency for ankylosis to occur.[29,32]

In a study of 13 patients with late-onset Still's disease, Medsger and Christy[35] noted that the carpometacarpal and intercarpal joints, particularly around the capitate, became indistinct and narrowed within 27 months of onset of the disease. The result was bony ankylosis without erosions within another year. This selective and rapid ankylosis seems to be characteristic of adult onset Still's disease (Table 15–7).

Alteration in carpal size is another feature of JRA. Because this can also occur in some of the congenital malformation syndromes, Poznanski and associates devised a useful method for the measurement of carpal length.[40] They measured the distance between the midradial epiphysis and the base of the third metacarpal in a standard x-ray of the wrist and hand. This was correlated with age, intermetacarpal width (MW) (distance between the most radial point on the base of the second metacarpal and the most ulnar point on the base of the fifth metacarpal), and

erosions particularly affect the bones involved in the radiocarpal joint (Fig. 15–5). Cyst formation is not a usual feature of JRA. Resorption with severe arthropathy leading to arthritis mutilans (opera glass hand) is not common in JRA. When it occurs, it is more often associated with the seropositive (RF-positive) JRA.

Complete loss of cartilage resulting in bony ankylosis of the carpal joints is a common sequela of systemic type JRA (Fig. 15–6).

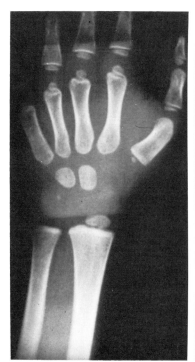
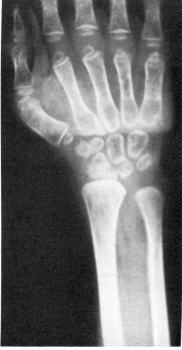

Figure 15–4. Pauciarticular JRA involving the right wrist of a 3-year-old boy. Note the advanced bone age of the involved wrist, with accelerated appearance of ossification of carpal bones.

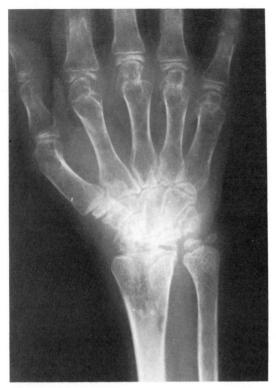

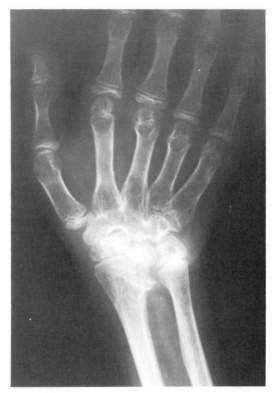

Figure 15–5. Severe destructive arthritis in a 10-year-old girl with seronegative polyarticular JRA. Note the severe erosions of the carpal bones, the ulnar styloid, the radius, and the base of the metacarpals.

Figure 15–6. Carpometacarpal ankylosis in a 12-year-old girl with systemic JRA.

maximum length of the second metacarpal (M2). A strong linear relationship was noted between carpal length and MW and between carpal length and M2. Using these relationships, the authors showed reduction in carpal length in JRA.

Fingers. Swelling and pain in joints with or without limitation of range of movement are the usual findings during the active early phase of the disease. Wasting of the muscles

Table 15–7. **Carpometacarpal and Intercarpal Ankylosis in Rheumatoid Arthritis Variants**

RA Variant	Number of Patients	Percentage
Late onset Still's disease	7/13	54
Juvenile Still's disease	2/9	22
Adult RA	4/38	22
Juvenile polyarticular RA	0/10	0

(From Medsger TA Jr, Christy WC. Carpal arthritis with ankylosis in late onset Still's disease. Arthritis Rheum 19:232–242, 1976 by permission.)

of the hand and poor grip also may be seen early. Deformities and disabilities in function are seen later with persistent synovitis.

Metacarpophalangeal (MCP) Joint. Involvement of the MCP joint is not common in patients with JRA except in the seropositive variety that resembles adult RA. The joint is visibly swollen in the presence of significant synovial hypertrophy or effusion or both. There may be redness over the dorsum, and the joint may feel warm. Synovial thickening of the MCP joints can commonly be appreciated with digital palpation.

The normal range of motion (ROM) at the MCP joint is 0° to 90° of flexion and 0° to 25° of abduction. There also is 5° to 15° hyperextension at the MCP joint, which is lost early in the course of synovitis. Later, there is limitation of flexion. Exaggerated lateral movements due to ligamental laxity and ulnar or radial deviations are common deformities.

Common deformities described in association with adult RA are ulnar deviation and volar subluxation of the MCP joints. In one large study, ulnar drift was noted in 63% of the fingers examined, and volar subluxation was observed in 68%.[50] In contrast, decreased flexion is the most common finding at the MCP joint in JRA.[16] Radial deviation is the next most common deformity. Volar subluxation, ulnar deviation, and tendon dislocation are seen only rarely.

X-ray changes include soft-tissue swelling, juxta-articular osteoporosis, and periostitis in early cases. Marginal erosions are usually seen in the metacarpal heads (Fig. 15–7) in association with narrowing of the joint space. In addition, premature fusion of the epiphysis of the metacarpals, overgrowth of the epiphyses, and loss of the normal biconcave shape of the phalanges and metacarpals are characteristically seen in JRA. The metacarpals may also be longer or shorter.

Proximal Interphalangeal (PIP) Joints and Distal Interphalangeal (DIP) Joints.

These joints are more commonly involved in the seronegative polyarticular and the systemic types of JRA. The usual findings are swelling, pain, limitation of range of movement, and bony deformities. The swelling often is diffuse and fusiform and difficult to detect because of associated tenosynovitis. The joints may be warm and tender. One can ascertain synovial thickening by palpating the dorsum of the joint on either side of the extensor tendon. Fluid in the joint may be appreciated by palpation of the lateral distention of the capsule when vertical pressure on the dorsum is applied.

The normal ROM at the PIP joint is 120° of flexion from neutral; that of the DIP is 0° to 80°. One can best demonstrate loss of flexion of these joints by asking the child to make a fist and looking at the distance between the fingertip and the palm. Limitation of flexion with poor grip is the most common functional deficit associated with involvement of these small joints of the hand. Later in the course of the disease, fixed flexion contractures may develop with extreme limitation in the range of movement in either direction.

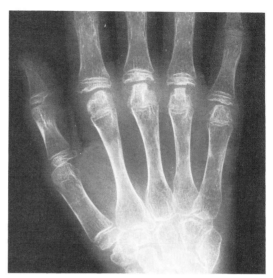

Figure 15–7. Erosion of heads of the second, third, and fourth metacarpals in a patient with seropositive polyarticular JRA. Note the erosions of the proximal phalanges.

In a large study involving 414 patients with JRA,[14] three common types of deformities were noted: boutonniere, swan-neck, and "flexion" at all joints (Table 15–8). The most common deformity was of the boutonniere variety, and swan-neck deformity was not as common in children as in adults. This is similar to our experience. In a study of 92 patients with JRA in our clinic,[3] finger involvement was noted in 30. Boutonniere deformity was the most common (seven patients), and only one child had swan-neck deformity. In contrast, both boutonniere deformity and swan-neck deformity are common in adults with RA.

Involvement of the DIP joints in adults with RA is not common, and involvement of DIP joints should lead one to consider other causes of arthritis (e.g., degenerative joint disease, psoriasis). However, involvement of the DIP is commonly seen in children with JRA. In one study of 100 children with JRA,

Table 15–8. **Incidence of Finger Deformity in Juvenile Rheumatoid Arthritis**

Age at Onset (Years)	Total Cases	Boutonniere Deformity		Swan-Neck Deformity		"Flexion" Deformity	
		Number of Cases	Percentage of Total	Number of Cases	Percentage of Total	Number of Cases	Percentage of Total
0–4	120	24	20	4	3	39	32
5–12	201	53	26	15	7	41	20
13–15	93	25	27	4	4	4	4

(From Chaplin D et al. Wrist and finger deformities in juvenile rheumatoid arthritis. Acta Rheum Scand 15:206–223, 1969 by permission.)

Table 15–9. **Incidence of Deviation of the Second Finger in JRA**

Age at Onset (Years)	Total Hands Considered	Percentage of Fingers With Ulnar Deviation		Percentage of Fingers With Radial Deviation	
0–4	90	Total:	4	Total:	34
		Males:	0	Males:	36
		Females:	5	Females:	28
5–12	182	Total:	15	Total:	21
		Males:	16	Males:	9
		Females:	14	Females:	23
13–15	98	Total:	35	Total:	18
		Males:	18	Males:	7
		Females:	46	Females:	23

(From Chaplin D et al. Wrist and finger deformities in juvenile rheumatoid arthritis. Acta Rheum Scand 15:206–223, 1969 by permission.)

the DIP was found to be affected in 18 children.[16] We noted DIP involvement in eight of 92 patients with JRA.[3]

Ulnar or radial deviations of fingers were noted in 16 fingers (five patients) in our group[3] and in 62 fingers by Cranberry and Mangum.[16] There is a reciprocal relationship between deviation of the wrist and of the fingers. The tendency seems to be to keep the axis of the 2nd metacarpal aligned with the radius. Since ulnar deviation at the wrist is more common in JRA than in adult RA, radial deviation of the fingers also is seen more frequently in children. Chaplin and colleagues[14] noted radial deviation to be most common in the 0 to 4-year onset group, and ulnar deviation was noted in the 13- to 15-year onset group (Table 15–9). They also documented the reciprocal relationship be-

tween wrist and finger deviations (Table 15–10).

Radiologic changes are similar to those seen in the MCP joints. Growth and postural abnormalities that occur in JRA are listed in Table 15–11.

Thumb. There is very little information on the frequency and pattern of involvement of the thumb in JRA. In a series of 84 patients with JRA in our clinic, 16 had involvement of the thumbs.[3] It is difficult to recognize involvement of the carpometacarpal joint of the thumb during the acute stage. Tenderness is the most frequent finding and may be the only clinical evidence. However, swelling, erythema, warmth, and tenderness of the metacarpophalangeal and interphalangeal joints of the thumb may also be seen.

Laxity of ligaments around the MCP joint resulting in volar subluxation is a common finding. Our observation suggests the following three stages in the evolution of deformities of the thumb:

(1) Laxity of ligaments: There is a tendency for volar subluxation of the MCP joint. This is reversible in the early stages (Fig. 15–8).

(2) Rotation of the thumb along its long axis (Fig. 15–9).

(3) Adduction contracture resulting in loss of web space (Fig. 15–10).

Once adduction contracture develops, there is difficulty with lateral pinch, and the pinching movement accentuates extension of the IP joints. This deformity is similar to the type I deformity of Nalebuff. Type II and III deformities in which the basic defect is at the carpometacarpal joint are not commonly seen in the hands of children with JRA, ex-

Table 15–10. **The Relationship Between Wrist and Finger Deviation in JRA**

Age at Onset (Years)	Direction of Wrist Deviation	Number of Cases	Average Deviation of Hand	Average Deviation of Second Finger
	Radial	27	13°	0°
0–4	Ulnar	36	17°	10° to radial side
	Neutral	53	—	0°
	Radial	64	14°	4° to ulnar side
5–12	Ulnar	87	11°	7° to radial side
	Neutral	96	—	0°
	Radial	29	13°	6° to ulnar side
13–15	Ulnar	54	9°	3° to radial side
	Neutral	41	—	0°

(From Chaplin D et al. Wrist and finger deformities in juvenile rheumatoid arthritis. Acta Rheum Scand 15:206–223, 1969 by permission.)

Table 15–11. **Patterns of Hand Involvement: Differences Between Adult and Juvenile RA**

	JRA	RA
Growth abnormalities	Common	Uncommon, except for loss of height
Advanced bone age	Common	Not applicable
Ulnar deviation of wrist	Common	Rare
Radial deviation of fingers	Common	Rare
MCP involvement	Uncommon	Common
DIP involvement	Common	Rare
Boutonniere deformity	Common	More common
Swan-neck deformity	Rare	Common

cept in those with long-standing seropositive JRA. Tendon ruptures are seldom seen in children.

Adduction contracture with problems in pinching interferes with essential activities of daily living, particularly holding large objects. The grip also becomes weaker.

Roentgenographic changes of the joints of the thumb include soft-tissue swelling, osteopenia, and volar subluxation in early stages. Later, marginal erosions, loss of joint space, and alterations in epiphyseal growth are seen. Ultimately, growth abnormalities, severe erosive changes, and deformities are seen in established long-standing arthritis.

Treatment

General medical management of JRA has already been described. Therapeutic techniques to maximize joint motion and muscle strength are the objectives of treatment. The physician coordinating the care of these children should be knowledgeable in the principles of physical and occupational therapy, splinting techniques, and coordination of care by multiple specialties. He should have a good understanding of the developmental level of the child, the emotional needs of the child, and the environment in which the child lives.

Such care requires a team. A pediatrician trained in rheumatology is the ideal coordinator of such a care team. A hand surgeon should be an essential part of this team. It is hard to define the role of physical and occupational therapists in treating these children. Do physical therapists work on shoulders and elbows? Do occupational therapists work on hands and fingers? Or do therapists take care of activities of daily living (ADL) and do physical therapists take care of range

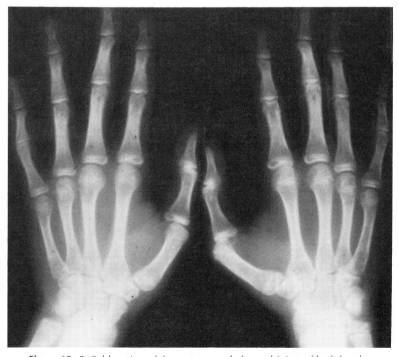

Figure 15–8. Subluxation of the metacarpophalangeal joints of both hands.

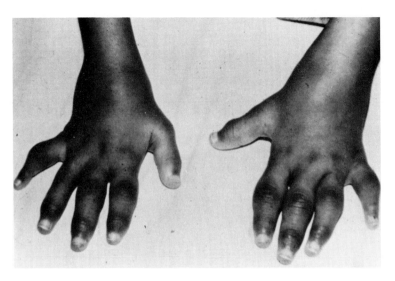

Figure 15–9. On the left hand, palmar surface of the thumb faces the other fingers. On the right, the axis has changed, so that the palmar surface of the thumb touches the table top.

of movement and muscle strengthening? Does an orthotist make the splint? What are the roles of the mother and the nurse? It is the author's personal opinion that these professional divisions of labor are arbitrary.

In children, most activities are developmentally related, and therapy techniques should be adapted to the child's developmental stage. To accomplish this goal, we need to educate the family, school staff, and nurses (e.g., school nurses) who spend more time with these children. Also, it is important that physical and occupational therapy procedures be incorporated into daily activities, such as carrying books to school—not only doing specific exercises twice a day.

At the completion of initial evaluation including documentation of degree of involvement, parents should have physical therapeutic techniques explained to them. If parents become part of the team, the chances for success are far better, although in certain families it may be better not to expect the parent to be responsible for therapy. Periodic supervision and suggestions for therapy should come from therapists. The physical and occupational therapists should be prepared to work together, yield to each other's role, and look at the therapy as a developmental therapy—not physical therapy and occupational therapy.

Initial evaluation should include the following:

I. Physical
   a. Extent of involvement
   b. Range of motion of joints
   c. Muscle strength
   d. Grip strength
   e. Pinch strength
   f. ADL evaluation (writing, grooming, feeding, dressing). (Standard forms are available.)
II. Developmental
   a. Motor development
   b. Intellectual development
   c. Emotional development and needs

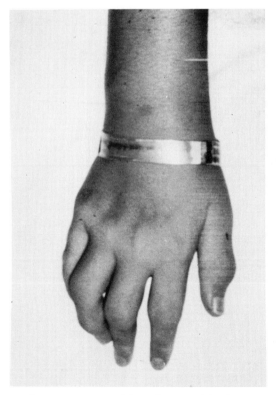

Figure 15–10. Loss of the web space of the thumb.

III. Environmental
   a. Family structure
   b. Family's financial level and needs
   c. Home structure and facilities
   d. School
   e. Friends/school activities/play

The aim of therapy should be to help the child achieve the maximum functional level given his developmental level, the demands of the environment, and the natural history of the disease.

Relief of Acute Pain and Spasm

During the acute phase of JRA, it is often necessary to splint the wrist joint for relief of pain. A resting splint should be worn for two or three days, except twice a day for 15- to 20-minute periods when the child should actively move the joint through a range of motion. Wrapping the flexor muscles of the wrist just below the elbow with a warm Turkish towel for 10 to 15 minutes often relieves muscle spasm and allows more extension at the wrist.

Injection of the wrist with steroid may be necessary occasionally.

Stiffness

Some of the simple measures that help reduce stiffness, particularly morning stiffness of the hands, are (1) sleeping in a sleeping bag, (2) wearing stretch gloves to sleep, and (3) upon awakening, immersing the hands in warm water in the sink followed by exercise. Deep heat in the form of paraffin dip is very useful, particularly in children with moderate to severe involvement of the joints of the hands. Portable units are available. In some children, cold is more effective than heat. These children may do better with special methods of applying ice to the extremities.

Use of a splint at night, particularly a splint that includes the fingers (pancake splint), may cause stiffness of the wrists and hands in the morning. Leaving the fingers out of the splint, and use of warmth and exercises in the morning, should help relieve this problem.

Preservation of Joint Alignment

The usefulness of the hand relies heavily on functioning wrists and thumbs. In JRA, the most common problems are flexion contrac-

ture at the wrist and adduction contracture of the thumb. The ability to flex and extend the wrist is essential to good grip strength. Also, it is necessary to maintaining the web space of the thumb. These goals are accomplished by the use of splints.

There are two categories of splints: *resting splints*, which are used during rest at night, and *functional splints*, which are used during activities. There is controversy about the factors causing loss of alignment at the wrist. The child keeps the wrists, elbows, and fingers in the flexed position for prolonged periods during sleep, and this is considered to be responsible for the deformities seen in the upper extremities. If one subscribes to this hypothesis, use of a resting splint at night is the logical way to avoid these deformities.

An alternative explanation for the cause of these deformities is the unusual postures that children with arthritis assume to protect their painful, stiff joints. These children use their hands in wrong positions, particularly when carrying books (Fig. 15–11), and when rising from a sitting position (Fig. 15–12). These dysfunctional activities may accentuate the deformities. If one accepts this explanation, functional splint is the answer.

In reality, both resting and functional positions contribute to these deformities. Whether resting or functional splints are used is often determined by the child's developmental level, age, and cooperation.

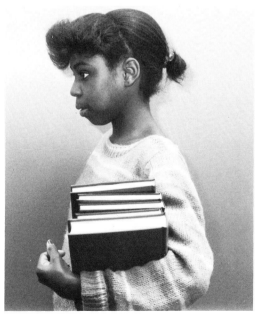

Figure 15–11. Improper technique for carrying books.

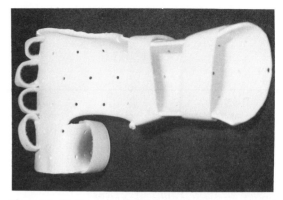

Figure 15–13. Resting splint with a C-bar for the thumb and loops to correct mild flexion deformities of the PIP joints.

Correction of Deformities

Correction of more established deformities may require serial casting. Three-point bracing may be needed for correction of ulnar deviation at the wrist.

Dynamic splinting becomes essential for the correction of finger deformities. For example, a knuckle-bending device may be necessary for improving flexion at the MCP joint. Splints with outriggers are used to maintain the MCP or PIP joints in extension while allowing active flexion. Simple splints made of synthetic material will help correct minor flexion deformities (Fig. 15–14) and deviations at the PIP joints. Hair curlers can be used effectively for early boutonniere deformities. For established boutonniere deformity, splints providing a three-point correction force are indicated. To prevent adduction contracture of the thumbs and to facilitate writing in school, a device can be fabricated that will both hold a pencil and

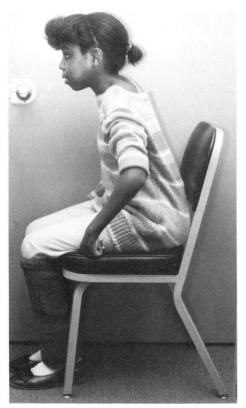

Figure 15–12. Improper technique in pushing-off from sitting position (use of flexed MCP joints instead of the heel of the palm).

Few adolescents will be willing to use a functional splint at school. No typical 3-year-old child will use a resting splint throughout the night.

A good functional wrist splint should be made of synthetic material and modified as needed. It should extend from the distal third of the forearm to the distal flexion crease of the hand, leaving the thenar eminence out. It must extend completely around the wrist to reduce motion. Easy-to-wear, ready-made splints with a ventral bar (Futura) are better accepted by older children and adolescents but will not be adequate for children with severe, complicated deformities.

Resting splints should reach from the middle of the forearm to the distal flexion crease. There should be about 10° to 15° of extension, of the wrist if possible, and the thumb web space should be maintained with a C-bar. If the fingers are included in the splint, a single strap may be used for routine use, or individual loops may be used around the fingers to correct deformities (Fig. 15–13).

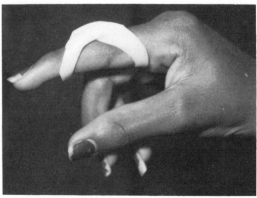

Figure 15–14. A simple splint to correct flexion deformity of PIP joints.

abduct the thumb to maintain an adequate web space.[37]

Maintenance of Function

Incorporation of therapy and joint protection techniques into the daily life of the child is essential. These activities must be adapted to the child's interests and developmental level.[24] Adaptive equipment, if needed to maintain function, must be introduced carefully and in such a way that the child will use it. Even if physicians, therapists, or parents think that the child needs a dressing aid, there is no guarantee that it will be used unless the child feels the need for it. Attempts to motivate children to use these aids are often futile.

Table 15–12 lists play exercises that are appropriate for different age groups. Joint protection techniques that are useful for daily activities are listed in Table 15–13.

Surgery in Juvenile Rheumatoid Arthritis

In spite of adequate splints, casts, traction, and exercise, many patients with JRA require operative procedures. The natural history of the disease is that children under 10 years of age rarely have enough loss of function to require surgery. The choice of a child for whom surgery is appropriate is based upon

Table 15–12. **Play Exercises by Age Groups**

Age	Activities
6 months–4 years	Playing in warm water with toys
	Playing with toys that pull apart (pop beads)
	Reaching for toys over the head
	Squeezing and rolling modeling clay
	Reversing handle of tricyle
5–8 years	Taking warm bath and playing with toys in water
	Swimming
	Pulling pieces of plastic (Dental Dam) into funny shapes
	Participating in arts and crafts
	Playing with modeling clay and squeeze toys
	Riding a tricycle or bicycle
9–13 years	Swimming
	Participating in arts and crafts
	Participating in gym activities
	Hitting and catching softballs

(From Giesecke LL et al. Home care guide for JRA—A manual for parents. Atlantic City, NJ, Children's Seashore House Publications, 1982 by permission.)

Table 15–13. **Instructions to Children on Joint Protection Techniques During Activities of Daily Living**

Activity	Instructions
Bathing	Squeeze your washcloth or sponge. *Don't* wring it.
Getting dressed	Use long-handled shoe horn, snap-on shirts, zipper pull, and elastic shoe strings. (Give child lots of time to get dressed.)
Drinking	Use both hands to hold your cup or glass and spread your fingers around it.
Carrying books	Use a back pack. If you carry them in your arms, shift them often; if you use a school bag with a handle, carry it on your forearm or change from one side to the other often.
Waiting with a load	Put your books and heavy packages down while waiting.
Writing	Use a fat pen or fat pencil if the thin ones are hard to hold; rest periodically when writing for a long time; use tape-recorder or typewriter for assignments.
Sitting still	Don't lean your head on your hands. Don't stoop. Sit in a comfortable chair with both feet on the floor and your back against the chair. When you are ready to get up, push down on the seat of the chair with the palm of your hand, not with the knuckles.

(From Giesecke LL et al. Home Care Guide for JRA—A manual for parents. Atlantic City, NJ, Children's Seashore House Publications, 1982 by permission.)

loss or impending loss of function. These cases can be divided into two general categories: prophylactic and reconstructive.

The following procedures have been performed in 40 cases of juvenile rheumatoid arthritis. These procedures fall into two general categories: prophylactic and reconstructive.

Prophylactic Surgery (Synovectomy). The objective of prophylactic surgery is to prevent progression of deformity that will ultimately compromise the function of the upper extremity. In juvenile rheumatoid arthritis, as in adult rheumatoid arthritis, the major area affected by the disease process is the synovium. Synovectomy is performed in order to increase the motion of gliding structures (joint and tendons) before fixed deformities develop and also to prevent tendon ruptures. Joint and tendon synovectomies have been observed to be beneficial to children who have edematous, progressive synovitis not helped by proper medical therapy. The indications for surgery are (1) persistence of synovitis for more than 18 months without x-ray evidence of joint destruction and without significant loss of passive motion, and (2) persistence of tendon synovitis with loss of active joint motion that those tendons control in the face of adequate conservative therapy. Large series with long clinical follow-ups are not available at this time, but it appears that a well-planned synovectomy in selected children can defer loss of function and in some cases improve extremity function after surgery. The results of synovectomy in children with nonedematous JRA (the dry type) have not been satisfactory.

Among one group of patients who had synovectomies and who were followed a year or longer postoperatively, 14 showed maintained joint position and improved motion following MCP joint synovectomy, one was unchanged, and three were worse. Two of the patients had less flexion deformity and improved motion following PIP joint synovectomy, one was the same, and one was worse. Those who had flexor tendon synovectomy showed improved motion and better digital flexion following the procedure. Four patients who had extensor tendon synovectomies had no ruptures and 80° of MCP joint extension at 18 months. It was observed that 50% of the patients had recurrent synovitis, but all had significantly less bulk tissue at 18 months than before surgery.

Reconstructive. Reconstructive surgery is aimed at improving function by decreasing deformities and pain, increasing motion of the tendons and joints, and improving power pinch and grip.

Tendon. Ruptured tendons occur more frequently on the dorsum of the hand and wrist than on the palmar side. Direct tenorrhaphy is not possible because the rheumatoid process compromises the tensile strength of the tendons, precluding satisfactory suture tendon anastomotic strength over the period of time required for tendon healing. Tendon transfer and tendon graft techniques have been used to restore satisfactory function after tendon rupture. The extensors to the small and ring fingers at the level of the distal ulna are the most frequent tendons ruptured, and an end-to-side anastomosis suturing the long and ring finger tendons to the long fin-

ger tendon is a reasonable technique for restoration of motion to the MCP joints of the long and ring fingers. Tendon transfer involving the extensor carpi ulnaris has been recommended, but this often leads to restriction of flexion of the wrist and MCP joints because the excursion of the extensor ulnaris is not sufficient to permit flexion at both joints at the same time. If the long finger extensor tendon has ruptured with the tendons to the small and ring fingers, one can perform a tendon graft, utilizing the palmaris longus in a loop fashion (Fig. 15–15) and reattaching the distal ruptured tendon segments to the proximal segments of the extensor communis of the respective fingers at a level near the muscle belly, where the tendon is of good substance. The flexor pollicis longus is the most frequently ruptured flexor tendon. With such ruptures, tendon transfer involving the superficialis of the ring finger provides satisfactory results.

Nerve. Median nerve compression is occasionally an early sign of tenosynovitis of the flexor tendons. The treatment is release of the transverse carpal ligaments in com-

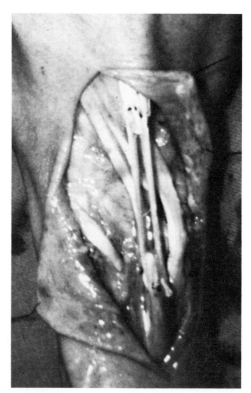

Figure 15–15. The palmaris longus tendon used to form a loop tendon graft for reconstruction of ruptured extensor tendons at wrist level.

bination with flexor tendon synovectomy. In our experience this has been helpful in lessening paresthesias in the median innervated fingers of the hand and in increasing finger flexion.

Bone. Pain, limited elbow motion, forearm rotation, and wrist motion are occasionally seen in juvenile rheumatoid arthritis. This combination can be treated by radial head excision and synovectomy with good results. Distal ulna resection is less predictable. In our series, elbows fixed at 90° had motion increased to 75° in the patients who had undergone radial head resection, and wrist extension increased from 0° to 35° in the patient who had had distal ulnar resection.

Joint. Intrinsic plus finger deformity with PIP extension contracture can be overcome by resection of the lateral bands, which releases the intrinsic muscles. In patients with MCP joint involvement, resection (in younger patients) or silastic implant arthroplasties (in patients with little growth remaining) are viable options. There is a tendency for finger deformities to recur after these procedures, but the overall alignment of the fingers relative to the metacarpals is usually improved for several years. When the two procedures are compared, there is no difference in terms of finger position or power pinch and grip at two years. In contrast, resection arthroplasties are usually unsatisfactory for PIP joint deformity. PIP fusion produces a more predictable result.

SYSTEMIC LUPUS ERYTHEMATOSUS

Systemic lupus erythematosus (SLE) is a multisystem disease in which genetic, endocrine, and environmental factors are involved in the production of various immunologic aberrations. SLE is less common than rheumatoid arthritis in children, and when it occurs, it usually manifests itself between ages 10 and 20. It is most common in females and in blacks.[13, 26, 27]

Clinical Features

Arthritis, low-grade fever, and rash are the most common early manifestations of SLE in children. Low-grade fever is more common than high fever. Arthritis is usually symmetric and polyarticular, involving large and small joints. Destructive changes and deformities of joints are not as common as in JRA. The rash can be of any clinical type: macular, papular, urticarial, petechial, nodular, or necrotic. The characteristic rash of lupus is scaly, erythematous, maculopapular, crusted, and often atrophic. This rash is frequently present over the forehead, the cheek and the bridge of the nose in a butterfly distribution. Palpable purpura is characteristic of any type of vasculitis. Erythema of the hard palate and ulcers over the palate and nasal septum are other common features of SLE. Additional general systemic features of SLE include arthralgia, myalgia, malaise, morning stiffness, loss of appetite, and loss of weight.

Other clinical manifestations of the disease depend on the systems involved. Proteinuria, hematuria, cylindruria, edema, hypertension, and renal failure are the usual manifestations of renal involvement. Chest pain, dyspnea, tachycardia, pericardial friction rub and effusion, and congestive heart failure suggest the presence of pericarditis or myocarditis. Seizures, peripheral neuropathy, headache, personality changes, and hallucinations are the most common features of central nervous system involvement. Anemia, leukopenia, and thrombocytopenia (all of autoimmune type) indicate involvement of the hematopoietic system.

The American Rheumatism Association (ARA) criteria for diagnosis of SLE are listed in Table 15–14. It is recommended that at least four of these 11 criteria be present before a diagnosis of SLE is made. This rule is most applicable to patients in research studies. In a clinical setting, the presence of a multisystem disease together with the dem-

Table 15–14. **Revised Criteria for the Classification of Systemic Lupus Erythematosus (SLE)**

Butterfly rash
Discoid lupus
Photosensitivity
Oral ulcers
Arthritis
Serositis (pleuritis, pericarditis)
Renal disorder
Neurologic disorder (seizures, psychoses)
Hematologic disorder
Immunologic disorder (anti-DNA, anti-Sm, false-positive STS, positive LE cells)
Antinuclear antibody

(From American Rheumatism Association (ARA), 1982.)

onstration of autoimmune phenomena in the serum (presence of antinuclear antibody or anti-DNA) is sufficient basis for the diagnosis of SLE, after exclusion of other possible causes.

Laboratory Features

Even in the absence of autoimmune hemolysis, mild to moderate anemia may be observed. The presence of reticulocytosis usually suggests an autoimmune process. Coombs' test is usually positive. Leukopenia and thrombocytopenia may be present independently or as part of pancytopenia. Erythrocyte sedimentation rate, C-reactive protein, and complement all may be elevated as evidence of a chronic inflammatory process. Urinalysis may be normal or may show proteinuria, hematuria, and cylindruria. Elevation of BUN and serum creatinine suggests more advanced renal involvement.

ANF is invariably present in the serum, and its measurement is a sensitive test for the diagnosis of SLE. Presence of anti-DNA antibody in high titer and Sm antibody is more specific. Elevated levels of anti-DNA antibody with low levels of complement correlate with active disease, particularly with active renal disease. Joint fluid in the arthritis of SLE is of the mild inflammatory type.

Leukocytoclastic vasculitis of small vessels in involved organs is characteristic of SLE. Immunoglobulins and complement have been demonstrated in the skin and the kidneys by immunofluorescence techniques. Major pathologic changes in various organs are secondary to vasculitis and vascular occlusion. Synovial biopsy in SLE shows diffuse lining cell proliferation, perivascular inflammatory infiltrate with predominance of mononuclear cells, and vasculitis.

Diagnosis

Multisystem disease in the presence of circulating ANA or anti-DNA or both is the hallmark of SLE. However, there are many overlap syndromes, particularly vasculitis syndromes, and it may be difficult for one to ascertain the diagnosis. Exclusion of other multisystem disorders, such as infectious diseases, is a necessary step in arriving at the correct diagnosis.

Treatment

The general features of the disease, such as fever and arthritis, are treated best with salicylates or one of the nonsteroidal anti-inflammatory drugs. For skin involvement, hydroxychloroquine is an effective drug, provided the dosage is controlled and the patient is closely monitored. For severe systemic disease and for moderate organ involvement (e.g., pericarditis, diffuse proliferative kidney disease, and hemolytic anemia), steroids are the drugs of choice. The usual starting dose is 2 mg/kg/day of prednisone, which is then tapered as rapidly as possible to alternate-day use.

Cytotoxic agents are used to treat severe disease unresponsive to steroids and rapidly progressive disease and in the presence of steroid toxicity. High-dose, single-bolus steroids ("pulse therapy") are used for rapidly progressive disease, particularly renal disease. Plasmapheresis is reserved at present for desperate situations.

Patterns of Involvement of Upper Extremity in SLE (Table 15–15)

Certain types of lesions involving the upper extremity give clues to the diagnosis of SLE. These are as follows:

1. Palmar erythema, although nonspecific, is often seen in SLE.
2. Subungual splinter hemorrhages, although characteristic of subacute bacterial endocarditis, can occur in SLE.
3. Erythema and telangiectasia of the posterior nail folds are more common than ne-

Table 15–15. **Clinical Features of SLE as Manifested in the Hand**

Lesions that give clues to the diagnosis of SLE:
    Palmar erythema
    Subungual hemorrhage
    Nail fold thrombosis
    Raynoud's disease
    Nodules
    Tenosynovitis
    Vasculitic ulcers
    Arthritis

Lesions secondary to SLE:
    Arthritis of large and small joints
    Jacoud's arthropathy
    Vasculitic ulcers
    Peripheral neuropathy
    Carpal tunnel syndrome

crosis of the nail folds. Nail-fold microscopy may show tortuous loops, decrease of superficial capillaries, and giant enlarged capillaries.

4. Raynaud's phenomenon occurs in approximately 3% of children with SLE. It is one of the major criteria for the diagnosis of SLE and can often be a major management problem. Raynaud's phenomenon may precede the onset of SLE by many years or may be one of the early manifestations. It is usually mild, characterized by discoloration and pain of the hands following exposure to cold. Rarely, this may be severe with intractable pain, intense color changes, numbness of fingers, gangrene, and vasculitic ulcers. Protective clothing and avoidance of cold are usually sufficient to control this symptom. Biofeedback may also have a role in controlling this symptom. In severe cases, intra-arterial reserpine or guanethidine, oral vasodilators, oral calcium-blocking agents, and intravenous prostaglandins also have been used with varying levels of success. Cervical sympathectomy must be considered in very severe cases in which loss of fingers is threatened.

Other lesions that may involve the upper extremity but are not characteristic of SLE are subcutaneous nodules, vasculitic ulcers at the tips of the fingers, and arthritis of the wrists and small joints.

Subcutaneous nodules are less common in childhood SLE compared with the adult form. When they occur, they are seen on the extensor aspect of the elbow along the ulna and on the extensor tendons of the wrists and hands. Histologically, the nodules of SLE show a marked chronic inflammatory reaction without the palisading of epithelial cells and central necrosis characteristic of rheumatoid nodules.

Vasculitic ulcers at the tips of the fingers are usually associated with involvement of medium-sized arteries, as opposed to the nail fold lesions associated with vasculitis of the small arteries. Early lesions are purplish, indurated, and tender at the tips of the fingers. These lesions are often associated with moderate to severe Raynaud's phenomenon and heal rather easily. Occasionally, there is loss of tissue with wasting of the pulp of the fingers and subcutaneous calcification. Early lesions are purplish, indurated, and tender at the tips of the fingers.

Wrists and small joints of the hand are commonly involved in the *arthritis* of SLE.[7] The arthritis may be acute and evanescent or chronic and persistent. It may wax and wane with systemic disease activity. Pain, stiffness, and limitation of range of movement are the common symptoms. On physical examination, the joints are often swollen with synovial hypertrophy or fluid. However, these joints, unlike those in JRA, are not markedly warm or tender. Periarticular swelling is also commonly seen, giving the appearance of joint enlargement. Tenosynovitis of flexor tendons may give rise to diffuse swelling of the entire finger.

In rheumatoid arthritis, active synovitis leads to erosion, destructive changes, and deformed joints. In SLE, synovitis is mild, and the joint changes that occur are due to laxity of supporting structures. Consequently, hyperextensible joints and lateral instabilities of the DIP are the most common findings. Correctable swan-neck deformities and ulnar drift of fingers, hyperextension at the IP joint of the thumb, and subluxation of the carpometacarpal joint of the thumb are the most commonly observed deformities. These correctable deformities of the hand are similar to those described with Jaccoud's arthropathy (Fig. 15–16). Jaccoud's arthropathy results from recurrent bouts of arthritis in acute rheumatic fever and SLE.[49] The characteristics of this arthropathy are: (1) flexion and ulnar deviation of all MCP joints, particularly of the 4th and 5th fingers; (2) hyper-

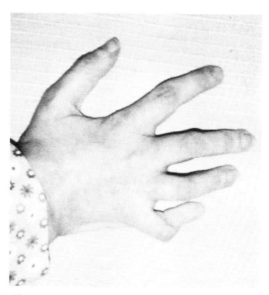

Figure 15–16. Jaccoud's arthropathy in a girl with SLE.

extension at PIP joints; (3) all deformities are correctable in the early stages.

Wrist drop and claw hand in patients with SLE may indicate neuropathy. Distal weakness, wasting, loss of tendon reflexes, and sensory changes are the other features of peripheral neuropathy. Diffuse interstitial disease of the lungs may give rise to clubbing of fingers. Carpal tunnel syndrome, which is common in adults with SLE, is rare in children.[7]

X-rays of the hands characteristically show minimal changes, even in the presence of chronic arthritis. Osteopenia, soft-tissue swelling with hyperextensible PIP joints, and absence of erosions should suggest SLE as a possible diagnosis. Occasionally, soft-tissue calcification may be seen at the tips of the fingers or in the periarticular tissues.

DERMATOMYOSITIS/ POLYMYOSITIS

Dermatomyositis (DM) is a chronic, nonsuppurative inflammatory disease of the muscles and skin.[13, 26, 44] In children, dermatomyositis is more common than polymyositis. Clinical clues and problems related to the hand are often associated with DM, and our discussion will be confined to this entity only.

The disease can occur at any age during childhood. Girls are more commonly affected than boys. There are wide variations in the clinical presentation, ranging from skin manifestations to severe, progressive paralysis of respiratory muscles.

Clinical Features

During the prodromal phase, the child may have aches and pains, nondescript rash, low-grade fever, and generalized weakness for many weeks before the classic features are evident. During this period, the child may have edema of the hands and feet. The acute phase is characterized by myositis and dermatitis. The classic triad of heliotrope rash (violaceous color of upper eyelids), periungual erythema, and dusky red, scaly lesions over the extensor aspects of the knees, elbows, and the small joints of the hand is seen during this acute phase.

Myositis is characterized by pain, tenderness, and weakness of the proximal muscles. The involvement is symmetric and often involves the anterior neck flexors. The disease may progress to involve respiratory muscles and muscles of the palate and pharynx, resulting in pooling of secretions in the mouth, nasal voice, and respiratory distress. Gastrointestinal hemorrhage may occur during the acute stage. This stage lasts for about 2 to 3 years.

During the next phase, there are exacerbations and remissions but no further progression. The rash over the extremities becomes atrophic. Acute muscle pain disappears, but weakness persists and contractures develop.

In the final phase, extensive subcutaneous calcification, muscle contractures, and pigmentary changes of the skin are the prominent features.

Laboratory Features

The most important investigations for the diagnosis of DM are (1) assessment of muscle enzymes, (2) electromyography (EMG), and (3) muscle biopsy. Serum levels of creatine kinase and aldolase are often elevated in DM, although not invariably so. If elevated, one of these enzymes can be used during the period of follow-up as a measure of disease activity. Electromyograms of proximal muscles may show a myopathic picture with polyphasic potential of short duration, positive sharp waves, and fibrillation. Muscle biopsy shows focal muscle degeneration and regeneration as well as intense perivascular and interstitial infiltration with lymphocytes, plasma cells, and perifascicular atrophy. Angiopathy involving small vessels of the skin, muscle fat, and gastrointestinal tract is considered typical of childhood DM but not of adult DM.

Radiologically, edema of the soft tissue of affected areas is seen in the early phase. Later, atrophy of the soft tissues can be appreciated. Generalized osteopenia may be seen that may be related to the disease or to the steroid therapy. Recurrent fractures are common. The most important finding is the subcutaneous calcification. Unlike the subcutaneous calcification of scleroderma, which is superficial and patchy, this calcification involves muscles and deeper tissue and is often extensive.

Treatment

Corticosteroids (2 mg/kg/day of prednisone) are used as the initial therapy. Most children show clinical response in 2 to 6 weeks. Once the muscle strength returns and serum muscle enzymes return to normal, the dose of steroids is gradually reduced to the lowest tolerated level. Steroids may have to be continued in low dosages for 2 to 3 years.

In children who do not respond to high-dosage steroids in 6 weeks and in those who develop steroid toxicity, cytotoxic agents (methotrexate, cyclophosphamide, and azathioprine) may have to be used. Intravenous "bolus" of large doses of methylprednisolone (pulse steroids) and plasmapheresis also have been used in severe cases.

Proper attention to palatal and respiratory functions is essential during the acute phase of the disease. Maintenance of good nutrition is an essential part of total management of these patients, particularly in the presence of palatal and pharyngeal weakness. It may be necessary to feed these children a high-calorie soft or liquid diet either by mouth or through a nasogastric tube.

As soon as the acute pain in the muscle has improved, active physical therapy should be initiated to improve muscle strength, improve range of motion, and maintain daily activities. When subcutaneous and muscular calcification starts, contractures become a severe problem in management. Aggressive physical therapy, dynamic splinting, and surgical release of contrac-

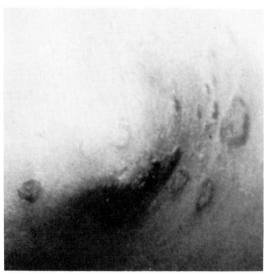

Figure 15–17. Gottron's patches in dermatomyositis.

tures are essential parts of the management of these problems.

Involvement of Upper Extremities

During the acute phase of dermatomyositis, the characteristic rash often involves the extensor aspect of the elbows (Fig. 15–17) and of the small joints of the hand (Fig. 15–18). Early lesions over large joints are red, warm, raised, and dry. These erythematous plaques are called Gottron's patches. The lesions over the knuckles are often atrophic and scaly. After the acute phase, the lesions over the knuckles are atrophic and depigmented.

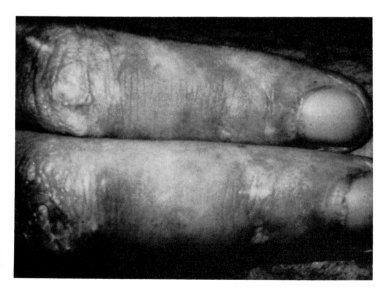

Figure 15–18. Rash over extensor aspects of the small joints of the fingers in dermatomyositis.

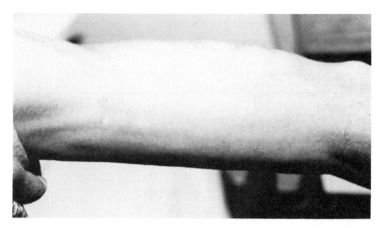

Figure 15–19. Subcutaneous nodules of calcium over upper arm in a girl with dermatomyositis.

The other important clinical feature of DM is periungual erythema with hyperkeratotic cuticles. Although subcutaneous calcification can occur anywhere in the body, it is rarely seen over the hands and fingers (Fig. 15–19).

Pain, tenderness, and weakness of the muscles around the shoulders are part of the proximal muscle involvement of this disease. During this stage, the child has difficulty with raising the arm above the head, combing the hair, or doing activities that involve raising the arm. Later, as atrophy develops, the problems of abduction at the shoulder may persist. Elbow flexion contracture may develop, particularly if there is subcutaneous calcification over the anterior aspect of the forearm. Open ulcers discharging calcium may develop over the elbow joint.

Tightness of finger flexors may result in spontaneous flexion of fingers as the wrist is extended (tenodesis). During the early phase, the child can be asked to hold the fingers in extension as the wrist is extended and perform this as an exercise twice daily while sitting and relaxing or watching television. If this deformity becomes a more difficult problem, an active program should be instituted and followed two or three times a week, and a static holding splint should be prescribed.

SCLERODERMA

Scleroderma is a generic term that includes a variety of conditions (Table 15–16). It is a relatively rare disorder in children, but when it occurs it involves the upper extremities in varying degrees.[1, 13, 26, 44]

Clinical Features

Localized forms of scleroderma are more common in children than progressive systemic sclerosis (PSS). The lesions may be one of three types:

1. Morphea. These are focal ivory-white patches with a violaceous rim. These are most commonly seen over the trunk, although they may be generalized.

2. Linear scleroderma. This often starts as

Table 15–16. **Classification of Scleroderma**

A. Systemic sclerosis
   1. Classic disease with bilateral symmetric diffuse involvement of the skin (scleroderma) affecting face, trunk, and proximal as well as distal portions of the extremities; associated with tendency toward relatively early appearance of visceral involvement
   2. Relatively limited involvement of skin; often confined to fingers and face; tendency to long delayed appearance of visceral involvement (CRST syndrome)
   3. "Overlap" syndromes, including sclerodermatomyositis and mixed connective tissue disease
B. Localized (focal) forms of scleroderma
   1. Morphea (plaque-like, guttate, or generalized; subcutaneous and keloid morphea)
   2. Linear scleroderma
   3. Scleroderma en coup de sabre, with or without facial hemiatrophy
C. Chemical-induced scleroderma-like conditions
   1. Vinyl chloride disease
   2. Pentazocine-induced fibrosis
   3. Bleomycin-induced fibrosis
D. Eosinophilic fasciitis
E. Pseudoscleroderma
   1. Edematous (scleredema, scleromyxedema)
   2. Indurative (amyloid disease, porphyria cutanea tarda, carcinoid syndrome, phenylketonuria, acromegaly)
   3. Atrophic (progeria, Werner's syndrome, lichen sclerosis et atrophicus)

(From Bull Rheum Dis 31:1–6, 1981 by permission.)

an erythematous, edematous patch and later becomes indurated, shiny, and atrophic. The lesions often involve only one extremity or one side of the body. They may enlarge and ultimately involve an entire extremity, with binding of the skin to subcutaneous tissue and to the bone. There may be contractures, limitation of growth of the affected extremity, and complete atrophy of the extremity. The involved areas may be hyper- or hypopigmented.

Children with linear scleroderma often present with sudden onset of flexion contracture of the fingers (Fig. 15–20). On examination, one can notice shiny, atrophic skin adherent to deeper structures with loss of tissue and thinning of the forearm. This type of involvement particularly affects the ulnar aspect of the forearm, the hypothenar group of muscles, and the ulnar fingers. Multiple small nodules along the flexor and extensor tendons of the hands and feet have been reported. Contractures may be secondary to these tendon nodules. The surgical correction of these cases by scar excision in the forearm has improved the functional position of the small and ring fingers.

3. Generalized scleroderma. This is characterized by lesions distributed over various parts of the body. The clinical characteristics of the lesions are similar to those of linear scleroderma. Fullness of the hands, arthritis, sclerodactyly, subcutaneous calcification,

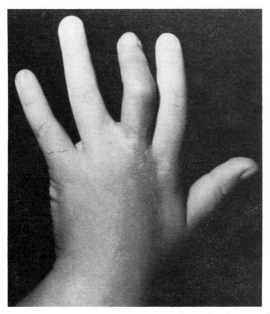

Figure 15–20. Linear scleroderma involving the dorsum of the left hand in a girl aged three and one half.

telangiectasia, and amputation of the fingers are some of the characteristic lesions that involve the hand.

Sclerodactyly (scleroderma of hands or feet) is not characteristic of scleroderma unless it is associated with skin changes over the proximal parts of the extremity. Early in the course of the disease, the hands and wrists may look puffy, and there may be symmetric diffuse swellings of the fingers, even in the absence of Raynaud's phenomenon. Later, there is stiffness of the fingers and inability to touch the palm with the finger tips, even on maximal flexion of MCP and IP joints.

The term "progressive systemic sclerosis (PSS)" denotes visceral involvement associated with features of scleroderma. The skin changes are symmetric and are characterized by hidebound skin with induration, atrophy, contractures, and pigment changes. Subcutaneous calcifications over the knuckles, telangiectasia, and spontaneous amputation are more common with this type of scleroderma. Fingertips show thinning of the pulp and are tapered. The disease may involve the GI tract (esophageal reflux with regurgitation and esophagitis), lung (interstitial fibrosis), heart (cardiomyopathy), and kidney (scleroderma kidney).

Raynaud's phenomenon may precede the onset of the disease by many years. These cases are usually precipitated by cold and due to emotional stress. Classically, there are periods of pallor of the finger (or fingers) associated with numbness followed by periods of intense cyanosis. This may be followed by a period of flushing or redness with a burning sensation. However, not all patients show all these clearly demarcated stages. If there are doubts in the history, the examiner can elicit an episode of vasospasm by having the patient immerse one hand in ice-cold water for 45 seconds and then look for cyanosis which is caused by vasospasm. Ideally, one should measure the time it takes for the fingers to rewarm following exposure to ice-cold water for 45 seconds.

During these attacks, some children have intense pain over the fingers with edema of the hands and induration. Sometimes the fingers become intensely blue and demarcate. Occasionally, this may progress to full gangrene and to spontaneous amputation. Fortunately, this is rare. More often, the vasospasm clears but leaves these patients with atrophy of the pulp or ulceration at the tip of the fingers or scars under the edge of the fingernails. Subcutaneous calcification around the pulp or around the knuckles may be other sequelae.

The arthritis of scleroderma is symmetric and polyarticular and may be acute or chronic with a slowly progressive course. It also involves the wrists and small joints of the hand.

Laboratory Features

Mild anemia, elevated sedimentation rate, and hypergammaglobulinemia are commonly seen. Presence of rheumatoid factor and antinuclear antibody in high titers is compatible with a diagnosis of scleroderma. Restrictive pattern of pulmonary function tests, diffusion abnormalities, and increased reticulation of the lung on x-rays are associated with pulmonary involvement. Hypertension, proteinuria, microangiopathic hemolytic anemia, and elevated levels of BUN and creatinine are associated with scleroderma kidney.

Microscopy of the nail fold is an excellent clinical tool and an easily performed procedure.[31, 49] Characteristic changes have been demonstrated in scleroderma including enlargement of capillary loops, loss of capillaries, disorganization of normal distribution of capillaries, and hemorrhages.[33]

Specimens from affected areas of the skin show increased density of collagen in the dermis with flattening of rete pegs, obliteration of appendages of the skin, hyalinization and fibrosis of arterioles, and infiltration of mononuclear cells around small vessels. Early lesions in synovium include lymphocytic infiltrations; in later stages there is fibrosis.

The most common x-ray features of the hand in scleroderma are sclerodactyly, flexion contractures, subcutaneous calcification, and digital tuft resorption (Fig. 15–21). Rare findings are narrowing of joint space, juxtaarticular demineralization, ankylosis, and marginal erosion.[8]

Treatment

There is no known specific therapy for scleroderma,[13, 26] although several studies indicate that D-penicillamine may be useful in controlling the progress if used early in the course. Treatment is symptomatic, particularly for visceral involvement.

Various simple measures used for the treatment of Raynaud's phenomenon include avoidance of exposure to cold, swing-

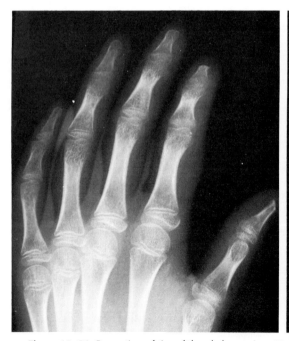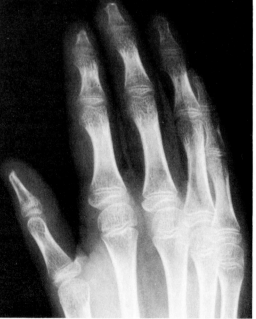

Figure 15–21. Resorption of tips of the phalanges in a 10-year-old girl with progressive systemic scleroderma.

ing the arm in an arc, and biofeedback. In established cases, various drugs have been tried, but without consistent effect. These include reserpine, tolazoline, (Priscoline), griseofulvin, and calcium-blocking agents. In intractable cases, intra-arterial reserpine and sympathetic blockade may have to be tried. Intravenous treatment with PGE_1 or PGE_2 also has been tried. If gangrene sets in, it is best to allow the finger to separate spontaneously because this is associated with less morbidity than surgical amputation.

Therapeutic measures for prevention of contractures must be aggressive. This is hard to accomplish in children who want to play and socialize and who are busy with their studies and do not wish to be bothered with daily stretching of the wrists and fingers.

Splints for the correction of wrist deformities should be worn both during activity and at rest. Finger flexion contractures are difficult to correct. Pancake splints with straps to tighten and extend the PIP and DIP joints and dynamic splints with dorsal outrigger devices may be needed to correct the flexion deformities. In severe cases, surgical correction may be required.

POLYARTERITIS NODOSA (PAN)

Polyarteritis nodosa is a relatively rare disorder. In children, there are two varieties of PAN: (1) infantile polyarteritis (in children younger than 2 years of age), and (2) childhood polyarteritis, which resembles the adult type.[13, 17, 22, 26]

Pathologically, there is necrotizing vasculitis of small and medium-sized arteries of various organs, including those of the skin, muscle, heart, and kidneys. These lesions skip segments of the vessel and are at different stages of inflammation and of repair. Thrombosis and aneurysms may occur in the tissues of these organs.

In infantile PAN, the usual clinical features are fever, conjunctivitis, maculopapular rash, and aseptic meningitis syndrome. Coronary artery disease occurs in 80% to 90% of infants, and sudden death may occur.

In childhood PAN, the course is variable. Fever, weakness, myalgia, maculopapular rash, abdominal pain, vomiting, hematuria, and hypertension are the common features. Central nervous system disease is heralded by seizures and hemiparesis or peripheral neuritis. Heart disease due to coronary artery involvement and renal failure secondary to involvement of renal vessels are the common causes of death.

The usual manifestations involving the upper extremity include discolored, painful, and tender lesions involving the tips of the fingers and of the palms. These lesions may ulcerate. Arthritis involving the larger joints of the hand and peripheral neuropathy involving one of the nerves of the upper extremities also may occur.

Aggressive treatment with steroids and cytotoxic agents has improved the prognosis associated with this disease.

KAWASAKI DISEASE (MUCOCUTANEOUS LYMPH NODE SYNDROME)

Kawasaki disease is characterized by prolonged fever, rash, conjunctivitis, lesions of the mucous membrane, and cervical lymphadenopathy. The course of the disease resembles infantile polyarteritis nodosa, and the lesions are pathologically identical in both these diseases.[26, 36]

The disease occurs predominantly in children: Few adults with this disease have been reported. There is a preponderance of children of Asian (Japanese) origin with this disease, and there may be an association with certain HLA types. Etiology is unknown, although many of the features of this disease suggest an infectious agent as the causative factor.

The importance of this disease lies in the fact that 10% to 20% of affected children develop cardiac disease, with 1% to 2% mortality due to coronary artery disease.

One of the most important clinical characteristics of Kawasaki disease involves the upper extremities, specifically the hands. During the acute phase (first 7 to 14 days of illness), there is a brawny, indurated swelling of the hands, including the fingers, which are held in flexion. Arthritis of the wrists and elbows also may develop. The arms, hands, and fingers are very painful to touch, so children with this disease do not use their hands for any activities.[25, 36]

Later in the course of the disease (third week of illness), there is peeling of the skin starting around the fingertips and nails (Fig. 15–22). Occasionally, severe vasculitis may develop, leading to gangrene of the fingers.

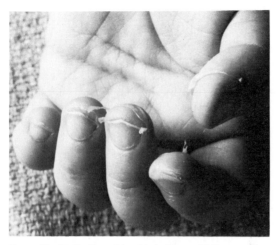

Figure 15–22. Peeling of the skin in Kawasaki disease. (Photograph courtesy of Jerry C. Jacobs, M.D.)

Careful investigation of the heart for the presence of myocarditis and coronary artery disease is essential to the management of children with Kawasaki disease. Long-term follow-up is necessary for detection of any aneurysms in the coronary artery or other large vessels, including brachial arteries.

The changes in the hand will disappear even without treatment. During the acute phase of the disease, aspirin is used in therapeutic doses for its anti-inflammatory effect. Once the fever and arthritis subside, aspirin in low doses may be indicated for its antiplatelet effect and possible beneficial effect on the coronary circulation.

MIXED CONNECTIVE TISSUE DISEASE (MCTD)

This is a syndrome characterized by clinical features of systemic lupus erythematosus, dermatomyositis, and scleroderma. Such an "overlap" syndrome has been known to clinicians for years. What distinguishes this entity is the presence of high titers of antibody to ribonucleoprotein (so-called RNP) in the sera.[13, 26, 48]

Clinically, children with MCTD develop polyarthritis, Raynaud's phenomenon, sclerodermatous skin changes, rash resembling DM or SLE, myositis, esophageal abnormalities, and lung disease. Renal disease is less common than in SLE.

Characteristic abnormalities described in the hand include diffuse, tense swelling of the dorsum of the hand and of the fingers, which is seen early in the course of the disease. The fingers often appear sausage-shaped. In addition, the arthritis associated with MCTD affects the MCP and PIP joints of the hand predominantly. Wrists and elbows also are involved, but not the shoulder and the DIP joints. Raynaud's phenomenon and the associated changes are similar to those described for scleroderma. Subcutaneous nodules may be seen near the elbows.[6, 42]

Changes on x-rays include joint space narrowing, erosions, and calcinosis. Most of these are seen around the MCP and PIP joints.

Treatment

Steroids have been known to be effective in controlling the systemic features of this disease. Physical therapy measures for control of flexion contractures of the fingers and therapy for Raynaud's disease are similar to those described for scleroderma.

MISCELLANEOUS DISORDERS

Hypertrophic Pulmonary Osteoarthropathy (HPOA)

This is a disorder characterized by clubbing of the fingers, increased sweating of the hands and feet, and swelling of various joints—notably the knees, ankles, elbows, and wrists. The joint fluid is not of the inflammatory type. Diagnosis is suggested by periosteal elevation along the phalanges and along the distal portion of the diaphysis of the bones of the forearm and leg.

In the pediatric age group,[4, 13, 26] this condition is commonly associated with cystic fibrosis and congenital heart diseases and is called secondary HPOA. Other conditions associated with secondary HPOA are inflammatory bowel disease, cirrhosis of the liver, and neoplasms such as neuroblastoma and osteogenic sarcoma. There are two types of primary HPOA, both of which are autosomal dominant. In one variety, progressive thickening of the skin of the face leading to leonine or acromegalic facies occurs in addition to the clubbing and periostitis (pachydermoperiostosis). In the second familial variety, skin thickening does not occur.[12]

Figure 15–23. Synovial granuloma in a patient with sarcoidosis (× 100).

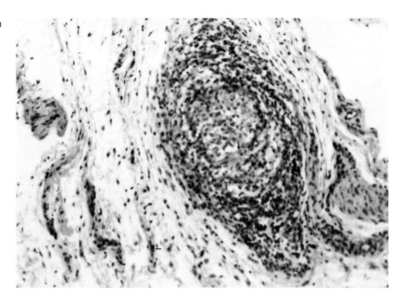

Sarcoidosis

Sarcoidosis is rare in children. When it occurs, there are two varieties.[13, 39] In children younger than seven years, the disease is characterized by painless effusions into the joints and by tenosynovitis, most marked over the extensor aspects of the wrists and of the ankles. These children do not usually have systemic features of sarcoidosis, except for iridocyclitis. Biopsy of the synovium should establish the diagnosis (Figure 15–23).

In older children and adolescents, the disease resembles adult-onset sarcoidosis. The arthritis may be acute and polyarticular or chronic and pauciarticular. The acute polyarticular form may involve the wrists and small joints of the hand, which may be stiff and painful. In the chronic form, granulomatous changes in various tissues may be apparent before joints are affected. Tenosynovitis, flexion contracture, and rheumatoid deformities of the fingers may occur in this variety. Bone lesions, particularly of the phalanges, are seen in the chronic variety.

Multicentric Reticulohistiocytosis

Multicentric reticulohistiocytosis is a rare, distinctive type of arthritis. There are less than six cases reported in the pediatric age group. In addition to the arthritis involving the large and small joints of the hand, one

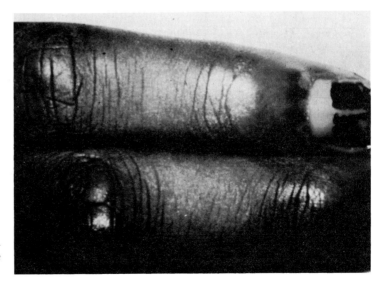

Figure 15–24. Multicentric reticulohistiocytosis: note the nodules at the base of the nail.

other finding characteristic of this disease occurs in the hand—namely, the presence of pearly nodules along the edge of the nails (Figure 15–24).

OTHER DISEASES PRODUCING DEFORMITIES OF THE UPPER EXTREMITIES

In addition to the specific diseases already described, one may also see:

A. Reducible deformities of the hand in the following conditions[19]:
  1. Marfan's syndrome. Long, thin extremities with long fingers in a tall person with arm span longer than total height, scoliosis, high arched palate, mitral valve prolapse, dislocated lens, and high myopia are the characteristic features.
  2. Wilson's disease. This is characterized by hepatic disease, Kayser-Fleischer ring, and occasionally an arthropathy.
  3. Jaccoud's arthropathy. This is described earlier, under Patterns of Involvement of the Upper Extremity in SLE.

B. Nonreversible deformities of the hand in the following conditions[19]:
  1. Mucopolysaccharidosis. There are various subtypes—the more common ones are Hurler's and Hunter's syndromes. Both types are characterized by growth retardation, coarse features, and corneal abnormalities.
  2. Diabetes. Limited mobility of small joints of the hand has been demonstrated in approximately 50% of children with insulin-dependent, or type

I, diabetes. This occurs most commonly between the ages of 10 and 20 years and is characterized by inability to approximate the palmar surfaces of interphalangeal joints (Figure 15–25). This was originally called "cheiroarthropathy" because the hand was the only area known to be affected. Now we know that this joint stiffness affects all other joints also and can predict the occurrence of microvascular complications later in life.[43, 46]

Another finding seen in association with juvenile onset diabetes mellitus is the palpable thickening and induration of the skin of the fingers of the hand. This affects the fingers distal to the PIP joints only and occasionally involves the dorsum of the hand.[46]

  3. Reflex sympathetic dystrophy syndrome (neurovascular dystrophy, Sudeck's atrophy) occurs in children, often without antecedent trauma.[13, 26] There is a large emotional component to this illness in children. Pain in the extremity is excruciating and interferes with sleep. The child will not allow even clothing to touch the limb. In addition to pain, there may be juxta-articular swelling accompanied by trophic changes. There is usually pallor or redness of the extremity, increased mottling, coldness, and excess sweating. The skin appears moist and shiny and is hyperesthetic. The child refuses to use the extremity. At later stages, there may be dystrophic changes with absence of sweating, shiny skin, and atrophy of the limbs. The laboratory tests are often normal. X-rays may show patchy demineral-

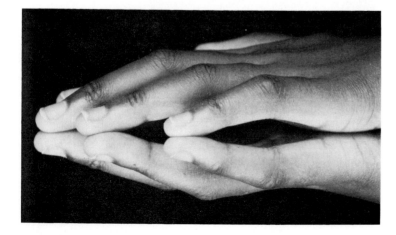

Figure 15–25. Inability to approximate the palmar surfaces of the PIP and DIP joints in diabetes. (Reprinted by permission of the New England Journal of Medicine 305: 191, 1981. Photograph courtesy of A. Rosenbloom, M.D.)

zation, and technetium bone scan may show increased or decreased flow.

It is best to treat these children with a positive approach and minimum medication. In most cases, one can handle the situation successfully with an explanation of the reasons for the pain followed by physical therapy, reassurance, and repetitive exercises. Psychological counseling may be needed in a few situations.

Hemoglobinopathies

Diffuse nonpitting swelling of the hands and feet with exquisite pain in a black child should make one think of sickle cell dactylitis and the hand-foot syndrome of sickle cell anemia.[13] Children with this syndrome are often febrile and anemic. The syndrome is not seen beyond the age of two years, and, although it is primarily associated with sickle cell disease, it may also be seen in SC disease and S-thalassemia. X-ray changes associated with the syndrome occur one to two weeks after the clinical attack and are characterized by periosteal elevation and motheaten appearance of the metacarpals. Analgesics and treatment of the crises are adequate management. Osteomyelitis must be considered in the differential diagnosis.

Migratory polyarthritis of sickle cell disease may involve joints of the upper limb and is often associated with sickle cell crises.[45] Elbow joints are the most commonly involved. Other problems associated with sickle cell disease include septic arthritis, osteomyelitis, and aseptic necrosis. Aseptic necrosis of the head of the humerus is usually associated with sickle cell disease but may also occur in association with hemoglobin–SC disease. Significant anemia, abnormal sickle cell preparation, elevated reticulocyte count, and leukocytosis are the usual laboratory abnormalities. Hemoglobin electrophoresis will establish the precise hemoglobin defect. There is no specific therapy, particularly when the humeral head is involved, except the usual management of sickle cell crises and supportive therapy for pain. Physical therapy measures may be needed to rest the joint during acute episodes of pain so that range of motion and muscle strength around the shoulder joint can be maintained.

Leukemia

Leukemia often presents with fever, hepatosplenomegaly, lymphadenopathy, severe aches and pains, and, in about 10% of affected children, with frank arthritis, which may be poly- or monarticular. Usually, patients are pale and the pain is out of proportion to the arthritis. The involved joints may include shoulders and elbows. Very rarely, small joints of the hand also may be involved. Pain and swelling of the hands, particularly in young children, may be due to dactylitis, and the hand may resemble what one sees in sickle cell crises and hand-foot syndrome. Clinical suspicion, repeated examination of blood smear, and bone marrow examination are needed for correct diagnosis because neuroblastoma can behave like leukemia. Urine should be examined for VMA also to rule out neuroblastoma.[13, 26]

Hemophilia and Other Bleeding Disorders

Hemophilia is characterized by episodes of hemorrhaging that may be either spontaneous or secondary to minor trauma. The condition is genetically determined and is due to a deficiency of a coagulation factor. Depending upon the specific factor deficiency, hemophilia may be classified as follows:

Hemophilia A. The defect in hemophilia A, also known as classic hemophilia, is a deficiency in the blood of Factor VIII (antihemophilic globulin), a substance that is essential to normal hemostasis and blood clotting. Factor VIII is a glycoprotein with a biologic half-life of 8 to 12 hours and is thought to be synthesized in the reticuloendothelial system. The genetic error in classic hemophilia is synthesis of an aberrant form of this glycoprotein, which lacks Factor VIII clotting activity.

Classic hemophilia, which accounts for approximately 75% of all inherited coagulation disorders, affects males and is genetically transmitted in a sex-linked recessive manner by apparently normal females. Theoretically, the female offspring of a hemophiliac father and a carrier mother can be affected, but this is extremely rare. The incidence of the severe form is approximately three to four per 100,000 population. If the less severe forms also are considered, the incidence of classic hemophilia rises to approximately six to eight per 100,000 population. In 30% of hemophiliac patients, there is no family history and the disorder is probably due to a spontaneous genetic mutation.

Hemophilia B. This condition, also known as Christmas disease, is due to a deficiency of Factor IX, the plasma thromboplastin component. Hemophilia B too is transmitted by a gene linked to the other chromosomes and is clinically identical with hemophilia A but has an incidence that is six to eight times lower than that of hemophilia A, accounting for approximately 12% to 15% of hemophilia cases.

Hemophilia C. This is a mild form of the disease that occurs in both males and females. It is due to a deficiency of Factor XI, the plasma thromboplastin antecedent. It is inherited as an autosomal dominant trait.

Von Willebrand's Disease. This is the third most common inherited coagulation disorder, caused not only by a variable lack of Factor VIII coagulant activity but also by a platelet functional problem. Von Willebrand's disease accounts for approximately 8% of all inherited coagulation disorders and is transmitted by an autosomal gene.

The severity of hemophilia A and B is constant in any one patient, but varies from patient to patient. In the mild form, the patient has a functional plasma level of 20% to 60% of Factor VIII or IX and may bleed excessively during surgery. In the moderate form, the plasma level is between 5% and 20%, and bleeding may occur during surgery or after trauma. Patients with moderately severe disease have plasma levels of between 1% and 5%, whereas those with severe disease have levels below 1%. With plasma levels below 5%, hemophiliacs may have spontaneous bleeding episodes and may bleed as a result of unrecognized mild trauma.

Although bleeding may occur in any area of the body, severe hemophiliacs demonstrate musculoskeletal involvement, either by soft tissue bleeding or intra-articular bleeding, in almost 80% of cases.[20, 28] The presence of residuals of hemorrhage in these areas is the most disabling consequence of hemophilia.

Hemarthrosis. Characteristically, hemarthrosis occurs in early childhood and tends to occur frequently and apparently spontaneously in those patients with severe disease. In the upper extremity, hemarthrosis most commonly affects the elbow joints. Oc-

casionally, the shoulder joints and the wrist joints are involved, but spontaneous hemarthrosis of the phalangeal joints is quite rare.

The essential aims of treatment in acute cases are to arrest hemorrhage, relieve pain, maintain and restore joint function, and prevent chronic joint changes. The methods used include replacement of clotting factor, occasional joint aspiration, immobilization of the affected joints, maintenance and restoration of joint function, and institution of a rehabilitation program.

Prompt replacement of deficient clotting factor by infusion of fresh frozen plasma, cryoprecipitate, or human antihemophilic globulin concentrate is essential. Cryoprecipitate or antihemophilic globulin in a dosage of 10 to 15 units of Factor VIII/kg of body weight is usually sufficient to elevate the patient's Factor VIII level to 15% to 20% of normal. This will control most joint bleeding. Small spontaneous hemarthroses treated within a few hours after onset can usually be managed on an outpatient basis with a single dose of Factor VIII. However, in severe hemarthrosis, especially when associated with trauma or when treatment is delayed beyond 12 hours, admission to the hospital is advised. Such patients with large, tense hemarthroses have considerable pain, muscle spasm, and loss of movement. Under these circumstances, joint aspiration is occasionally recommended. However, an intravenous effusion of cryoprecipitate or antihemophilic globulin must be available and given simultaneously with the aspiration. If factor is infused prior to aspiration, rapid clotting of the hemarthrosis may occur. Conversely, if factor infusion is given after aspiration, there may be considerable additional bleeding. Factor replacement is subsequently administered daily for 2 to 3 days or until bleeding is controlled. Reliable indications that bleeding has stopped are pain relief and a decrease in joint circumference. Immobilization and splinting are advised for several days following an acute hemorrhage and for 2 or more weeks at night.

Prolonged immobilization results in muscle atrophy with subsequent risk of joint instability. A rehabilitation program consisting of exercise and mobilization at the earliest safe opportunity is an important part of management.

Repeated episodes of hemarthrosis cause synovial hypertrophy followed by a chronic inflammatory reaction. The inflamed synovium produces reactive granulation tissue, which forms a pannus extending over and absorbing the articular cartilage and its margins. The subsequent erosion of the articular cartilage can lead to a secondary degenerative arthritis. Early proper treatment is therefore needed to delay this result.

In chronic hemarthrosis, as in acute hemarthrosis, the elbow joint is the most commonly affected joint in the upper extremity. The wrist and shoulder joints are less commonly affected. Treatment of chronic upper extremity arthropathy includes use of orthotic appliances, corrective plaster casts, traction, and various surgical options.

Synovectomy has been advocated for the treatment of joints in which repeated bleeding has been associated with chronic thickening of the synovial membranes. Removal of this hyperplastic vascular membrane should theoretically reduce hemarthrosis and protect the articular cartilage from further enzymatic destruction. Although an occasional synovectomy of the wrist or elbow joint may be indicated, findings on the long-term effect of synovectomy in reducing the extent of hemophilic arthropathy are not conclusive.

When painful fixed contractures become permanent and functionally disabling, arthrodesis or arthroplasty may be indicated.

Soft-Tissue Hemorrhage. The flexor surface of the forearm appears to have the highest incidence of subcutaneous bleeding, permitting sizable volumes of blood to accumulate in the forearm. A volar hematoma may compress ulnar or median nerve branches, producing motor and sensory deficits of the palm, thumb, or fingers. If severe, a carpal tunnel or ulnar tunnel release with evacuation of hematoma may be indicated. If left untreated, severe complications can result. Hey Groves (1907)[25] was the first to describe a Volkmann's contracture in association with untreated hemophilia. Lancourt and colleagues (1977)[31] reported 34 complications of untreated hemophilia in the hand and forearm, four of which involved a Volkmann's contracture. These authors recommended fasciotomy in cases of impending Volkmann's contracture.

In forearm hemorrhages seen early, the wrist usually assumes a flexed position with the fingers held in varying amounts of flexion. Active finger motion is impaired. Pain is usual and may be accompanied by tingling, itching sensations or varying degrees of numbness. During this initial period, one should apply a well-padded volar splint without attempting to change the position of the hand and wrist. As the hemorrhage resolves, frequent splint changes are utilized to maintain the hand and wrist in a more functional position. As active wrist, finger, and thumb function returns, the splint is removed. With early treatment and prompt correct evaluation of the problem, complete recovery without functional deficit is usual.

Psoriasis and Arthritis

Psoriatic arthritis is defined as an inflammatory arthritis that is associated with psoriasis, which either precedes the onset of the arthritis or occurs subsequently. In patients with this condition, both the psoriasis and arthritis develop before the age of 16 years. In adults, this type of arthritis belongs to the general category of seronegative spondyloarthropathies and is characterized by atypical polyarthritis, sausage-shaped digits, involvement of DIP joints, and a destructive arthropathy with or without sacroiliitis. Such typical arthritis of psoriasis is rare in children, and it is very difficult for one to differentiate between psoriatic arthritis and psoriasis with coincidental JRA.

In children, psoriatic arthritis is characterized by monarticular presentation progressing to asymmetric polyarthritis, and there is usually a strong family history of psoriasis.[30, 47] Destructive, resorptive arthropathies seen in adults are rare in children, but sausage digits are common. Pitted nails and scaly lesions over the dorsum of the hand are other features of psoriasis characteristically evident on examination of the hand (Figure 15–26). The nails may show pitting, ridging, hyperkeratosis, and subungual atrophy. X-rays in children characteristically show asymmetric polyarthritis, growth abnormalities similar to those described for pauciarticular JRA (e.g., advanced bone age and elongation of bones), and periostitis. Marginal erosions of phalanges, erosions of the tufts of the terminal phalanges, resorptive arthropathy, sacroiliac disease, and ankylosis are not common.

Because psoriatic arthritis is an inflammatory arthropathy, many children with this condition will require treatment with one of the nonsteroidal anti-inflammatory drugs.

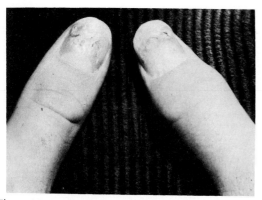

Figure 15–26. Psoriasis and arthritis in a 13-year-old boy. Note the nail changes and the swelling of distal interphalangeal joint of the right thumb. (Photograph courtesy of William M. Bason, M.D.)

Rarely, these children may require injections of steroids into the affected joints and tendon sheaths. Intramuscular gold injections and oral steroid therapy are very rarely indicated. Surgical correction of deformities of the joints may be needed, as in JRA.

Nonspecific Nodules

Two types of nodules may be seen on the hands and wrists: granuloma annulare and erythema nodosum.

The lesions of granuloma annulare are infiltrative plaques seen over the arms, legs, and trunk. They are reddish-brown and of varying sizes and shapes. Most of them have a ring shape and a rolled edge. These lesions may be triggered by trauma, such as insect bites. Histologically, the lesions resemble rheumatoid nodules, except that these lesions are located deeper. Occasionally, this condition may be associated with arthritis, so differentiation between JRA and granuloma annulare becomes difficult. No specific treatment for this condition is necessary.

Erythema nodosum[9] is characterized by the sudden appearance of painful subcutaneous nodules that are indurated, warm, and tender. Associated systemic symptoms—such as fever, malaise, arthralgia, and arthritis—also are common. Females are affected more than males, and the usual location is the anterior surface of the leg (pretibial); occasionally, however, these lesions may occur in the upper extremities.

In erythema nodosum, crops of nodules appear for approximately three to six weeks, and individual lesions undergo characteris-

tic progression. After the initial sudden appearance of small nodules, the lesions become bigger and indurated and display various colors; eventually, they become smaller and induration becomes less prominent and disappears. They leave a brownish discoloration but no scars. Primary pathology of erythema nodosum is vasculitis of deeper blood vessels of the skin and septal panniculitis. This condition is probably a hypersensitivity response and is seen in association with various infectious agents, such as *Streptococcus, Leptospira, Yersinia,* and *Mycobacterium*; with fungal infections such as histoplasmosis and coccidioidomycosis; with granulomatous conditions such as sarcoidosis; with drug reactions, such as those due to sulfa and birth control pills; and with various rheumatic diseases, including JRA, lupus, and inflammatory bowel disease. In children, one of the most common associated conditions is inflammatory bowel disease. Laboratory investigations to be ordered in cases of erythema nodosum include various tests for exclusion of the aforementioned conditions. However, in a number of cases, specific etiology may not be identified. Therapy with salicylates is adequate for control of systemic symptoms. Treatment of the primary condition is obviously necessary. Very rarely, steroids may be indicated.

Bibliography

1. Ansell BM, Nasseh GA, Bywaters EGL. Scleroderma in childhood. Ann Rheum Dis 35:189–197, 1976.
2. Arden G, Ansell BM. Surgical Management of Juvenile Chronic Arthritis. London, Academic Press, 1978.
3. Athreya BH. The hand in juvenile rheumatoid arthritis. Arthritis Rheum 20(suppl 2):573–574, 1977.
4. Athreya BH, Borns P, Rosenlund ML. Cystic fibrosis and hypertrophic osteoarthropathy in children. Am J Dis Child 129:634–637, 1973.
5. Babbitt DP, Sty JR, Kohler EE. A complication of JRA—spontaneous biceps tendon rupture. Wis Med J 78(3):32–33, 1979.
6. Bennett RM, O'Connell DJ. The arthritis of mixed connective tissue disease. Ann Rheum Dis 37:397–403, 1978.
7. Bleifeld CJ, Inglis AE. The hand in systemic lupus erythematosus. J Bone Joint Surg 56(a):1207–1215, 1974.
8. Blocka KLN, Bassett LN, Furst DE, et al. The arthropathy of advanced progressive systemic sclerosis. A radiographic survey. Arthritis Rheum 24:874–884, 1981.
9. Blomgren SE. Erythema nodosum. Semin Arthritis 4:1–24, 1974.
10. Brewer EJ, Giannini EH, Person DA. Juvenile Rheumatoid Arthritis. Major Problems in Clinical Pediatrics, Vol. 6. Philadelphia, WB Saunders, 1982.

11. Brewerton DA. Hand deformities in rheumatoid disease. Ann Rheum Dis 16:183–196, 1957.

12. Calabro JE, Marchesano JM, Abruzzo JL. Idiopathic hypertrophic osteoarthropathy (pachydermoperiostitis); onset before puberty. Arthritis Rheum 9:496, 1966.

13. Cassidy JT. Textbook of Pediatric Rheumatology. New York, John Wiley & Sons, 1982.

14. Chaplin D, Pulkki T, Saarimaa A, et al. Wrist and finger deformities in juvenile rheumatoid arthritis. Acta Rheum Scand 15:206–223, 1969.

15. Costello PB, Kennedy AC, Green FA. Shoulder joint rupture in juvenile rheumatoid arthritis producing bicipital masses and a hemorrhagic sign. J Rheum 7:563–566, 1980.

16. Cranberry WM, Mangum GL. The hand in the child with juvenile rheumatoid arthritis. J Hand Surg 5:105–113, 1980.

17. Cupps TR, Fauci AS. The vasculitides. Major Problems in Internal Medicine Series, Vol. 21. Philadelphia, WB Saunders, 1981.

18. Dabrowski W, Fonseka N, Ansell BM, et al. Shoulder problems in juvenile chronic polyarthritis. Scand J Rheum 8:49–53, 1979.

19. Dorwart B, Schumacher HR. Hand deformity resembling rheumatoid arthritis. Semin Arthritis Rheum 4:53–71, 1974.

20. Duthie RB, Rizza CR. Rheumatological manifestations of the hemophilias. Clin. Rheum Dis 1(1):53–93, 1975.

21. English CB, Nalebuff EA. Understanding the arthritic hand. Amer. J. Occup. Ther. 25:352–359, 1971.

22. Fink C. Polyarteritis and other diseases with necrotizing vasculitis in childhood. Arthritis Rheum 20 (suppl.):378–384, 1977.

23. Forrester DM, Brown JC, Nesson JW. The Radiology of Joint Disease, 2nd Ed. Philadelphia, WB Saunders, 1978.

24. Giesecke LL, Athreya BH, Doughty RA. Home care guide for JRA—A manual for parents. Atlantic City, Children's Seashore House Publications, 1982.

25. Hey Groves EW. A clinical lecture upon the surgical aspects of hemophilia with especial reference to two cases of Volkmann's contracture resulting from this disease. Br Med J 1:611–614, 1907.

26. Jacobs JC. Pediatric Rheumatology for the Practitioner. New York, Springer-Verlag, 1982.

27. King KK, Kornreich HK, Bernstein BH, et al. The clinical spectrum of systemic lupus erythematosus in childhood. Arthritis Rheum 20(Suppl. 2):287–294, 1977.

28. Kisker T, Perlman AW, Benton C. Arthritis in hemophilia. Semin Arthritis Rheum 1:220–235, 1971.

29. Laaksonen AL. A prognostic study of juvenile rheumatoid arthritis. Analysis of 544 cases. Acta Paediatr Scand 166(Suppl.):1–168, 1966.

30. Lambert JR, Ansell BM, Stephenson E, et al. Psoriatic arthritis in children. Clin Rheum Dis 2:339–352, 1976.

31. Lancourt JE, Gilbert MJ, Posner MA. Management of bleeding and associated complications of hemophilia in the hand and forearm. J Bone Joint Surg 59A:451–460, 1977.

32. Maldonado-Cocco JA, Garcia-Morteo O, Spindler

33. Maricq HR. Widefield capillary microscopy: technique and rating scale for abnormalities seen in scleroderma and related disorders. Arthritis Rheum 24:1159–1165, 1981.

34. Martel W, Holt JF, Cassidy JT. Roentgenologic manifestations of juvenile rheumatoid arthritis. Am J Roentgenol 88:400–423, 1962.

35. Medsger TA Jr, Christy WC. Carpal arthritis with ankylosis in late onset Still's disease. Arthritis Rheum 19:232–242, 1976.

36. Melish ME. Kawasaki syndrome (mucocutaneous lymph node syndrome). Pediatr Rev 2:107–114, 1980.

37. Nalebuff EA. Diagnosis, classification, and management of rheumatoid thumb deformities. Bull Hosp Joint Dis 29:119–137, 1968.

38. Nalebuff EA, Yeria A, Millender L. The incidence and severity of wrist involvement in juvenile rheumatoid arthritis. J Bone Joint Surg 54A:905, 1972.

39. North AF, Fink CW, Gibson WM, et al. Sarcoid arthritis in children. Am J Med 48:449–455, 1970.

40. Poznanski AK, Hernandez RJ, Guire KE, et al. Carpal length in children—a useful measurement in the diagnosis of rheumatoid arthritis and some congenital malformation syndromes. Radiology 129:661–668, 1978.

41. Pulkki T. Rheumatoid deformities of the hand. Acta Rheum Scand 7:85–88, 1961.

42. Ramos-Niembro F, Alarcon-Segovia D, Hernandez-Ortiz J. Articular manifestations of mixed connective tissue disease. Arthritis Rheum 22:43–51, 1979.

43. Rosenbloom AL, Silverstein JH, Lezotte DC, et al. Limited joint mobility in diabetes mellitus of childhood. Natural history and relationship to growth impairment. J Pediatr 101:874–878, 1982.

44. Schaller JG, Hanson V, eds. Proceedings of the First American Rheumatism Association Conference on the rheumatic diseases of childhood. Arthritis Rheum 20(Suppl. 2):145–628, 1977.

45. Schumacher HR. Rheumatological manifestations of sickle cell disease and other hereditary hemoglobinopathies. Clin Rheum Dis 1(1):37–52, 1975.

46. Seibold JR. Digital sclerosis in children with insulin-dependent diabetes mellitus. Arthritis Rheum 25:1357–1361, 1982.

47. Shore A, Ansell BM. Juvenile psoriatic arthritis—an analysis of 60 cases. J Pediatr 100:529–535, 1982.

48. Singsen BH, Bernstein BH, Kornreich HK, et al. Mixed connective tissue disease in childhood—a clinical and serological survey. J Pediatr 90:893–900, 1977.

49. Spencer-Green G, Schlesinger M, Bove KE, et al. Nailfold capillary abnormalities in childhood rheumatic diseases. J Pediatr 102:341–346, 1983.

50. Swanson AB, deGroot GA, Hehl RW, et al. Pathogenesis of rheumatoid deformities in the hand. In Cruess RL, Mitchell NS, eds. Surgery of Rheumatoid Arthritis. Philadelphia, JB Lippincott, 1971:143–158.

51. Zvaifler NJ. Chronic post-rheumatic fever (Jaccoud's) arthritis. N Engl J Med 267:10–14, 1962.

AJ, et al. Carpal ankylosis in juvenile rheumatoid arthritis. Arthritis Rheum 23:1251–1255, 1980.

Heritable and Endocrine Disorders of Connective Tissue Metabolism

FREDERICK KAPLAN

Heritable Disorders

The hand of the adult is a mirror of heritable and systemic disease. The hand of the child, however, is more like a reflecting pool, projecting the dynamic changes of growth and development. The diagnosis and treatment of heritable and endocrine-related hand disorders consists primarily of the diagnosis and treatment of the underlying condition.

The child's hand is a structural organ that reflects the metabolic status of the growing organism. There are numerous conditions and disordered states of skeletal homeostasis, and a separate consideration of each will shed light on only a small portion of the complex physiology that underlies normal growth and development.

Before we tamper, we must attempt to understand. Any consideration of bodily form during the childhood years must incorporate the concepts of growth, development, and change. The hand in childhood not only *is* but also *is becoming*. In addition, there is concern not only for the limb at the moment but also for its ultimate structure and function at the time of skeletal maturity.

SKELETAL DYSPLASIAS[7-9, 11, 13, 15-17]

The largest category of heritable disorders of connective tissue consists of the skeletal dysplasias, or the osteochondrodystrophies. The surgeon focusing on hand problems in skeletal dysplasia is like a lost person mesmerized by an individual tree in a vast forest. Attention to specific clinical concerns will eventually be required, but never before a full comprehension of the location and natural history of the clinical "forest." Enthusiasm must be tempered by an overall understanding of the conditions involved. The panoply of radiographic anomalies, often helpful in diagnosis, may be confusing, causing one to presume the presence of a clinical disability that does not in reality exist.

Although our major focus will be on hand and upper limb abnormalities associated with a wide variety of disorders, one should remember that the major risk is in the loss of clinical perspective. The interested reader is referred to the references for sources of broader discussions of these conditions.

In considering these disorders categorically, the reader should keep in mind several general principles:

1. The growth plate, the site of endochondral bone formation, is the organ responsible for the longitudinal growth of the appendicular skeleton and is the site of the numerous genetic disorders that give rise to the skeletal dysplasias.

2. Intramembranous ossification, responsible for the growth in width of the long bones, is often less disturbed in the skeletal dysplasias than is endochondral ossification.

3. The particular clinical presentation and radiographic appearance of the hand in the various skeletal dysplasias involve not only a decrease in size as compared to normal, but also an abnormality in shape, brought about by the discrepancy between endochondral and intramembranous ossification.

4. The high rate of skeletal turnover at all bone remodeling surfaces in the child (periosteal, haversian, endosteal, and trabecular) can bring about rapid morphologic changes.

5. The distinctive radiographic appearance of the skeletal dysplasias often allows a diagnosis to be made on radiographic appearances alone.

6. The child's adaptability to a congenital disorder involving an abnormality in the shape and interrelationship of the parts of the upper limb is greater than might be expected from the clinical presentation and radiographic appearance of the anomalous parts.

The first step in the evaluation of a child with short stature involves the determination of whether the short stature is normal or abnormal. Thorough family and social histories are critical in the detection of specific cultural or environmental factors that may predispose the child to short stature and be normal in the situation in question. For instance, it is important that one know the height of the child's parents and grandparents because correction for parental height can now be made with revised growth charts. Although the third percentile is defined as the lower limits of normal, 3% of normal children will, by definition, fall below this percentile.

After determining that the stature is abnormal according to familial and social standards, one must next decide whether the decreased height is proportionate or disproportionate. At birth, the head and trunk are disproportionately larger than the limbs, whereas after birth, the growth of the appendicular skeleton increases relative to the growth of the skull and trunk, so that by the time the child is approximately 8 years of age, the upper segment is equal in length to the lower segment. In the past, measurements of sitting heights were used to determine relative body proportion, but because it is difficult to obtain standardized sitting height measurements, the upper segment:lower segment ratio—an accurate measurement that can be reproduced with precision—is more commonly employed. One determines the length of the lower segment by measuring the vertical distance from the symphysis pubis to the floor while the child is standing upright. The length of the upper segment is defined as the total length minus the length of the lower segment. The upper segment:lower segment ratio ranges from 1.7 to 1.8 at birth; it declines to approximately 1.1 by 4 years of age, to 1.0 by 8 years of age, and to 0.95 at the time of skeletal maturity. The upper segment:lower segment ratio is slightly lower in blacks at the time of skeletal maturity. Significant deviations from normal (greater than two standard deviations) in upper segment:lower segment ratios are diagnostic of disproportionate stature.

The two major categories of disproportionate short stature are short-trunk dysplasia and short-limb dysplasia. In the disproportionate short-trunk skeletal dysplasias, the child's height is below normal, and the upper segment:lower segment ratio is abnormally low. In the disproportionate short-limb dysplasias, the upper segment:lower segment ratio is abnormally high. The upper segment length, as in achondroplasia, is characteristically normal, but the lower segment length is abnormally low, and thus the upper segment:lower segment ratio is high.

One may make a simple diagnostic confirmation of short limb versus short trunk skeletal dysplasia by observing the level of the fingertips with the child in the standing position. Under normal conditions of growth and development, fingertips should reach the midthigh level with the child in a standing position and the hands at the sides. In short-trunk dysplasia, the limbs are relatively long compared with the trunk. The fingertips may reach below the midthigh level and, in some conditions, to the level of the knee and below. In the short-limb dysplasias, the limbs are disproportionately short compared with the trunk segment, and the fingertips will often reach no farther than the proximal thigh crease.

After making the distinction between disproportionate short-trunk and disproportionate short-limb dysplasia, one must next ascertain whether the disproportion in the short limb dysplasia is in the proximal, middle, or distal segment of the limb.

When the relative shortening in the disproportionate short-limb dysplasia occurs in the proximal segments (i.e., the shoulder and arm segment or the hip and thigh segment), the disorder is referred to as rhizomelic dysplasia. The prefix "rhizo" is derived from the Greek word meaning "root," and the suffix "melos" refers to the "limb." Thus, "rhizomelic" refers to the root of the limb and thus the proximal segment. The prototype of disproportionate short-limb rhizomelic skeletal dysplasia is achondroplasia.

When the predominant shortening occurs in the middle segment of the limb (forearm or leg segment), the condition is referred to as mesomelic dysplasia. The prefix "meso" refers to the middle portion of the limb. Léri-Weill dyschondrosteosis with its accompanying Madelung's deformity is an example of disproportionate short-limb mesomelic dysplasia.

When the predominant shortening occurs in the distal segment of the limb (the hand or the foot), the condition is referred to as acromelic dysplasia, or disproportionate short-limbed acromelic dysplasia. The prefix "acro" is derived from the Greek word meaning "tip" or "end"; again, the suffix "melos" refers to the limb. Ellis–van Creveld's syndrome, a chondroectodermal dysplasia, is an example of disproportionate short-limbed acromelic dysplasia.

In one skeletal dysplasia, there is a short-limb dysplasia at birth, but that changes to short-trunk dysplasia later in childhood. This particular dysplasia is referred to as metatropic dwarfism, or metatropic dysplasia. The word "metatropic" is derived from Greek and refers to the changing proportions seen with this very severe and often lethal form of skeletal dysplasia. Although almost all of these disorders have a genetic basis, many occur sporadically as a result of a spontaneous mutation. Most of these sporadic cases may be passed on as autosomal dominant disorders, indicating that the abnormal phenotype is expressed when only a single allelic mutation occurs in the genome. Metatropic dwarfism is thought to be the result of an autosomal recessive disorder; that is, both abnormal alleles must be present for the disorder to be expressed. The risk of recurrence with the autosomal recessive disorders is one in four for all future births to the same parents. The risk of recurrence following the birth of a child with a sporadic mutation is virtually nil if the parents are not similarly affected and if the mutation has not occurred in the parental germ cell line. The importance of genetic counseling cannot be overestimated, not only following the birth of a child with a nonlethal skeletal dysplasia but also after the birth of a child who dies early in infancy. The importance of the establishment of an accurate diagnosis may be critical for future family planning.

Although the skeletal dysplasias are heritable, not all are congenital. For instance, the congenital form of spondyloepiphyseal dysplasia may be identifiable at birth, whereas the similar appearing mucopolysaccharide disorder, Morquio's syndrome (MPS IV), may not be detectable clinically until the child is 3 to 4 years of age. It is remembered that not all heritable disorders are congenital and that not all congenital disorders are heritable.

So far, we have discussed some general principles in the diagnostic approach to the complex skeletal dysplasias. Table 16–1 may be of further help.

For the next part of the evaluation of a child with skeletal dysplasia, x-rays of the spine and extremities must be obtained. In reviewing the x-rays of the extremities, one will find it helpful to determine what portions of the tubular bones are most severely affected in any limb segment. For instance, is the skeletal abnormality predominately metaphyseal or epiphyseal? If the abnormality is predominately in the metaphysis, the roentgenographic abnormality would be called a metaphyseal dysplasia. If the abnormality predominately involved the epiphysis, the dysplasia would be referred to as

Table 16–1. **Evaluation of Short Stature**

I. Normal short stature
II. Abnormal short stature
   A. Proportionate short stature (think of endocrine disorders)
   B. Disproportionate short stature (osteochondrodysplasia)
      1. Short-trunk dysplasia
      2. Short-limb dysplasia
         (a) Rhizomelic dysplasia
         (b) Mesomelic dysplasia
         (c) Acromelic dysplasia

an epiphyseal dysplasia. If both were involved to a similar extent, one would call the disorder an epimetaphyseal dysplasia.

One of the characteristic abnormalities of growth disturbance involving the spine in the skeletal dysplasias is the appearance of platyspondyly. The prefix "platy" means flattened and the suffix "spondyly" refers to the spine; thus, "platyspondyly" refers to a flattening of the vertebral segments, specifically a flattening of the vertebral body. There are often concomitant abnormalities in the anterior vertebral ring apophyses, resulting in the appearance of beaking on the anterior aspect of the vertebral body. If the spine is roentgenographically involved with the skeletal dysplasia, the disorder is called a spondylodysplasia. The roentgenographic combination of an epiphyseal abnormality in the appendicular skeleton and a dysplasia in the spine would be referred to as a spondyloepiphyseal dysplasia. The combination of a metaphyseal disorder in the appendicular skeleton with spine involvement is known as a spondylometaphyseal dysplasia.

Thus, achondroplasia is considered a disproportionate short-limb rhizomelic epiphyseal dysplasia. The prototype of short-trunk dwarfism would be the congenital form of spondyloepiphyseal dysplasia. Although the epiphyses would be affected in all the tubular bones of the appendicular skeleton, the abnormalities of growth are more notable in the spine, thus contributing to the short-trunk dwarfism.

With these principles of diagnosis and terminology in mind, we can now focus on the individual upper limb abnormality seen with the various forms of skeletal dysplasia.

Achondroplasia

Achondroplasia is the most common and prototypic form of rhizomelic short-limb dysplasia. Its genetic transmission is autosomal dominant, but it often arises sporadically as a result of a spontaneous mutation.

The condition is easily recognizable at birth, with disproportionate short-limb short stature and an upper segment:lower segment ratio that is abnormally high.

The apparently enlarged head, frontal boss, and depressed nasal bridge are the result of a disproportionate growth between the intramembranous bones that form the calvarium and the endochondral bones that form the face and the base of the skull.

The growth plate abnormality results in a striking disturbance in the longitudinal growth of the long bones, but the width of the long bones and the relative cortical thicknesses are essentially undisturbed.

Although the limbs are most severely involved, the abnormality in the growth centers in the spine results in both a narrow interpedicular distance and a foreshortened pedicle. This growth abnormality may lead to spinal stenosis later in life, secondary to central canal narrowing or neural foraminal narrowing. Any secondary degenerative changes that may occur would tend to exacerbate the clinical symptoms of spinal stenosis. Thoracic kyphosis and lumbar hyperlordosis are common.

The hand in achondroplasia has a characteristic trident configuration. The middle three digits (the index, long, and ring fingers) are identical in length, and apposition is difficult because of asymmetric growth on the ulnar and radial sides of the long and ring fingers, respectively. The distal phalanges all have a squat, broad appearance on x-rays, and the proximal and middle phalanges have a broad conical shape. A ball-in-socket appearance of the metacarpophalangeal region of the digits is seen.

Paradoxically, the most severe upper limb problems seen in achondroplasia occur at the elbow. This is the result of asymmetric growth about the elbow and consequent subluxation of the radial head. Nearly all children with achondroplasia have this problem to a variable degree, and in the severe forms the child may have difficulty with activities of daily living because of the resultant flexion contractures. Physical therapy may be of some help in certain instances, but surgery is rarely indicated. No controlled studies are available for assessment of the efficacy of the various forms of treatment for radial head subluxation in this condition.

As in most of the skeletal dysplasias, the characteristic x-ray findings seen early in life are less striking once skeletal maturity has been reached. When longitudinal growth ceases and the physis no longer exists, the difference between epiphyseal and metaphyseal regions blur to indistinction, and it is often impossible for one to reconstruct the aberrant temporal and spatial dynamics of the skeletal dysplasias.

A great deal of clinical heterogeneity may exist in the heritable dysplasias, especially in the autosomal dominant forms. Variable expressivity and incomplete penetrance are common. The former refers to the wide range of clinical expression of a heritable disease within a given kindred. The latter refers to the apparent skipping of a generation as far as the phenotypic expression of the disease is concerned.

Hypochondroplasia

This disorder is distinct from classic achondroplasia. In marriages between individuals with hypochondroplasia and achondroplasia, segregation of the genes is evident in the clinical appearance of the offspring. Hypochondroplasia, like achondroplasia, either is inherited as an autosomal dominant trait or arises sporadically as the result of a spontaneous allelic mutation. A mild disproportionate rhizomelic short-limb dysplasia is seen. It may be difficult to detect the milder forms unless upper segment:lower segment ratios are obtained. Unlike achondroplasia, hypochondroplasia does not involve the skull and face. In hypochondroplasia, as in achondroplasia, the long bones of the fingers are characteristically short, but there is no trident configuration to the hand, and the fingers can be apposed without difficulty.

Pseudoachondroplasia

Pseudoachondroplastic spondyloepiphyseal dysplasia is a form of severe disproportionate rhizomelic short-limb dysplasia that is inherited either as an autosomal dominant (most common) or as a recessive trait. Unlike achondroplasia, this disorder is not apparent at birth and is not manifest until the child is 3 to 4 years of age. The skull is uninvolved, and the face may have a cherubic appearance. Although the spine is less involved than the limbs, resulting in an upper segment:lower segment ratio that is characteristic of a short-limb dysplasia, x-rays of the spine reveal mild to moderately severe platyspondyly. Early degenerative joint disease of the hips is common, and progressive scoliosis may be a clinical problem.

The clinical presentation and radiographic appearance of the hands in this condition are more severe than in achondroplasia. The long tubular bones are short and squat, and the metaphyses are irregular. The ball-in-socket appearance of the epiphyses also is

seen in this condition, but trident configuration of the hand is absent.

Thanatophoric Dysplasia and Achondrogenesis

Thanatophoric (Greek, "thanatos," meaning "death-bearing") dysplasia and achondrogenesis are two of the most severe forms of short-limb dysplasia. Both are diagnosable at birth and incompatible with life. The affected children are stillborn or die shortly after birth. The inheritance pattern is not known for either form, but in achondrogenesis it is thought to be autosomal recessive because of a report of two affected siblings born at different times to normal parents. These two forms of severe dysplasia are often confused with achondroplasia, but the distinction is important, especially with regard to genetic counseling. The clinical presentation and radiographic appearance of both conditions are characteristic and have been well documented by McKusick[9] and by Smith.[13]

A clearer understanding of these two fatal conditions—and of all the other skeletal dysplasias—awaits elucidation of the genetically determined biochemical cartilage abnormality. Until such information is available, diagnosis of all the skeletal dysplasias must be based on careful clinical and radiographic evaluation and phenotype-matching with previously described "classic cases." For detailed explanation of the radiographic appearance of the upper limb in the skeletal dysplasias, the reader is referred to the book by Steinbach and colleagues.[15]

Mesomelic Dysplasia

The mesomelic dysplasias are characterized by short-limbed short stature with disproportionate shortening of the middle limb segments. The upper limbs are more severely involved than the lower limbs. Dyschondrosteosis (Léri-Weill syndrome) is the prototype of mesomelic dysplasia. Although shortening predominates in the middle portions of the limb segments (the forearms and legs), it is present in all other long bones.

In 1878, Madelung described an isolated skeletal abnormality characterized by posterior subluxation of the distal radius, with lateral radial bowing. Although this may be seen in other conditions such as Turner's syndrome or in association with acro-osteolysis, Madelung's deformity is an invariable feature of dyschondrosteosis.

The adult height of affected individuals is less than 1.5 m (5 ft). The middle segment deformity does not become clinically evident until later in adolescence, with marked shortening and lateral bowing of the radius. Severe deformities exist within the carpus. Abnormal cone-shaped epiphyses are seen in the proximal phalanges (Fig. 16–1).

The middle segment of the lower limb is affected in dyschondrosteosis, but the tibial and fibular abnormalities with their associated deformities about the ankle are much less severe than those seen in the forearm and wrist.

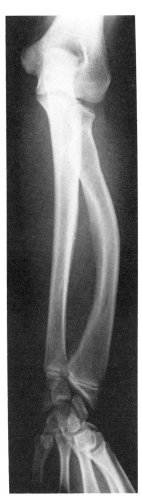

Figure 16–1. Madelung's deformity in a 13-year-old with Léri-Weill dyschondrosteosis (disproportionate mesomelic short-limb short stature).

Acromelic Dysplasia

The prototype of acromelic dysplasia was described by Ellis and van Creveld in 1940. This rare disorder, carefully studied by McKusick in the Amish of Lancaster County, Pennsylvania, is characterized by mild disproportionate short-limb short stature with malformation of the hair, teeth, and nails and associated polydactyly and congenital heart disease. Family studies have revealed that this disorder is transmitted as an autosomal recessive trait.

The most consistent finding is polydactyly. The disorder can be diagnosed at birth and usually occurs in the hands. The extra finger is always postaxial and is often well formed and functional. Polydactyly is uncommon in the feet.

Occasionally, one may observe duplication of the phalanges of the extra digits. Ossification centers in the hand and carpus are delayed in maturation. Malformations of the nails and teeth are common. Atrioseptal defect is the most common cardiac anomaly and is present in as many as 60% of affected individuals. When congenital heart disease is absent, life expectancy is normal.

Metatropic Dysplasia

Metatropic dysplasia, which means "changing form," is a disproportionate short-limb rhizomelic short stature that is recognizable at birth. Grotesque metaphyseal swellings and a pathognomonic radiographic halberd appearance to the pelvis along with dumbbell-shaped femora and humeri are characteristic. The thorax is long and narrow at birth, and many children die early in infancy as the result of respiratory complications of their small chest or lethal C1–C2 subluxations.

Those who survive will develop a severe recalcitrant kyphoscoliosis and a morphologic pattern that changes to that of a short-trunk dysplasia, reminiscent of the severe forms of spondyloepiphyseal dysplasia. Although most of the shortening is proximal, the hands are affected with severe contractures, as are other joints in the appendicular skeleton. Passive stretching exercises are indicated for the flexion contractures, which may involve the fingers (Fig. 16–2).

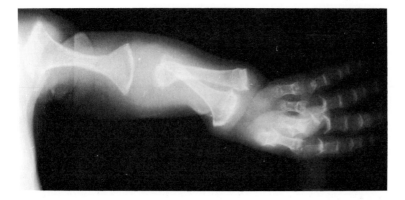

Figure 16–2. X-ray of the upper limb of a neonate with metatropic dysplasia.

Diastrophic Dysplasia

In 1960, Lamy and Maroteaux described a rare form of autosomal recessive inherited disproportionate short-limbed short stature that is recognizable at birth. The severe kyphoscoliosis that affected children develop early in life reminded these authors of the forces that throw the earth's crust into upheaval—thus the term "diastrophic."

The "hitchhiker's thumb," present at birth in many children with this autosomal recessive form of short-limb short stature, heads the long list of profound axial and appendicular disorders seen in this condition. Soon after birth, the clinical features of severe appendicular joint contractures appear, as do resistant club feet, deformed ears, and

severe kyphoscoliosis. The children develop cystic cauliflower-like swelling of the ears and calcification of the pinnae. The skull is normal except for the variable presence of cleft palate. Intelligence is normal. There is characteristic short stature and symphalangism of the proximal and distal phalanges of the thumb (Fig. 16–3).

In diastrophic dysplasia, as in most of the skeletal dysplasias, the underlying biochemical abnormality is presently unknown, but histopathology of the physeal regions reveals a chondrocytopenia throughout the reserve, proliferative, and hypertrophic zones of the growth plate. An abnormality in type II collagen production has been postulated.[14a]

Although life expectancy may be normal, severe joint contractures are often resistant to simple management.

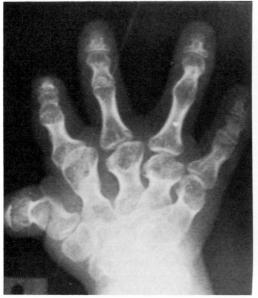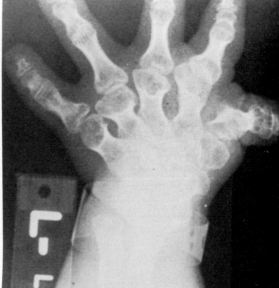

Figure 16–3. X-rays of the hand of a child with diastrophic dysplasia. Note the hitchhiker's thumbs.

Chondrodysplasia Punctata (Conradi's Disease)

This severe dysplasia, transmitted in an autosomal recessive pattern, is detectable at birth or during early infancy. It is characterized by disproportionate short-limb rhizomelic short stature with stippling of the epiphyses, disordered growth, mental retardation in as many as 50% of affected children, cataracts and blindness, congenital heart defects, and fascial hernias.

Characteristic abnormalities occurring in the axial skeleton include craniosynostosis, hypertelorism, micrognathia, and hypoplasia of the nasal bones.

Joint contractures are common throughout the appendicular skeleton. There is a high infant mortality rate associated with this condition secondary to bronchial pneumonia. Those children who survive infancy have an improvement in their musculoskeletal condition, and the stippling disappears by the time they are 3 to 4 years of age.

Appendicular abnormalities most consistently include joint contractures, polydactyly, and syndactyly as well as short-limbed rhizomelic dysplasia.

Pyknodysostosis

Toulouse-Lautrec was thought to have this rare autosomal recessive form of disproportionate short stature with increased bone density. Skeletal fragility with pathologic fractures is seen in this rare dysplasia, and the radiographic appearance of the skeleton may resemble that seen in osteopetrosis.

The average adult height achieved in this dysplasia is less than 1.5 m (5 ft). The histopathology in this condition is similar to that seen in osteopetrosis, but there is always evidence of normal intramedullary hematopoiesis, and the medullary canal can be seen on x-rays. Pancytopenia and cranial nerve disorders do not develop in this condition as they do in osteopetrosis.

Abnormalities in the appendicular skeleton are notable with dysplasia or absence of the acromial ends of the clavicles. The digits are short, especially the terminal phalanges, and fragmentation of bone in the distal phalanges similar to that seen in idiopathic acroosteolysis (Hajdu-Cheney syndrome) may be

present. The prognosis of the disorder is based on the presence and recurrence of pathologic fractures due to the abnormally fragile bone.

De Lange's Syndrome (Amsterdam Dysplasia)

A chromosomal defect has been implicated in this rare sporadic form of short stature with structural limb defects. The disorder is recognizable at birth. Associated features include mental retardation, a characteristic facies, prominent eyebrows with low hairline, small nose, congenital heart disease, undescended testicle, and hypospadias. The children are microcephalic and have a high, arched cleft palate.

A variety of limb defects can be seen in the appendicular skeleton, including absent ulna, dislocated radial head, flexion contracture of the elbow, syndactyly, and short metacarpals (especially the thumb metacarpal, which results in a proximally placed thumb). Intercarpal fusion may be present, and phocomelia is commonly seen.

Most affected children have an intrinsic failure to thrive and do not survive infancy.

Acrocephalosyndactyly (Apert's Syndrome)

Apert's syndrome is the prototype of the head-hand syndromes. This disorder either arises as a sporadic mutation or is inherited in an autosomal dominant pattern. Characteristic clinical features include a tower-shaped skull with premature fusion of the sutures and subsequent mental retardation. Syndactyly is the most common hand anomaly in this condition. The middle three digits are fused and often share one nail. This gives the characteristic mitten appearance to the hand. Esophageal atresia and renal anomalies may complicate this disorder, but it is the cranial anomaly that accounts for high infant mortality. Early surgery of cranial synostosis has met with limited success.

Syndactyly of the index, long, and ring fingers is present and may involve the feet as well as the hands. Synostosis of the radius and ulna and dislocation of the radial head also have been reported.

Acrocephalopolysyndactyly (Carpenter's Syndrome)

This disorder is similar to Apert's syndrome, but the syndactyly in Carpenter's syndrome is not as severe or deforming. One may also note preaxial polysyndactyly in the toes in this disorder. Family pedigrees indicate that Carpenter's syndrome, unlike Apert's syndrome, is inherited as an autosomal recessive trait.

Focal Dermal Hypoplasia (Goltz's Syndrome)

Nearly all cases of focal dermal hypoplasia are sporadic and seen in females. This condition is likely an X-linked dominant disorder that is lethal in males. Atrophy and pigmentation of the skin with structural limb and hand defects are evident at birth. The skin disease is characterized by linear pigmentation with telangiectasia and subdermal herniation of fat. Papillomas are seen on the skin and mucous membranes. A variety of ocular disorders, including strabismus and microphthalmos, may occur.

Although syndactyly in the hands is the most common finding in this disorder, polydactyly and flexion contractures of the digits also are common.

Holt-Oram Syndrome

Holt-Oram syndrome is the prototype of the heart-hand syndromes. The congenital heart defect in this disorder is most often a septal defect, and arrhythmias are likely to arise.

A nonopposable triphalangeal thumb is present, or the thumb may be totally absent. Also, there is either an absent radius (a similar deformity is present in Fanconi's syndrome) or a radial club hand. The lower limbs are not involved in Holt-Oram syndrome.

Although controversy exists as to the mode of inheritance of this condition, at least one form of the disorder is inherited as an autosomal dominant trait.

Onycho-Osteodysplasia (Nail-Patella Syndrome)

Genetic linkage studies reveal that this autosomal dominant disorder is linked with the A, B, and O blood groups. Clinically, the disorder is characterized by hypoplastic or absent nails and hypoplastic or absent patellae. Other skeletal disorders include small scapulae, hypoplasia of the lateral epicondyle, hypoplasia of the humeral capitellum, and a small radial head. Congenital subluxation or dislocation of the radial ulnar joint is common.

Short-Trunk Dysplasia

All the short-trunk dysplasias are characterized by disproportionate short stature and a decrease in the upper segment:lower segment ratio.

The prototype and most severe form of short-trunk dysplasia is spondyloepiphyseal dysplasia congenita. This disorder is detectable at birth, with short-trunk disproportionate short stature and a normal face and skull. Severe involvement of the epiphyses of the proximal segments (hips and shoulders) develops early in life, with coxa vara and genu valgum. The disorder is inherited as an autosomal dominant trait.

Radiographic features of the disorder in the newborn infant include delay in ossification of the epiphyses and platyspondyly with hypoplasia of the anterior segment of the vertebral body.

During adolescence, the thoracic kyphosis and lumbar lordosis may become severe, whereas the odontoid process, although incompletely ossified, rarely poses severe clinical problems. Nevertheless, there have been rare reports of symptomatic C1–C2 subluxation, and lateral flexion-extension x-rays should be obtained.

During childhood, the phenotypic features of spondyloepiphyseal dysplasia (SED) congenita and Morquio's syndrome (MPS IV) are often similar but warrant differentiation. The clinical manifestations of spondyloepiphyseal dysplasia congenita are present at birth; in Morquio's syndrome, they do not appear until the child is 2 to 3 years of age. Deficient ossification of the pubic bone is present in SED congenita, but it is absent in Morquio's syndrome. The femoral neck in SED congenita is in varus, whereas in Morquio's syndrome it is in valgus. The hands and feet are minimally involved in SED congenita but are severely involved in Morquio's syndrome. Ophthalmologic abnormalities are seen in both conditions; severe myopia is common in SED congenita, whereas corneal clouding is seen in Morquio's syndrome. Mucopolysacchariduria is absent, of course, in SED congenita but present in Morquio's syndrome. The symptomatic C1–C2 subluxation common in Morquio's syndrome is an indication for atlantoaxial fusion. Although present in SED congenita, it is most often asymptomatic and rarely causes clinical problems. Finally, the mode of inheritance is autosomal dominant in SED congenita, whereas it is recessive in Morquio's syndrome.

Spondyloepiphyseal dysplasia tarda is a mild chondrodystrophy that is not manifest until late childhood or early adolescence. It is characterized by a mild form of short-trunk dysplasia and is often confused with Legg-Calvé-Perthes disease because it presents with bilateral anterior thigh and groin pain. Radiographic appearance may be confused with that of idiopathic avascular necrosis of the hips if upper segment:lower segment ratios are not carefully evaluated. Spondyloepiphyseal dysplasia tarda should be suspected in all individuals with bilateral Legg-Calvé-Perthes disease. The differentiation is important because, in SED tarda, precocious degenerative arthritis of the hips is likely to develop despite any intercurrent treatment modalities.

Mild shortening of the tubular bones of the hand will be inapparent clinically, and therefore it is unlikely that x-rays of the hands will be taken during early childhood prior to closure of the growth plates. Following skeletal maturity, early degenerative arthritis may exist in the joints of the hand and carpus.

Mucopolysaccharide Dysostoses[1, 2, 7–9, 11, 13–15, 17]

The genetic mucopolysaccharidoses are true skeletal dysplasias resulting from an inborn error in the metabolic degradation of mucopolysaccharide with mucopolysaccharide deposition in numerous organ systems, including the skeleton. The mucopolysaccharidoses are listed in Table 16–2 (MPS I to MPS VIII). Many of these disorders share similar clinical features, and the mode of inheritance in most is autosomal recessive, characteristic of the defined enzyme deficiency, with the exception of Hunter's syndrome (MPS II-A, II-B), in which X-linked recessive transmission occurs. The deficient enzyme has been identified for each of the mucopolysaccharide disorders, although some conditions such as Morquio's syndrome (MPS IV) probably represent more than one allelic form of the disorder. Characteristic excessive urinary mucopolysaccharide has been identified for each of the seven major types and subtypes.

Clinically, children with mucopolysaccharide disorders have disproportionate short-trunk dysplasia. Of all of the mucopolysaccharidoses, Hurler's syndrome presents with the most severe clinical involvement, with severe skeletal deformation resulting from intracellular deposition of mucopolysaccharides in bone. Progressive heart failure from coronary artery disease and endocardial and myocardial disease from intracardiac deposition of mucopolysaccharides are seen.

Although detectable biochemically, the mucopolysaccharide disorders are not diagnosed clinically at birth. The children spend their first year of life asymptomatic, with the stature becoming disproportionate only during the end of the first or second year. Deposits of mucopolysaccharides in the liver cause the appearance of an enlarged or bloated abdomen.

In Hurler's syndrome (MPS I-H) death usually occurs before the age of 10 years. In Scheie's syndrome (MPS I-S), stiff joints, cloudy cornea, and mitral regurgitation are seen in the presence of normal intelligence. The Hurler-Scheie compound (MPS I H/S) is a phenotypic intermediate between classic Hurler's syndrome and classic Scheie's syndrome.

The severe hand abnormalities noted in the mucopolysaccharide disorders are best reflected in Hurler's syndrome (MPS I-H). McKusick notes broad, stubby fingers with flexion contractures and hypoplastic terminal phalanges. A claw hand deformity may be seen later in childhood, resulting from the flexion contractures and the abnormal mucopolysaccharide deposition in the subcutaneous and integumentary tissues.

Radiographically, the hand deformities seen in classic Hurler's syndrome are severe. However, changes are not evident before the end of the first year of life. By the age of 2 years, flexion contractures are apparent clinically. Widening of the medullary cavities of the long bones secondary to intramedullary mucopolysaccharide deposits cause cortical osteopenia and increased endosteal resorp-

Table 16–2. **The Genetic Mucopolysaccharidoses**

Number	Eponym	Clinical	Genetics	Urinary MPS	Enzyme-Deficient
MPS I-H	Hurler	Clouding of cornea; grave manifestations; death usually before 10 years of age	Homozygous for MPS I-H gene	Dermatan sulfate; heparin sulfate	α-ʟ-iduronidase
MPS I-S	Scheie	Stiff joints; cloudy cornea; aortic valve disease; normal intelligence and (?) lifespan	Homozygous for MPS I-S gene	Dermatan sulfate; heparin sulfate	α-ʟ-iduronidase
MPS I H/S	Hurler-Scheie	Intermediate phenotype	Genetic compound of MPS I-H and MPS I-S genes	Dermatan sulfate; heparin sulfate	α-ʟ-iduronidase
MPS II-XR, severe (30990)	Hunter, severe	No corneal clouding; milder course than MPS I-H; death before 15 years of age	Hemizygous for X-linked gene	Dermatan sulfate; heparin sulfate	Iduronate sulfatase
MPS II-XR, mild	Hunter, mild	Survival to 30s to 60s, fair intelligence	Hemizygous for X-linked allele	Dermatan sulfate; heparin sulfate	Iduronate sulfatase
?MPS II-AR (25285)	?Autosomal Hunter	Same as mild or severe MPS II-XR	Homozygous for autosomal gene	Dermatan sulfate; heparin sulfate	Iduronate sulfatase
MPS III-A (25290)	Sanfilippo A	Indistinguishable phenotype: mild somatic effects; severe central nervous system effects	Homozygous for Sanfilippo A gene	Heparin sulfate	Heparin N-sulfatase
MPS III-B (25292)	Sanfilippo B		Homozygous for Sanfilippo B gene	Heparin sulfate	N-acetyl-α-D-glucosaminidase
MPS III-C (25293)	Sanfilippo C		Homozygous for Sanfilippo C gene	Heparin sulfate	α-glucosaminidase?

MPS IV-A (25300)	Morquio A	Severe, distinctive bone changes; cloudy cornea; aortic regurgitation	Homozygous for Morquio A gene	Keratan sulfate	Galactosamine-6-sulfate sulfatase
MPS IV-B (25301)	Morquio B	Mild bone changes, cloudy cornea, hypoplastic odontoid	Homozygous for Morquio B gene	Keratan sulfate	β-galactosidase
MPS V					
MPS VI, severe (25320)	Maroteaux-Lamy, classic severe	Severe osseous and corneal changes; valvular heart disease; striking WBC inclusions; normal intellect; survival to 20s	Homozygous for Maroteaux-Lamy (M-L) gene	Dermatan sulfate	Arylsulfatase B (N-acetylgalactosamine 4-sulfatase)
MPS VI, intermediate	Maroteaux-Lamy, intermediate	Moderately severe changes	Homozygous for allele at M-L locus or genetic compound	Dermatan sulfate	Arylsulfatase B (N-acetylgalactosamine 4-sulfatase)
MPS VI, mild	Maroteaux-Lamy, mild	Mild osseous and corneal changes; normal intellect; aortic stenosis	Homozygous for allele at M-L locus	Dermatan sulfate	Arylsulfatase B (N-acetylgalactosamine sulfatase)
MPS VII (25322)	Sly	Hepatosplenomegaly dysostosis multiplex; mental retardation variable; WBC inclusions	Homozygous for mutant gene at β-glucuronidase locus	Dermatan sulfate; heparin sulfate	β-glucuronidase
MPS VIII (25323)	DiFerrante	Short stature; mild dysostosis multiplex; ring-shaped metachromasia of lymphocytes	Homozygous for MPS VIII gene	Keratan sulfate; heparin sulfate	Glucosamine-6-sulfate sulfatase

(From McKusick VA. Mendelian Inheritance in Man. Catalogs of Autosomal Dominant, Autosomal Recessive and X-linked Phenotypes, 5th ed. Baltimore, The Johns Hopkins University Press, 1978.)

tion. This is most prominent in the fifth metacarpal. Abnormalities in funnelization of the bones are seen. The trabecular pattern in the cancellous trabecular bone is coarse. Abnormalities are evident in the distal radial and ulnar ossification centers. Hypoplasia of the ossification centers of the carpal bones is noted. Similar findings are found in the feet but are less striking than those in the hand.

The most common mucopolysaccharide disorder is Morquio's syndrome (MPS IV). (See discussion under "spondyloepiphyseal dysplasia congenita.")

Early diagnosis of Morquio's syndrome is possible during infancy before the characteristic clinical deformity appears. There are diagnostic radiographic changes in both the axial skeleton and the appendicular skeleton. Vertebra plana is seen throughout the spine. There is anterior beaking of the vertebral bodies secondary to abnormalities in the ring apophyses. Hypoplasia of the odontoid is seen in Morquio's syndrome. Thoracolumbar kyphosis is present and may be severe. Many secondary epiphyseal growth centers are delayed in appearing.

The radiographic changes seen in the hand in Morquio's syndrome are less severe than those seen in classic Hurler's syndrome. The bases of the metacarpals are cone-shaped. Unlike Hurler's syndrome, Morquio's syndrome does not involve flexion deformities. Brachydactyly is common, with the most severe shortening in the metacarpals. Clinically, the hand has a thickened, flaccid appearance (Fig. 16–4).

Although the dysostosis seen with the mu-copolysaccharide disorders may be severe and life-threatening (especailly MPS I), the hand abnormalities do not present clinical management problems. Affected children adapt well to the abnormalities seen in the limb musculature. In the disorders in which flexion contractures are common, hand therapy with passive range of motion exercises may be helpful and can often be performed at home by the parents.

The Mucolipid Dysostoses[9, 15]

The genetic mucolipid dysostoses are rare storage disorders of acid mucopolysaccharide and glycolipid. Clinically, these disorders are characterized by short stature, joint stiffness, pudgy coarsened facies, and spondyloepiphyseal dysplasia. Unlike the mucopolysaccharide disorders, these conditions are not characterized by increasing urinary excretion of mucopolysaccharide.

Severe flexion contractures are seen in nearly all the genetic mucolipid dysostoses. The long bones of the hand are short and broad, and a delay in carpal ossification is noted. The interested reader is referred to McKusick[9] for further description of these rare storage disorders.

CYTOGENETIC DISEASES[4, 10, 15]

The clinical application of chromosome analyses and sophisticated quinacrine and Giemsa banding techniques have allowed prenatal karyotyping in many of the cytogenetic and dysmorphic conditions.

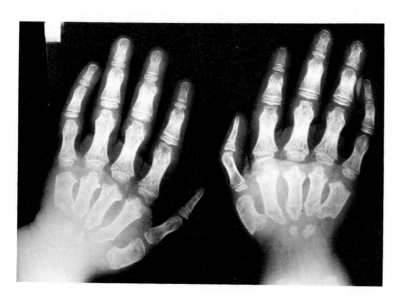

Figure 16–4. Hand X-rays of a child with the Morquio syndrome. (MPS IV)

All four major autosomal trisomy syndromes (trisomy 21 or Down syndrome; trisomy 18; trisomy 13; and trisomy 8) are associated with abnormalities of the hands and feet.

Trisomy 21 is characterized by short broad hands with prominent simian crease and clinodactyly of the little finger. There is often a wide gap between the first and second toes. Trisomy 18 is distinguished by a clenched hand with the index and little fingers overriding the middle and ring fingers, respectively. The clenched hand with overlapping digits may also be seen in trisomy 13 along with severe flexion contractures. Joint immobility in the fingers and toes and limited supination in the forearm are commonly seen in trisomy 8, along with an exacerbation of the joint stiffness and flexion contractures over time. Clinodactyly of the little fingers, club feet, and vertebral column abnormalities are common.

Experimental animal models suggest that the inborn errors in morphogenesis are more likely to interfere with different developmental processes than are those in the familial metabolic disorders. By considering the complex stages of cell migration, inductive interaction between ectoderm and mesoderm, anteroposterior differentiation of the limb, proximodistal organization of the limb bud (controlled by specialized positional information with autonomous timing), and programmed cell death, one can begin to appreciate the phenotypic complexity of the morphologic disorders seen with the cytogenetic syndromes. This is exemplified most prominently in the trisomy conditions but is also present in the deletion syndromes (4p− syndrome; 5p− syndrome, or cri du chat; 13q− syndrome; and 18q− syndrome). Abnormalities in the development of the appendicular skeleton also can be seen in Turner's and Klinefelter's sex chromosome anomaly syndromes, but these tend to be less severe than those of the autosomal trisomy and deletion syndromes. The reader is referred to two excellent review articles by Holmes and Nyhan.[4,10]

EHLERS-DANLOS SYNDROMES[1, 8, 9, 14, 15, 17]

Ehlers-Danlos syndromes comprise a large group of heritable disorders of collagen metabolism (Table 16–3). Clinically, the Ehlers-Danlos syndromes are characterized by variable degrees of joint laxity. It is often difficult to establish the boundary between normal and pathologic joint laxity with little information available on regional and racial differences. Excessive joint laxity may be characterized by recurrent or habitual subluxations or dislocations without any significant history of trauma. Fascial hernias are common in many of the joint laxity syndromes.

In the well-established Ehlers-Danlos syndromes, underlying disorders of posttranslational collagen metabolism have been identified in several of the genotypes. Loose-jointedness and capillary fragility with easy bruisability are common features of some of the disorders. Life-threatening complications including dissecting aortic aneurysms, aortic rupture, and gastrointestinal bleeding can occur in the more severe disorders.

Wynne-Davies[17] established criteria for generalized joint laxity, including (1) hyperextension of the wrist, (2) hyperextension of the carpometacarpal joint of the thumb, (3) hyperextension of the metacarpophalangeal joints, (4) excessive dorsiflexion of the ankle, and (5) hyperextension of the elbows and knees. Genetic heterogeneity may account for the variability seen within families with the various Ehlers-Danlos genotypes, and the clinician must exercise care in establishing the pattern of laxity throughout the appendicular skeleton. McKusick notes that hyperextension of the thumb can occur as an isolated heritable phenomenon. Individuals who have chronically dislocated or subluxed interphalangeal, metacarpophalangeal, or carpometacarpal dislocations may be at higher risks for developing early degenerative changes. The presence of generalized joint laxity is often a valuable clinical clue to an underlying heritable disorder of connective tissue and rarely, if ever, represents an isolated phenomenon for the clinician's therapeutic prowess.

THE MARFAN SYNDROME[1, 8, 9, 13, 15, 17]

This generalized disorder of connective tissue was first described by Antoine Marfan in 1896. Ironically, what Marfan described was not Marfan's syndrome, but congenital contractural arachnodactyly.

The Marfan syndrome is transmitted as an

Table 16–3. **Ehlers-Danlos Syndromes**

Number	Name	Clinical Features	Genetics	Biochemical Defect
E-D I (13000)	E-D, gravis type	Classic features, all severe	Autosomal dominant	Unknown
E-D II (13000)	E-D, mitis type	Classic features, all mild	Autosomal dominant	Unknown
E-D III (13000)	B-D, benign hypermobile type	Generalized marked joint hypermobility without skeletal deformity; skin features minimal	Autosomal dominant	Unknown
E-D IV (22535, 13005)	E-D, ecchymotic, arterial, or Sack-Barabas type	Severe bruisability; very thin skin; rupture of bowel; rupture of large arteries; minimal joint laxity (e.g., limited to fingers)	Autosomal recessive (autosomal dominant in some families)	Deficient synthesis of type III collagen
E-D V (30520)	E-D, X-linked type	Stretchable skin striking; joint hypermobility minimal; skin fragile; bruisability variable	X-linked recessive	?Deficiency of lysyl oxidase
E-D VI (22540)	E-D, ocular type; lysyl hydroxylase deficiency; hydroxylysine-deficient collagen disease	Scoliosis, severe; skin features, moderate; blindness from retinal detachment or ocular rupture	Autosomal recessive	Deficiency of protocollagen lysyl hydroxylase
E-D VII (25241)	Arthrochalasis multiplex congenita; procollagen peptidase (or protease) deficiency	Short stature; severe joint laxity with congenital dislocations; moderate skin stretchability and bruisability	Autosomal recessive	Deficiency of procollagen protease (or peptidase)
E-D VIII (13008)	E-D, periodontosis type	Fragile skin, especially on shins; mild to moderate loose-jointedness; severe periodontosis with early loss of teeth	Autosomal dominant	Unknown

(From McKusick VA. Mendelian Inheritance in Man. Catalogs of Autosomal Dominant, Autosomal Recessive and X-linked Phenotypes, 5th ed. Baltimore, The Johns Hopkins University Press, 1978.)

autosomal dominant trait. In this disorder, as in any of the autosomal dominant conditions, a great variability in expressivity of the phenotype may be seen. The major organ systems involved in the Marfan syndrome include the skeleton, the cardiovascular system, and the eye. Current research in the Marfan syndrome has identified abnormalities in collagen solubility that may reflect abnormalities in posttranslational collagen metabolism.

Clinically, patients with the Marfan syndrome appear Lincolnesque. They may suffer from lens dislocation and myopia with strabismus. Aortic root aneurysm may be present. Arachnodactyly with excessive joint laxity is common. Kyphoscoliosis may be severe. Pectus excavatum or the reverse (pigeon breast abnormality) is present.

It is likely that the individual with the Marfan syndrome is brought to clinical attention by the progressive kyphoscoliosis, the ocular abnormalities, or the cardiac dysfunction. If untreated, the aortic aneurysm can prove fatal with spontaneous rupture of the aorta or progressive dissection with subsequent rupture. Sudden precipitous fatalities are common in individuals with the Marfan syndrome. Beta-adrenergic blockers may be used to control the cardiac afterload and pulse pressure and thereby decrease the risk of untimely dissection of the aorta. In certain instances, life-saving surgery is required.

Progressive kyphoscoliosis can lead to severe spinal deformity with restrictive chest disease and subsequent pulmonary compromise.

Arachnodactyly is characteristically seen in the Marfan syndrome but is not specific because it may also be seen in homocystinuria. The arachnodactyly seen in the Marfan syndrome is even more striking in congenital contractural arachnodactyly and may be quite noticeable at birth. The congenital arachnodactyly seen in the latter condition likely reflects the excessive growth of the long bones in comparison with the growth of the musculature and may account for the dichotomy of joint laxity along with flexion contractures. The bone age is greatly accelerated with respect to chronologic age in congenital contractural arachnodactyly (Fig. 16–5). A striking feature of the Marfan syndrome is a disproportionately tall stature with excessively long limbs compared with the size of the trunk and a consequent tall, thin, Lincoln-like appearance; the upper segment to

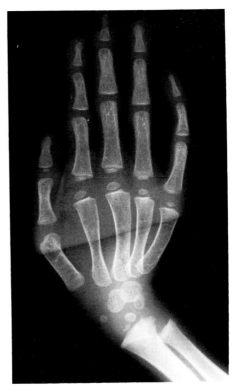

Figure 16–5. Hand x-ray of a 2-year-old child with congenital contractural arachnodactyly. Note the advanced carpal bone age.

lower segment ratio is below normal despite the above normal height.

HOMOCYSTINURIA[6, 8, 9, 13, 14, 15]

Homocystinuria is a heritable, congenital disorder of methionine metabolism and results from a deficiency of the enzyme cystathionine synthase. Homocystine accumulates in the tissues and is excreted in the urine. A simple screening test for homocystine in the urine is specific for this rare metabolic disorder.

Both homocystinuria and the Marfan syndrome share phenotypic characteristics, although they are unrelated genetically. Each disorder poses its own life-threatening vascular risk—the Marfan syndrome with its cardiovascular and aortic complications, and homocystinuria with its microvascular thrombosis. Whereas the former may be managed with beta-adrenergic blockers, the latter may be successfully managed with pyridoxine.

Both the Marfan syndrome and homocystinuria present clinically with excessive height, overgrowth of the long bones, excessive joint laxity, scoliosis, arachnodactyly, and dislocation of the ocular lens. Homocystinuria, unlike the Marfan syndrome, is commonly associated with mental retardation and osteopenia, although the pathophysiology of these complications is unknown.

Although several carpal abnormalities have been described in homocystinuria— specifically malformation of the capitate and a small lunate—the clinical distinction between the Marfan syndrome and homocystinuria is best established on the basis of less subtle differences.

OSTEOGENESIS IMPERFECTA[6, 8, 9, 12, 15]

Osteogenesis imperfecta is the most common heritable form of osteoporosis and refers to a group of at least four diseases that are often congenital and always heritable. They are manifested by either autosomal dominant or autosomal recessive inheritance. These disorders, phenotypically similar, are characterized by a number of signs and symptoms of varying severity, including generalized appendicular and axial osteopenia, marked skeletal fragility, multiple pathologic fractures, scoliosis, dentinogenesis imperfecta, blue sclerae, and deafness. Specific disorders in collagen metabolism have been identified in only a few of the more severe and rare recessive forms of the disorder.

Classification of osteogenesis imperfecta as congenita and tarda forms is obsolete and has been replaced by a more useful empiric classification.[12]

Severe osteopenia is evident radiographically in both the axial and appendicular skeletons. Appendicular osteopenia is characterized by excessively thin cortices, decreased metacarpal-cortical index, and decreased combined cortical thickness throughout all the long bones. Appendicular fractures are more commonly seen in the proximal and middle limb segments. However, they are not limited to these areas and may be seen in the hands and feet as well. Radiographically, fractures are commonly noted in various stages of healing and generally heal without difficulty. The risk of fracture decreases with increasing age, although the ravages of accumulated deformity

are registered in the crumpled, shortened, and distorted frame (Fig. 16–6).

OSTEOPETROSIS[9, 15]

Osteopetrosis, or marble bone disease, was first described by Albers-Schoenberg in 1904. The congenital and fatal form of the disorder is transmitted by autosomal recessive inheritance. It is radiographically diagnosable at birth but often does not become clinically manifest until the first or second month of life, when the child presents with anemia, thrombocytopenia, leukopenia, hepatosplenomegaly (as a secondary manifestation of extramedullary hematopoiesis), blindness, and deafness.

The basic disorder is a dysfunction of the circulating monocyte, an osteoclast precursor. Although osteoclasts may be present and their specialized ruffled borders and clear zones may be noted on electron micrographs, they are dysfunctional. As a result, endochondral bone formation may proceed normally down through the hypertrophic zone and the zone of provisional ossification, but the matrix clasts (osteoclasts) are unable to resorb the primary calcified cartilage bars and thus are unable to prepare the primary spongiosum for osteoblast activity. Thus, the primary cartilaginous bars persist down into the metaphysis, crowding out the marrow elements and precipitating a severe myelophthisic anemia. Extramedullary hematopoiesis results, and a peripheral pancytopenia is seen. The increase in infection rate observed in this condition results not only from the peripheral leukopenia and the presence of immature cells in the peripheral circulation but also from an abnormality in the circulating monocyte line, associated abnormalities in leukocyte chemotaxis, and intracellular killing of bacteria. The severe cranial nerve dysfunction arises as a result of the inability to form normal neural foramina for the passage of the cranial nerves.

If untreated, affected children succumb to a bleeding disorder or to recurrent infection. Several centers have reported successful heterologous HLA-matched bone marrow transplantation, with survival now at 5 years.

The radiographic features of osteopetrosis are impressive, with the entire skeleton appearing radiopaque. No distinction can be made between the medullary cavity and the

Figure 16–6. X-ray of 2-month-old child with severe perinatal type III osteogenesis imperfecta. Note the severe axial and appendicular osteopenia and the fractures in various stages of healing.

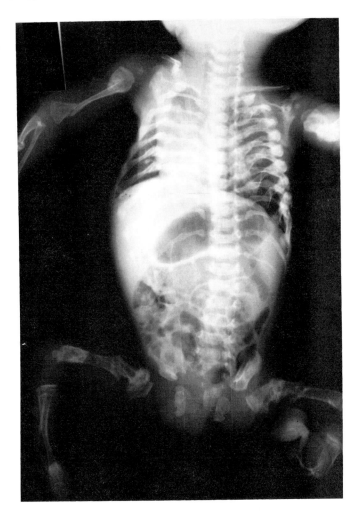

cortices of the long bones, and the axial skeleton appears uniformly dense. There is also metaphyseal splaying and abnormalities in funnelization secondary to the disordered osteoclastic bone remodeling normally found in the metaphyseal region. The uniform sclerosis of the skeleton is due not to an increase in bone formation but to the persistence of calcified cartilage. Radiographic features in the hand are no different from those of other parts of the skeleton, and a uniform sclerosis is present throughout the carpal bones and the long tubular bones (Fig. 16–7).

The tarda form of osteopetrosis is a distinct heritable disorder that shares some radiographic and clinical features with the more severe congenita form. The tarda form of osteopetrosis may not be diagnosed until late childhood or even adulthood, when x-rays are obtained either for routine assessment (e.g., preoperative chest x-ray) or for the diagnosis of a fracture following minimal trauma. Osteopetrotic bone, although more radiodense, is less strong than normal bone, which is obvious when one considers the fact that the skeleton in this condition is composed predominately of calcified cartilage rather than bone and that what bone is formed cannot properly remodel.

X-rays of the skeleton in the tarda form of the disorder may reveal alternating radiopaque zones with bone of relatively normal density. This may reflect the evanescent nature of the tarda disorder and result in the radiographic appearance of a bone within a bone or a skeleton within a skeleton. Such features may be seen in either the axial skeleton or the appendicular skeleton and also may be manifest in the cancellous and tubular bones of the hand.

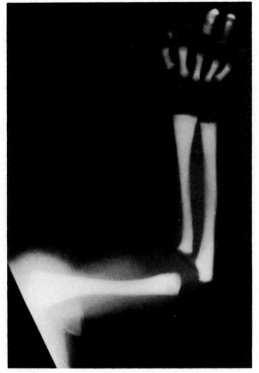

Figure 16–7. X-ray of an upper limb of a child with severe neonatal autosomal recessive osteopetrosis.

Endocrine Disorders[1, 3, 5, 6, 14, 15, 17]

In the growing child as in the adult, the body regulates few parameters with greater fidelity than the ionized serum calcium. Indeed, the survival of the organism depends on the maintenance of ionized serum calcium within a very narrow range for the purposes of (1) intercellular enzymatic kinetics, (2) cell-membrane integrity, (3) inter- and intracellular communication, (4) interneuronal transmission, (5) neuromuscular transmission, (6) muscular contraction, (7) axonal transport, and (8) blood clotting mechanisms.

Consequently, with its great metabolic investment in calcium, the body has many interrelated endocrine control systems to ensure this critical homeostasis. When the body's calcium supply is in jeopardy, the skeleton, the major storage depot of 99% of the total body calcium, is the first to suffer, and the ravages are magnified throughout the dynamic spectrum of growth. The organs that are most sensitive to disorders of mineral homeostasis in the growing individual are the growth plates (physes), especially those deep within the hypertrophic zone and in the subzone of provisional calcification. The diagnosis and treatment of endocrine-related hand disorders consists of the diagnosis and treatment of the underlying endocrinopathy.

GIGANTISM

Human growth hormone (HGH) extracted from the eosinophilic cells of the anterior lobe of the pituitary gland is a polypeptide hormone that induces the formation of intermediary growth-promoting factors known generically as somatomedins. Human growth hormone, through its intermediary somatomedin, has a role in the growth and development of all mesenchymal tissue. Somatomedin has a specific stimulatory effect on the replication of the stem cell in the proliferative zone of the growth plate. Human growth hormone has a stimulatory effect on cartilage via its intermediary somatomedin.

The French neurologist, Pierre Marie, observed the increased abnormal stature relating to hyperfunctioning of the pituitary gland. However, it was not until the early twentieth century that Harvey Cushing discovered the connection with the eosinophilic cells in the pituitary that were related to this extraordinary overgrowth of the skeleton.

Pituitary gigantism is a rare condition that results from hyperfunctioning of the eosinophilic cells of the pituitary gland prior to skeletal maturity. The condition is defined as excessive endochondral growth beyond a total body height of 2 m (6 ft 8 in). Affected individuals have been known to exceed 2.5 m (8 ft) in height. The excess of the growth-stimulating substances causes overgrowth of the bone, cartilage, and fibrous tissues, resulting in a proportionate increase in the length and mass of the skeleton and its supporting tissues.

When hyperfunctioning of the eosinophilic cells of the anterior pituitary occurs in adolescence near the time of growth plate closure, an abnormal pattern results that is a combination of increased endochondral growth and articular cartilage stimulation. When hyperfunctioning of the eosinophilic cells of the anterior lobe of the pituitary occurs completely following skeletal maturity, pure acromegaly results.

Characteristic hand abnormalities include wide phalanges with thick cortices and enlargement of the tufts of the distal phalanges (acromegaly). The skin is coarsened and thick not only in the hands but also throughout the body. Tufting of the distal ends of the digits is seen in the feet as well as in the hands.

In pituitary gigantism, the hands appear grossly and radiographically normal and reveal an accentuation of the normal growth patterns.

Treatment of the disorder consists of treatment of the underlying pituitary disorder. This may be approached either by limited surgical hypophysectomy or by extirpation of the pituitary with irradiation.

HYPOTHYROIDISM

Thyroid hormone plays a critical role in the growth and development of the skeleton. The growing skeleton is sensitive to small amounts of thyroid hormones, and a rather severe deficiency must be present early in life for skeletal growth to be retarded. Cretinism, or thyroid dwarfism, is the most severe form of hypothyroidism. It is caused by a congenital lack of formation of the thyroid gland. Mild disproportionate short-trunk stature, mental lethargy, a low basal metabolic rate, myxedema, and skeletal immaturity with respect to chronologic age are characteristic features of cretinism. This disorder is one of the few endocrinopathies that leads to disproportionate rather than proportionate short stature. Postnatal endochondral growth in the long bone does not accelerate normally and catch up with the prenatal growth of the cranium, which results in a head size that appears abnormally large for the extremities.

There are severe abnormalities in collagen and osteoid metabolism resulting in increased free water binding by the collagen of mesenchymal tissues. This water is firmly bound, unexpressible with extrinsic pressure, and decidedly distinct from edema fluid. The characteristic myxedematous appearance of a child with disproportionate short stature is often a valuable clue to the eventual diagnosis of thyroid dwarfism in distinction to the proportionate dwarfism seen in juvenile renal osteodystrophy or pituitary dwarfism.

The skin of a child with cretinism has a characteristic dry, scaly appearance, and the subcutaneous tissues are thickened throughout the body and are particularly noticeable in the hands. A child with cretinism has mild mental retardation.

The growth and maturation of the skeleton are often severely retarded. There is discrepancy in the maturation of intramembranous and endochondral bone formation. Intramembranous bone formation proceeds at a relatively normal rate, whereas endochondral bone formation is severely retarded. The long bones appear abnormally wide compared with their length. However, unlike achondroplasia, the disorder in chondrocyte maturation is seen throughout the zones of the growth plate and is not limited specifically to the cells in the proliferative zone.

Radiographically, there is a delay in appearance of the secondary epiphyseal ossification centers. In addition to the delay in ossification, the secondary growth centers appear smaller than usual and have irregular spotty calcifications. The delay in cartilage mineralization in the zone of provisional calcification is a manifestation of the delay in maturation in all areas of the growth plate.

X-rays of affected hands show a striking delay in skeletal maturation when compared with x-rays of hands of normal, age-matched controls.

A common metabolic disturbance in severe hypothyroidism is hypocalcemia. The skeletal turnover of calcium is diminished in hypothyroid states. It has been postulated that the absence of calcitonin, a polypeptide hormone manufactured and secreted by the parafollicular cells of the thyroid gland, may have a significant role in the development of hypocalcemia. Athyrotic children who receive appropriate replacement doses of thyroxine continue to manifest abnormalities in the skeletal turnover of calcium and an abnormal response to the intravenous infusion of calcium despite a normal parathyroid–vitamin D endocrine axis.

Treatment of hypothyroidism consists of administration of thyroxine and assiduous monitoring of thyroid hormone levels.

HYPERTHYROIDISM

Hyperthyroidism, either idiopathic or iatrogenic, causes a condition in the growing skeleton quite opposite to that of hypothyroidism. Skeletal maturation is accelerated, and x-rays of affected hands reveal an increased bone age with respect to the corresponding chronologic age. Increased bone turnover rates are seen with resorption exceeding formation, and the net result is generalized osteopenia, which is more apparent in the appendicular skeleton than in the axial skeleton.

Some individuals with hyperthyroidism will develop thyroid acropachy, characterized by cortical metacarpal striations, generalized periosteal new bone formations, irregularities in the periosteal and endosteal margins of the cortical bones, and severe soft-tissue swelling in the hands. Acro-osteolysis also may be seen in the distal phalanges. A more descriptive term for thyroid acropachy is "acropachydermoperiostitis." This term incorporates the findings of soft-tissue swelling ("pachydermo"), new bone formation ("periostitis"), and involvement of the distal tufts of the fingers ("acro").

Treatment of the skeletal disorders resulting from hyperthyroidism is essentially treatment of the underlying endocrinopathy.

OSTEOPOROSIS

Unlike the normal mature adult skeleton that is in a state of euskeletal homeostasis with net bone formation equaling net bone resorption, the child's skeleton is growing in volume and increasing in mass. In the most common osteopenic condition, postmenopausal osteoporosis, net bone formation rates are relatively small, whereas net bone resorption rates are increased above normal. In the child with osteopenia, however, if bone formation equals bone resorption, a plateau in bone mass will occur, and the relative density for age will decrease as the child grows older.

The growth and development of the skeleton begin in utero and continue throughout adolescence in a series of well-timed events. New bone formation occurs either through intramembranous ossification via direct mineralization of osteoid formed by mesenchymal osteoblasts or through a well-orchestrated sequence of endochondral ossification from a preliminary cartilaginous model. The long bones grow in length by a combination of cartilage proliferation and an elaborate process of endochondral ossification. The growth in width of the long bones proceeds by a combination of periosteal new bone for-

mation and endosteal bone resorption. The periosteal bone formation is responsible for the growth in width of the long bone, and the endosteal resorption is responsible for the growth in width of the medullary canal.

Once modeled, bone is remodeled by bone cells (osteoblasts and osteoclasts) on the four bone surfaces, or remodeling bays: periosteal, haversian, endosteal, and trabecular. The greatest surface area and the highest metabolic activity of the skeleton are in trabecular bone.

Although trabecular bone remodeling proceeds at a greater rate than cortical remodeling, the rate of cortical remodeling during the first 2 years of life is approximately 50%. For instance, the diameter of the medullary canal in the midshaft of the femur in a 2-year-old child is equal to the diameter of the entire shaft of the bone at birth. Thus, the entire thickness of the cortical bone is remodeled in the midshaft of the femur in the first 2 years of life. This represents a 100% remodeling rate over 2 years, or a 50% remodeling rate per year.

In early adolescence, the length and mass of the skeleton increase at variable rates: Where there is a rapid spurt in longitudinal growth, there is only a moderate increase in mineral content of the bones. It is not until late adolescence, when skeletal maturity is reached and longitudinal growth ceases, that the bone mineral content rapidly increases. The bone mass reaches a peak following skeletal maturity and remains relatively constant throughout early adult life. Genetic, racial, nutritional, endocrine, and physical factors play a large role not only in the growth and development of the skeleton but also in the attrition that occurs later in life.

When considering osteopenic conditions in childhood, one should remember that it is as important to focus on the peak bone mass achieved as it is to consider the rate of bone loss. In conditions such as idiopathic juvenile osteoporosis, the skeleton never achieves its normal peak bone mass, and this may be due as much to the decrease in formation rates below normal as to the increase in resorption rates. Thus, we derive the definition of "osteoporosis"—a decrease in the mass per unit volume of normally mineralized bone as compared with bone of controls matched for age and sex. ·

The causes of osteoporotic conditions in childhood can be divided into those that are congenital and those that are acquired. The most common congenital causes of osteopenia are the osteogenesis imperfecta syndromes, which are heritable as well as congenital. The congenital myotonic dystrophies, which lead to states of severe disuse, are complicated by the presence of disuse osteoporosis. In children, as in adults, disuse osteoporosis represents a state of high metabolic activity and skeletal turnover with net bone resorption greater than net bone formation, resulting in a net decrease in skeletal mass compared with that observed in normal, age-matched controls.

Perhaps the most intriguing forms of childhood osteopenia are seen in the progeria syndromes. In these genetic syndromes (Hutchinson-Guilford and Werner's syndromes), early senescence in all tissue and organ systems is noted, and the skeleton is not excluded from the nefarious effects of the premature aging process. Osteopenia with multiple vertebral compression fractures, thoracic kyphosis, and hip and distal radial fractures all may be seen in individuals whose chronologic age may be no more than 15 years but whose skeletal age may be well into the eighth or ninth decade.

Acquired forms of osteopenia in childhood may be secondary to chronic disease, malnutrition, hyperthyroidism, hypercortisolism (either idiopathic or iatrogenic), hypogonadism, or juvenile onset diabetes. Focal or regional causes of osteopenia may be related to prolonged immobilization secondary to trauma or chronic illness.

As in most forms of severe osteopenia, radiographs may provide a baseline screening test but are inadequate in distinguishing the normal state of bone mass from that of mild osteopenia. Depending on the region of the skeleton in question, between 40% and 60% of the bone mineral must be removed before osteopenic changes can be detected on plain films. Thus, profound osteopenia must result before radiographic documentation is available. In its early stages, osteopenia is a silent condition; it is only after the skeletal mass has decreased to the point at which spontaneous fractures may occur that the osteopenia becomes clinically evident.

One can estimate osteopenia in the appendicular skeleton by assessing the combined cortical thickness in the midshaft of a long bone. Standardized age-matched control data are available for the second metacarpal as assessed by plain AP x-rays of the hand. Measurements of combined cortical thickness of the second metacarpal in children and adults are available.[3] The measurements are higher for males than for females in all age groups. The combined cortical thickness takes into account the relative periosteal new bone contribution as well as endosteal resorption and accounts for two of the three remodeling bays in cortical bone. However, intracortical porosity, which occurs with bone loss from remodeling in the haversian canals, will not be detected by combined cortical thickness measurements.

Newer methods for assessing bone mass in the more metabolically active trabecular bone are available, but controls have not been obtained for children. These methods include single- and dual-energy quantitative computed tomography and the dual-photon radioisotope absorption technique. Newer developments in computed tomographic scanning and radioisotope technology will permit rapid, safe scanning at low energy levels. These techniques will provide accurate methods for assessing the degree of skeletal mass in the axial skeleton in a growing child who is at great risk for developing an osteopenic condition or in a child who already has an osteopenic disorder. Combined with the method already described for measuring the bone mineral contents in the appendicular skeleton, these new techniques will allow a more rational approach to the diagnosis and management of osteopenic disorders in children.

In osteopenia, as in all metabolic disorders affecting either the axial skeleton or the appendicular skeleton, treatment must be based on treatment of the underlying condition. When definitive treatment of the underlying condition is not possible, every attempt must be made to slow the untimely loss of bone mass and to allow for the normal age-related increase in bone mass that typically accompanies growth and development of the skeleton. Proper attention must be paid both to recommended daily allowances of calcium throughout growth and development and to weight-bearing physical activities. When ambulation is not possible, the upright posture may be facilitated through use of tilt-tables or standing boards. The ravages of disuse osteopenia in the child may be far greater than those seen in the adult skeleton because of the increased metabolic turnover of the immature skeleton. Proper rehabilitation is essential if fractures are to be prevented following immobilization in the child; otherwise, the vicious cycle of immobilization–osteopenia–fracture–immobilization–osteopenia will result.

RICKETS AND OSTEOMALACIA

Although a comprehensive view is essential to total understanding of the disease process, mysteries can be discovered both in the smallest bone and growth plate and in the largest.

Osteomalacia is defined as a skeletal condition characterized by an increased, normal, or decreased mass of insufficiently mineralized bone. Rickets is the disease process that occurs in the growing skeleton and is characterized by mineralization abnormalities in endochondral ossification, widened growth plates, and hypomineralization or absent mineralization in the zone of provisional calcification in the physis. In rickets, in contrast to states of osteoporosis in which there is a decreased mass per unit volume of normally mineralized bone, there is an insufficient mineralization of normally produced bone matrix and an abnormality in mineralization of the intercolumnar cartilaginous bars in the growth plates.

The two major categories of rickets involve those conditions associated with disorders in vitamin D metabolism and those conditions associated with disorders in phosphate recruitment and metabolism. The sources of vitamin D are extrinsic (the diet) and intrinsic (production by the skin). The major dietary sources of vitamin D are fish-liver oil and vitamin D added to milk and milk products. In the skin, the vitamin D precursor, 7-dehydrocholesterol, is converted to cholecalciferol by a photocatalytic reaction with ultraviolet light. Cholecalciferol (vitamin D_3) is converted in the liver to a vitamin D metabolite, 25-OH-D_3. The final conversion to the active hormone, 1,25-$(OH)_2$-D_3, occurs in the mitochondria of the proximal tubular cells in the kidney under the influence of the 1-alpha-hydroxylase enzyme. This enzyme is directly stimulated by the presence of parathyroid hormone (PTH), which is manufactured and released under the influence of hypocalcemic conditons. Then 1,25-$(OH)_2$-D_3, the active hormone, circulates systemically and acts on the two end organs, the jejunum and the bone. In the jejunum, the active hormone is a potent stimulator of calcium and inorganic phosphate absorption. In bone, the active hormone is a potent stimulator of osteoclastic bone resorption. The net effect of 1,25-$(OH)_2$-D_3 is an increase in the serum levels of both calcium and phosphate. This differs from parathyroid hormone, which has a net effect of increasing the serum calcium while decreasing the serum inorganic phosphate. It is at the level of the 1-alpha-hydroxylase enzyme in the kidney, the metabolic gateway to the hormonally active vitamin D, that the two systems are intrinsically linked.

It is important to remember that simple calcium deficiency does not lead to a mineralization defect but to secondary hyperparathyroidism. At times, when the serum calcium rises above normal, the body's "calcium stat" causes a decrease in the formation and secretion of the parathyroid hormone, a decrease in the conversion of 25-OH-D_3 to 1,25-$(OH)_2$-D_3, and an increase in the 24,25-$(OH)_2$-D_3. So, under conditions of transient hypercalcemia, the kidney preferentially hydroxylates the 25-OH-D_3 in the 24 position, thus producing the inactive metabolite 24,25-$(OH)_2$-D_3.

A clear comprehension of the pathways involved in vitamin D metabolism allows one to understand the major categories that can produce osteomalacia in the adult and rickets in the child. Classic nutritional or vitamin D deficiency rickets can result when there is a deficiency of vitamin D in the diet combined with inadequate synthesis of vitamin D in the skin due to lack of sunlight. This condition, which was common in industrial England during the nineteenth century, is prevented today by sufficient intake of vitamin D through ingestion of dairy products and by adequate exposure to sunlight.

Malabsorption of vitamin D is another major cause of both rickets and osteomalacia and can be seen with the numerous conditions that are involved with fat malabsorption, including celiac disease, sprue, regional enteritis, amyloidosis, chronic pancreatic disease, and ileal loops or blind pouches.

Severe end-stage liver disease also can produce rickets or osteomalacia, but even with minimal functional reserve of the liver, the 25-hydroxylation step of cholecalciferol is preserved. In premature infants, however, the ability of the liver to 25-hydroxylate cholecalciferol is impaired, and severe neonatal rickets may result, presenting as severe osteopenia with appendicular and axial fractures. If recognized, the disorder is easily treated with oral vitamin D_3 or with calciferol (25-OH-D_3).

Medications containing phenytoin or phenobarbital or drugs metabolized to phenobarbital (primidone) may induce a state of rickets if ingested over a long period of time. The mineralization defect from the anticonvulsants is secondary to the increased hepatic breakdown of the vitamin D metabolites by the same enzyme systems that are stimulated to breakdown the anticonvulsants. Rickets is likely to develop in children on long-term anticonvulsant therapy, especially if the children have meager dietary intake of vitamin D or if they are sequestered in institutions where they have little exposure to sunlight. The dietary supplementation of vitamin D in these children is essential if severe mineralization defects are to be avoided. The peripheral requirements for vitamin D are increased in these children because of the increased breakdown of the vitamin D metabolites.

One of the metabolic manifestations of severe chronic renal failure is rickets, which arises as a result of the decreased conversion of 25-OH-D_3 to 1,25-$(OH)_2$-D_3. The end result of all forms of vitamin D deficiency is a net decrease in availability of both calcium and phosphorus for osteoid and cartilage mineralization. A rare autosomal recessive disorder known as vitamin D pseudodeficiency rickets arises as a result of an abnormality in the 1-alpha-hydroxylase enzyme in the kidney. The vitamin D cascade is blocked at the second hydroxylation step in the kidney, and the disease is readily treated by the administration of the active hormone 1,25-$(OH)_2$-D_3.

The vitamin D deficiency states are characterized by low 24-hour urine calcium and phosphorus levels with normal 24-hour urine creatinine levels. The serum calcium and phosphorus levels are low to low-normal. The alkaline phosphatase level is markedly elevated in all forms of vitamin D deficiency rickets, as is the parathyroid hormone level. In fact, the serum calcium may be normal, but at the expense of the extremely high PTH levels. In states of nutritional vitamin D deficiency (which are now quite rare in the United States, except in several religious sects in which the children are kept heavily clothed and are not fed milk fortified with vitamin D), the vitamin D metabolite levels would be characteristically low.

In the rare pseudodeficiency syndrome, the 25-OH-D_3 level is normal, whereas the 1,25-$(OH)_2$-D_3 level is low.

The other major forms of rickets involve renal tubular defects in which the primary problem occurs not in the vitamin D metabolic cascade but in the renal tubular reabsorption of inorganic phosphate. These conditions are characterized by hypophosphatemia with normocalcemia. The most characteristic of these conditions is X-linked dominant familial hypophosphatemic vitamin D resistant rickets. In this condition, the serum phosphate is low, but the serum calcium is normal. The alkaline phosphatase, as in all forms of rickets, is elevated, but the parathyroid hormone level is likely to be normal because there is no hypocalcemic stimulus for increased PTH secretion. Many soft-tissue tumors may induce a state of hypophosphatemia owing to peripheral phosphate utilization by the tumors or the production of a phosphaturic factor. This may be seen with neurofibromas, hemangiomas, and other benign mesenchymal tumors. Extirpation of the soft-tissue tumor results in a cure of the underlying rachitic condition.

Familial hypophosphatemic rickets also results in short stature. The hypophosphatemic conditions are treated primarily with phosphate repletion. Vitamin D therapy is necessary to block the secondary hyperparathyroidism that results from phosphate repletion.

The renal tubular defects resulting in the Fanconi syndromes also result in the development of rickets.

Despite the myriad causes of rickets, the phenotypic expression is similar in all forms of the disorder. In the most flagrant disease state, rickets manifests with severe bone pain and tenderness, proximal muscle weakness, and clinical signs of hypocalcemia with tetany and laryngeal stridor. Because of the muscle weakness and bone pain, ambulation may be delayed in afflicted infants. If the disease develops after the child is walking, ambulation may decrease and all ambulatory activities may cease. The severe weakness and manifestations of hypocalcemia are not seen in the rachitic disorders due to hypophosphatemia alone. When rickets develops early in infancy or childhood, the clinical disease is more severe. The child is irritable. Craniotabes and frontal bossing of the skull are present. Harrison's groove is seen at the attachment of the diaphragm to the inferior ribs. Rachitic rosary is noted and represents an enlargement of the growth plates at the costochondral junctions. Bowing of the long bones and characteristic widening of the metaphyses are easily noticed and are most prominent at the wrist with involvement of the distal radius and ulna and at the ankle with involvement of the distal tibia and fibula, although all long bones are involved.

The radiographic appearance of the skeleton in the rachitic disorders is distinct from that of the skeleton in any other major metabolic disease process and is characterized by metaphyseal irregularities, a decrease in the radiographic density of the zone of provisional calcification along with observed irregularities, and cupping and widening of the metaphyses. The growth plate appears widened owing to a proliferation of unmin-eralized or hypomineralized cartilage in the zone of provisional calcification. The mineralization abnormalities are not confined to the growth plate, as noted previously, and may be seen in the shafts of the long bones as well. The cortices of the long bones often appear irregular and bowed. There is a mild coarsening of the trabecular pattern in the medullary canal and a blurring of the medullary canal–endosteal border (Figs. 16–8 and 16–9).

Pseudofractures commonly occur in the outer cortex of the long bones but may also extend through the cortex to the endosteum and into the medullary canal. There are often radiographic signs of an abortive attempt at callus formation and mineralization at the sites of these transverse pseudofractures. They occur most commonly in adults but may also be seen in children. Soft-tissue swelling is noted on physical examination, and the bone is point-tender, as would be expected in any fracture. The ^{99}Tc methylene diphosphonate bone scan shows increased activity in the area of the pseudofracture. Treatment of the pseudofracture consists of treatment of the underlying osteomalacic

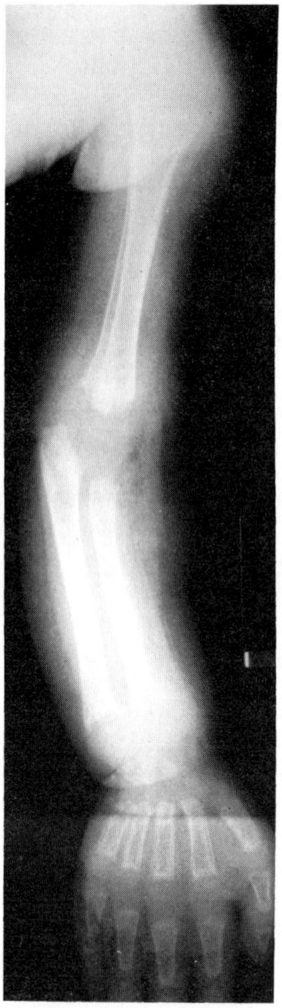

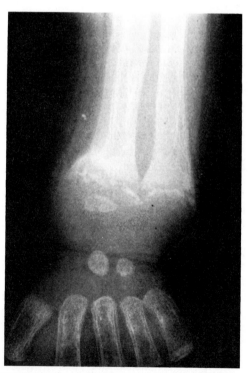

Figure 16–8. X-ray of the upper limb of a one-year-old child with newly diagnosed and untreated vitamin D deficiency rickets.

Figure 16–9. The child in Figure 21–8 one month after vitamin D replacement therapy. Note the appearance of secondary growth centers and mineralization at the zone of provisional ossification in the physes.

condition combined with recommendations for decreased weight-bearing until the pseudofracture is healed clinically and radiographically.

PRIMARY HYPERPARATHYROIDISM

Primary hyperparathyroidism in children is a rare and often fatal disorder. Primary hyperplasia of the parathyroid is seen only in infancy and very early childhood. It is often detected in the neonatal period. Parathyroid adenomas are not found in children younger than 4 years of age. Neonatal parathyroid hyperplasia is a fatal disease if parathyroidectomy is not promptly performed. The disorder is familial, and a careful family history may indicate relatives who died during the neonatal period. The disorder is generally inherited as an autosomal recessive trait, but in some families an autosomal dominant pattern or a sporadic mutation explains the genetic picture. The clinical symptoms are severe, and the hypercalcemia is often untreatable except by total ablative parathyroidectomy. There is failure to thrive. The neonates are febrile and dehydrated, and hypercalcemia in the range of 15 to 20 mg% is common. As expected, hypophosphatemia is seen. X-rays of the appendicular skeleton reveal profound osteopenia with numerous pathologic fractures, a coarsening of the bony trabeculae, and flagrant subperiosteal bone resorption. The majority of long bone fractures are metadiaphyseal rather than diaphyseal, as in the osteogenesis imperfecta syndromes. Once the diagnosis of hyperparathyroidism has been made, parathyroidectomy should be performed. Following surgery, intravenous administration of calcium may be necessary owing to the precipitous fall in serum calcium. However, the skeletal response to the definitive treatment is rapid, and the radiographic appearance of both the appendicular skeleton and the axial skeleton will revert to normal within several months of the surgery. The cause of death in untreated neonatal primary hyperplasia of the parathyroid is cardiac arrest secondary to malignant hypercalcemia. For infants who undergo total parathyroidectomy, subsequent management is similar to that used for hypoparathyroid patients.

Parathyroid adenomas are more common than glandular hyperplasia. Parathyroid adenomas are not seen before several years of age and are most likely to occur in late childhood or early adolescence. Common physical findings in adenomatous hyperparathyroidism are weakness, fatigue, anorexia, vomiting, constipation, polyuria, polydipsia, bone pain, and pathologic fractures. Less commonly seen are nervousness, depression, and irritability. Radiographically, subperiosteal erosions are common, especially in the phalanges in both the hands and the feet. Although nephrolithiasis is uncommon, the bone disease in children is often more severe than that in adults and is commonly ascribed to the increased rate of bone turnover in the years prior to skeletal maturity. Adenomatous hyperplasia is less severe than the rampant, fatal neonatal parathyroid hyperplasia and rarely results in death. In adenomatous hyperplasia in children, as in the symptomatic disorder in adults, parathyroid ablation with subcutaneous implantation of normal parathyroid tissue often leads to cure.

PSEUDOHYPOPARATHYROIDISM

This rare, perplexing disorder was first described by Fuller Albright in 1942 and represents an end-organ insensitivity to parathyroid hormone. Exogenously administered parathyroid hormone fails to reverse the abnormalities in this condition and fails to return the serum calcium to normal. Exogenously administered parathyroid hormone also fails to elicit a phosphaturic effect. Circulating levels of C-terminal parathyroid hormone are extremely high in this condition; thus, paradoxically, this represents a state of hyperparathyroidism with insensitivity of the end organs (the kidney and the bone) to the calcemic and phosphaturic effects of the hormone.

In 1969, Chase, Melson, and Aurbauch tested Albright's theory by measuring the urinary excretion of cyclic AMP in response to exogenously administered parathyroid hormone. Cyclic AMP is normally stimulated in both the kidney and the bone by the presence of parathyroid hormone. The investigators found that individuals with pseudohypoparathyroidism had decreased excretion of cyclic AMP in the urine, as compared with normal individuals and individuals with hypoparathyroidism. In 1980, investigators showed that the primary molecular defect in pseudohypoparathyroidism occurs in a protein (N-protein) that couples the target-organ membrane receptor to the adenylate cyclic enzyme. The N-protein activity in individuals with pseudohypoparathyroidism was reduced well below normal. This helps to describe the molecular defect in the more prevalent type of pseudohypoparathyroidism (pseudohypoparathyroidism type I). In pseudohypoparathyroidism type II, an extraordinarily rare disorder, the urinary cyclic AMP response to exogenously administered parathyroid hormone is normal, but the phosphaturic response is abnormal. Thus, although the disorders of pseudohypoparathyroidism may appear phenotypically similar, there is likely a heterogeneity in the genotypes.

The major clinical and biochemical characteristics of the disorder are (1) hypocalcemia and hyperphosphatemia, which is in response to administration of parathyroid hormones; (2) shortening of the fourth metacarpal and metatarsal; and (3) the clinical syndrome of short stature, shortened metacarpals, and round facies.

High doses of vitamin D are used to treat the condition and to keep the serum calcium in a normal range. Albright described family members who had all of the previously mentioned physical features of pseudohypoparathyroidism but lacked the biochemical abnormalities. He called this syndrome pseudopseudohypoparathyroidism.

RENAL OSTEODYSTROPHY

The inability of the failing kidney to excrete phosphate and to make the final conversion to the active vitamin D metabolite is thought to be the primary cause of the numerous bone disorders seen in patients with renal osteodystrophy.

Individuals with this disorder manifest a florid hyperparathyroidism and hyperphosphatemia. A transient decrease in serum calcium stimulates the parathyroid glands to increase the secretion of parathyroid hormone. Because the kidney, one of the two primary target organs for parathyroid hormone, is unresponsive to its presence, the primary effect of the circulating parathyroid hormone is to resorb bone. Osteoclastic bone resorption and recruitment of preosteoclasts occur. This results in a radiographic appearance of severe subperiosteal bone resorption and osteitis fibrosa cystica and a histologic

appearance of osteoclast-mediated bone resorption with peritrabecular fibrosis. Severe osteomalacia is likely to result because the kidney, in severe renal failure, can no longer make the final conversion from 25-OH-D$_3$ to the active hormone 1,25-(OH)$_2$-D$_3$. Normally, this final step in active hormone D synthesis is under the control of parathyroid hormone, but the presence of the parathyroid hormone goes unheralded by the failing kidney. The serum calcium is maintained at a low-normal to normal level at the expense of profound bone resorption. Gastrointestinal absorption of calcium and phosphorus are, of course, minimal because of the low circulating levels of 1,25-(OH)$_2$-D$_3$.

The combination of hyperphosphatemia and a normal serum calcium may lead to an increase in the calcium-phosphate product in the serum and to metastatic calcification and osteosclerosis. Thus, one may see in chronic renal failure combinations of the following: (1) hyperparathyroid bone disease with osteitis fibrosa cystica, (2) rickets, (3) osteosclerosis with metastatic calcification in muscles and tendons as well as the joint capsules, and (4) regional osteopenia (Fig. 16–10).

Treatment in renal osteodystrophy should be aimed at (1) decreasing the serum phosphate with phosphate-binding antacids, (2) maintaining the serum calcium at a normal level, and (3) managing the rachitic component of the disorder with 1,25-(OH)$_2$-D$_3$. This will also help to suppress the secondary hyperparathyroidism. Compliance with the phosphate-binding antacids is often difficult, especially in children. In those situations in which vigilant attention is not directed to the underlying pathophysiology of the numerous bone lesions, the subsequent bone disease may be severe. Parathyroidectomy is often necessary prior to renal transplantation, especially when refractory hyperparathyroidism occurs (tertiary hyperparathyroidism). Bone pain is a common feature of renal osteodystrophy due either to the rachitic and osteomalacic component or to the hyperparathyroid component of the disease. Transiliac bone biopsy following double tetracycline labeling is often necessary to properly assess the various components of the disease process in any particular individual. The presence of aluminum in hemodialysate fluid, or the heavy use of aluminum-containing phosphate binders may lead in some to a state of

Figure 16–10. Hand x-rays of an 11-year-old child with renal osteodystrophy. Note the osteitis fibrosa cystica, subperiosteal bone resorption in the phalanges, irregularity of the epimetaphyseal regions, osteosclerosis, and focal appendicular osteopenia.

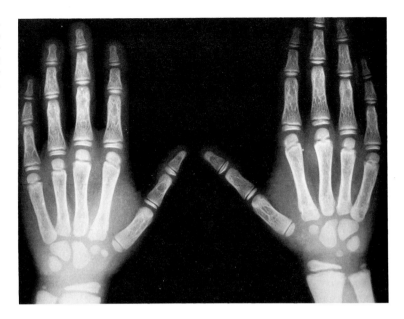

pure "aluminum-associated" osteomalacia. Special stains identify aluminum at the mineralization fronts on a bone biopsy specimen. When identified, the disease may be treated with desferoxamine, an agent that chelates aluminum.

HYPOPHOSPHATASIA

Hypophosphatasia represents a group of rare, heritable autosomal recessive disorders of mineralization, all characterized by deficiencies in the skeletal alkaline phosphatase isoenzyme. The disorder was first described by Rathbun in 1948. Clinically, the disease may resemble rickets becasue it results from a deficiency of deposition of skeletal mineral in bone matrix and in growth plate cartilage. The levels of alkaline phosphatase in both serum and bone are low compared with normals and the urinary excretion and plasma levels of phosphoethanolamine and inorganic pyrophosphate are increased above normal. Phosphoethanolamine is believed to be a substrate for alkaline phosphatase and may play a role in the normal inhibition of mineralization. The hypophosphatasia syndromes, unlike the vitamin D deficiency rickets syndrome, are associated with no known abnormalities of vitamin D metabolism. Hypophosphatasia frequently involves hypercalcemia and hypercalciuria. The direct cause of the hypercalcemia seen in hy-

pophosphatasia is unknown, although it has been postulated that the defect in mineralization overwhelms the body's ability to compensate for such a huge shift in its metastable calcium pool.

Determination of the clinical hypophosphatasia syndromes is based on the time of appearance of the bone lesions, and three distinct clinical periods of emergence have been recognized.

Infantile Form. The characteristic feature of hypophosphatasia in all clinical syndromes is the generalized inadequacy of mineralization in the mature bone. Thus, the earlier the disorder appears, the more severe the clinical disease is manifested. Failure to thrive, severe rickets and hypercalcemia, and a high mortality rate (approximately 50%) are seen in the infantile form of the disease.

Childhood Form. The childhood form presents a less severe picture than the infantile form. In addition to presenting with mild hypercalcemia, these children have premature loss of deciduous teeth. As in all forms of the disorder, they have a decreased level of serum alkaline phosphatase compared with age-matched normal children and have an increased concentration of urinary phosphoethanolamine.

Adult Form. The mildest forms of the disease occur when onset appears in adult life. Decreased levels of alkaline phosphatase and mild bone fragility may be the only noted features. In many individuals who come to medical attention for the first time in adulthood, a childhood history of rickets may be elicited. Many of these patients have generalized osteopenia and pseudofractures, very similar to those in classic osteomalacia. The distinction between rickets and hypophosphatasia can be made on the basis of the serum alkaline phosphatase measurements. The alkaline phosphatase will be elevated in all forms of rickets, except hypophosphatasia in which it is decreased.

In addition to the characteristic triad of decreased serum alkaline phosphatase levels, premature loss of deciduous teeth, and excessive urinary excretion of phosphoethanolamine, other features that might be seen include premature synostosis of the cranium, spontaneous fractures secondary to qualitative bone fragility, and hypercalcemia, hypercalciuria, and nephrocalcinosis.

Within a given kindred with known hypophosphatasia, individuals may be present who have all of the associated findings but who have a normal alkaline phosphatase level. These individuals are described as having pseudohypophosphatasia. The hypophosphatasia syndromes, much like the hemoglobinopathies, may represent numerous closely related chemical and structural disorders in the same molecule.

Attempts at treatment of patients with hypophosphatasia have been unsuccessful. This disease is not responsive to vitamin D; and glucocorticoid therapy has been tried in numerous individuals without much success. Attempts at treatment with high-dose oral phosphatase have been promising. With a rise in plasma phosphate concentration, an increased excretion of pyrophosphate in the urine is seen, and some improvement in the mineralization process is noted radiographically.

References

1. Aegerter E, Kirpatrick JA, Jr. Orthopaedic Diseases. Philadelphia, WB Saunders Co, 1975.
2. Edmonson AS, Crenshaw AH. Campbell's Operative Orthopaedics. St Louis, CV Mosby Co, 1980.
3. Garn SM, Poznaski AK, Nagy JM. Bone measurement in the differential diagnosis of osteopenia and osteoporosis. Radiology 100:509, 1971.
4. Holmes LB. Inborn errors of morphogenesis—a review of localized hereditary malformations. N Engl J Med 291(15):763–773, 1974.
5. Isselbacher KJ, Adams RD, Braunwald E, et al., eds. Harrison's Principles and Practice of Internal Medicine, 9th ed. New York, McGraw-Hill Book Co, 1980.
6. Kaplan FS. Osteoporosis. Ciba Clin Sympos 35(5):1–32, 1983.
7. Kopits SE. Orthopaedic complications of dwarfism. Clin Orthop Rel Res 114:153–179, 1976.
8. McKusick VA. Heritable Disorders of Connective Tissue. St. Louis, CV Mosby, 1972.
9. McKusick VA. Mendelian Inheritance in Man. Catalogs of Autosomal Dominant, Autosomal Recessive and X-Linked Phenotypes, 6th ed. Baltimore, The Johns Hopkins University Press, 1983.
10. Nyhan WL. Cytogenetic disease. Ciba Clin Sympos 35(1):1–32, 1983.
11. Saldino RM. Radiographic diagnosis of neonatal short-limbed dwarfism. Med Radiogr Photogr 49(3):61–95, 1973.
12. Sillence D. Osteogenesis imperfecta: an expanding panorama of variants. Clin Orthop Rel Res 159:11–25, 1981.
13. Smith DW. Recognizable Patterns of Human Malformation, 2nd ed. Philadelphia, WB Saunders Co, 1976.
14. Stanbury JB, Wyngaarden JB, Fredickson DS. The Metabolic Basis of Inherited Disease, 4th ed. New York, McGraw-Hill Book Co, 1978.
14a. Stanescu V, Stanescu R, Maroteaux P. Pathogenic mechanisms in osteochondrodysplasias. J Bone Joint Surg 66(A):817–836, 1984.
15. Steinbach HL, Gold RH, Preger L. Roentgen Appearance of the Hand in Diffuse Disease. Chicago, Year Book Medical Publishers, 1975.
16. Thompson DW. In Bonner JT, ed. On Growth and Form. Cambridge, Cambridge University Press, 1961.
17. Wynne-Davies R. Heritable Disorders in Orthopaedic Practice. Oxford, Blackwell Scientific Publications, 1973.

CHAPTER ○ 17

Cerebral Palsy

RICHARD H. GELBERMAN

Cerebral palsy includes a range of nonprogressive neurologic disorders caused by a central motor deficit dating to events occurring in the prenatal, perinatal, and postnatal periods. It is not a specific disease but a grouping of disorders characterized by paralysis, weakness, and loss of coordination. There may be associated manifestations of organic brain damage (e.g., seizures and mental retardation), sensory and learning defects, and behavioral and emotional problems.

It is estimated that cerebral palsy affects 300,000 children in the United States. The incidence rose to a maximum in the 1950s but subsequently has been falling steadily. There has been an increase in the number of children with spasticity and in the small group of atonic patients, but there has been a dramatic decrease in athetosis. A striking change in associated etiologic factors has occurred with a marked decrease in erythroblastosis, which dropped to almost zero in the 1970s. Lesser decreases in encephalitis, dystocia, and idiopathic cases have been reported.[42]

The relationship between cerebral palsy and neonatal anoxia was first established by Little in 1843. Cerebral anoxia, currently considered the most likely etiologic factor, is often complicated by intraventricular and subependymal hemorrhages. Mechanical trauma to the brain at birth also is a cause and is particularly implicated in patients with spastic hemiplegia. More than one third of children with cerebral palsy weigh less than 2500 gm at birth.[2, 9]

A useful classification of cerebral palsy is based on the nature of the observed motor deficit.[2, 39, 40] The most common types are spasticity (tetraplegia, paraplegia, hemiplegia, and monoplegia); extrapyramidal cerebral palsy (athetosis and dystonia); atonic cerebral palsy (atonic diplegia, ataxia); and mixed types.

Spastic hemiplegia accounts for approximately one third of cerebral palsy cases.[42] There is often an associated homonymous hemianopsia and a hemisensory deficit on the side of the hemiplegia. Seizures occur at some stage in life in 25% of patients, and significant visual problems develop in 20%. Hearing problems are seen in many, particularly in those with athetosis. The level of the patient's intellect depends largely on whether the brain lesion is confined to one hemisphere.[39, 40] Learning problems are significant in many, and at least 50% of patients with cerebral palsy are retarded.[44]

The neurophysiologic mechanisms that cause spasticity are not fully known.[6, 28, 52] There have been several recent studies investigating the pathophysiologic mechanisms; however, they have little relevance insofar as management of the upper extremity is concerned.[3, 36] Electromyographic activity recorded from agonist and antagonist muscles during passive involuntary alternating flexion and extension movements has demonstrated resistance to passive movements that increases linearly with the frequency of flexion and extension. There is a diversity of patterns varying from a completely reciprocal relationship between flexion and extension, through partial overlap, to complete synchrony.[36] In patients with mildly affected limbs, it has been noted that normal alternating activity is preserved between flexors and extensors during voluntary movements. In patients with moderate deficits, normal patterns are seen in movements of low frequency, but reciprocal patterns break down as the movements become more rapid. In severely affected limbs, continuous muscle firing is noted at any frequency of flexion and extension.

The occurrence of continuous muscle firing as the degree of involvement increases has resulted in the paradox of treatment in patients with spastic cerebral palsy. Operative management is more predictable and useful in those patients who are least severely affected. In addition, unpredictable results occur more frequently in patients with spasticity of the upper limb when there is a strong admixture of motion disorders—ataxia, athetosis, dyskinesia, and tremors.[24, 26] These observations have resulted in a pessimistic view toward operative reconstruction and have led to a conservative attitude, reflected by the fact that only 3% to 5% of patients with cerebral palsy undergo upper extremity surgery.[30, 31]

EVALUATION OF THE PATIENT WITH SPASTIC HEMIPLEGIA

There are several categories of assessment essential to planning upper extremity management. These include the patient's intelligence, sensation, muscle strength and control, age, extent of involvement, and mo-

tivation.[14] The parents, nurse, teacher, and physical and occupational therapists can provide information about the patient's ability to perform daily activities, his motivation, and his capacity for learning. The treating physician must then assemble a large field of specific information based on a detailed evaluation of each of these factors.

Intelligence

A specific intelligence level has not been established as a prerequisite for the operative treatment of the upper extremity in cerebral palsy. Goldner has used a 70 IQ as a general level for obtaining patient assistance in postoperative care. In special circumstances, with specific indications, he found that an IQ as low as 50 was not a contraindication. Green has also noted that a greater proportion of patients with higher intelligence showed improvement after operative treatment.[23] No patient in his series with an IQ of less than 80 achieved an excellent result. Samilson, however, pointed out that intelligence, measured by the standard means, may be misleading because of the patient's significant motor impairment.[48, 49] In general, the closer the intelligence rating to normal, the greater the improvement that can be expected; however, a high intelligence level is not essential to obtaining significant improvement from surgery. The intelligence quotient should be known and considered in prescribing treatment, but the IQ should not be the sole determining factor.

Sensation

Tachdjian performed sensory evaluations of 96 children with cerebral palsy, all with average intelligence and over the age of 5 years.[57] He found sensory deficits in almost half. The most common defects were astereognosis (30 of 96), abnormal two-point discrimination (22 of 96), and loss of position sense (10 of 96). A correlation has been established between the functional status of the patient with cerebral palsy and the presence of these deficits, with a high incidence of sensory loss in the most functionally disabled hands. There are two potential explanations for the diminished sensation in cerebral palsy: (1) organic brain lesions in the parietal cortices, and (2) lack of patient experience in using the hand. It is generally accepted that the motor and mental handicaps are due to organic brain lesions and that the sensory handicap is more closely related to the organic lesion than to lack of use. There is no current evidence that surgical treatment influences the sensation in any way. Peripheral nerve compression syndromes have not been shown to play a role in the diminished sensation in these patients.

The sensory examination should be performed in a specific and organized manner, concentrating on stereognosis, two-point discrimination, and proprioception.[15]

Stereognosis. The patient should close his eyes and raise his hand over his head. A square block, round peg, ball, safety pin, pencil, and a key should be placed in his hand and his fingers moved over the surface of the object. The patient should describe the size, shape, consistency, and surface characteristics of the various objects.

Two-Point Discrimination. This should be determined with a paper clip applied along the longitudinal axis of the digit. The two points should be depressed just to the point of blanching of the skin. The normal value for the median and ulnar distribution is 6 mm, and a grading of good is less than 10 mm. Absent two-point discrimination is defined as greater than 15 mm.

Proprioception. This is determined by having the patient correctly identify his index finger when it is positioned while his eyes are closed. The patient is asked to touch the examiner's finger in space and then to touch his nose, or to move his hand from the top of his head to his opposite knee and then back to the top of his head. Other sensory tests such as sharp/dull, light touch, weighing perception, vibration, hot/cold, location of tactile stimuli, and wet/dry are less helpful in cerebral palsy.

In younger patients, sensory examination is more difficult. If the child can follow directions, one may find it possible to assess, by observing the child playing, his ability to differentiate square from round and identify other common shapes and sizes.

Particular attention should be devoted to detecting the child with dissociation or denial. The child with poor stereognosis and denial will usually not benefit from reconstructive efforts. Denial is the only absolute contraindication to operative treatment based on the sensory examination.

Although the results of sensory testing, aside from denial, will not limit the indications for operative treatment, they do influence the expectations. Green found that the results of surgery correlated closely with stereognosis.[23] Of 14 patients with considerable improvement following surgery, only two had astereognosis. Of the 16 patients with very little improvement following tendon transfer, 14 showed significant disturbances in sensory function.

Muscle Strength and Control

There has been considerable controversy about the optimal method of muscle testing in patients with cerebral palsy. Certainly, the better the determination of existing voluntary and tenodesis function, the more effective the treatment plan. Baker has commented that when the spastic muscle is in need of correction, one must study that muscle and its antagonist before deciding on the extent and method of correction.[1] But how can one best evaluate muscle control and strength in the presence of spasticity? One can obtain a gross evaluation by observing the patient grasp and release objects and transfer objects from one hand to another. The effectiveness of grasp and release can be noted, and a major problem with one or the other can usually be determined. Release may be difficult owing to overactivity of the finger flexors, and grasp may be difficult as a result of weak wrist extensors, persistent thumb-in-palm deformity, weakness of the flexor digitorum profundi, or a combination of these problems.

It is also possible to determine the strength of the individual wrist and digital flexors and extensors. The patient will frequently have to be observed on three or four occasions and reexamined following periods of splinting and stretching. One must attempt, however, to perform an adequate muscle test and grade muscles 0 to 5 according to the American Orthopaedic Association criteria for muscle power. The findings should be recorded as for extremities affected by peripheral nerve injuries.[20]

It is frequently difficult to examine the strength of the wrist and digital extensors if the hand and wrist are in a position of marked flexion. By weakening the flexor muscles, however, the examiner can often determine the strength and voluntary control of the extensors. He accomplishes this by blocking the median nerve at the elbow with 10 ml of 1% lidocaine without epinephrine. After 15 to 20 minutes, the wrist, fingers, and thumb extensors may demonstrate active voluntary activity that was not present previously. In addition, the examiner should determine the presence and severity of associated joint contractures. He should compare the range of passive and active motion of the hand or digits before and after selected nerve block. This information helps one make decisions concerning soft tissue release and the necessity of contracture release.[14, 20]

Another method of determining the patient's control of muscle function is dynamic electromyography. Hoffer considers muscle control and the phasic activities of various muscles the most important factors in the evaluation of the cerebral palsy patient.[25] He uses standard electromyographic techniques and video analysis of patients performing various activities. Based on the data obtained, decisions are made regarding the optimal muscles for transfer. Hoffer performed a series of transfers in 17 patients based on the concept that cerebral palsy muscles are phase-dependent and are not capable of changing phase. It was considered important, therefore, to transfer muscles that operated in the same phase as the muscles to which they were transferred. His best results were obtained when both the physical examination and the electromyographic results agreed with respect to the type of transfer needed. In addition, he found that the majority of patients with cerebral palsy had a problem with weak release rather than weak grasp. Thus, tendon transfers that improved finger extension were needed more often than those improving wrist extension alone.

These observations on the basic characteristics of spastic muscles are not uniformly accepted, however.[48, 49] Samilson performed electromyograms after tendon transfer and showed some restoration of asynchronous, or phasic, activity in muscles that had previously been synchronous.[49] He found that even the synchronous activity of the flexor carpi ulnaris was beneficial if that muscle was transferred to either the extensor carpi radialis brevis or the extensor digitorum communis. Goldner has stated that the individual muscle test and the repeated observation of the patient's activities in grasp and release are most important. He has noted that an effective series of transfers can be outlined

from the physical examination and that preoperative electromyography is not essential.

Dynamic electromyography has been used in our laboratory as an adjunct to decision making for tendon transfer in cerebral palsy patients since the late 1970s. Although we think it is of some benefit, there are several questions that have not yet been answered. It is clear that predominantly phasic muscles in patients with spasticity can be predictably transferred and will continue to function phasically. It has not been determined, however, whether spastic muscles can become more phasic after transfer. It also has not been determined conclusively whether muscles that fire continuously are useless for transfer or, as Samilson has noted, become phasic following transfer.

The most effective tendon transfers in cerebral palsy are those that utilize grade 5 muscles that are under good voluntary control and that are phasic with the activity for which they are transferred.[4] Muscles that are less phasic or that fire continuously also may be useful, however, when transferred in specific circumstances. A clearer understanding of the capability of the spastic muscle should be provided as investigators continue to explore this area with a variety of the techniques now available.

Age

Goldner has pointed out that the limitations of age are flexible as far as reconstructive surgery of the upper extremity is concerned. A four-year-old child with a thumb-in-palm deformity and a hypermobile metacarpophalangeal joint not controlled by bracing can be effectively treated by arthrodesis of the metacarpophalangeal joint of the thumb. If the epiphysis is spared, no significant shortening of the thumb will result. A teenager with wrist and digital flexion deformities can also benefit both functionally and cosmetically from reconstructive surgery.

In the first few years of life, the cerebral palsy patient is best managed by thumb abduction splints worn at all times and wrist and digital splints used at night. At 4 years of age, the patient with resistant deformities can first be evaluated for operative treatment. The thumb-in-palm deformity may be corrected, and tendon transfers to provide grasp and release can be considered at this age. The optimal time for tendon transfer and reconstruction, however, is between 6 and 12 years of age.

Extent of Involvement

It is important that the patient's existing function and extent of involvement are determined prior to selection of a course of treatment. A grading system based on hand function was introduced by Green and Banks[23] and has been useful in evaluating patients pre- and postoperatively.

An *excellent* classification connotes good use of the hand in dressing and eating, effective grasp and release, and excellent control. Dorsiflexion of the wrist is possible to at least 45°, and full active extension of the fingers is possible with the wrist extended 30° or more. There is no ulnar deviation deformity, and there is active supination of the forearm to at least 50°.

A *good* classification refers to a hand that is used as a helper in dressing and eating, has effective grasp and release with good control, and exhibits active dorsiflexion of the wrist in the range of 15° to 45°. Active extension of the fingers is possible with the wrist dorsiflexed from 0 to 30°. There is minimal or no ulnar deviation deformity, and active supination of 10° to 50° is possible.

A *fair* classification is used for a helper hand that is not effective in dressing. Moderate grasp and release are possible with fair control when dorsiflexion of the wrist is 0. Active extension of the fingers with the wrist in neutral is possible, and there is an ulnar deviation deformity of the wrist. Active supination to a neutral position is possible.

A *poor* grade is given to hands used as paper weights, in which grasp and release are absent and the wrist is fixed in flexion. Finger extension is impossible unless the wrist is held in maximum palmar flexion. There is an ulnar deviation deformity of the wrist and a pronation contracture.

In addition to the assessment of the patient's level of hand use, determination of the overall severity of involvement is important. Severe spasticity of all four extremities accompanied by athetosis or major sensory deficits or both limits the benefits of surgery unless one or two specific goals can be accomplished. Also, significant athetosis is a contraindication to tendon transfer. Determining the presence of athetosis may be difficult; it may be perceptible only after the

patient is observed performing a variety of activities on several occasions. Tendon transfers in athetoid patients are unpredictable and usually do not improve function.

SURGICAL TREATMENT

Many of the early operative procedures recommended for cerebral palsy were modifications of operations used in polio. Most of the procedures were ineffective in the hemiplegic, however, and the poor results led to increasing pessimism about the benefits of surgery for this condition. Experience with 500 operations on 242 patients led one investigator to conclude that tendon transfers always failed in cerebral palsy because the injury did not involve individual muscles as in polio or other lower motor neuron problems but affected total joint function mediated through the upper motor neurons.[45]

Through extensive experience and careful follow-up, others have found that planned surgical procedures in patients with adequate sensibility and motivation are predictable and do improve overall function.[1,5,7,8,16,20,29, 34, 35, 38, 41, 46, 47, 50, 51, 53, 56]

Most Frequently Indicated Upper Extremity Procedures for Spastic Hemiplegia

The Thumb-in-Palm Deformity

Instability of the Metacarpophalangeal Joint. If the thumb metacarpophalangeal joint is unstable and hyperextensible, stabilization by capsulodesis[11] or arthrodesis[12, 14, 16, 17, 20] is indicated as part of an overall correction of the thumb-in-palm deformity.

Capsulodesis. In this procedure, the metacarpal attachment of the palmar plate is moved proximally on the metacarpal to prevent hyperextension of the metacarpophalangeal joint.

Technique. A volar zigzag incision is made along the palmar aspect of the metacarpophalangeal joint of the thumb. The A-1 pulley is incised, and the flexor pollicis longus is exposed and retracted. The neurovascular bundles are isolated. The palmar plate is then incised at its proximal attachment and along its medial and lateral borders. The strong distal attachment is left intact. The intrinsic muscles that insert onto the palmar plate are divided. The metacarpophalangeal joint is then positioned in 30° to 35° of flexion, and the proximal margin of the palmar plate is inserted into a slot created in the metacarpal neck. A pull-out wire is tied over a button on the dorsal aspect of the thumb metacarpal. The joint is pinned in flexion with a 0.045-inch Kirschner wire. Postoperatively, the thumb is maintained in abduction with a palmar plaster splint. The pull-out wire is removed at 6 weeks, and both the plaster splint and Kirschner wire are removed 8 weeks postoperatively.

Metacarpophalangeal Joint Fusion. Fusion of the metacarpophalangeal joint of the thumb is preferred if the metacarpophalangeal joint is unstable in flexion and extension or if the hyperextension deformity exceeds 20°. It is more predictable than capsulodesis and, when properly performed, does not interfere with the growth of the thumb. It provides great stability when other transfers are being done about the thumb to correct a marked thumb-in-palm deformity.

Technique. A radial midlateral incision is made, and the radial collateral ligament and lateral band are isolated. The incision is carried through the capsule and radial collateral ligament, and the joint is dislocated manually. A small rongeur is used to remove only the cartilaginous surface of the metacarpal head; the underlying subchondral bone is left intact. The articular surface of the proximal phalanx is then denuded of its cartilage in a similar fashion. The physes of the metacarpal and phalanx are not disturbed. The joint is positioned in 10° of flexion and 10° of internal rotation, which allows the thumb

to be brought easily to the radial side of the index finger. Two 0.045-inch Kirschner wires are used to stabilize the joint. The capsule is closed with 4-0 braided Dacron suture, and a thumb spica cast is applied. Immobilization is continued until firm union has occurred.

Adduction Contracture. Release or lengthening of the adductor pollicis is indicated in a patient with palpable adductor spasticity and a contracted thumb web. The web is first deepened with a conventional or four quadrant Z-plasty (Fig. 17–1). Then the transverse head of the adductor is released (1) at its insertion into the ulnar base of the proximal phalanx, (2) through its midsection, or (3) from the long finger metacarpal.[32, 33] This author prefers partial myotomy of the adductor muscle performed at the time of Z-plasty of the web. An overzealous adductor release may result in weakness of pinch.

Technique. After release of the thumb web by Z-plasty, the fascia overlying the adductor and the first dorsal interosseous are located. The surgeon incises the fascia over both muscles using dissection scissors. The superficial fibers of both muscles are then incised sharply until the thumb metacarpal can be easily brought into extension. Only in rare instances is a palmar incision necessary to release the transverse head of the adductor from the long finger metacarpal. Z-plasty lengthening of the insertion of the adductor is difficult, and tenotomy will produce weakness of pinch.

Weakness of Thumb Abduction and Extension. A number of operative procedures may be necessary to maintain the thumb out of the palm. These include extensor pollicis

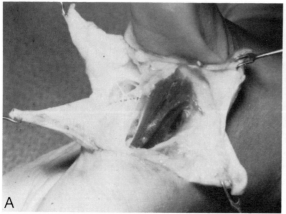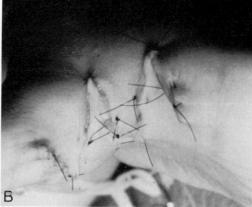

Figure 17–1. *A,* Elevation of four flaps for thumb-web deepening and adductor release. *B,* The four-quadrant Z-plasty closure gives a smooth, round, well-contoured web space.

longus rerouting with or without addition of a motor, imbrication of the abductor pollicis longus and extensor pollicis brevis, or tendon transfer, brachioradialis into the abductor pollicis longus and extensor pollicis brevis.

Extensor Pollicis Longus Rerouting

Technique. Rerouting of the thumb extensor is accomplished through a longitudinal incision over the dorsoradial aspect of the wrist. The third dorsal compartment is entered, and the extensor pollicis longus is located. The tendon is freed proximally and isolated distally up to the point at which it joins the dorsal hood of the thumb. The tendon is removed from its groove and displaced radially (Fig. 17–2). Frequently, a tendon transfer into the thumb extensor will be needed, and, if the brachioradialis is of sufficient strength and active in digital extension, it is an ideal choice for transfer. The tendon of the brachioradialis is released from its insertion into the radius in the floor of the first dorsal compartment and then mobilized into the proximal forearm to allow adequate excursion (Fig. 17–3). The surgeon then sutures the tendon into the extensor pollicis longus using a side-weave with 4-0 braided Dacron suture.

Abductor Pollicis Longus and Extensor Pollicis Brevis Shortening.
When the thumb metacarpal has been maintained in marked flexion in the palm, shortening of the ab-

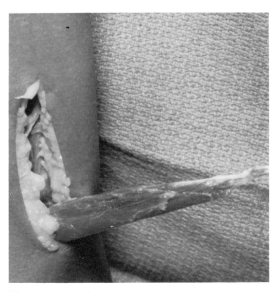

Figure 17–3. The brachioradialis must be mobilized into the proximal forearm to provide adequate excursion.

ductor pollicis longus provides reinforcement to keep the thumb out of the palm. Shortening alone will usually not be successful when the thumb-in-palm deformity is severe. For the mild to moderate thumb deformity, however, imbrication of both tendons is effective (Fig. 17–4).

Technique. A longitudinal, curved incision is made over the first dorsal compartment, and the extensor retinaculum is incised longitudinally after the superficial branches of the radial nerve have been protected. The abductor pollicis longus frequently has two to four slips. Occasionally, one of the slips may insert into the floor of the first compartment. The tendons may be shortened in one of two ways. They may be incised transversely 2 cm proximal to the abductor insertion site at the base of the metacarpal, and the proximal segment is advanced distally and anchored into the base of the metacarpal with a 3-0 or 4-0 Dacron suture. The distal stump is then sutured over the proximal tendon. The alternative is to roll the tendon without incising it and suture it in a shortened position (Fig. 17–4). The metacarpal is then immobilized in extension for 4 to 6 weeks.

If the thumb-in-palm deformity is severe, transfer of the flexor digitorum superficialis of the long or ring finger around the radial aspect of the wrist or of the brachioradialis into the abductor pollicis longus should be carried out.

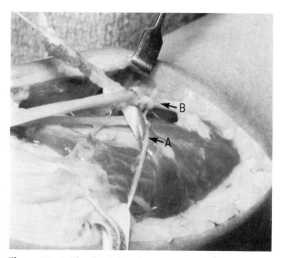

Figure 17–2. The third dorsal compartment is incised, and the extensor pollicis longus (A) is removed from its groove around the dorsal radial tubercle and is displaced radially. The extensor pollicis longus is reinforced here by the brachioradialis (B).

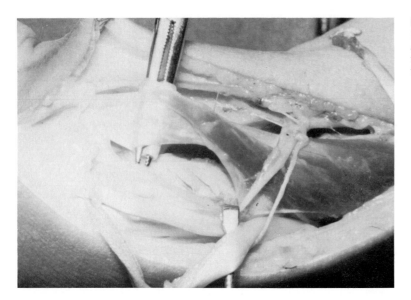

Figure 17–4. The abductor pollicis longus and extensor pollicis brevis are imbricated by rolling and suturing the tendons without incising them.

Inadequate Digital Extension

If a patient has poor digital extension, and thus a poor release in the presence of an effective grasp, transfer of the flexor carpi ulnaris into the extensor digitorum communis is indicated.

Technique. The flexor carpi ulnaris is exposed through an anteromedial incision beginning at the palmar wrist crease and extending to the junction of the proximal and middle thirds of the forearm. One detaches the tendon at its insertion into the pisiform and mobilizes it by proximal dissection as far as possible without disturbing the neurovascular bundle. A straight longitudinal incision is then made over the fourth dorsal compartment, the extensor retinaculum is divided, and the extensor digitorum communis is isolated. The flexor carpi ulnaris is passed around the ulna through a subcutaneous tunnel created by a large Kelly clamp. It is transferred in a straight line toward the extensor digitorum communis tendons at the wrist level. With the wrist and metacarpophalangeal joints in neutral position, the flexor carpi ulnaris is sutured into each of the extensor digitorum communis tendons. The wrist is held in 30° of extension, and the metacarpophalangeal joints are stabilized at neutral for 6 weeks in a plaster cast.

Inadequate Wrist Extension

Less frequently, the patient demonstrates inadequate grasp and requires a strong transfer to a wrist extensor. In a number of patients with inadequate grasp, the popular Green procedure,[21–23] transfer of the flexor carpi ulnaris to the extensor carpi radialis brevis, is used. A strong, spastic flexor carpi ulnaris can lead to excessive dorsiflexion force which can result in having the wrist in a fixed extension posture, which will not improve hand function. In such cases, a muscle that will often provide better balance is the extensor carpi ulnaris, transferred either totally or partially, into the extensor carpi radialis brevis, as described by Goldner.[13, 18, 19]

Extensor Carpi Ulnaris Transfer

Technique

A longitudinal incision is made over the extensor carpi ulnaris from a point distal to the styloid process of the ulna to the region of the musculotendinous junction. The tendon sheath is incised, and an umbilical tape is placed around the tendon for identification. The distal segment of the tendon is incised, and the tendon is mobilized to the proximal extent of the incision (Fig. 17–5). The extensor carpi radialis brevis is isolated through a longitudinal incision over the second dorsal compartment. The extensor carpi ulnaris is passed into the second incision through a straight subcutaneous tunnel and sutured into the extensor carpi radialis brevis just proximal to that tendon's insertion into bone (Fig. 17–6). This is performed in a side-weave fashion with a 4-0 braided Dacron suture. The wrist is immobilized in 30° of extension in a plaster cast for 6 weeks.

Figure 17–5. The extensor carpi ulnaris is mobilized to the level of its mid–muscle belly.

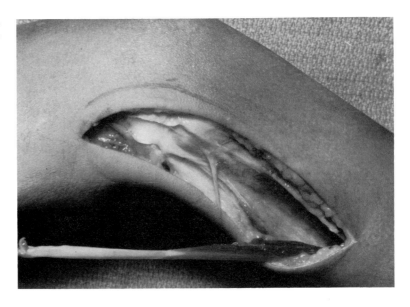

Flexor Carpi Ulnaris Transfer

Technique

A longitudinal palmar-ulnar incision begins in the proximal forearm and extends to the pisiform. The flexor carpi ulnaris muscle and the ulnar nerve are located. The nerve is tagged with a rubber drain, and the tendon is transected just prior to its attachment to the pisiform. The muscle is then mobilized into the proximal forearm. A second longitudinal incision is made over the wrist in line with the index metacarpal. The extensor retinaculum is incised over the second dorsal compartment, and the extensor carpi radialis brevis is located. A subcutaneous tunnel is made extending from the proximal flexor carpi ulnaris incision to the dorsal-radial incision. The flexor carpi ulnaris is passed through the tunnel and sutured into the extensor carpi radialis brevis in a side-weave fashion with tension sufficient to maintain the wrist in 20° extension. A long arm cast with the elbow at 90° and the forearm in supination is maintained for 4 weeks. Active exercises are then begun. The bivalved cast or a polypropylene splint is worn between exercise periods for 2 to 3 months, and a night brace is worn for 6 months.

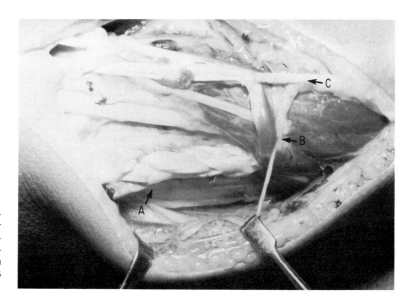

Figure 17–6. The extensor carpi ulnaris (A) is woven into the extensor carpi radialis brevis by the Pulvertaft side-weave technique. The extensor pollicis longus (B) has been reinforced by the brachioradialis (C).

Alternatives

1. Pronator teres transfer to the extensor carpi radialis brevis.[10]
2. Flexor digitorum superficialis transfer to the extensor carpi radialis brevis.[12]

Wrist and Digital Flexion Deformities

If a growing child has contracted wrist and digital flexors, lengthening by Z-lengthening, fractional lengthening, or flexor/pronator origin release is indicated. The flexor/pronator release will be considered in the subsequent discussion of elbow flexion contracture. The author prefers individual Z-lengthening to correct flexion contractures of the wrist and digits.

Technique. The wrist flexors are exposed along the palmar aspect of the wrist through a curved carpal tunnel incision. The flexor carpi radialis may be lengthened 2 to 3 cm proximal to its insertion. The wrist and digits are extended maximally. If the proximal interphalangeal joints are contracted, the flexor digitorum superficialis tendons are lengthened by coronal step-cut incisions at the musculotendinous junction. The incisions are repaired with 4-0 braided Dacron suture. The flexor digitorum profundi are tested in the same manner, and each tendon is lengthened in such a way that the digits are flexed to about 45° when the wrist is placed in dorsiflexion. The flexor pollicis longus is lengthened in a similar fashion. It is important to avoid overlengthening because this will diminish flexor tendon power.

Elbow Flexion Contracture

Patients with marked flexion deformities of the elbow (greater than 60°, exaggerated on walking and running) can be managed by isolated lengthening of the biceps brachii, myotomy of the brachialis, and release of the origin of the wrist flexors and pronator teres.[27, 37, 43, 58]

Technique. A curved incision is made just anterior to the medial epicondyle of the humerus. The ulnar nerve is tagged with a rubber drain. The muscle origin of the flexor carpi ulnaris is released from the medial epicondyle and from its attachment to the proximal ulna. The pronator teres muscle is released by sharp dissection, as is the flexor carpi radialis. The median nerve and biceps tendons are isolated. The median nerve is tagged with a rubber drain and retracted. The biceps tendon is lengthened by coronal Z-lengthening, and a myotomy of the brachialis muscle is performed. If the ulnar nerve is under tension in the newly extended position of the elbow, the nerve is transferred anteriorly. The elbow is immobilized in 160° for 4 weeks in a plaster cast. A polyurethane elbow extension splint is then molded and is used at night for an additional 3 months.

Swan-Neck Deformity

Swan-neck deformities of the fingers are caused by chronic overpull of spastic intrinsic muscles and by the tenodesis effect of the extensor digitorum communis when the wrist is in flexion (Fig. 17–7). The central slip is relatively short compared with the lat-

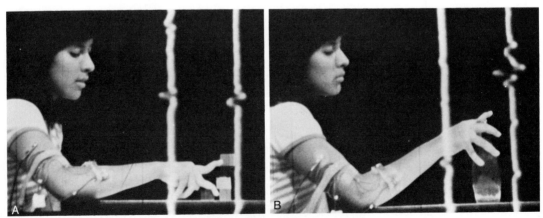

Figure 17–7. *A* and *B,* Fingers can lock in the hyperextended position, making pinch and grasp difficult.

eral bands. Thus, the proximal interphalangeal joint hyperextends, and the distal interphalangeal joint flexes. Superficialis tenodesis of the proximal interphalangeal joint, as described by Swanson, will restrict extension of the proximal interphalangeal joint.[54, 55]

Technique. A midlateral incision is carried from the midportion of the middle phalanx to the base of the proximal phalanx. The flexor sheath is incised, and the flexor tendons are located. The distal aspect of the palmar surface of the proximal phalanx is exposed subperiosteally on the proximal aspect of the palmar plate. Two drill holes 1 cm apart are made in the neck of the proximal phalanx in a palmar to dorsal direction. The two drill holes are then connected, and the bone is roughened to give a raw surface for attachment of the tendon. The superficialis is scarified and firmly anchored to bone, maintaining the interphalangeal joint in 20° to 30° of flexion. The flexed position of the joint is secured with a 0.045-inch Kirschner wire. A long arm cast extending to the tips of the fingers is maintained for 6 weeks. The Kirschner wires are removed at that time. Aluminum finger splints, holding the proximal interphalangeal joints in flexion, are then taped to the digits and worn, except for

exercise periods, for an additional 4 to 6 weeks (Fig. 17–8).

CASE STUDIES

Case 1. T.G., a 17-year-old female with right spastic hemiplegia, presented with the complaint of inability to pick up and hold objects with the right hand. She could stabilize large objects and could help lift and carry objects with the dorsum of her wrist but could not effectively grasp or release (Fig. 17–9).

Examination. The patient was intelligent and was planning to enter college the following year.

Posture. She carried her forearm in pronation, her wrist in flexion, and her digits in extension. The thumb was in the palm. On maximal passive wrist extension, there was a mild metacarpophalangeal joint extensor lag, and the thumb-in-palm deformity became worse.

Sensory Testing

Two-Point Discrimination. Thumb 10 mm, index finger 20 mm, long finger 20 mm, ring finger greater than 20 mm, and little finger 15 mm.

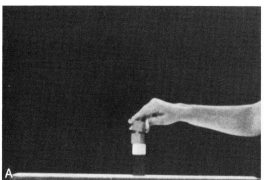
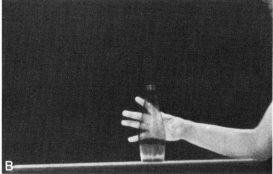
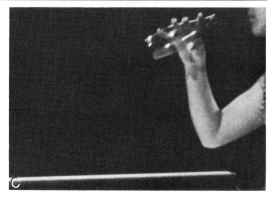

Figure 17–8. A–C, Stabilization of the proximal interphalangeal joints by tenodesis can significantly improve prehension.

Stereognosis. The patient was able to recognize size and shape correctly but could not identify common objects by name.

Proprioception. Position sense was good.

Motor Testing of Selected Muscles. Triceps 5, biceps 5, extensor carpi radialis brevis and longus 0, extensor carpi ulnaris 4 +, flexor carpi radialis 3, flexor carpi ulnaris 3, pronator teres 4, brachioradialis 4 +, extensor digitorum communis 3, extensor pollicis longus 2, flexor pollicis longus 3 +, flexor digitorum superficialis 3 to 4, and flexor digitorum profundus 2 to 3 +.

The patient had difficulties with grasp. With her wrist passively brought to neutral, her grasp improved considerably.

She was highly motivated and had an understanding, stable family.

Functional Classification.[23] Fair.

Dynamic Electromyography. The extensor carpi ulnaris was phasic and fired with wrist extension and digital flexion. The brachioradialis fired continuously but more actively with digital extension (Fig. 17–9).

Surgery

1. The extensor carpi ulnaris was transferred to the extensor carpi radialis brevis.

2. The brachioradialis was transferred to the extensor pollicis longus.

3. The abductor pollicis longus and the extensor pollicis brevis were imbricated.

4. The thumb index web was deepened with a four-quadrant Z-plasty, and the adductor pollicis was released in its midportion.

5. The metacarpophalangeal joint palmar plate of the right thumb was advanced, proximally stabilizing the metacarpophalangeal joint in flexion, and the interphalangeal joint was fused.

Postoperatively, the patient was maintained in a palmar wrist splint, which maintained the wrist in 30° of extension and the thumb in abduction. At 6 weeks, the cast was replaced by a molded polypropylene wrist and thumb splint, which was removed for periods of active exercises daily.

On follow-up at 3 years, the patient was using the hand to carry trays and glassware and to grasp and release large and small objects (Fig. 17–10). She could transfer a large rubber ball and small block from hand to hand and felt that she had improved appearance and considerably improved function. Her functional classification according to the criteria of Green and Banks[23] improved from fair to good.

Case 2. R.T., a 13-year-old male with left spastic hemiplegia, presented with the complaint of inability to use the left hand. The patient manipulated the hand as an assist and had some grasp for small objects but experienced great difficulty with release. He helped lift and carry objects with the side of his hand and wrist or in a markedly pronated position (Fig. 17–11).

Examination. The patient had an IQ of 90 and was doing average work in the 7th grade.

Posture. He carried his elbow in mild flexion, forearm in marked pronation, wrist in flexion, and thumb in the palm. He could extend his wrist to 20°.

Sensory Testing by Two-Point Discrimination. Thumb 15 mm, index finger 15 mm, long finger 15 mm, ring finger 10 mm, and little finger 5 mm.

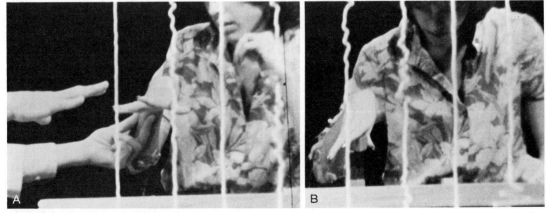

Figure 17–9. T.G. maintained her wrist in 45 to 60 degrees of flexion for all activities. The extensor carpi ulnaris (channel 1) fired with digital flexion (*A*) and was silent on release (*B*). The brachioradialis (channel 2) fired continuously.

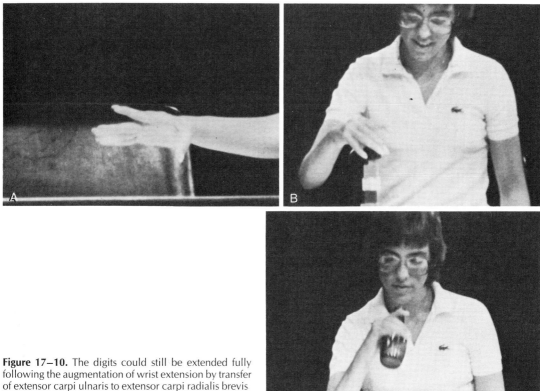

Figure 17–10. The digits could still be extended fully following the augmentation of wrist extension by transfer of extensor carpi ulnaris to extensor carpi radialis brevis (*A*). Grasp, release, and appearance were considerably improved (*B* and *C*).

Stereognosis. Fair. The patient could correctly identify most shapes, sizes, and textures, and he could name half the objects.

Proprioception. Excellent. He demonstrated very good position sense and control.

Motor Testing of Selected Muscles. Triceps 4 +, biceps 5, extensor carpi radialis brevis and longus 3 +, extensor carpi ulnaris 3 +, extensor digitorum communis 2, extensor pollicis longus 2 +, flexor carpi ulnaris 2, flexor carpi radialis 3, flexor digitorum profundi 4, flexor digitorum superficialis 4 to 4 +.

The patient had difficulties with release. With his wrist passively brought to neutral or slight dorsiflexion, he had difficulty extending his digits.

He was motivated and had good family support.

Functional Classification.[23] Poor.

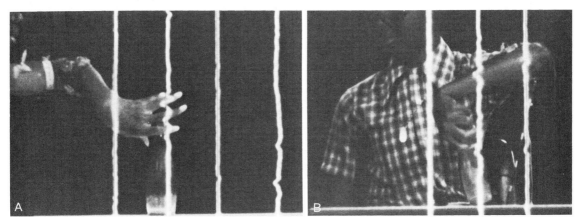

Figure 17–11. *A* and *B*, R.T. grasps a bottle with the forearm in marked pronation and the wrist in flexion. He is unable to bring it to his mouth.

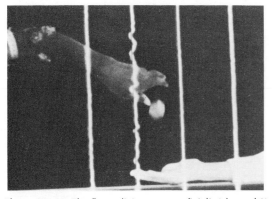

Figure 17–12. The flexor digitorum superficialis (channel 2) fires on release.

Dynamic Electromyography. The flexor digitorum superficialis fired continuously but fired more actively with wrist flexion and release (Fig. 17–12).

Surgery. The flexor digitorum superficialis of the ring finger was transferred to the extensor digitorum communis of the index, long, ring, and little fingers with the wrist in neutral and the metacarpophalangeal joints maintained at neutral. The flexor digitorum superficialis of the long finger was transferred subcutaneously around the radial aspect of the forearm into a rerouted extensor pollicis longus. The metacarpophalangeal joint of the thumb was fused in 10° of flexion

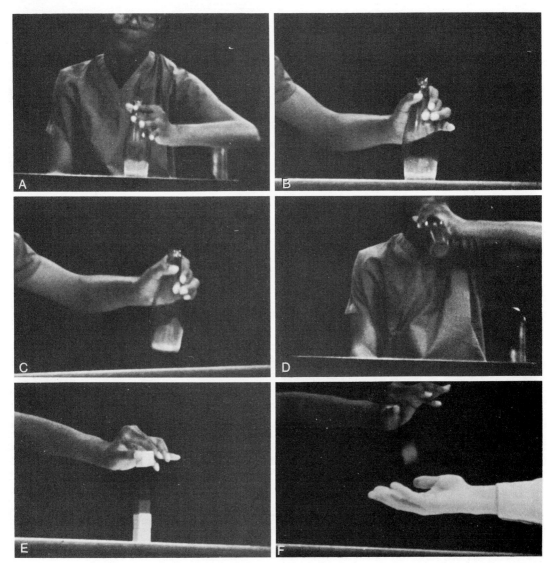

Figure 17–13. *A* to *F,* Grasp and release are improved following tendon transfer.

and internal rotation, and the abductor pollicis longus and extensor pollicis brevis were imbricated. The patient was placed in a bulky long arm dressing with plaster splints that was changed to a cast that maintained the wrist at neutral, the digits extended, and the thumb in abduction and extension. The cast was replaced at 6 weeks by a polypropylene splint that was removed intermittently for active exercises. At 12 weeks, immobilization was discontinued.

On his last follow-up examination, the patient continued to have active control of his wrist and demonstrated good flexion and extension of his digits. He had mild hyperextension of his proximal interphalangeal joints. His functional classification according to the criteria of Green and Banks[23] had improved from poor to fair (Fig. 17–13).

References

1. Baker LD. A rational approach to the surgical needs of the cerebral palsy patient. J Bone Joint Surg 38A:313, 1956.
2. Barnett HL, Einhorn AH. Pediatrics. New York, Appleton-Century-Crofts, 1972.
3. Barolat-Ramona G, Davis R. Neurophysiological mechanisms in abnormal reflex activities in cerebral palsy and spinal spasticity. Neurol Neurosurg Psychiatr 43:333–342, 1980.
4. Boyes JH. Selection of a donor muscle for tendon transfers. Bull Hosp Jt Dis Orthop Inst 23:1, 1962.
5. Braun RM, Vise GT. Sublimis to profundus transfers in the hemiplegic upper extremity. J Bone Joint Surg 55A:873, 1973.
6. Burman MS. The spastic hand. J Bone Joint Surg 20:133–145, 1938.
7. Carroll RE, Craig FS. Surgical treatment of cerebral palsy—the upper extremity. Surg Clin North Am 30:385–396, 1951.
8. Carroll RE, Craig FS. The treatment of cerebral palsy in the upper extremity. Bull NY Orthop Hosp 3:3–9, 1958.
9. Churchill JA, Musland RL, Naylor AA, et al. The etiology of cerebral palsy in pre-term infants. Dev Med Child Neurol 16:143–149, 1974.
10. Colton CL, Ransford AO, Lloyd-Roberts GC. Transposition of the tendon of pronator teres in cerebral palsy. J Bone Joint Surg 58B:220–223, 1976.
11. Filler BC, Stark HH, Boyes JH. Capsulodesis of the metacarpophalangeal joint of the thumb in children with cerebral palsy. J Bone Joint Surg 58A:667–670, 1976.
12. Goldner JL. Reconstructive surgery of the hand in cerebral palsy and spastic paralysis resulting from injury to the spinal cord. J Bone Joint Surg 37A:1141–1154, 1955.
13. Goldner JL. Upper extremity reconstructive surgery in cerebral palsy or similar conditions. AAOS Instructional Course Lectures, vol 18, St. Louis, CV Mosby, 1961:169–177.
14. Goldner JL. Reconstructive surgery of the upper ex-

tremity affected by cerebral palsy or brain or spinal cord trauma. Curr Pract Orthop Surg 3:125–138, 1966.
15. Goldner JL, Ferlic DC. Sensory status of the hand as related to reconstructive surgery of the upper extremity in cerebral palsy. Clin Orthop Rel Res 46:87–92, 1966.
16. Goldner JL. Cerebral palsy: Part I. General principles. AAOS Instructional Course Lectures, vol 20. St. Louis, CV Mosby, 1971:20–34.
17. Goldner JL. Outline of operative procedures for reconstruction of the upper extremity in cerebral palsy. In Keats OO, ed. Operative Orthopaedics in Cerebral Palsy. Springfield, Ill, CC Thomas, 1971:50–99.
18. Goldner JL. Upper extremity tendon transfers in cerebral palsy. Orthop Clin North Am 5:389–414, 1974.
19. Goldner JL. The upper extremity in cerebral palsy. Orthopedic aspects of cerebral palsy. In Samilson R, ed. Philadelphia, JB Lippincott, 1975:221–257.
20. Goldner JL.: Upper extremity surgical procedures for patients with cerebral palsy. AAOS Instructional Course Lectures, vol 28. St. Louis, CV Mosby, 1979:37–66.
21. Green WT. Operative treatment of cerebral palsy of spastic type. JAMA 118:434, 1942.
22. Green WT. Tendon transplantation of the flexor carpi ulnaris for pronation-flexion deformity of the wrist. Surg Gyn Obstet 75:337–342, 1942.
23. Green WT, Banks HH. Flexor carpi ulnaris transplant and its use in cerebral palsy. J Bone Joint Surg 44A:1343–1352, 1962.
24. Hoffer MM. The upper extremity in cerebral palsy. In Fredericks S, Brady GS, ed. Neurological Aspects of Plastic Surgery, vol 17. St. Louis, CV Mosby, 1978:133–137.
25. Hoffer MM, Perry J, Melkonian GJ. Dynamic electromyography and decision-making for surgery in the upper extremity of patients with cerebral palsy. J Hand Surg 4:424–431, 1979.
26. Hoffer MM. Cerebral palsy: patient I. In Green DP, ed. Operative Hand Surgery, New York, Churchill Livingstone, 1982:185–194.
27. Inglis AE, Cooper W. Release of the flexor-pronator origin for flexion deformities of the hand and wrist in spastic paralysis. J Bone Joint Surg 48A:847–857, 1966.
28. Jensen GD, Alderman ME. The prehensile grasp of spastic diplegia. Pediatrics 31:470–477, 1963.
29. Kaplan EB. Surgical treatment of spastic hyperextension of the proximal interphalangeal joints accompanied by flexion of the distal phalanges. Bull Hosp Jt Dis 23:35, 1962.
30. Keats S. Surgical treatment of the hand in cerebral palsy: correction of the thumb-in-palm and other deformities. Report of 14 cases. J Bone Joint Surg 47A:274–284, 1965.
31. Keats S. Operative orthopaedics in cerebral palsy. Springfield, Ill., CC Thomas, 1970.
32. Matev I. Surgical treatment of spastic "thumb-in-palm" deformity. J Bone Joint Surg 45B:703–708, 1963.
33. Matev I. Surgical treatment of flexion-adduction contracture of the thumb in cerebral palsy. Acta Orthop Scand 41:439–445, 1970.
34. McCarrol HR. Surgical treatment of spastic paralysis. AAOS Instructional Course Lectures, vol 6. St. Louis, CV Mosby, 1949:134–151.

35. McCue FC, Honner R, Chapman WC: Transfer of the brachioradialis for hands deformed by cerebral palsy. J Bone Joint Surg 52A:1171–1180, 1970.

36. Milner-Brown HS, Penn RD. Pathophysiological mechanisms in cerebral palsy. J Neurol Neurosurg Psychiatr 42:606–618, 1979.

37. Mital MA. Lengthening of the elbow flexors in cerebral palsy. J Bone Joint Surg 61A:515–522, 1979.

38. Moberg IE. Reconstructive hand surgery in tetraplegia, stroke and cerebral palsy: some basic concepts in physiology and neurology. J Hand Surg 1:29–34, 1976.

39. Nelson WE, et al. Textbook of Pediatrics, 9th ed. Philadelphia, WB Saunders, 1969.

40. Nelson WE, Behrman RE, Vaughan VC. Textbook of Pediatrics, 12th ed. Philadelphia, WB Saunders, 1983:1571.

41. Omer GE, Capen DA. Proximal row carpectomy with muscle transfers for spastic paralysis. J Hand Surg 1:197–204, 1976.

42. O'Reilly DE, Walentynowicz JE. Etiology factors in cerebral palsy. Dev Med Child Neurol 23:633–642, 1981.

43. Page CM. An operation for the release of flexor contracture in the forearm. J Bone Joint Surg 5:233, 1923.

44. Paine RS. Early recognition of cerebral palsy and prognostic signs. Instructional Course Lecture, Am Acad for Cerebral Palsy, Cleveland, 1965.

45. Phelps WM. Long-term results of orthopaedic surgery in cerebral palsy. J Bone Joint Surg 39A:53–59, 1957.

46. Pollack GA. Surgical treatment of cerebral palsy. J Bone Joint Surg 44B:68, 1962.

47. Sakellarides HT, Mital M. Treatment of the pronator contracture of the forearm in cerebral palsy. J Hand Surg 1:79, 1976.

48. Samilson RL, Morris JM. Surgical improvement of the cerebral palsied upper limb. Electromyographic studies and results of 128 operations. J Bone Joint Surg 46A:1203–1216, 1964.

49. Samilson RL. Principles of assessment of the upper limb in cerebral palsy. Clin Orthop Rel Res 47:105–125, 1966.

50. Sarkin TL. Surgery of the hand in infants with cerebral palsy. S Afr Med J 45:655–657, 1972.

51. Sherk HH. Treatment of the severe rigid contractures in cerebral palsied upper limbs. Clin Orthop Rel Res 125:151–155, 1977.

52. Steindler A. Pathokinetics of cerebral palsy. AAOS Instructional Course Lectures, vol 9, St. Louis, CV Mosby, 1952:118.

53. Stelling FH, Meyer LC. Cerebral palsy, the upper extremity. Clin Orthop Rel Res 14:70, 1959.

54. Swanson AB. Surgery of the hand in cerebral palsy and the swan-neck deformity. J Bone Joint Surg 42A:951–964, 1960.

55. Swanson AB. Surgery of the hand in cerebral palsy and muscle origin release procedures. Surg Clin North Am 48:1129, 1968.

56. Tachdjian MO. Pediatric Orthopedics, vol 2, Philadelphia, WB Saunders, 1972:830–857.

57. Tachdjian MO, Minear WL. Sensory disturbances in the hands of children with cerebral palsy. J Bone Joint Surg 40A:85, 1958.

58. White WF. Flexor muscle slide in spastic hand. J Bone Joint Surg 54B:453–459, 1972.

CHAPTER ○ 1 8

Arthrogrypo-sis Multiplex Congenita

W. P. COONEY
ANN H. SCHUTT

Arthrogryposis is an uncommon, occasionally hereditary syndrome that is characterized by joint contractures at birth.[1, 38] It is not a disease entity per se but presents as a *syndrome* with variable expressions of joint deformities, both multiple and protean, that are determined by abnormalities of the muscle and nerves that supply them.[18, 22] It is nonprogressive but, because of muscle imbalance and soft tissue fibrosis, can be recurrent. It can be mild, moderate, or completely disabling.

ETIOLOGY

Arthrogryposis literally means "curved joint."[19] The specific etiology remains unknown.[17, 24] The joint itself, however, is not at fault. Normal joint development requires movement of limbs up through the third to fourth month of fetal life. If such movements do not occur, articular surfaces and joint cavities do not form properly.[13]

Both primary muscle[1, 17, 28, 32] and nerve pathology[3, 12, 16, 21] have been implicated in the etiology of arthrogryposis. Whitten[37] demonstrated in calves a primary lesion within anterior horn cells secondary to viral insult that produced early destruction of muscle fibers in utero, loss of muscle tone, and secondary joint contractures. Drachman and Banker[12] presented a clinical case of arthrogryposis that demonstrated at necropsy a marked decrease in anterior horn cells in two patients with neurogenic arthrogryposis.[33] Drachman also produced fibrous ankylosis associated with anterior horn cell degeneration by tubocurarine injection.

Primary muscle disease was noted by Sheldon,[28] who termed it amyoplasia congenita and found postpartum cases that simulated progressive muscular dystrophy. Middleton[33] experimentally produced an autosomal recessive condition in sheep with primary muscle atrophy, fatty infiltration, and fibrosis.

Prenatal factors such as infection (rubella, measles), toxins, and increased intrauterine pressure have been implicated in the etiology of arthrogryposis.[13] A hereditary basis remains controversial because the majority of cases occur spontaneously, with normal siblings and no family history. However, primary myopathic arthrogryposis appears to be an inherited condition in animals, and clinical cases have demonstrated a variably expressive syndrome in members of the same family.

CLASSIFICATION AND PATHOGENESIS

Evidence indicates that clear differences exist between the neuropathic and myopathic types of arthrogryposis (Table 18–1).[3] Neuropathic types present as distinct patterns of deformity, with loss of muscle activity correlating with specific levels of segmental patterns. Myopathic types appear hereditary and simulate progressive muscular dystrophy.

From either primary muscle, primary nerve, or the rare arthrogenic disorders, a syndrome of joint contractures develops that begins in utero and causes muscle atrophy, periarticular joint fibrosis, and incomplete joint formation. Classification into *myopathic* or *neuropathic* types can be established by muscle biopsy, peripheral nerve biopsy, and electromyographic studies and can help determine both the prognosis and the appropriate methods of treatment. Joint contractures in arthrogryposis are the result of muscle pathology or nerve pathology or both, and if primary congenital joint involvement is present, one can exclude the diagnosis of arthrogryposis.[33]

The incidence of arthrogryposis varies. A rate of three per 10,000 live births has been reported from Helsinki.[4] Gibson[18] reviewed 114 patients over 15 years at the Hospital for Sick Children in Toronto; Lloyd-Roberts[22] had 58 patients over 13 years at Sick Children's Hospital in London; and Jones and colleagues[21] studied 40 patients over 10

years at the Mayo Clinic. Wynne-Davies and Lloyd-Roberts,[39] in their epidemiologic survey of 66 sporadic cases of arthrogryposis, were impressed by the similarity of this syndrome to a poliomyelitis-like intrauterine infection. Associated congenital anomalies are common, with single or multiple congenital defects or both. Twenty-eight of 40 patients in the Mayo Clinic series[21] and 77 of 82 patients in the Toronto series[18] demonstrated that the syndrome has a high association with congenital anomalies.

DIAGNOSIS

The diagnosis of arthrogryposis is based on the presentation of a number of clinical features that typify the disease syndrome. The patients characteristically have thin, atrophic limbs with adducted and internally rotated shoulders; knees and elbows fixed in either flexion or extension; and dislocated hips (Fig. 18–1A). Hands and wrists have flexion contractures. The fingers are stiff in extension, and the thumbs are adducted into the palm (Fig. 18–1B).

To make a clear diagnosis of arthrogryposis, however, one must establish the presence of two or more of the following classic criteria[21]:

1. Joint abnormality present at birth; often symmetric
2. Decreased or absent joint motion
3. Absent muscles or fibrous muscle groups
4. Associated joint dislocations, with webbed joint spaces
5. Involvement in three or more joints

Characteristic features include limitation of both *active* and *passive* joint motion (unique to this condition); dimpling of skin around ankylosed joints; absent skin creases with webbing; and port-wine stains on the affected extremities. Tachdjian[33] observes that a "wooden doll" appearance of thin, featureless extremities with limb atrophy, cylindrical limbs, and stiffened knees and elbows can be diagnostic of this condition (Fig. 18–2). Sensation is usually normal, and, most importantly, the children have normal intelligence.

The syndrome can present with different grades of severity and varies in amount of limb involvement. Most cases have mixed upper and lower limb contractures. In our series of 40 patients, 32 had generalized joint

Table 18–1. **Classification of Arthrogryposis**

Neuropathic	Myopathic
More common	Rare
Anterior horn cell	Muscle atrophy
Type I C5–C6	Progressive muscle
Type II C5, C6, C7	dystrophy
Neurosegmental	Nonsegmental muscle
involvement	changes
Extension contracture	Flexion contracture
	Deformities of chest and
	spine
Nonhereditary	Hereditary
Normal sensation	
Normal intelligence	Normal intelligence

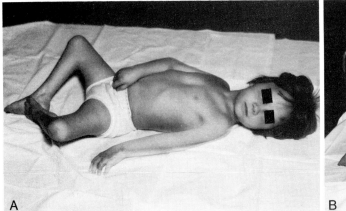
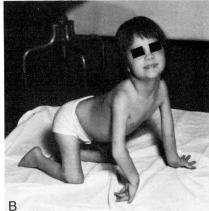

Figure 18–1. *A* and *B*, Classical features of arthrogryposis include flexion contractures of the hips and the knees, with internally rotated "club feet." The upper extremity deformities include internally rotated, adducted shoulders; extended elbows; and flexion deformities of the wrist and the hand.

involvement, four had upper limb involvement, and four had lower limb involvement (Table 18–2). Joint involvement consisted of complete ankylosis with varying degrees of muscle imbalance and, especially in lower

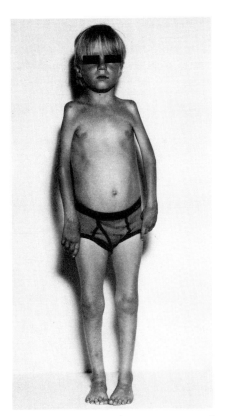

Figure 18–2. Atrophic "featureless" extremities with cylindrical shaped limbs are the hallmark of myopathic arthrogryposis. Note the symmetrical involvement, proximal muscle wasting, lack of joint flexion creases, and webbed joint spaces with normal hands and wrists.

extremities, joint dislocations. The more distal joints (i.e., hands and feet) are involved to a greater degree than the more proximal joints. Clubfoot deformities and contractures of the hand and wrist (club hands) are commonly seen in the same patient. The wrist and finger MCP and PIP joints are in flexion, and the thumb is fixed in adduction. In mild cases, deformities are limited to the hands and wrists, with finger MCP flexion contracture, wrist flexion–ulnar deviation contracture, and thumb-in-palm deformities.

Differential diagnosis at birth can occasionally be difficult.[3, 13, 15] Spinal dysraphism, osteogenesis imperfecta, diastrophic dwarfism, congenital muscular dystrophy, and benign hypotonia should be ruled out by appropriate physical findings, by skeletal limb and spine x-rays, and by muscle and nerve biopsy.[17] Other syndromes[26, 32, 34] (Table 18–3) should be excluded by appro-

Table 18–2. **Distribution of Joint Involvement in 40 Patients with Arthrogryposis Multiplex Congenita**

Joint Involved	Side Involved (No. of Patients)	
	Right	*Left*
Shoulder	14	13
Elbows in flexion	13	15
Elbows in extension	10	9
Wrist in flexion	15	16
Finger involvement	23	23
Hip dislocation	14	14
Hip deformity	12	11
Knee involvement	23	21
Clubfeet	31	32

Table 18–3. **Conditions and Syndromes That Simulate Arthrogryposis**

Spinal dysraphism
Congenital muscular dystrophy
Benign hypotonia
Sacral agenesis
Cerebral palsy
Spina bifida
Birth palsy
Mieter's syndrome
Jensen's syndrome
Intrauterine postural malformation

priate genetic and pediatric investigation and counseling.

Muscle biopsy, nerve biopsy, and serum muscle enzyme studies are helpful in the diagnosis and classification of arthrogrypotic conditions.[14, 27, 32] Electromyography and nerve conduction studies also help distinguish neurogenic conditions from myopathic ones.[21] Of 15 patients who were studied with electromyography, eight (50%) had confirmed anterior horn cell disease, three (20%) had myopathic disease, one had peripheral neuropathy, and only three were not diagnostic. Muscle biopsy was performed in eight patients and revealed type I fiber atrophy in four patients. This was not routinely performed in milder cases. Of the eight patients with anterior horn cell disease, none had familial arthrogryposis; however, of

those with hereditary patterns, three of eight had myopathic patterns on EMG, suggesting primary muscle pathology present. Electromyography and muscle biopsy should be performed as part of the diagnostic work-up because both can be used to distinguish neurogenic arthrogryposis from the myogenic type (see Table 18–1) and can help physicians plan genetic counseling and treatment programs.

TREATMENT: ARTHROGRYPOSIS OF THE UPPER EXTREMITY

The treatment of arthrogryposis involving the upper extremity is difficult because patterns of deformity and weakness are variable, multiple joints are affected, and treatment is often delayed until after lower extremity deformities are corrected.[2] Principles of treatment and long-term goals require close understanding and cooperation that involve the parent, the child, the physician, and the physical therapist.[21] Because affected children have normal intelligence and great ability to adapt to their disabilities, definitive treatment steps must be undertaken cautiously and with careful planning (Figs. 18–3A and B). The general goals of treatment of upper limb deformities include the following:

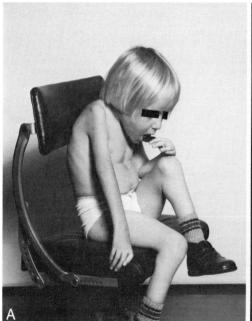
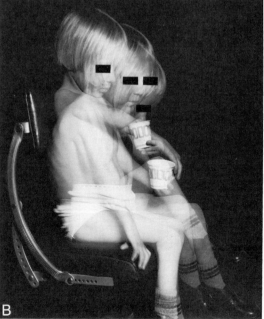

Figure 18–3. Arthrogrypotic children have normal intelligence and demonstrate considerable adaptability in increasing their functional capacity. These factors make surgical options difficult and delay decisions for tendon transfers.

1. Increased functional range of joint motion

2. Correction of disabling deformity

3. Improvement of adaptive use of the hands

Specific functional goals that apply to the upper extremity include the following:

1. Independence in feeding

2. Attention to toilet

3. Object handling in activities of daily living

Although upper limb surgery should, according to some, be used sparingly and generally is less urgent than surgery of the lower extremity, upper extremity function in activities of daily life may often be more essential than lower limb straightening and ambulation. The lower extremity requires straight, stable, strong, and moderately mobile limbs for ambulation. The upper extremity, however, is more complex, requiring multiple functions that primarily involve limb positioning and, in turn, functioning of the hands in a wide variety of self-sustaining activities. Although the joints of the lower extremity can be treated individually, the upper extremity *must* be approached as a whole.[13, 22] Shoulder, elbow, and wrist joints must function to serve the hand, and surgery on one joint should not limit function in the others.

Principles of treatment in the upper extremity include variations of the following[38]:

1. Early surgical joint release

2. Prolonged splinting to maintain correction

3. Tendon transfers (especially elbow) to replace the ineffective muscles and restore balance

In the upper extremity, early stretching and splinting can help prevent severe contractures and joint deformity. Forced stretching and manipulation, however, are contraindicated and ineffective because they can cause greater fibrosis and fracture or crushing of fragile bones.[22] If joints are not mobilized, adaptive cartilage and bone changes occur as growth occurs, and they in turn limit joint motion.

Surgical release of contracted joint capsule, muscle-tendon lengthening, and muscle transfer have proved more effective than corrective osteotomies in treatment of the arthrogrypotic. The latter procedures are associated with recurrence of deformity and progression of the joint articular changes. One directs early treatment at the joint itself to release contracture and to increase joint mobility.

THE HAND AND THE WRIST IN ARTHROGRYPOSIS

The condition of the hand determines what, if any, treatment is required at the elbow or shoulder.[13] If arthrogrypotic hands are supple with finger mobility and reasonable muscle strength, aggressive treatment can be initiated. Stiff, spider-like fingers with contracted wrists and thumbs, however, are bad prognostic signs and serve as specific contraindications to *any* upper extremity surgery.[33] Hands that bend toward each other—even with stiff, flexed wrist and thumbs—can provide bimanual manipulation skills that could be lost with premature or unwarranted surgical intervention.

In Lloyd-Robert's series,[22] 46 of 52 children with arthrogryposis had hand deformities. Treatment of thumb and wrists deformities is undertaken first if the hand is relatively supple. Thumb-in-palm contracture (Fig. 18–4A)[9] requires adductor myotomy (Fig. 18–4B) from the third metacarpal, tendon transfer for opposition and extension, and occasionally thumb MCP fusion or chondrodesis. *Chondrodesis* involves joint stabilization by partial resection of the articular cartilage. This technique provides fibrous tissue fixation with limited motion and does not interfere with bone growth. Finger flexion deformity can be improved by separation of syndactyly (Fig. 18–4C) and capsulotomy of PIP and MCP joints so that finger position is better aligned for prehensile pinch and grasp.[29] Intrinsic and extrinsic muscle (and tendon) release or lengthening also may be necessary. To improve joint position, we prefer muscle releases in the hand, and tendon lengthening at the wrist or forearm (Fig. 18–4D) rather than osteotomies. The joints should be pinned in corrected position for 2 to 3 weeks and maintained with intermittent orthoplast splinting for 1 to 2 years (Fig. 18–4E). Tendon transfers for extrinsic extensor weakness and thumb opposition can be performed, provided their antagonist muscles function to maintain proper balance.

The wrist usually presents in flexion and ulnar deviation (37 of 48 wrists in the Lloyd-Jones series). If hand function is limited, the wrist is left in this position so that it acts as a "hook" or cup for bimanual function. Grasping a shovel or rake, for example, can be accomplished with a bent wrist and can provide fairly good strength. Releasing such

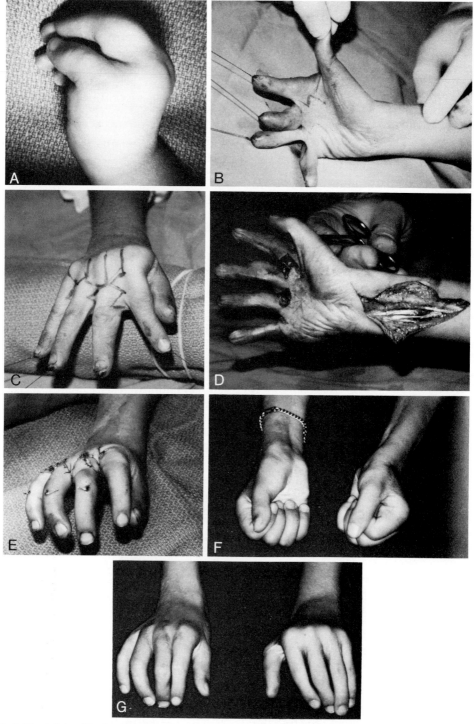

Figure 18–4. Hand deformities in arthrogryposis: *A,* Thumb with adducted flexed contracture; finger with MCP flexion and PIP extension contractures; wrist with extension contracture. *B,* Thumb adductor myotomy; *C,* surgical correction of syndactyly; *D,* flexor tendon lengthening at the wrist; *E,* postoperative stabilization of repositioned PIP and MCP joints; *F* and *G,* 5-year results of surgical correction of bilateral arthrogrypotic hand deformity with excellent flexion and improved extension of both fingers and thumb.

a wrist by tendon lengthening could jeopardize such activities and reduce strength.

If the hand is supple and amenable to reconstructive surgery, we prefer release of wrist flexion contractures by a volar capsulorrhaphy. The joint should be pinned in neutral to slight extension and maintained in this position with a cast and then with orthoplast splints. After the wrist flexion deformity is overcome, transfer of the flexor carpi ulnaris to an extensor eliminates the need for a holding splint.[22, 25]

Wrist contractures that are more fixed may require proximal row carpectomy to improve the functional position, which is generally the treatment of choice. Proximal row carpectomy has been effective in both spastic and fixed wrist flexion contractures.[38] Neither osteotomies of radius and ulna nor carpal corrective osteotomies[25] have been effective in the long term and are not recommended. Proximal row or subtotal carpectomy combined with wrist fusion should be the last option considered in the extremity with a severely contracted wrist. This procedure provides stability, improves cosmesis, and may free tendons for appropriate transfer.

The goal of hand-wrist surgery is the creation of a functional end organ for pinch and grasp so that objects used for activities such as feeding can be handled. Release of contractures for hygiene reasons is an acceptable (secondary) goal. Serial casting and splinting can help prevent the more serious deformities in the severely involved hand and wrist if started early. Passive stretching of the infant's hand and wrist by the parents immediately after birth is helpful until dynamic splints can be applied. Even if hand motor control is limited, these procedures will benefit the patient by preventing secondary contractures. Although some question the benefit of any hand surgery in the arthrygrypotic child, we feel that independent function levels have been improved in selected cases (Figs. 18–4F and G).

THE ELBOW IN ARTHROGRYPOSIS

Surgical treatment of the elbow has received the most attention of reconstructive procedures in the upper extremity.[11, 38] Elbow extension contractures predominate, with range of motion varying from 5° to 50°. The triceps muscle is usually normal, although it can be contracted. The biceps and brachialis muscles are either absent or markedly atrophic. The muscles of the forearm flexor-pronator group may be present but often have function too poor to be considered for transfer.

Treatment of newborns should start with passive stretching and progressive splinting. Bayne[2] recommends an elastic harness and passive assisted flexion splints. As the child gets older (4 years and up), one can apply commercially available dynamic flexion assist splints to increase joint mobility.

When conservative treatment fails to mobilize joints or the patient presents late with a fixed extension contracture, surgical release and lengthening of contracted tissues such as posterior capsule and triceps should be performed. The triceps tendon may be lengthened by a step-cut or by the V-Y technique with freeing of the olecranon from the posterior capsule. These procedures are best considered early (age 2 to 3 years or sooner) so that optimal opportunity for normal joint development is provided. Following surgical release, passive joint mobilization must be achieved with custom-designed orthoplast hinged splints,[23] hinged external fixaters,[10, 35] or combinations of these with the recently available passive elbow motion machines.[8] Static splinting in flexion both during the day and at night should accompany the passive motion program.

Tendon transfers for restoration of elbow flexion are delayed until maximal passive motion is present.[20] Of the three transfers commonly described, pectoralis major transfer (Clark technique)[6, 7] is preferred (Fig. 18–5A). In this procedure, rectus femoris fascia is raised with the distal muscle edge of the pectoralis muscle and inserted into the ulna for elbow flexion.

Anterior transfer of the triceps[5] is a good second choice for elbow flexion, but it does leave the patient with only passive (gravity) extension. The triceps tendon is transferred laterally around the elbow after the muscle is freed halfway up the arm and the aponeurosis is tubulated (Fig. 18–5B). The surgeon must include periosteum from the olecranon and proximal ulna to ensure that there is enough length for a tendon for insertion into the proximal radius or remnant of the biceps tendon (often absent). Tendon tension should be set in over 100° of elbow flexion.

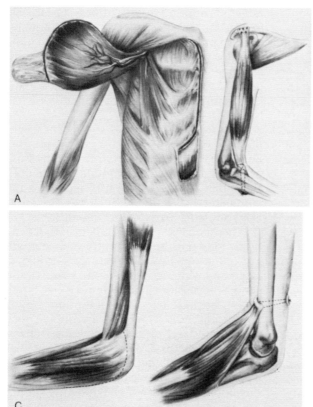

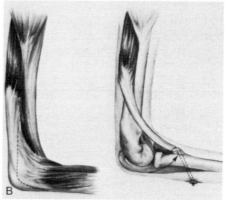

Figure 18–5. Tendon transfers for elbow flexion include release of the posterior capsule and step-cut lengthening of the triceps. *A,* Transfer of the pectoralis major. The muscle insertion on the humerus becomes the new origin, with clavicle attachment, and the pectoralis fascia serves as new insertion into the proximal radius. *B,* Anterior transfer of triceps (Carroll) with distal insertion into the radial tuberosity or the remnant of biceps tendon. *C,* Proximal transfer of the flexor-pronator origin (Steindler plasty) to the distal humerus. (*A, B,* and *C,* reprinted from Doyle JR et al. J Hand Surg 5:149–152, with permission.)

Bilateral triceps transfers should never be performed in the arthrogrypotic patient.

Anterior transfer of the flexor-pronator origin[30] onto the shaft of the humerus is another option (Fig. 18–5C). It has been recommended as the procedure of choice in cases in which the flexor-pronator group has normal strength. In our experience, however, this transfer has been unsatisfactory because it results in an arm with short flexion and requires active wrist extension to balance wrist flexion overpull. We do not recommend this transfer for the complex problems seen in arthrogrypotic patients.

A fourth option for arthrogrypotic children is transfer of the latissimus dorsi.[31] This muscle, with accompanying skin and subcutaneous tissue, can provide excellent flexor strength and excursion as well as soft tissue and skin cover.

Nonoperative treatment of elbow extension contractures has been recommended in children under 2 years of age in the hope of preventing joint deformity. If the elbow joint has 20° to 30° of passive flexion, dynamic splinting[23] with a constant gentle stretch can be beneficial. When this treatment is used, static splints at night are needed to maintain correction. Both cast wedging and forced manipulation are unlikely to be successful and are not recommended because they may result in cartilage damage, including chondrolysis.

Flexion contractures of the elbow are less common and require no operative treatment. Physical therapy including passive stretch, dynamic splints, and occupational therapy modalities improve elbow motion. Affected children use ingenious ways of overcoming their disability, and, because children are usually independent, most should be left alone.

THE SHOULDER IN ARTHROGRYPOSIS

Shoulder deformity involves medial rotation with varying degrees of adduction contracture. In the London Sick Children's series,[22] 33 of 48 patients had medial rotation deformity, and 29 had limited abduction. Rotation is the more disabling of the two deformities because it directs a flexed elbow to the opposite shoulder instead of toward the mouth.

Treatment of the shoulder is determined by its position and the integrated function of the elbow, forearm, wrist, and hand in the child's self-care and other activities of daily living. Either external derotation osteotomy or nothing[22, 38] is the treatment. If the hand is rigid, the wrist in flexion, the elbow in extension, and shoulder in adduction and medial rotation, a functional extremity may be an impossible goal. If the hand is supple and amenable to surgery, however, restoration of hand to mouth function may be provided by elbow extension release, a tendon transfer for active elbow flexion, and a corrective derotation osteotomy of the humerus. If the hands face each other back-to-back because of bilateral medial rotation of the upper extremities, derotational osteotomy through a medial incision adjacent to the axillary fold and fixation with a plate can provide bimanual prehensile grasp.[22]

SUMMARY

Arthrogryposis multiplex congenita is a complex clinical syndrome caused by myopathy or anterior horn cell neuropathy, which impairs muscle activity, leading to incomplete joint development and fixed joint contracture. In the upper extremity, shoulder internal rotation-adduction contractures combined with fixed elbow extension contractures limit extremity positioning of the hands. Conservative therapy—including passive stretching, dynamic splints, and serial casts—may decrease deformities, improve joint mobility, and increase extremity function. Hand and wrist deformities vary from stiff contracted joints in flexion without intrinsic or extrinsic muscles to hands that are more supple and whose function may be improved by surgery. The treatment objective is self-care, and the decision as to which children will benefit from surgery is usually evident by the second year of life.

A careful evaluation of the child's function should be carried out by the physician, therapist, and parents so that the potential gains versus the possible losses can be assessed before upper extremity surgery is performed.[21] One upper extremity should be treated at a time, and the results should be evaluated with overall function (e.g., crutch-walking and the ability to rise from a sitting position) before additional surgery is considered.

References

1. Banker BQ, Victor M, Adams RD. Arthrogryposis multiplex due to congenital muscular dystrophy. Brain 80:319–334, 1957.
2. Bayne LG. Arthrogryposis. In Green DP, ed. Operative Surgery of the Hand. New York, Churchill Livingstone, 1982.
3. Brown LM, Robson MJ, Sharrard WJW. The pathophysiology of arthrogryposis multiplex congenital neurologica. J Bone Joint Surg 62B:291–296, 1980.
4. Caitinen O, Hiruensalo M. Arthrogryposis multiplex congenita. Ann Paediatr Fenn 12:133, 1966.
5. Carroll RE, Hill NA. Triceps transfer to restore elbow flexion. J Bone Joint Surg 52A:239–244, 1970.
6. Carroll RE, et al. Pectoralis major transplantation to restore elbow flexion to the paralytic limb. J Hand Surg 4:501–507, 1979.
7. Clark JMP. Reconstruction of biceps brachii by pectoral muscle transplantation. Br J Surg 34:180, 1946.
8. Cooney WP. Contractures and burns of the elbow. In Morrey BF, ed. The Elbow and Its Disorders. Philadelphia, WB Saunders, 1985:433–451.
9. Danglis CJ, et al. Surgical correction of thumb deformity in arthrogryposis multiplex congenita. Hand 13(1):55–58, 1981.
10. Deland JT, Walker PS, Sledge CB, Farberov A. Treatment of post-traumatic elbows with a new hinged distractor. Orthopedics 6:732, 1983.
11. Doyle JR, James PM, Larsen LJ, Ashley RK. Restoration of elbow flexion in arthrogryposis multiplex congenita. J Hand Surg 5:149–152, 1980.
12. Drachman DB, Banke BQ. Arthrogryposis multiplex congenita. A case due to disease of the anterior horn cells. Arch Neurol 5:77–93, 1961.
13. Drennan JC. Neuromuscular disorders. In Lovell WW, Winter RB, eds. Pediatric Orthopedics, 2nd ed. Philadelphia, JB Lippincott, 1986.
14. Drummond DS, Seller TM, Cruess RL. Management of arthrogryposis multiplex congenita. AAOS Instructional Course Lectures 23:79, 1974.
15. Ferguson AB, Jr. Orthopedic Surgery in Infancy and Childhood. Baltimore, Williams & Wilkins, 1957:438–441.
16. Fowler M. A case of arthrogryposis multiplex congenita with lesions in the nervous system. Arch Dis Child 34:505–510, 1959.
17. Friedlander HL, Westin GW, Wood WL. Arthrogryposis multiplex congenita. J Bone Joint Surg 50A:89–112, 1968.
18. Gibson DA, Urs NDK. Arthrogryposis multiplex congenita. J Bone Joint Surg 52B:483–493, 1970.
19. Hansen OM. Surgical anatomy and treatment of patients with arthrogryposis. J Bone Joint Surg 43B:855, 1961.
20. Holtmann B, Wray RC, Lowrey R, Weeks P. Restoration of elbow flexion. Hand 7:256–261, 1975.
21. Jones LE, Schutt AH, Sawtell RR. Arthrogryposis multiplex congenita. A review of 40 cases (unpublished data).
22. Lloyd-Roberts GC, Lettin AWF. Arthrogryposis multiplex congenita. J Bone Joint Surg 52B:494–508, 1970.
23. McMasters WC, Tivnon MC, Waugh TR. Cast brace for the upper extremity. Clin Orthop 109:126–129, 1975.
24. Mead NG, Lithgow WC, Sweeney HJ. Arthrogryposis multiplex congenita. J Bone Joint Surg 40A:1285–1309, 1958.

25. Meyn M, Ruby L. Arthrogryposis of the upper extremity. Orthop Clin North Am 7:501–507, 1976.
26. Mirise RT, Shear S. Congenital contractural arachnodactyly. Arthritis Rheu 22:542–546, 1979.
27. Shapiro F, Bresnan MJ. Orthopedic management of childhood neuromuscular disease. J Bone Joint Surg 64A:949–953, 1982.
28. Sheldon W. Amyoplasia congenita. Arch Dis Child 7:117–135, 1932.
29. Smith RJ. Treatment of congenital deformities of the hand and forearm. N Engl J Med 300:402–407, 1979.
30. Steindler A. Arthrogryposis. J Int Coll Surg 12:21–25, 1949.
31. Stern P. Latissimus dorsi musculocutaneous flap for elbow flexion. J Hand Surg 7:25, 1982.
32. Swinyard CA, Magora A. Multiple congenital contractures (arthrogryposis). An electromyographic study. Arch Phys Med Rehabil 43:36–41, 1962.
33. Tachdjian MO. Pediatric Orthopedics. Philadelphia, WB Saunders, 1972.
34. Triguiros AP, Vasquez JLV, and DeMiguel GFD. Larsen's Syndrome. Acta Orthop Scand, 49:582–588, 1978.
35. Volkov MV, Oganesian OV. Restoration of function in the knee and elbow with a hinge-distractor apparatus. J Bone Joint Surg 57A:591, 1975.
36. Weeks PM. Surgical correction of upper extremity deformities in arthrogrypotics. Plast Reconstr Surg 36:459, 1965.
37. Whitten JH. Congenital abnormalities in calves: arthrogryposis and hydrencephaly. J Pathol 73:375–387, 1957.
38. Williams P. The management of arthrogryposis. Orthop Clin North Am 9:67–88, 1978.
39. Wynne-Davies R, Lloyd-Roberts GC. Arthrogryposis multiplex congenita—search for prenatal factors in 66 sporadic cases. Arch Dis Child 51:618–623, 1976.

PART IV

Special Conditions of the Upper Extremity

CHAPTER ○ 1 9

Dermatologic Disorders

JAMES J. LEYDEN

The same skin disorders are found in both children and adults—the difference is the frequency of each disorder within the two age groups. For example, atopic dermatitis, a form of eczema, is more prevalent in children than in adults. Congenital skin problems such as pachyonychia congenita and nail patella syndrome are seen in the adult years, even though they can be first observed in childhood.

ANATOMY

Hands and nails are commonly involved with various dermatologic disorders, both in a localized fashion and as part of more generalized processes. The anatomy of the skin on the hand is similar to that of the skin on other body areas, with only a few, but important, differences. The outer portion of the skin, or epidermis, consists of a viable epithelial tissue that undergoes a series of cellular differentiation processes designed to manufacture the final membrane that interfaces with our environment. This membrane, known as the stratum corneum, consists of various structural proteins called keratins, which are immersed in an intrakeratin matrix termed filaggrin. This layer consists of proteinaceous cells that are tightly bound to each other by intercellular polar lipids and is the outer membrane with which we interface with our environment. In most body areas, the stratum corneum membrane is only 10 to 15 cell layers thick. On the hand, the palmar stratum corneum is 50 times thicker than other body areas. This difference is beneficial to children whose hands are exposed to the mechanical shear and frictional forces of sports. The mid portion of the skin, known as the dermis, primarily consists of the proteins collagen and elastin, which are immersed in a matrix of glycosoaminoglycans, particularly hyaluronic acid. In addition, various appendages such as eccrine and apocrine sweat glands and terminal and sebaceous follicles along with lymphatic, arterial, and venular vessels are found in most body areas. On the palms, there is an increased number of eccrine sweat glands, which, unlike eccrine sweat glands on other body areas, function continuously, increase their output mainly as a result of mental and emotional stimuli, and respond little to thermal stress. Eccrine sweat glands on other body areas respond to heat stimuli, and inactive glands are recruited when body temperature increases. Increased sweating is necessary for stabilization of body temperature. The increase in the number of eccrine sweat glands that continuously produce sweat serves a purpose in that hydration of skin increases the coefficient of friction and facilitates the gripping of objects. Apocrine sweat glands, terminal hair follicles (e.g., those on the scalp, beard area, trunk, and extremities), and sebaceous follicles (i.e. follicles with attached oil-producing glands that are found primarily on the head and trunk) are not found on the palm.

Because the hand frequently comes into contact with numerous surfaces, it is a very common site for dermatitis, despite the increased thickness of the stratum corneum outer membrane. The increased exposure of hands in play situations and other stresses that can result in breaks in the integrity of the skin appear to be important factors in the development of infection in and around the fingernails. In addition to being sites for fungal infections and contact dermatitis, the hands and nails often are involved in psoriasis, lichen planus, viral verrucae, and genetic disorders in which the process of differentiation of skin and nails (keratinization) is disturbed.

CONTACT DERMATITIS

Contact dermatitis (i.e., dermatitis arising from contact with a chemical) is clearly the most common dermatitic process involving the hands of children. Contact dermatitis can be broadly divided into two major varieties: contact irritant dermatitis and contact allergic dermatitis. Contact irritant dermatitis is more prevalent than contact allergy, yet far more is known about the pathophysiology of the latter.

In contact irritant dermatitis, a direct toxic effect of a chemical on cell membranes, cytoplasm, or nucleic acids leads to cell damage and death followed by a host inflammatory response of vasodilation and ingress of polymorphonuclear leukocytes. The clinical picture is that of erythema and scaling, often accompanied by fissures. The inflammation of contact irritation is often accompanied by itching, and usually there also are symptoms of pain or "irritation," such as tightness. On the hand, the dorsum is char-

acteristically more intensely involved than the palm. The thicker stratum corneum of the palm is protective. Once the integrity of the skin is compromised, further exposure to environmental factors (e.g., soaps, detergents, acidic food juices, and sport gloves) intensify the problem. A common error that parents make is to try and keep their children's hands clean "so they won't become infected." This and fear of contagion lead to overwashing, which only results in further damage. The inflammation of contact irritant dermatitis usually will respond to topical corticosteroid creams and ointments: e.g., (1) fluocinalone cream and ointment, 0.25%, b.i.d. or t.i.d.; (2) betamethasone valerate cream and ointment, 0.1%, b.i.d.; (3) hydrocortisone cream and ointment, 1%, b.i.d. Although ointments are less acceptable than creams from an aesthetic point of view, they are preferable when excessive scaling and fissuring are prominent features. It should be remembered that chronic use of corticosteroid preparations can result in cutaneous atrophy, which makes skin more vulnerable to further toxic injury. One can successfully manage contact irritant dermatitis by using potent corticosteroid preparations to dampen the acute phase of inflammation and then by administering less potent agents in combination with lubricating creams and ointments to minimize excessive scaling and to provide adequate protection against further damage.

Contact allergic dermatitis is much less common than contact irritant dermatitis but is better understood from the standpoint of basic mechanisms of pathophysiology. Contact allergy is a cell-mediated cytotoxic process in which epidermal dendritic cells of monocyte-macrophage origin, known as Langerhans cells, process antigens and present them to regional nodes, where a specific clone of T-lymphocytes is induced. Specific T-lymphocytes hone in on antigens in epidermal Langerhans cells, release lymphokines, and damage cells. Clinically, contact allergic dermatitis is more inflammatory than contact irritant dermatitis and is characterized by intense erythema, vesicles that rupture, ooze, and then crust over, and by intense itching (Fig. 19–1). The dorsum of the hand is usually more obviously involved in contact allergic dermatitis, again demonstrating the protective nature of the thick stratum corneum of the palm. On the palm, deep-seated vesicles can be appreciated by close inspection. Poision ivy dermatitis,

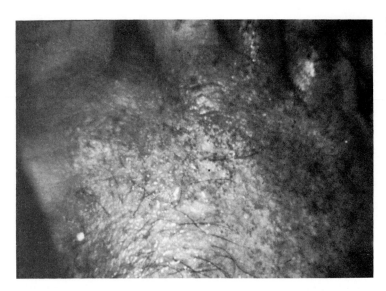

Figure 19–1. Acute contact dermatitis with vesicles, erythema, and edema.

found commonly in children, is an example of an acute allergic contact dermatitis. Contact allergy thus represents an example of an immunologically mediated dermatitis, in contrast to contact irritant dermatitis, which is a direct cytotoxic nonimmunologically mediated process. Treatment of contact allergic dermatitis involves administration of topical corticosteriods or systemic steriods for extremely severe cases coupled with avoidance of further contact with the allergen. Topical drugs—either fluocinolone, 0.025%, or betamethasone valerate, 0.1% can be given t.i.d.; a systemic steroid—prednisone, 1 mg/kg—can be given for 2 weeks, then tapered off over the next week. When the allergen is not evident, patch testing with a battery of allergens is very useful. Application of an allergen under an occlusive dressing for 48 hours enhances penetration of the allergen, which then evokes a localized contact dermatitis.

DYSHIDROTIC ECZEMA

Dyshidrotic eczema is a condition of recurrent, acute, or chronic vesiculation of the hands, usually associated with intense itching. In the most prevalent variety, small vesicles occur along the sides of each finger. Larger blisters can occur on the fingers and palms but this finding is less common. Children may have associated hyperhidrosis, a finding that caused earlier authors to propose that the blisters represented sweat retention vesicles. Studies have shown, however, that these vesicles are not related to eccrine sweat ducts but are exuberant examples of inter- and intracellular edema of the epidermis. Children with an underlying background of atopy (e.g., allergic rhinitis, asthma, and atopic dermatitis) appear to be more susceptible to this condition, particularly in the summer months. Atopic dermatitis is more prevalent in children than in adults. Atopic dermatitis will classically be expressed as thickened plaques with erythema, scaling, and lichenification (tree-bark appearance) as is frequently found in the anticubital fossa. Similar lesions can occur elsewhere, and the skin over the flexor surfaces is most commonly involved. Contact allergic dermatitis can also present as an acute vesicular eruption on the sides of the fingers and should be particularly suspected in children who have an isolated attack in the absence of a strong history of atopic disease. Treatment consists of applying cool compresses until the vesicles have crusted over and the crusts have fallen off. After the crusts are gone, topical corticosteroids are recommended. Patch testing to exclude contact allergic dermatitis is desirable. Treatment of atopic dermatitis involves application of topical steroids of mid to high potency for acute eczema followed by use of low-strength steroids, such as hydrocortisone. Systemic steroids such as hydroxyzine (dose: children under age 6, 50 mg/day in divided doses; children over age 6, 50–100 mg/day) are used to suppress itching in severe cases that are unresponsive to topical therapy and are used for only a brief period.

HYPERHIDROSIS

There are children who appear perfectly normal except for profuse sweating from the palms or soles or both. This condition, known as hyperhidrosis, does not occur in response to thermal stimuli but is clearly aggravated by emotional stimuli. At times, the degree of hyperhidrosis can be so intense that an affected child cannot shake hands without extreme embarrassment. Anticholinergic agents delivered by iontophoresis can control hyperhidrosis but are cumbersome. Soaking in 20% to 30% aluminum chloride solution daily for 20 to 30 minutes until sufficient reduction in sweating occurs is currently the best approach.

INFECTIOUS DISORDERS

Viral Infections (Warts, Molluscum Contagiosum, Herpes Simplex)

The human papilloma virus is responsible for inducing benign papillomatous proliferation of the epidermis, a disorder known as warts. This condition is common in adolescents. A DNA virus that is relatively contagious is responsible, and autotransmission and transfer to individuals who are not immune are common. When this virus induces growths in and around the nail plate and lateral nail folds (see further on), treatment can be particularly difficult.

Another viral infection, called molluscum contagiosum, is due to a member of the poxvirus group and produces umbilicated papular lesions.

Both the common wart and molluscum contagiosum are frequently seen in children and can be easily treated by a variety of approaches, including destruction with liquid nitrogen, use of various acids (e.g., salicylic and lactic acids), or removal by surgery.

Viral infections due to herpes simplex can occur on the hand. A first or primary attack of herpes simplex is usually associated with fever and adenopathy. When the distal finger is infected, the host response generates inflammation that is sufficient to produce edema and pain in this small compartment. Clinically, herpetic infections produce grouped vesicles that usually show central umbilication. Vesicles develop into pustules with ingress of polymorphonuclear leuko-

cytes. Treatment consists of cool compresses, topical antiviral agents such as Acyclovir, (5% ointment: cover all lesions q 4 hr, 6 times/day, for 7 days) and then topical steroids once the vesicles have crusted over, which usually coincides with the death of virus particles.

Fungal Infections

Dermatophytic fungi can cause infection of the hand. The clinical picture is normally that of a slowly expanding scaling erythema with associated pruritis. Often, one or more nails will commonly be involved (see further on). Typically, only one hand will be involved and both feet will show infection—the so called two feet, one hand syndrome. The reason that only one hand becomes involved is not clear. One possibility is that there may be significant differences in the amount of eccrine sweating in the two hands and that these variations are important in the ecology of fungal colonization of skin. Fungi require moisture for spores to develop into filaments, which can then penetrate the stratum corneum because of the production of various keratinolytic enzymes. The clinical picture tends to be one of relative symbiosis in which fungi proliferate, invade the stratum corneum, and evoke a mild host reaction that results in low-grade scaling and erythema. The usual organism is *Trichophyton rubrum*. Antigenically, more active species such as *T. mentagrophytes* rarely colonize the hand, and acute vesicular eruptions due to fungal infection are uncommon on the hands. Fungal infections of the hand are less common in children than in adults.

Acute vesicular eruptions on the palms can develop in a child who is experiencing an intense host reaction to fungal infection on the feet. *T. mentagrophytes* infection of the feet can result in a T-cell–mediated cytotoxic contact dermatitis that results in an acute vesicular dermatitis on the feet. Concomitant with this host reaction to fungal infection on the feet, a vesicular eruption can develop on the palms in the absence of fungi in that site. This was formerly referred to as an *id* reaction, short for dermatophytid reaction. This dermatophytid reaction on the palms is viewed as an immune complex–mediated immunologic reaction in which the antigen is a fungal antigen.

Treatment of dermatophytic infections of

the hand can be successfully achieved with any of the topical imidazole formulations such as miconazole nitrate (Micatin) or clotrimazole nitrate (Fotrimin). For more resistant infections and for those that involve the nail, systemic antifungal therapy in the form of griseofulvin (250 mg b.i.d.) or ketoconazole (200 to 400 mg once daily) is required. Dermatophytid reactions are treated with topical compresses and topical corticosteroid creams.

Hand Signs in Bacterial and Other Infections

Bacterial infections due to *Staphylococcus aureus* and *S. pyogenes* can occur on the hands but rarely do so in the absence of lesions elsewhere. There are certain infections that commonly express their presence with lesions on the hands. These include gonococcemia, meningococcemia, subacute bacterial endocarditis, and syphilis. In these infections, lesions on the hand are important signs of significant systemic infection.

Gonococcemia presents as slightly painful pustules appearing in crops on the distal fingertips, wrists, ankles, and toes. Commonly, there is an associated tenosynovitis or a swollen joint. In young girls, the usual site of primary infection is the pelvis; in boys, infection is most common in the prostate. Hand lesions are the result of bacteremia. Treatment consists of administration of systemic antibiotics.

Similar lesions appear in aubacute endocarditis, with most appearing distally as hemorrhagic, painful, subungual lesions in a patient with generalized malaise and recurrent fever.

Meningococcemia is a fulminating infection in an acutely or critically ill child. Coalescent hemorrhagic lesions commonly appear on the palms.

Infectious syphilis in the so-called secondary stage, associated with dissemination of the spirochete and early immune reactivity, typically results in numerous copper- or ham-colored papules on the palm, which resolve with intense hyperpigmentation.

HAND SIGNS IN COLLAGEN DISEASE

The hand is a common site for the cutaneous expression of systemic disease processes. This is particularly true of the so-called col-

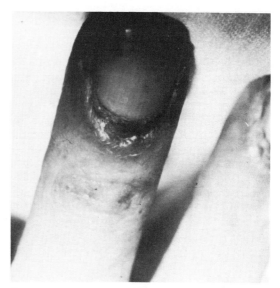

Figure 19–2. Periungual erythema and telangiectasia of "collagen vascular" disease.

lagen vascular disorders. Both specific and nonspecific changes commonly occur on the hands. The most frequent nonspecific changes involve periungual erythema with telangiectasia and punctate and confluent erythema of the palms (Fig. 19–2). The mechanism for vasodilatation and telangiectasia formation is unknown. Specific changes occur in systemic sclerosis in which the first changes consist of diffuse swelling of digits followed by a dense sclerosis and tapering of the fingers (Fig. 19–3), as seen in scleroderma. Characteristic telangiectasias consisting of flat, circular dilatations without ra-

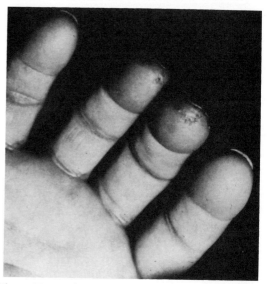

Figure 19–3. Sclerotic fingertips with calcinosis cutis that are seen in scleroderma.

Figure 19–4. Atrophic scarring papules and plaque of dermatomyositis.

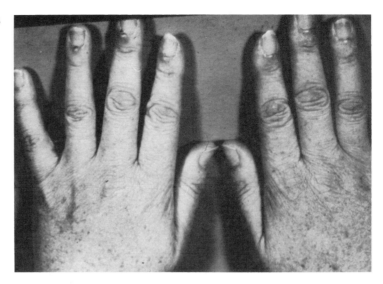

diating reticulated projections (as seen in "spider" telangiectasias) develop on the palmar and plantar surfaces as well as on the tongue and lips. In children with dermatomyositis, typical erythematous, slightly atrophic scarring papules develop over phalangeal joints, whereas in those with lupus erythematosus the lesions appear between joints (Fig. 19–4).

PSORIASIS AND LICHEN PLANUS

Three common dermatologic conditions that involve the child's hands are psoriasis, lichen planus, and drug-induced cutaneous eruption.

Psoriasis most commonly occurs as sharply defined, annular, erythematous plaques with a thick, silvery scale (Fig. 19–5). Characteristically, removal of the scale results in pinpoint bleeding. Because the hands are used so frequently, the classic morphology may be distorted by trauma, contact irritation, and use of various home remedies. The appearance of typical lesions elsewhere and the frequently associated typical nail changes are helpful in diagnosis. Other, less common expressions of psoriasis are the variant in which circumscribed plaques are studded with pustules and the diffuse pustular psoriasis in which numerous pustules with one circumscribed plaque occur over the palms, soles, and even the entire body surface (Fig. 19–6). The inflammation of psoriasis is extremely difficult to control (Fig. 19–7). Potent topical steroids (such as Lidex

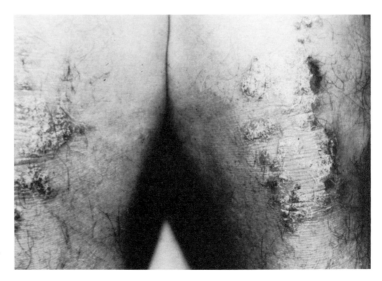

Figure 19–5. Typical plaques of psoriasis, in the knees.

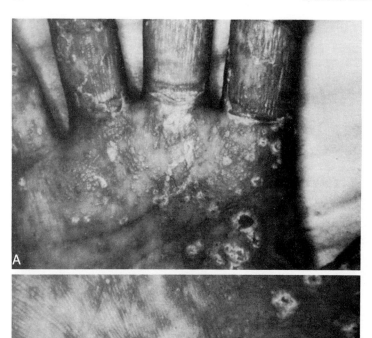

Figure 19–6. *A* and *B*, Pustular psoriasis.

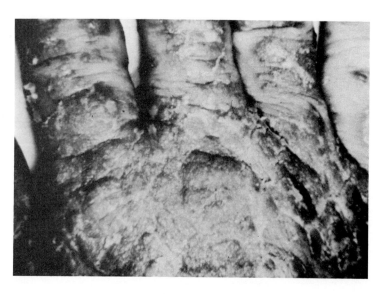

Figure 19–7. Psoriasis with inflammation.

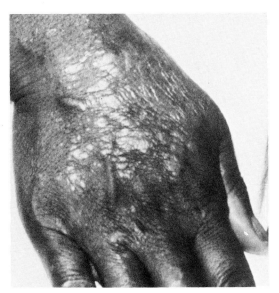

Figure 19–8. *A,* Flat-topped violaceous papules of lichen planus.

0.05% b.i.d. or Diprosone cream 0.05% q.i.d.), topical tar preparations, and photochemotherapy are useful therapeutic modalities.

Lichen planus is a disorder of unknown etiology except for occasional cases in which a drug eruption assumes the characteristic pattern of this disease. Flat-topped, polygonal papules with a purplish hue are the hallmark lesions of lichen planus (Fig. 19–8). These are typically found on the wrists and not infrequently occur on the palms. Typically, atrophic nail plate changes are also present. Lichen planus is particularly resistant to therapy and commonly runs a course of several years before spontaneously clearing. Potent topical steroids and systemic corticosteroids (prednisone 20–40 mg/day) can temporarily suppress symptoms such as pruritis, but steroids do not shorten the course of the disease process. In children, a syndrome called twenty-or-ten nail dystrophy is an expression of lichen planus in which nail plate atrophy develops in all fingernails and toenails or only on the hands or feet.

FINGERNAIL ANATOMY AND GROWTH

The nail plate, commonly referred to as the nail, is a collection of highly differentiated, tightly coherent cells produced by the nail matrix. The matrix is found beneath the cuticle, or proximal nail fold, and consists of a pool of dividing, germinative cells that pro-

duce daughter cells that undergo cellular differentiation and result in cells primarily containing protein that are tightly bound to each other. The principal component of protein in the nails is similar to that found in hair and skin. The protein fibers lay parallel to the surface of the nail and are perpendicular to the direction of nail growth in the nail matrix. The distal end of the nail matrix corresponds to the semicircular white area, or lunula, which is seen just distal to the cuticle. Fingernails grow at different rates, with growth rate being faster for the fingers than for the thumb. It takes 3 to 4 months for the nail plate to regrow. The average rate of growth for the thumbnail is 0.10 to 0.12 mm per day. Nail thickness depends on the size of the germinative pool in the nail matrix. The nail bed extends from the lunula and forms a bond with the overlying nail plate. The typical pink color of this region results from blood flowing through blood vessels in the nail bed.

Accurate diagnosis of nail disorders requires identification of the area of the nail involved, the type of abnormality present, and the correlation with known patterns of disease process.

Patterns of Nail Disease

Typical patterns of disease exist for disorders that affect the nail matrix, the nail folds, and the nail bed.

Matrix Disorders

Atrophy. As a result of a decrease in the size of the matrix or the proliferative activity of the germinative cells in this compartment, the final product, or nail plate, may become thinned, such as typically occurs in lichen planus as a result of an inflammatory infiltrate in the nail matrix (see further on). When a child is acutely ill, temporary disturbance of the nail matrix can occur, resulting in production of cells that maintain their nuclei. These cells refract and disperse light, producing a white band. If the process is severe enough (i.e., associated with an acute childhood disease), the nail plate is temporarily thinned, resulting in a depressed, atrophic band of furrows called Beau's lines.

Hypertrophy. Thick nails result from chronic injury or inflammation in the matrix. Chronic infection of the cuticular area, for example, commonly results in a thickened nail plate. Chronic inflammation of the skin of the proximal nail fold, such as commonly occurs in atopic dermatitis and in chronic contact dermatitis, can extend to the matrix and result in a thickened nail plate. Psoriasis commonly results in nail matrix inflammation and a thickened nail plate. Invasion of the nail plate by dermatophytic fungi also can result in a thickened dystrophic nail plate.

Nail Fold Disorders

Paronychia, or infection of the nail folds, results in tender, erythematous swelling of the proximal and lateral nail folds. When the proximal nail fold is extensively involved, extension to the matrix area can result in thickened nails.

Nail Bed Disorders

Onycholysis, or separation of the nail plate from the underlying nail bed, is a common disorder that is frequently misdiagnosed as fungal in origin. When the nail plate separates from the underlying nail bed, light is dispersed, resulting in a yellowish color rather than the normal pink. This usually occurs in older children. Use of nail files or tooth picks only further aggravates onycholysis and is to be avoided at all costs. Psoriasis and fungal infections also can produce onycholysis.

Nail Disorders Associated with Skin Disease

Psoriasis

Nails are involved in psoriasis in as many as 50% of cases. The typical lesions are pits in the nail matrix, onycholysis with discoloration, subungual thickening, and thickened dystrophic nail plates.

Pits result from focal psoriatic lesions in the nail matrix that produce areas of parakeratotic cells that fall off as the nail plate emerges from under the proximal nail fold (Fig. 19–9). The size and shape of the pit depend on the size, shape, and duration of the psoriatic process in the matrix.

Onycholysis results from psoriatic involvement of the nail bed. Subungual thickening results from prolonged involvement of the nail bed, which produces increased

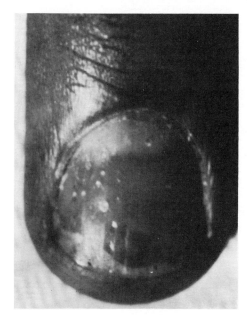

Figure 19–9. Nail pitting in psoriasis.

amounts of keratinous material as a result of the inflammation of the psoriatic process.

Thickened nails result from prolonged, extensive involvement of the nail matrix, which results in a parakeratotic nail plate that crumbles easily.

Lichen Planus

In lichen planus, the intense inflammation consisting of a dense infiltrate of lymphocytes results in severe impairment of the nail matrix. Very thinned atrophic nails are typical, and often all nails on both hands are severely involved (Fig. 19–10). With extensive, severe inflammation, loss of the nail plate with an overgrowth of tissue from the proximal nail fold, or pterygium unguis, develops. Treatment is extremely difficult, with intralesional steroid therapy the most successful.

Onychomycosis

Infection of the nail plate by dermatophytic fungi is an extremely common disorder. Typically, the process involves one or more nails and gradually spreads to other fingers. Infection starts distally or at the lateral folds and moves proximally or centrally. Progressive destruction of the nail plate results in a thickened, crumbling nail plate. Extension to the nail bed can result in onycholysis with extensive subungual debris. Treatment consists of systemic therapy with griseofulvin (250 mg b.i.d.) or ketoconazole (200–400 mg

Figure 19–10. Atrophic nail plates in lichen planus.

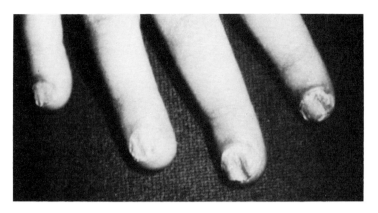

once daily), because topically applied antifungal agents cannot penetrate the nail plate sufficiently to eradicate fungi.

Congenital and Hereditary Disease

There is a wide variety of inherited disorders in which the skin, hair, and nails are compromised by production of abnormal proteins.

Pachyonychia Congenita Syndrome

Jaddassohn and Lewandowsky[1] described an ectodermal dysplasia of excessive keratin formation. Its transmission is autosomal dominant, and its expression is extremely variable.[2] This disorder is predominantly found in Slavs and Jews of Slavonic origin. The nail appears grotesque, showing thickness, color changes, and abnormal texture (Fig. 19–11). Surgical removal is recommended and must be radical and include the nail, the nail bed, the nail matrix, and the periosteum on the dorsum of the distal phalanx (Fig. 19–12).

Nail-Patella Syndrome (Hereditary Osteo-Onychodysplasia)

More than 200 cases of this disorder have been reported since it was first described by Little in 1879. Transmission is autosomal dominant and there is always some expression.[5] There is a close linkage with the genetic dominants of the ABO blood group.[3, 6] Deformities of the knee, elbow, and distal interphalangeal joint are found in the syndrome. When these joints are involved, they show limited mobility or dislocation or both. In some cases, the distal interphalangeal joint is absent. The patella may be hypoplastic or absent and is sometimes associated with hypoplasia of the lateral femoral condyle. The elbow may demonstrate a hypoplastic capitellum and a small radial head. Osteoarthritis of these joints usually occurs earlier in patients with this syndrome than in the general population. Over 80% of the ilia show spurring, which is not reported in any other species or associated human condition and is pathognomonic as an expression of this mutant gene.[4]

Hypoplasia of the scapula and delayed ossification of the secondary centers of ossification may be seen. Other organ systems involved include the central nervous system, eyes, and specific muscle groups. Albuminuria is the first indication of renal dysfunction, although renal failure is rare prior to the fourth decade.

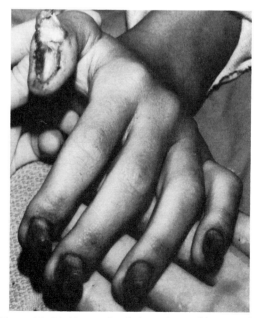

Figure 19–11. Abnormal nails in pachyonychia congenita.

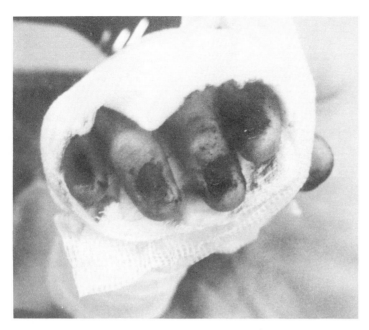

Figure 19–12. Radial excision of nail tissue for pachyonychia congenita.

Paronychia

Paronychia is an infection of the cuticle in children whose hands are exposed to water. The lateral fold of the nail is the most common structure affected. Chronic hydration results in a lifting upward of the proximal and lateral nail folds, which provides a portal of entry for bacteria and yeasts. Once microorganisms colonize these compartments, growth is promoted by the warmth and moisture under nail folds. The primary clinical feature of paronychia is usually the same regardless of the causative organism—namely, acute, painful erythematous swelling. One must assess cell cultures before determining therapy. Frequently, mixed flora including yeasts, gram-negative bacteria such as *Proteus* and *Pseudomonas*, and gram-positive bacteria such as *Staphylococcus aureus* will be present. When *Proteus* is present, there often will be a black discoloration in and under the nail plate. *Pseudomonas* frequently will produce a greenish discoloration (Fig. 19–13). Compression with a broad-spectrum antimicrobial agent such as 1% acetic acid is a practical way of protecting against a wide range of organisms. Specific topical and systemic antimicrobial therapy must be determined by culture results. A critical aspect of management is protection from further excessive exposure to water.

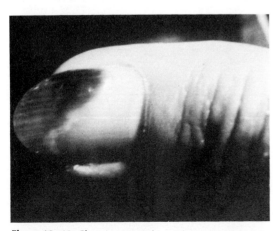

Figure 19–13. Chronic paronychia with green pigment, indicating *Pseudomonas* infection.

REFERENCES

Pachyonychia Congenita Syndrome

1. Jadassohn J, Lewandowsky F. Pachyonychia congenita, keratosis disseminata circumscripta tylomata; leukokeratosis linquae. Ikonographica Dermatologica, Tab. 629, 1906.
2. Soderquist NA, Reed WB. Pachyonychia congenita with epidermal cysts and other congenital dyskeratoses. Arch Dermatol 97:31, 1968.

Nail-Patella Syndrome

3. Beals RK, Eckard AL. Hereditary onycho-osteodysplasia. A report of nine kindreds. J Bone Joint Surg (Am) 51:505, 1969.
4. Darlington D, Hawkins CF. Nail-patella syndrome with iliac horns and hereditary nephropathy. Necropsy report and anatomical dissection. J Bone Joint Surg (Br) 45B:164, 1967.
5. Little EM. Congenital absence or delayed development of the patella. Lancet 2:781, 1879.
6. Lucas GL, Opitz JM. The nail-patella syndrome. Clinical and genetic aspects of five kindreds with 38 affected family members. J Pediatr 68:273, 1966.

CHAPTER ○ 20

Infections of the Upper Extremity

J. P. LEDDY

Upper extremity infections in children are common and may result in serious consequences if proper treatment is not given. Because a good history is often unobtainable and the physical examination may be difficult to interpret, a high index of suspicion is essential.[1, 11, 12, 40]

Every attempt to identify the specific organism prior to initiation of antibiotic therapy should be made. This may require wound, blood, synovial fluid, or bone cultures. Once the appropriate specimens for Gram stain and culture have been obtained, antibiotic treatment can begin. A change can be made at a later date, depending on the organism identified and its sensitivity. The type of organism can sometimes be inferred from the age of the patient, the nature of the injury, or the characteristics of the underlying disease.[28] For example, *Staphylococcus aureus* is the most common cause of hematogenous infection in children of all ages. The high incidence of resistance to penicillin with this organism is well known.[36] *Haemophilus influenzae* is more common in joint infections in patients under the age of 2 years, and *Salmonella* is seen more frequently in those with sickle cell disease.[40] *H. influenzae*, *Staphylococcus*, and *Diplococcus pneumoniae* are frequently seen following otitis media.[31] A human bite produces a mixed flora, whereas a dog or cat bite commonly produces *Pasteurella multocida*.[2, 6] Injuries in homes result in colonization by gram-positive organisms, whereas farm injuries often result in mixed gram-positive and gram-negative infections.[13] Appropriate antibiotics and tetanus toxoid booster or hyperimmune gamma globulin or both can be administered, depending on the immunization status of the child and the nature and extent of the injury. Other general principles include evaluation and splinting of the affected part and incision and drainage of pus.

CELLULITIS

Cellulitis can result from a small scratch or puncture wound. It may or may not be accompanied by lymphangitis or lymphadenitis. X-rays, including xeroroentgenograms, help detect a foreign body.[9] If any drainage is present, a Gram stain and wound culture and sensitivity should be obtained. Blood cultures are taken if there are systemic signs of infection, such as chills or fever. Treatment consists of elevation, splinting, warm soaks, and systemic antibiotics. Incision and drainage are not beneficial unless and until there is abscess formation.[33]

PARONYCHIA

Paronychia is a collection of pus beneath the paronychial fold of the skin around the nail. This disorder is termed eponychia if it affects the eponychium and is known as a runaround if it goes all the way around the nail.[9] It can result from a hangnail, nail biting, or improper trimming of the nails, and it is very common in children.[3] The early, acute stage is manifested by pain, swelling, and erythema in the paronychial fold. Treatment consists of warm soaks and splinting. Antibiotics are usually not necessary. In the more advanced stage, the nail fold is bulging owing to purulent material under pressure. The pain is often intense. In these cases, after producing a digital block, one uses a no. 11 blade to incise and drain the pus by elevating and separating the paronychial fold from the nail[9, 33] (Fig. 20–1). If there is pus under the eponychium, two short longitudinal incisions are made in the edges of the eponychial fold and this tissue is retracted proximally. One excises the proximal portion of the nail, being careful not to damage the germinal center of the nail bed[4, 30] (Fig. 20–2). The eponychium is tacked back into position with

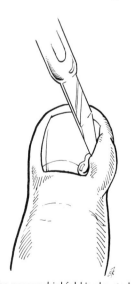

Figure 20–1. The paronychial fold is elevated and separated from the nail, allowing the pus to drain.

5-0 plain catgut. Soaks are started after 24 hours. The nail, if lost, will grow back in 3 to 6 months. The pus should be sent for Gram stain, culture, and sensitivity. The patient can be started on a broad-spectrum antibiotic while awaiting the culture results. *S. aureus* is the most common organism encountered in acute paronychia. In infants, *Candida albicans* can cause an acute paronychia[33] but is less painful. This organism is frequently seen in dental technicians and in other people whose fingers are constantly wet. This infection presents as small vesicles that can coalesce to form bullae. The diagnosis is made by culture of the vesicular fluid or by measurement of immunofluorescent titers of serum antibodies to herpes simplex antigens 2 to 3 weeks after onset. Treatment consists of keeping the affected fingers clean and dry. Incision and drainage can lead to secondary bacterial contamination[27] and is not recommended. Chronic paronychia is also more common in adults than in children. The diagnosis can be made by a microscopic examination of the scrapings, which usually reveals fungus or yeast. Treatment is nonsurgical.

SUBCUTICULAR ABSCESS

Subcuticular abscess is a collection of purulent material beneath the epidermis surrounded by erythema. It is not uncommon in the hands of children. An x-ray helps one ascertain that a foreign body is not present. If soaks fail, incision and drainage with insertion of a small wick may be necessary. One must drain the entire infection to ensure that a collar button abscess is not present. After surgery, soaks are recommended. Antibiotics are not necessary.

FELON

A felon is a closed-space infection of the soft tissues of the terminal phalanx.[9] The thumb and index finger are most commonly affected. The pain may seem out of proportion to the physical findings, and there are no systemic signs. Fibrous septa extend from the distal phalanx to the skin. The pain results from an increase in pressure in this closed space. The pus can destroy the soft tissues of the pulp, and the infection may also lead to osteomyelitis of the distal phalanx, epi-

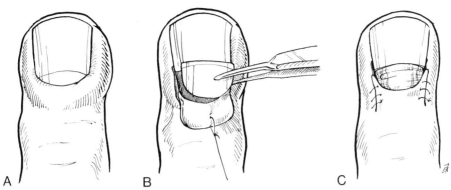

Figure 20–2. A, Pus bulges the eponychial fold. B, Two longitudinal incisions made at the edges of the eponychial fold, which is retracted. The proximal third of the nail is removed. C, Nonadherent gauze is placed over the defect, and the skin incisions are closed.

physeal injury, septic arthritis, or suppurative tenosynovitis if it is not treated early and properly. A felon should be treated with immediate incision and drainage[4] following local digital block anesthesia without epinephrine. General anesthesia may be necessary in the uncooperative child. Several incisions have been advocated for drainage of a felon. A midline incision is often inadequate, and a fishmouth incision is unnecessary and can cause problems such as a painful scar and flap necrosis.[9, 26, 32] Incisions over the volar pad also can result in

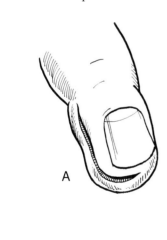

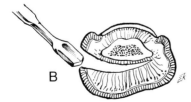

Figure 20–3. A, "J," or hockey stick, incision, dorsal to midline. The neurovascular bundle stays with the volar flap. B, The fibrous septum is completely detached from the distal phalanx.

painful scars and are not recommended unless the abscess is pointing or has already broken through the skin in this area. A longitudinal incision should not cross the skin crease at the distal interphalangeal joint because a scar contracture may develop. I recommend a **J** incision,[9] which extends along the distal phalanx dorsal to the midline halfway across the tuft just beneath the nail (Fig. 20–3). The distal phalanx is visualized, and the fibrous septa are separated from the bone completely to the opposite side. After the incision, all purulent and necrotic tissue should be evacuated and the wound packed open with gauze. A smear and cultures are obtained, and systemic antibiotics are given. Soaks are begun within 24 hours. One gradually removes the packing, allowing the wound to close from the base. Antibiotics should be continued until the infection is controlled (usually within 72 hours).

ACUTE SUPPURATIVE TENOSYNOVITIS

This is an infection within the flexor tendon sheath that can destroy the tendons if it is not properly treated. The tendon sheath then contracts and fills with scar and adhesions, and fixed joint contractures develop. The infection may start with a penetrating injury, spread from a contiguous structure, or begin by hematogenous seeding. The most common organism is S. aureus. The physical signs of this infection were reported by Kanavel:[24]

1. The finger held in a semiflexed position
2. Pain with passive extension of the finger

3. Tenderness over the flexor tendons
4. Swelling of the finger and palm

If the patient is seen early with only mild or moderate pain and good motion of the finger, parenteral antibiotics, splinting, and elevation should be started.[33] The patient must be carefully monitored. If there is no significant improvement within 24 hours or if the condition worsens, operative treatment is indicated. If the infection is well established when the patient is first seen, immediate surgical drainage is required.[4] A thorough knowledge of the flexor tendon sheath, the bursae, and their common variations is mandatory (Fig. 20–4). In the "open" method, a midlateral incision is made on the ulnar side of the affected finger or the radial side of the thumb. The neurovascular bundle is left with the volar flap, and the sheath is opened at multiple levels between the annular pulleys, which are preserved. A transverse incision in the midpalmar crease is used to drain the proximal portion of the sheath (the cul-de-sac) of the index, middle, ring, and little fingers if they are involved. If pus in the tendon sheath of the little finger spreads to the ulnar bursa, drainage is through an incision proximal to the wrist crease (Fig. 20–5). If the thumb is involved, an incision should be made along the thenar crease to drain the sheath of the flexor pollicis longus tendon.

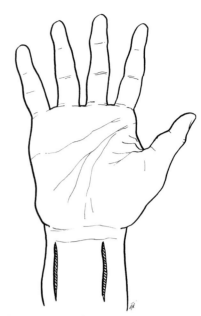

Figure 20–5. Incisions for drainage of the radial and ulnar bursae.

Care must be taken to avoid damage to the motor branch of the median nerve. If pus from the thumb extends to the radial bursa, it should be drained through an incision proximal to the wrist crease (Fig. 20–5). If the radial and ulnar bursae join proximally to the wrist, allowing the infection to spread from one side to the other, a "horseshoe" abscess occurs.[26] In such cases, both bursae must be drained. If the infection extends through the radial and/or ulnar bursa at the wrist, Parona's space may be involved,[4, 14, 15] This space is bordered dorsally by the pronator quadradus muscle, volarly by the flexor digitorum profundus and flexor pollicis longus tendons, radially by the flexor carpi radialis, and ulnarly by the flexor carpi ulnaris tendon.[25] If the infection spreads proximally into the forearm from this space, it should be treated by a volar wrist incision and drainage of all necrotic tissue, and the wound should be thoroughly irrigated with saline solution. The wounds are packed with nonirritating gauze, and the hand and wrist are splinted. The splint and packing are removed on the first or second postoperative day. A supervised program of saline soaks and range of motion exercises is begun.

Closed techniques also have been described for tendon sheath infections.[7, 32, 33] An incision is made in the palm. A polyethylene catheter is placed under the A$_1$ pulley and inserted 1.5 to 2 cm distally into the ten-

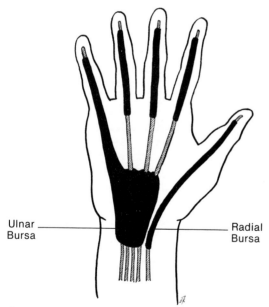

Ulnar Bursa

Radial Bursa

Figure 20–4. The "normal" arrangement of the flexor tendon sheaths and their bursae. The radial bursa is formed at the proximal end of the flexor pollicis longus sheath, and the ulnar bursa at the proximal end of the little finger flexor tendon sheath. There are many variations.

don sheath. A second incision is made on the ulnar midlateral side of the finger overlying the middle and distal phalanges. The sheath is resected distal to the A_4 pulley. A drain is inserted from the skin wound into the tendon sheath and the wound closed. The catheter is irrigated with saline until the returns are clear. The wound in the palm is then closed, and the catheter under the A_1 pulley sutured to the skin. Infections in the radial and ulnar bursae also can be treated in this manner. The hand is splinted, and the sheath is flushed manually with 50 ml of sterile saline every 2 hours for 48 to 72 hours, depending on the clinical situation. The catheters are removed after the infection is controlled, and supervised motion exercises are begun. In the "closed" method, the wounds may heal with less scar. If the infection is severe, the "open" method is preferable.

DEEP INFECTION OF THE HAND

There are two deep palmar spaces beneath the flexor tendons, separated by a fascial septum which originates from the sheath of the long finger profundus tendon and inserts along the entire length of the long finger metacarpal. On the radial side of this septum is the thenar space. The dorsal boundary is the fascia of the adductor pollicis muscle. The volar border is composed of the thin fascial extension of the midpalmar septum, the index flexor tendons, and the thenar fasciae. The radial border is formed by the junction of the thenar and adductor fasciae, and on the ulnar border of the midpalmar septum is the midpalmar space. Dorsally lies the fascia covering the metacarpals of the long, ring, and little fingers and their volar interossei. This fascia joins with the fasciae of the hypothenar muscles to form the ulnar border of this space. The flexor tendons of the middle, ring, and little fingers, the long and ring lumbrical muscles, and the thin interconnecting fasciae of these structures form the anterior boundary. Proximally, there is a thin fascial septum at the distal end of the transverse carpal ligament. Distally, the space ends 2 cm proximal to the webs, where vertical septa of the palmar fascia extend to the fascia anteriorly.[14, 15, 25] There is a hypothenar space ulnar to the midpalmar space within the fascia of the hypothenar muscles.[4, 33] Infection here is quite rare and usually the result of a penetrating injury. Deep-

space infections in the hand were surgical emergencies prior to the antibiotic era. If seen early, they may respond to splinting, elevation, and parenteral antibiotics. If not, surgical incision and drainage constitute the procedure of choice.

Thenar Space Infections

Thenar space infections present with swelling and tenderness in the first web space and over the thenar muscles and the dorsum of the hand. The infection may arise from a penetrating wound or from a pre-existing infection in the thumb or index finger. If conservative treatment does not cause rapid improvement or if the infection is first seen at a late stage, surgical incision and drainage are necessary.

Flynn and others advocate open drainage through a longitudinal incision over the dorsum of the first web space, starting midway between the thumb and index metacarpal heads.[14, 15] The interval between the adductor pollicis longus and first dorsal interosseous is explored. A hemostat is then placed over the lateral edge of the adductor to drain the abscess that lies on the anterior surface of this muscle. A drain is left in place for 24 to 48 hours while the hand is immobilized and elevated in a splint. When the drain is removed, soaks and supervised range of motion exercises are begun. The abscess may also be drained by an incision along the thenar crease, but one must take care to avoid injury to the recurrent motor branch.[30] A combined dorsal and volar approach can be utilized.

Neviaser prefers a closed method combining a dorsal longitudinal and a thenar crease approach.[33] After the abscess has been drained and irrigated, a 16-gauge polyethylene catheter is placed in the thenar wound and sutured to the skin that is closed. The dorsal wound is then closed around the drain, and the hand is splinted and elevated. Sterile saline is used to irrigate the wound at the rate of 100 ml/hour for a 48-hour period. The drains are then removed and range of motion exercises are begun.

Midpalmar Space Infections

In midpalmar space infections, marked swelling and tenderness occur both in the palm and on the dorsum of the hand. The middle and ring fingers are held in a partially flexed position. Pain occurs with both active and passive range of motion.[4, 14, 15] The infection may result from a direct wound to the palm or from extension of a pre-existing infection in the long, ring, or—rarely—the little finger. If conservative treatment fails or if the infection is well established when first seen, surgical incision and drainage are indicated.

Several incisions have been recommended and work well.[33] A transverse incision paralleling the distal palmar crease can be made that curves proximally for a short distance between the metacarpals of the ring and little fingers (Fig. 20–6). The palmar fascia is incised, and the flexor tendon sheaths of the middle and ring fingers are identified. The dissection is then carried down on either side of the ring finger flexor tendons, and the abscess cavity is entered and drained.[30] After thorough débridement and irrigation, the wound may be packed open or closed over a catheter and then irrigated. The drains and packing or catheter are removed after 48 hours, and soaks and range of motion exercises are begun.

Web Space Abscess

Swelling and tenderness in the web space between adjacent fingers suggest a web space infection. The fingers may be abducted. The

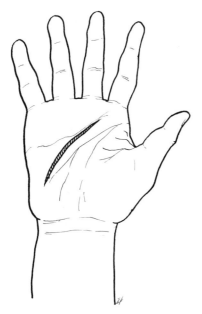

Figure 20–6. Incision for drainage of a midpalmar space abscess.

infection may extend in both palmar and dorsal directions to the deep transverse metacarpal ligament and the natatory ligaments; in such cases the infection is called a collar button abscess.[26] The infection results from a penetrating injury or a split in the skin of the web space or over a palmar callosity.[4] If conservative treatment fails or if the infection is well established when first seen, surgical incision and drainage are indicated. A transverse incision should not be made in the web because it may lead to a late contracture. The recommended incision is on the palmar aspect of the hand proximal to the web space and ending at the distal palmar crease. This may be longitudinal, curved, or zig-zag. The abscess is drained, and if pus extends dorsally to the deep transverse metacarpal ligament and/or to the natatory ligaments, a separate longitudinal incision is made in the dorsum of the web space so that the remainder of the infection can be drained.[4, 30]

Dorsal Subaponeurotic Space

The dorsal subaponeurotic space lies beneath the aponeurosis of the extensor tendons and the fascial layer covering the interosseous muscles and the metacarpals.[4] An infection in this space causes tenderness and marked swelling on the dorsum of the hand, with swelling also present in the palm. The fingers are partially flexed, and any motion is painful. This space infection is difficult to distinguish from a midpalmar space infection in a child because it can arise from a penetrating wound or from spread of an adjacent infection in the fingers, the web spaces, or the wrist. If conservative treatment fails or if the abscess is well developed when first seen, incision and drainage are indicated. A longitudinal incision is made on the dorsum of the hand overlying the long finger metacarpal. The surgeon divides the aponeurosis between the extensor tendons, exposing the abscess. The cavity is drained, débrided, irrigated, and packed open or closed over a catheter. The catheter is removed when drainage stops.

HUMAN BITES

Human bite infections often result from clenched fist injuries and have a mixed flora[10, 29, 37, 39] requiring both aerobic and anaerobic cultures. *Eikenella corrodens,* a common pathogenic agent in these infections, frequently is not sensitive to penicillinase-resistant penicillins or to cephalosporins alone.[16, 17] Antibiotic coverage after human bites therefore should include a penicillinase-resistant penicillin (or cephalosporin) in combination with penicillin.[16, 17] Tetanus immunization should be updated. These wounds should never be closed primarily.[29] They should be thoroughly débrided and packed open. Small puncture wounds may have to be enlarged.[26] If the wound is located directly over a joint, with or without tendon involvement, exploration of the joint may be required for adequate débridement, irrigation, and removal of an osteochondral fracture or of any foreign body that may be present.[10, 29] In such cases, a drain is placed in the wound and the hand is splinted and elevated. The drain is removed at 48 hours, and joint motion is started when the infection is under control.

ANIMAL BITES

Domestic animal bites and scratches are common in children. These wounds should be débrided, irrigated, and left open. Cultures should be obtained, and tetanus immunization should be updated. The animal should be inspected for rabies. Wounds directly over joints should be carefully explored, débrided, irrigated, and left open. The extremity should be splinted and elevated. A cephalosporin is given until results of the culture and sensitivity are available. *Pasteurella multocida* is a frequent pathogen in these wounds,[2, 6, 26] and the treatment of choice for this infection is penicillin.[6]

ARTHRITIS

Acute Suppurative Arthritis

Hematogenous septic arthritis is rare in the upper extremity, especially in the small joints of the hand and wrist. Infection in these joints usually follows a penetrating injury, a bite, or spread of infection from a contiguous structure.[40] If infection is suspected in the small joints of the hand, immediate aspiration for Gram stain, culture, and sensitivity should be obtained.[31, 40] If pus is present, immediate incision and drainage may prevent enzymatic destruction of the articular cartilage.[31] One approaches the interphalangeal joint through a midlateral incision and enters the joint by dividing the collateral ligament. A boutonnière deformity can develop, requiring extensor tendon reconstruction after the infection has been satisfactorily treated and good passive joint motion is present. If a joint is destroyed, fusion may be necessary, but an open growth plate should not be violated. The MP joint is approached through a dorsal incision, and the joint is entered through the extensor hood and joint capsule. The cord portion of the collateral ligament can be released from its metacarpal origin if more exposure is needed. The pus is drained and the joint irrigated, and the wound is left partially open with a drain. An alternative method involves suturing a small catheter in place at one end of the wound and a Penrose drain at the other. The wound is closed, and the joint is irrigated with sterile saline for 48 to 72 hours. Appropriate parenteral antibiotics are administered, and motion is begun when the infection is controlled. Loss of motion is common in joints following infection.

Arthritis of the Wrist, Elbow, and Shoulder

Septic arthritis of the wrist, elbow, and shoulder is rare. It can occur at any age but is more frequently seen in infants and children 2 years of age or younger. If the infection is seen early, intravenous antibiotics, traction, and repeated joint aspirations may be successful. If pus is present, the diagnosis can be confirmed by joint aspiration with a large bore needle followed by surgical incision and drainage of the joint.[23] The wrist is usually drained through a dorsal incision, the elbow through a lateral incision, and the shoulder through an anterior and/or posterior incision. The joint is débrided and irrigated, a drain is inserted, and the wound is left partially open and drained or closed over a catheter which is used for postoperative irrigation. Drains and catheters are removed at 48 hours, and motion is started when the infection is controlled. Proper parenteral antibiotics are given. Irrigation and débridement by arthroscopy may be beneficial in shoulder infections in older children.

Gonococcal Arthritis

Gonococcal arthritis can affect young children. Females are more often afflicted than males, and upper extremities are more frequently affected than lower ones. The wrist is the most common site. More than one joint may be involved, and polyarthralgia is common.[6, 19] Genitourinary symptoms may or may not be present. Joint aspiration is not always positive and should be cultured on chocolate agar because the organism is difficult to grow. The white blood cell count averages about 50,000[19] but may be as low as 20,000. Aspirations of the joint may be of benefit by removing infected synovial fluid, and distention of the synovium by injecting sterile saline helps prevent postinfection scarring. Surgical incision and drainage are usually not necessary. The antibiotic of choice is penicillin.[40] Although there is a gonococcal strain resistant to this antibiotic, it usually does not cause arthritis.[19]

OSTEOMYELITIS

Acute hematogenous osteomyelitis occurs most frequently in infants and children but can occur at any age. It is more common in the lower extremity but, when seen in the upper extremity, usually occurs in the metaphyseal regions of the humerus, the distal radius,[40] and the proximal ulna. It is rare in the bones of the hand and wrist.[26] Systemic signs of infection are usually present, and there is swelling and tenderness to digital pressure over the involved metaphysis. The sedimentation rate and white blood cell count are elevated. S. aureus is the most common infecting organism.[35, 40, 41] Bone changes appear on x-rays at 7 to 10 days.[18, 35, 40] Gallium scan is accurate in diagnosing osteomyelitis, but it takes 24 to 48 hours to complete and is therefore of limited value. Technetium bone scanning is not 100% accurate in the diagnosis of acute hematogenous osteomyelitis.[18, 35]

Differential diagnosis includes acute rheumatic fever, septic arthritis, rheumatoid arthritis, acute leukemia, and Ewing's sarcoma.[1, 11, 12, 40] If an adjacent joint is painful or swollen, one should aspirate it first to differentiate a septic joint effusion from a sympathetic one. The periosteal region is then aspirated; following this, the needle is pushed through the cortex into the metaph-

ysis and the aspirate from this region sent for Gram stain, culture and sensitivity.[40] Blood and other appropriate specimens should be sent for bacteriologic investigations. After all these specimens have been obtained, acute hematogenous osteomyelitis should be treated with the parenteral antibiotics that seem appropriate on the basis of the information available at that time.[40] If the patient fails to improve or worsens while waiting for a bacteriologic diagnosis, surgical incision and drainage are recommended. Antibiotic therapy can be adjusted as soon as culture and sensitivity results are available. Late infections with x-ray changes showing destruction require surgical débridement. An opening is made in the overlying cortex, and all purulent and necrotic material is removed. The wound should be packed open. Drainage tube systems have been reported to be satisfactory in treating osteomyelitis, and, in these cases, the system should be removed after 72 hours. Each case should be individualized regarding the duration of treatment with antibiotics.[31] It has been reported that those treated early in the course of their dis-

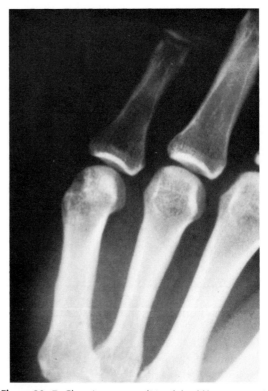

Figure 20–7. Chronic osteomyelitis of the fifth metacarpal head and neck in a 16-year-old following a clenched fist injury at age 11. Intermittent swelling, erythema, and drainage are present.

ease do well with 1 to 3 weeks of intravenous antibiotics followed by 3 to 6 weeks of oral antibiotics. We recommend 6 weeks of intravenous antibiotics for all documented bone infections.

Chronic osteomyelitis may present with sequestrum formation (Fig. 20–7) with a constant or intermittent drainage through an established sinus. When surgery is indicated in such cases, the entire sequestrum and all necrotic and purulent material should be removed. The skin is closed over an irrigation-drainage system when possible. In some instances, one may need to delay closure by packing the wound open and allowing it to heal by secondary intention. If there is a large defect in the skin following control of the infection, skin grafting may be necessary. This is accomplished with split skin grafts, local or distant pedicle flaps, or a free microvascular flap, depending on the location and size of the defect.

TUBERCULOSIS

The incidence of tuberculosis in the United States continues to decrease.[38] Bony involvement in the hand is more frequent in children than in adults. Tuberculous dactylitis in children that causes characteristic x-ray changes in the phalanges and metacarpals is known as spina ventosa.[4, 26, 28] This consists of expansion of the cortex together with a mottled, lytic area in the medullary cavity. The infection may break through the cortex, causing a periosteal reaction and an associated soft-tissue swelling. Involvement of more than one finger in the same hand is not unusual. Appropriate antibiotics (see below) and splints can control local infections, but soft-tissue abscesses and sinus tracts may require surgical débridement.[38] Tuberculous tenosynovitis and arthritis of the upper extremity are not common in children. Occasionally, however, synovectomy of a joint or of the extensor tendons on the dorsum of the wrist or of the flexor tendons with an associated release of the carpal tunnel will be indicated. The wounds can be closed primarily, and drug therapy should be started before the operation. The diagnosis is confirmed with culture or biopsy or both. The drugs currently recommended for use in this disease are isoniazid and rifampin. Occasionally, a third drug, such as ethambutol, streptomycin, or pyrazinamide, may be added. At one time, the standard triple therapy consisted of isoniazid, para-aminosalicylic acid (PAS), and streptomycin.

ATYPICAL MYCOBACTERIAL INFECTIONS

These infections occur in adults, but none has been reported in children.[20] M. marinum is the most common organism infecting the hand and upper extremity, but M. kansasii, M. avium, M. intracellularis, and M. terrae[20, 21] also have been reported. M. marinum infections follow abrasions or puncture wounds sustained in warm marine environments such as beaches, rivers, lakes, pools, and fish tanks.[8, 43] The clinical course is usually benign, with chronic skin ulceration or localized swelling occurring along the flexor tendon sheath, the carpal canal, or the extensor tendons on the dorsum of the wrist. Diagnosis is confirmed by biopsy and culture on Lowenstein-Jensen medium at 30° to 32° C.[8, 43] Treatment consists of surgical synovectomy and antituberculous medication. Recommended drugs are isoniazid, ethambutol, and rifampin for up to 24 months.[8, 20, 21, 43]

FUNGAL INFECTIONS

Fortunately, fungal infections are rare in children.[5, 40] Systemic fungal infections, such as blastomycosis and coccidioidomycosis, can involve bone. Surgical biopsy is for diagnostic purposes only, and the recommended treatment is with an antifungal agent such as amphotericin B.[34] Sporotrichosis usually causes cutaneous infections but can become disseminated. Amphotericin B and potassium iodide are recommended for treatment.[34] Fungal soft-tissue and bone infections are known as mycetoma.[5] These infections originate from a penetrating wound or compound fracture. Diagnosis is confirmed by biopsy and cultures, although the organisms are very difficult to grow in the laboratory.[34] Radical débridement of infected bone and soft tissue is indicated because antifungal agents are not effective against mycetoma.

Opportunistic fungi can cause serious systemic infections in children being treated for malignancies with various chemotherapeutic agents.[5] Bacterial infection in these cases can often be controlled with antibiotics, but fungal infections are difficult to control in this group and should be treated with antifungal agents such as amphotericin B. Surgery is usually not recommended.

PYOGENIC GRANULOMA

This infection is characterized by the projection of exuberant, "proud" granulation tissue that can appear serious[9, 26] (Fig. 20–8) but is actually a local problem for which systemic antibiotics are not indicated. Topical antibiotics and cauterization may be helpful, but if they are not, the lesion should be excised. The closure technique depends on the skin defect following granuloma excision. Small wounds are left open to granulate and epithelialize, moderate wounds (0.5 mm by 0.5 mm) are closed primarily, and larger wounds are covered with a split-thickness skin graft.

TETANUS

Tetanus is uncommon in the United States. The incidence is higher in underdeveloped countries in which adequate prophylaxis is not readily available.[42] *Clostridium tetani*, the causative agent, can enter the body either through a seemingly minor puncture wound or through a major wound such as a compound fracture. Seizures and other neurologic symptoms are caused by tetanospas-

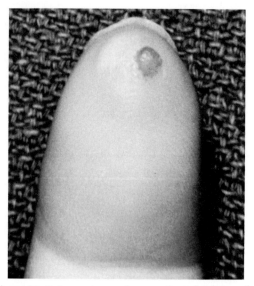

Figure 20–8. Pyogenic granuloma on the index finger of a child.

min, a neurotoxin produced by the organism.[42] The mortality rate is as high as 50%. Treatment includes specific antitoxin, antibiotics (penicillin G), surgical excision of the necrotic tissue in the wound, maintenance of electrolyte balance, and intensive supportive care.[36, 42]

GAS GANGRENE

Gas gangrene occurs after soft-tissue injuries or compound fractures contaminated with soil. The most common cause is *Clostridium perfringens*, although other organisms are usually present. The recommended treatment is adequate surgical irrigation and débridement with the wound left open and appropriate antibiotic therapy.[22, 36] Once gas gangrene is present, all devitalized tissue should be surgically removed and appropriate fasciotomies performed. Wounds should be left open, and intravenous antibiotics given in massive doses. Hyperbaric oxygen may be beneficial.[36] Amputation is sometimes necessary.[22] Other nonclostridial organisms can produce gas-forming infection.[13, 36]

NECROTIZING FASCIITIS

Hemolytic streptococci can undermine the skin from the subcutaneous tissue and cause soft tissue necrosis and gangrene. Meleney's "progressive synergistic gangrene" is caused by a nonhemolytic, microaerophilic *Streptococcus* in combination with *S. aureus* or strains of *Proteus*. Surgical débridement of the infected skin and subcutaneous tissue down to the fascia is often necessary.[9, 13] Systemic antibiotics are started prior to surgery and are adjusted if necessary after the results of the culture and sensitivity are obtained.

References

1. Aegerter E, Kirkpatrick JA Jr. Ewing's tumor. In Aegerter E, Kirkpatrick JA Jr, eds. Orthopaedic Diseases, 3rd ed. Philadelphia, WB Saunders, 1968:696–708.
2. Arons MS, Fernando L, Polayes IM. *Pasteurella multocida*—The major cause of hand infections following domestic animal bites. J Hand Surg 7:47–52, 1982.
3. Bell MS. The changing pattern of pyogenic infections of the hand. Hand 8:298–302, 1976.
4. Boyes JH. Infections. In Boyes JH, ed. Bunnell's Sur-

gery of the Hand, 5th ed. Phildelphia, JB Lippincott, 1970:613–642.

5. Brown H. Fungus infections of the hand. In Flynn JE, ed. Hand Surgery, 3rd ed. Baltimore, Williams & Wilkins, 1982:739–756.

6. Cahill JH. Special infections of the hand. In Flynn JE, ed. Hand Surgery, 3rd ed. Baltimore, Williams & Wilkins, 1982:706–718.

7. Carter SJ, Burman SO, Mersheimer WL. Treatment of digital tenosynovitis by irrigation with peroxide and oxytetracycline. Ann Surg 163:645–650, 1966.

8. Chow SP, Stroebel AB, Lau JH, Collins RJ. Mycobacterium marinum infection of the hand involving deep structures. J Hand Surg 8:568–573, 1983.

9. Crandon JH. Lesser infections of the hand. In Flynn JE, ed. Hand Surgery, 3rd ed. Baltimore, Williams & Wilkins, 1982:676–688.

10. Cuinard RG, D'Ambrosia RD. Human bite infections of the hand. J Bone Joint Surg 59A:416–418, 1977.

11. Dahlin DC. Bone Tumors, 2nd ed. Springfield, IL, Charles C Thomas, 1967.

12. Dick HM, Francis KC, Johnston AD. Ewing's sarcoma of the hand. J Bone Joint Surg 53A:345–348, 1971.

13. Fitzgerald RH Jr, Cooney WP III, Washington JA, et al. Bacterial colonization of mutilating hand injuries and its treatment. J Hand Surg 2:85–89, 1977.

14. Flynn JE. Grave infections of the hand. N Engl J Med, 229:898–905, 1943.

15. Flynn JE. The grave infections of the hand. In Flynn JE, ed. Hand Surgery, 3rd ed. Baltimore, Williams & Wilkins, 1982:688–706.

16. Goldstein EJ, Barones MF, Miller TA. Eikenella corrodens in hand infections. J Hand Surg 8:563–567, 1983.

17. Goldstein EJ, Miller TA, Citron, DM, Finegold SM. Infections following clenched-fist injury: a new perspective. J Hand Surg 3:455–457, 1978.

18. Green NE. The use of bone scans for the detection of osteomyelitis; Part III: Musculoskeletal infections in children. AAOS Instructional Course Lectures 32:40–43, 1983.

19. Green NE. Disseminated gonococcal infections and gonococcal arthritis; Part VI: Musculoskeletal infections in childern. AAOS Instructional Course Lectures 32:48–50, 1983.

20. Gunther SF. Nontuberculous mycobacterial infections of the hand. In Flynn JE, ed. Hand Surgery, 3rd ed. Baltimore, Williams & Wilkins, 1982:730–739.

21. Gunther SF, Elliot RC, Brand RL, et al. Experience with atypical mycobacterial infection in the deep structures of the hand. J Hand Surg 2:90–96, 1977.

22. Gustilo RB. Management of infected fractures; Part IV: Orthopaedic Sepsis and Osteomyelitis. AAOS Instructional Course Lectures 31:18–29, 1982.

23. Huskisson EC. The arthroses and diseases and injuries of the soft tissues. In Wadsworth TG, ed. The Elbow. Edinburgh, Churchill-Livingstone, 1982:283–302.

24. Kanaval AB. Infections of the Hand. A Guide to the Surgical Treatment of Acute and Chronic Suppurative Processes in the Fingers, Hand and Forearm, 7th ed. Philadelphia, Lea and Febiger, 1943.

25. Kaplan EB. Functional and Surgical Anatomy of the Hand, 2nd ed. Philadelphia, JB Lippincott, 1965.

26. Linscheid RL, Dobyns JH. Common and uncommon infections of the hand. Orthop Clin North Am, 6:1063–1104, 1975.

27. Louis DS, Silva J Jr. Herpetic whitlow; herpetic infections of the digits. J Hand Surg 4:90–93, 1979.

28. Mandel MA. Immune competence and diabetes mellitus: pyogenic human hand infections. J Hand Surg 3:458–461, 1978.

29. Mann RJ, Hoffeld TA, Farmer CB. Human bites of the hand: twenty years of experience. J Hand Surg 2:97–104, 1977.

30. Milford LW. The hand. In Edmonson AS, Crenshaw AH, eds. Campbell's Operative Orthopaedics, 6th ed. St. Louis, CV Mosby, 1980:385–417.

31. Morrissey RT. Bone and joint sepsis in children. AAOS Instructional Course Lectures 31:49–61, 1982.

32. Neviaser RJ. Closed tendon sheath irrigation for pyogenic flexor tenosynovitis. J Hand Surg 3:462–466, 1978.

33. Neviaser RJ. Infections. In Green DP, ed. Operative Hand Surgery. New York, Churchill-Livingstone, 1982:771–791.

34. Peterson HA. Fungal osteomyelitis in children; Part V: Musculoskeletal infections in children. AAOS Instructional Course Lectures 32:46–48, 1983.

35. Peterson HA. Hematogenous osteomyelitis in children; Part I: Musculoskeletal infections in children. AAOS Instructional Course Lectures 32:33–37, 1983.

36. Pruitt BA Jr, Lindberg RB, McManus WF. Infections: bacteriology, antibiotics and chemotherapy. In Flynn JE, ed. Hand Surgery, 3rd ed. Baltimore, Williams & Wilkins, 1982:636–676.

37. Robson MC, Schmidt MD, Heggers JP. Cefamandole therapy in hand infections. J Hand Surg 8:560–562, 1983.

38. Smith RJ, Leffert RD. Tuberculosis of the hand. In Flynn JE, ed. Hand Surgery, 3rd ed. Baltimore, Williams & Wilkins, 1982:718–730.

39. Stern PJ, Staneck JL, McDonough JJ, et al. Established hand infections: a controlled prospective study. J Hand Surg 8:553–559, 1983.

40. Tachdjian MO. Pediatric Orthopedics. Philadelphia, WB Saunders, 1972.

41. Weinstein AJ. Selection of antimicrobial therapy; Part III: orthopaedic sepsis and osteomyelitis. AAOS Instructional Course Lectures 31:14–18, 1982.

42. Weinstein L. Tetanus. In Flynn JE, ed. Hand Surgery, 3rd ed. Baltimore, Williams & Wilkins, 1982:756–765.

43. Williams CS, Riordan DC. Mycobacterium marinum (atypical acid-fast bacillus) infections of the hand. J Bone Joint Surg 55A:1042–1050, 1973.

CHAPTER ○ 21

Tumors of the Upper Extremity*

JOSEPH M. LANE
RICHARD R. McCORMACK, JR.
BRIAN HURSON
DALE GLASSER

The diagnosis and treatment of upper extremity tumors are based on well-established oncologic principles. Great strides have been achieved in the care of both benign and malignant conditions with improved survival and function. In this chapter, we will discuss the current general concepts of diagnosis, tumor staging, and treatment options, including limb preservation, and will then provide specific discussions of the most common malignant and benign bone tumors. The treatment of pathologic fracture due to primary and metastatic lesions of bone in the upper extremity is also considered. Although the thrust of this book is directed toward the pediatric population, this chapter will include a more general discussion. Many children and adolescents have tumors that occur more frequently in an older population; therefore, treatment principles for these lesions will be included for completeness.

After a history is obtained and physical examination is performed, basic radiologic assessment is always utilized. With these basic tools, the physician must then decide if further investigation or treatment is warranted. Treatment possibilities for these tumors and tumorlike lesions range from reassurance and observation to radical ablative surgery with reconstruction, depending on the diagnosis.

CLINICAL FINDINGS

The most common presenting symptoms in patients with bone tumors are progressive pain and increasing mass.[18, 20] Classically, the pain is unrelieved by position and can occur at night. Occasionally, lesions may not be active enough to cause symptoms and will be diagnosed incidentally on an x-ray for an unrelated problem. A small group of patients presents following a pathologic fracture. The medical history is usually not helpful in patients with primary disease, although it may reveal the location of a primary malignancy in metastatic lesions. There is a history of trauma in approximately 30% of cases, but evidence suggesting trauma as an etiologic factor is scant. Physical examination is usually nonspecific; a mass, if present, may not be tender. Lymphadenopathy is rare with

* Supported in part by The Greenwall Foundation.

primary bone tumors. The general examination should be directed toward looking for a primary cancer in cases of metastatic disease.

DIAGNOSTIC STUDIES

The single most useful test in the diagnosis of bone lesions is the conventional biplane x-ray.[15] It usually suggests the diagnosis of a benign or malignant process and offers a differential diagnosis.

The location of a lesion (epiphyseal, diaphyseal, metaphyseal) is of diagnostic importance. Epiphyseal location suggests giant cell tumor in the adult and chondroblastoma in the adolescent. The round cell tumors (myeloma, Ewing's lymphoma) tend to originate at a diaphyseal location, whereas osteogenic sarcoma, chondrosarcoma, and fibrosarcoma are found in the metaphysis.

The radiographic appearance of the solitary lesion can reveal much about its eventual growth or activity.[18, 20] Benign lesions are suggested by small size, elongated shape, and well-defined margination (Fig. 21–1). A sclerotic edge at the lesion's periphery indicates a slow process to which the normal bone outside the lesion is building a reactive layer. Malignant pathology is suggested by large size, a wide zone of transition with cortical breakthrough, and soft-tissue involvement, which may elevate the periosteum (Codman's triangle; Fig. 21–2). The presence or absence of calcification, reactive bone, sarcomatous bone formation, and pure lysis may help one differentiate the specific type of tumor. There are enough exceptions to the rules to force the surgeon to obtain a bone biopsy to provide a definitive diagnosis. However, some lesions, such as osteochondroma and fibrous cortical defects, can be diagnosed radiographically with 98% certainty.

Serologic, biochemical, and immunologic evaluations of these patients have limited diagnostic value.[15] The sedimentation rate is nonspecific, although it may be elevated in round cell tumors such as Ewing's sarcoma and non-Hodgkin's lymphoma of bone. The alkaline phosphatase is commonly elevated in patients with osteoblastic osteogenic sarcoma and in patients with Paget's disease. Protein immunoelectrophoresis is diagnostic for multiple myeloma. Bone marrow biopsies may assist in the diagnosis of metabolic bone

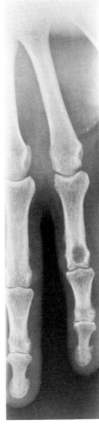

Figure 21–1. An AP x-ray of an enchondroma in the proximal phalanx exhibits the characteristics of a benign lesion of the bone: small size, with well-defined margins and without expanding the contours of the bone.

disease, multiple myeloma, or leukemia. Patients with chondrosarcoma may have a normal blood glucose level in the face of a diabetic glucose tolerance test.[28]

If at this stage the diagnosis of the lesion may be made with confidence—particularly if it is benign—further investigations may not be required. If, however, major surgery is required to remove the lesion, further radiographic and nuclear imaging may help one determine the extent of the tumor and its relationship to the neurovascular structures. Tomography may be used for accurate localization of the nidus of an osteoid osteoma or the presence of cortical penetration in a giant cell tumor, which may not have been detected on plain x-rays. Biplane peripheral arteriography (Fig. 21–3) will outline the extent of the accompanying soft-tissue mass and the relationship of the tumor to the major vessels and nerves. The extent of soft tissue involvement can be distinctly demonstrated by computed axial tomogra-

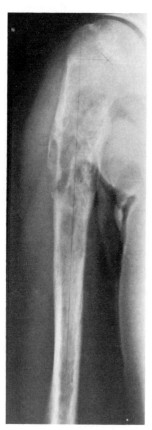

Figure 21–2. An x-ray of an osteosarcoma of the proximal humerus revealing a moth-eaten, poorly marginated, lytic lesion with endosteal scalloping, subperiosteal bone elevation, formation of a Codman's triangle, and a pathologic fracture—all indicative of malignant disease.

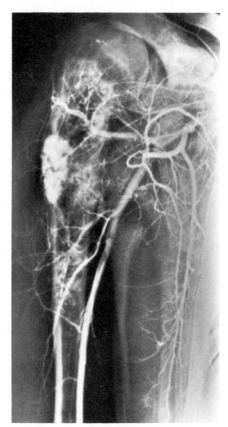

Figure 21–3. An arteriogram of an osteogenic sarcoma of the proximal humerus (the patient in Figure 21–2). The arterial phase of this angiogram shows an abnormal vascular supply to a malignant tumor from the circumflex humeral and profundus arteries with a large tumor blush indicating an arteriovenous (A-V) malformation at the lateral cortex of the humerus. The discrete distance between the brachial artery and the main tumor mass within the humerus as indicated on this arteriogram allowed a limb-sparing resection to be performed.

phy (CT) with or without contrast (Fig. 21–4), and, more importantly, the relationship of the tumor to the neurovascular structures can be assessed. In tumor staging (see further on), the CT scan is significantly superior to arteriography in 82% of cases. Lymphangiography is generally not indicated for primary bone tumors, except for lymphoma of bone to help in staging.

The search for distant or multiple bone disease should include a technetium-99m polyphosphate bone scan.[39] In addition to detecting distant disease, this scan helps one accurately localize the primary lesion and detect skip lesions (Fig. 21–5). Gallium scans (Fig. 21–6) are helpful in the assessment of the soft-tissue component of the tumor and in the clarification of the contribution of disuse osteoporosis to a "positive bone scan." Whole-lung tomography helps one detect pulmonary metastases so that appropriate staging can be accomplished. CT lung scans

may be too sensitive; in certain centers, they have provided false-positive findings in 25% of cases. Technologic advances in scanners and more experience may significantly improve accuracy.

Surgical Staging

With data from investigations to this point, it should be possible to determine a surgical stage for malignant tumors. Enneking and associates have devised a system for the staging of musculoskeletal sarcomas.[8] In this system, neoplasms are histologically graded on the basis of their biologic aggressiveness as low grade (I) or high grade (II). In general, low-grade lesions have a low risk for metastasis

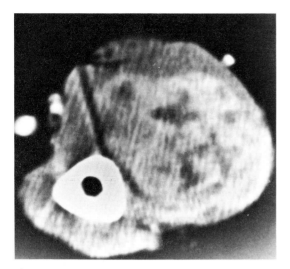

Figure 21–4. A CT scan of a 59-year-old female with a fibrohistiocytoma arising along the lateral surface of the distal humerus. CT scan with contrast revealed the proximity of the tumor mass to the brachial artery.

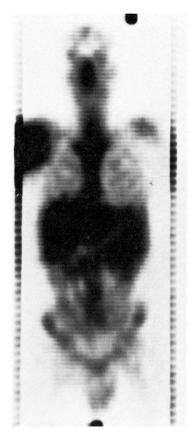

Figure 21–6. A gallium scan of another patient, showing uptake in the soft tissues associated with the tumor.

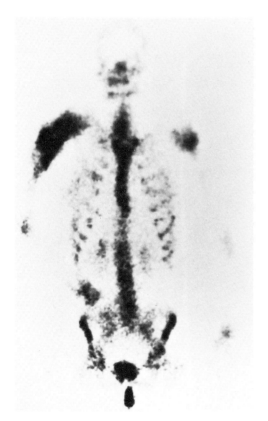

Figure 21–5. A 14-year-old girl with a primary osteogenic sarcoma of the right humerus. In this bone scan, evidence of metastatic sarcoma in the throacic and the lumbar spine is noted.

(less than 25%) and the 5-year survival rate among patients with these tumors is higher than that among patients with high-grade lesions. They can usually be managed by relatively conservative procedures. High-grade lesions have a significantly higher incidence of metastasis, and one must therefore use more aggressive procedures with these tumors to achieve local control. In addition to grading the neoplasm, one must assess its anatomic extent. If the tumor is confined to a well-defined anatomic compartment, it is designated intracompartmental, or *A*. A lesion in two or more anatomic compartments is designated *B*. An example of the latter would be an intraosseous lesion that lifts the periosteum from cortical bone. A superficial lesion that penetrates the deep fascia is also extracompartmental. Staging of the tumor is based on these two considerations—grading and anatomic extent. The stages are subdivided as *IA*—low-grade tumor within a compartment; *IB*—low-grade tumor in two or more functional compartments; *IIA*—high-grade tumor and intracompartmental; *IIB*—

high-grade tumor in two or more compartments; and *III*—any grade tumor with regional or distant metastasis. Lesions in the midfoot and hindfoot, popliteal space, groin, femoral triangle, intrapelvic area, midhand, antecubital fossa, axilla, periclavicular, intraspinal area, and head and neck are extracompartmental[18] and are therefore all *B*.

Benign tumors can be staged into three levels of activity. Stage 1 (latent) tumors (e.g., fibrous cortical defects) are intracompartmental, with little or no chance of expansion. Stage 2 (active) benign tumors (e.g., lipoma and unicameral bone cyst) are intracompartmental, with a tendency for slow continuous growth. Stage 3 (aggressive) lesions are benign, with a tendency to extend beyond the anatomic compartment and recur frequently, and they can occasionally transport cells to the lungs, as seen in giant cell tumors and chondroblastomas. In general, the treatment for stage 1 tumors is observation or incisional curettage; for stage 2 lesions, curettage or marginal excision is employed; for stage 3 lesions, excision or curettage beyond the pseudocapsule or reactive bone margin is used.

Biopsy

In many circumstances, one can confidently diagnose certain benign lesions (e.g., fibrous cortical defects and osteochondromas) from their clinical and radiographic appearances. If these lesions are found incidentally and are not the source of the patient's complaints, neither further investigation nor surgery is indicated. If, however, a lesion does not have one of the classic benign radiographic appearances or locations or if it is growing or causing symptoms, a biopsy is mandatory.[24, 38]

One may treat symptomatic osteochondromas by *excisional* biopsy, taking care to excise the perichondrium completely to minimize recurrence. Excisional biopsy is also adequate treatment for other lesions that have little or no potential for recurrence (e.g., osteoid osteoma).

An *incisional* biopsy is the most commonly employed type of open biopsy.[18, 20, 24, 38] It is the procedure of choice for open biopsy of most malignant tumors. The placement of the biopsy incision is crucial because the biopsy scar together with the biopsy tract must be excised en bloc with the malignant tumor at the definitive surgical procedure. The biopsy incision should be longitudinal along the lines of extensile exposure. Poorly placed biopsy scars may jeopardize further exposure for an en bloc resection; indeed, a large transverse scar may preclude the possibility of performing a limb-sparing resection and necessitate amputation. The smallest incision that allows one to obtain an adequate tissue specimen should be employed. The periphery of any tumor offers the best and most representative tissue in malignant tumors. The center may be necrotic. A small segment of bone may be carefully excised with a sharp osteotome or multiple small drill holes and then an osteotome. The biopsy of bone should be round or oval so that local stress concentrations are minimized. In addition to specimens for permanent sections, one should obtain frozen sections to confirm accurate location and adequacy of the biopsy. Special studies such as electron microscopy, lymphoma typing, and estrogen binding may be necessary and can be suggested by the frozen examination. Multiple cultures for aerobic, anaerobic, and acid-fast bacilli and for fungi should be obtained. Antibiotics should not be given prior to biopsy. Tumor blood also can be sent for biochemical analysis (e.g., acid and alkaline phosphatase). Very high values of alkaline phosphatase may be seen in osteosarcomas. One must take care to minimize tumor spillage. Meticulous hemostasis during wound closure is paramount because the larger the postoperative hematoma, the greater the contamination of soft tissues with neoplastic cells. Gelfoam with thrombin and microcrystalline collagen may be necessary. The use of a tourniquet during biopsy is not essential but may be useful if preferred. There is no evidence that a tourniquet prevents dissemination of tumor cells into the bloodstream. However, on no account should an Esmarch bandage be employed to drain the limb. Following biopsy, it is important that the limb be protected so that a pathologic fracture is avoided.

Percutaneous needle biopsies may be performed in some specialized centers, but again the placement of the needle should be carefully planned so that the needle tract can be excised en bloc.[30] It should be remembered that the accuracy associated with percutaneous needle biopsies is approximately 80%, compared with the 98% accuracy associated with open biopsies, as the former is just a small, open biopsy. The accuracy and methodology of the biopsy significantly affect the outcome.

Once the histologic grade of the tumor is determined by the pathologists, the tumor may be staged as *IA, IB, IIA, IIB,* or *III.*[8] This system of surgical staging helps one decide whether a limb-sparing procedure is feasible or an amputation is required. Stage III lesions with pulmonary metastasis may be considered for limb-sparing procedures because in many circumstances the pulmonary metastasis may be amenable to chemotherapy followed by surgical excision.[20]

TREATMENT OF BONE TUMORS

Benign Lesions

Benign lesions showing indisputable diagnostic radiographic characteristics (e.g., asymptomatic nonossifying fibroma or asymptomatic osteochondromas) do not require surgical treatment or even a biopsy.[15, 18, 20] If, however, any doubt about the benign nature of the lesion exists, a biopsy should be performed. Symptomatic osteochondromas may be treated by excisional biopsy (i.e., marginal excision). Most of the other benign grade 1 and 2 tumors are adequately treated by standard procedures such as curettage and packing with bone chips or by small en bloc excisions. Simple curettage can be extended for aggressive benign lesions (e.g., giant cell tumors and aneurysmal bone cysts) with cryosurgery, phenolization, and thermal cautery with methylmethacrylate. (A more detailed discussion follows later in this chapter for specific tumors.) Unicameral bone cysts have been successfully treated by repetitive intralesional injection with 40 to 80 mg of crystalline methyl prednisolone acetate. More will be said later in a discussion of pathologic fractures associated with these benign bone lesions.

The most common benign soft-tissue tumors in the hand and fingers include ganglia and giant cell tumors of the tendon sheath. These are considered under separate headings in the discussion of soft-tissue tumors.

Benign Bone-Forming Tumors

The two lesions in this class that affect the upper extremity are the osteoid osteoma and the osteoblastoma.[3, 15, 20] Approximately 25% of osteoid osteomas involve the upper

extremity. They are evenly distributed in location. The lesion is characterized by a nidus measuring approximately 1 cm in diameter that is surrounded by a sclerotic rim of varying thickness. Pain at night (which can be relieved with aspirin) has been the "classic" presentation, but this combination of symptoms and response to non-steroidal medications is not found in the vast majority of cases. The lesion is found predominantly in children and young adults between 10 and 25 years of age.

Osteoid Osteoma. The radiographic appearance of osteoid osteoma is quite helpful for diagnosis (Fig. 21–7). A nidus with a diameter of approximately 1 cm is surrounded by a rim of reactive sclerotic cancellous bone in the spongiosa or reactively thickened periosteal new bone if it occurs in the cortex. The nidus is a clear, radiolucent area that may become radiopaque as the nidus matures. The excessive, reactive bone may obscure the nidus. Bone scanning and tomography may be helpful in such cases.[39]

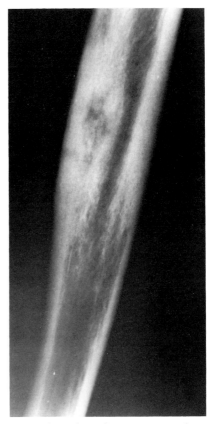

Figure 21–7. The radiographic appearance of an osteoid osteoma in a 14-year-old child reveals characteristic lucencies located eccentrically in the humerus, with a surrounding zone of sclerotic bone and with abundant periosteal new bone formation.

Angiography will demonstrate an intense blush because of the hypervascularity of the nidus. Osteoid osteomas in juxta-articular situations may be difficult to diagnose and may give rise to an inflammatory arthritis. Synovial biopsy in such cases may show chronic inflammatory changes.

The treatment of osteoid osteomas is surgical en bloc excision of the nidus with the surrounding rim of perilesional sclerotic bone and curettage of the adjacent bone. X-ray localization of the area of the nidus is mandatory. Drill holes or needle markers are commonly used with intraoperative x-rays so that exact placement of the incision is ensured. Commonly, if the lesion is cortical, the periosteal reactive bone will appear as a roughened, raised surface over the nidus. The intact en bloc excision of the nidus and surrounding bone may be examined radiographically during surgery so that complete removal of the nidus is ensured. Recently, the use of intraoperative radionuclide localization of the tumor has been helpful in identifying the prospective site of resection and confirming that the tumor has been resected.

Osteoblastoma. Osteoblastoma[3, 15, 20] is a benign bone-forming lesion, occurring in the upper extremity in approximately 15% of cases, and is related histologically to the osteoid osteoma. However, it is larger than the 1-cm nidus of osteoid osteoma, does not have as much perilesional reactive bone, and does not cause as much pain. This uncommon lesion is found in children and young adults, usually in the metaphysis or diaphysis. The lesions are well circumscribed, 2 to 12 cm in diameter, expansile, and radiolucent, with differing amounts of mottled calcification. Bone scans and angiography often help delineate the extent of the lesion. The treatment of choice is resection of the lesion, as for osteoid osteoma. Curettage is associated with a recurrence rate of 25%.[20] A small percentage of tumors become malignant (<2%).

Benign Cartilage-Forming Tumors

The benign cartilage-forming tumors affecting the upper extremity include osteochondroma, enchondroma, chondroblastoma, and chondromyxoid fibroma.[3, 15, 20]

Osteochondroma. The osteochondroma is a bony mass, either sessile or pedunculated, whose growth is produced by enchondral ossification of a cartilaginous cap (Fig. 21–8).

This is the most common benign bone tumor. Approximately one third occur in the upper extremity. The proximal humerus and distal radius are the most common sites. This benign growth is usually asymptomatic and is not seen or treated by the physician. Others may be palpable beneath the skin. A few may give rise to symptoms secondary to pressure on nearby structures, such as nerves and vessels. Patients over 30 years of age with symptomatic osteochondromas should be carefully evaluated for malignant transformation, particularly when the lesions are proximally located. Excisional biopsy should include the perichondrial lining layer.

Enchondroma. Enchondromas are benign cartilage tumors that probably represent developmental cartilage rests (see Fig. 21–1).[3, 15, 20] The most common primary tumors arising in the bones of the hand are enchondromas. They are benign but have a history of local recurrence after inadequate excision. When they do recur they often present with a more aggressive biologic behavior which makes treatment more difficult. Pathologic fracture or extension into soft tissues may be seen. They are frequently found incidentally following routine chest x-rays or investigation of shoulder arthralgias. Enchondromas are characterized by calcified cartilage within the metaphysis. Endosteal scalloping, cortical breakthrough, and localized pain all are suggestive of malignant degeneration. Bone scans will remain positive well into early adulthood. Benign enchondromas require no surgical treatment unless associated with pathologic fractures, as in the phalanges and metacarpals (Fig. 21–9A). In these cases, curettage with bone grafting should be curative. Very low grade chondrosarcomas and aggressive (recurrent) enchondromas can be cured with extensive curettage and cryosurgery. One should take care to prevent pathologic fracture, which can occur following cryosurgery. The bone should be protected until osseous remodeling has occurred.

At Memorial Sloan–Kettering Cancer Center, we have begun using a modified cryosurgery technique developed by Marcove for small osseous lesions of the phalanges and metacarpals (Fig. 21–9B).[29] Because of the skin and soft-tissue complications of the "pour" technique with liquid nitrogen, we use the Brymill "cryospray" unit, which enables us to ensure accurate control of the application of liquid nitrogen to the walls of the cystic lesion and to spare the nearby neu-

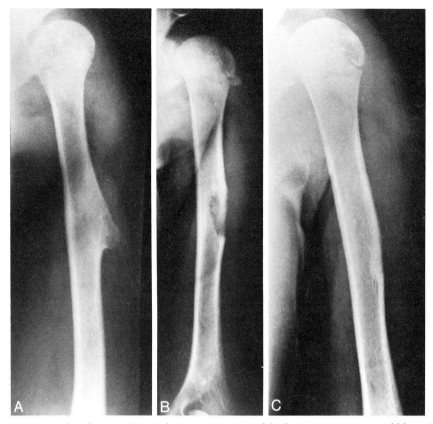

Figure 21–8. *A*, An osteochondroma arising in the posterior aspect of the humerus in a 13-year-old boy. The lesion was sessile and was closely associated with the radial nerve, causing pain that radiated into the forearm. *B*, An x-ray taken immediately following resection of the osteochondroma. *C*, X-ray 4 months after resection, with reconstruction of the humeral cortex.

rovascular structures and skin. The lesion is then filled with autogenous cancellous bone. The bone that has been made necrotic by freezing must be protected for an extended period of time against pathologic fracture. The use of cancellous autogenous bone speeds the incorporation and revascularization process.

Chondroblastoma. Chondroblastomas occur in the epiphysis (Fig. 21–10) during late adolescence. They are rarely present in individuals over 25 years of age. The lesion may be associated with an aneurysmal bone cyst component in 20% to 25% of cases. Treatment consists of thorough curettage and bone graft. Occasionally, chondroblastoma can be transported to the lung; in these cases, the tumor needs to be resected with thoracotomy. Rarely, the chondroblastoma can degenerate into a sarcoma.

Chondromyxoid Fibromas. Chondromyxoid fibromas rarely involve the upper extremity. They are usually located in the di-

aphysis and metaphysis. Curettage should cure the lesion.

Benign Noncartilaginous Lesions

Fibrous Dysplasia. Fibrous dysplasia is a benign developmental condition that may be monostotic or polyostotic. The disease begins in childhood but usually becomes clinically apparent in adulthood during an incidental radiographic examination. In the humerus and forearm, the appearance is usually that of a radiolucent cystic lesion (Fig. 21–11) with possible deformity and diffuse enlargement of the bone contour. Treatment is indicated for pathologic fracture or progressive deformity. Curettage, bone grafting, and stabilization either with bracing or internal fixation are required until osseous remodeling has been completed.

Myositis Ossificans. Myositis ossificans (heterotopic ossification) is a nonneoplastic condition usually associated with trauma.

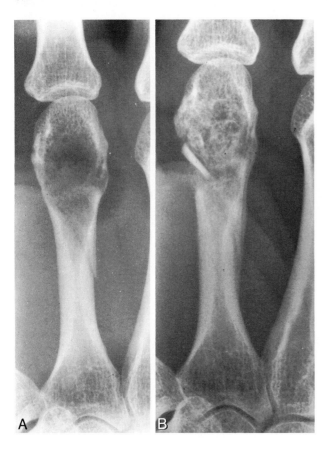

Figure 21–9. *A*, Pathologic fracture through an enchondroma in the metacarpal of an 18-year-old male. Note the calcified lytic lesion in the metacarpal head and a fracture extending into the diaphysis, with minimal displacement. *B*, Postoperative x-ray following curettage, cryosurgery, and bone grafting of the same lesion. Note the incorporation of the cancellous graft within the metacarpal head and the healed fracture.

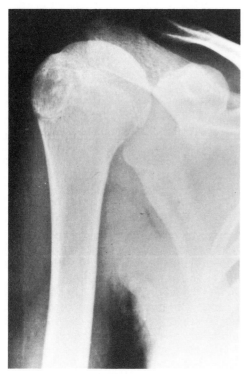

Figure 21–10. X-ray of a chondroblastoma in the proximal humerus of a 20-year-old male.

The most common complaint is a localized, painful swelling associated with limited shoulder or elbow motion. It can be seen in 3% of cases following dislocation of the elbow.[42] Over a period of several weeks following trauma, a bony mass will be seen developing within a muscle. Eventually, a well-circumscribed, rounded lesion with a radiolucent core and surrounding calcified zone will be seen separate from the bone (Fig. 21–12). The differential diagnosis should include juxtacortical osteogenic sarcoma. Myositis ossificans occurs some distance from an intact bony cortex, whereas osteogenic sarcoma violates and is in contact with the cortex. In myositis ossificans, a zonal pattern is present in which the radiographic and pathologic findings of peripheral calcified maturity are seen. Osteogenic sarcoma shows immaturity of cells and an indistinct radiographic periphery, with more central mineralization of the tumor.

Treatment is indicated for pain or dysfunction and should be postponed until the process has matured so that it is less likely to recur after excision. Often, a bone scan can help one determine the activity of an area of

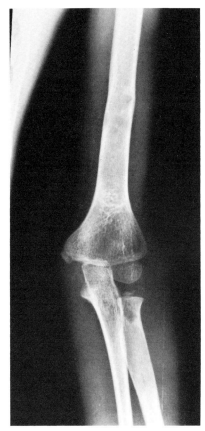

Figure 21–11. X-ray of a 9-year-old female with fibrous dysplasia in the distal humerus and proximal radius. Note the characteristic ground-glass appearance and two flame-shaped advancing margins in the radius.

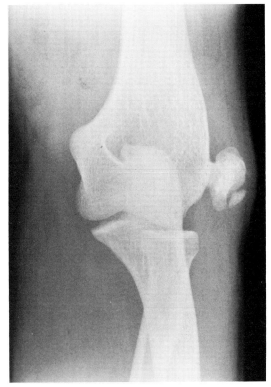

Figure 21–12. An x-ray of a myositis ossificans arising after a traumatic dislocation of the elbow. Note the mature appearance of the bone trabeculae.

myositis. Most of these lesions can be treated with physical therapy and graded, active range of motion exercises. Passive manipulation of the elbow or shoulder in this condition is to be condemned. If the tumor is resected, the patient should be treated with diphosphonate, 20 mg/kg/day for 1 month preoperatively and 3 months postoperatively.

Epidermoid Cysts. Epidermoid cysts, or inclusion cysts, of bone are traumatic in origin. Implantation of normal-growing epithelial cells into deep structures occurs and is usually seen in the fingers (most commonly in the terminal phalanx) and the palm. A history of a deep penetrating wound can sometimes be elicited. The lesion presents as a firm, rubbery mass that is intermittently painful, and it may be associated with changes in the nail plate. A radiographic picture of a radiolucent lesion with cortical thinning in the distal phalanx in a manual worker is classic.

Fibrous Cortical Defects. Fibrous cortical defects occur in approximately one third of all children. Spontaneous regression of this asymptomatic focus of periosteal fibrous tissue is usual.

Malignant Lesions

The surgical staging system for musculoskeletal sarcomas is linked to a planning system with four surgical procedures for obtaining local control.[8] Each has a well-defined surgical margin based on the relationship of the surgical margin to the neoplasm. An intralesional margin is made when an incision passes through the lesion. Incisional biopsies and curettage of a benign lesion are examples of intralesional procedures that are adequate only for benign lesions. A marginal excision is usually described as an excisional biopsy around the pseudocapsule. It usually leaves microscopic disease at the margin of the defect. In a wide excision or a wide amputation, the lesion is removed with a surrounding cuff of normal tissue. A radical margin is obtained by removal of the tumor en bloc or by amputation together with all potentially contaminated planes and all structures that pass through the involved anatomic compartment or compartments, as in a forequarter amputation.

Advances in the treatment of malignant lesions have been made since the mid 1970s. They include the use of multidrug chemotherapy and the refinement of the technique of en bloc, or wide, resection.

Chemotherapy

With modern multidrug chemotherapy, more than 75% of patients presenting with malignant bone tumors are now expected to be disease-free survivors following amputation or en bloc resection. In earlier reports, the 5-year cure rates of patients with osteogenic sarcoma ranged from 15% to 20%; for Ewing's sarcoma these rates were between 5% and 15%, regardless of whether amputation was performed or high-dose radiation was used.[4, 15, 26] Formerly, all patients with malignant lesions of the upper extremity were treated by forequarter or above-elbow amputation. Since the 1970s, the number of tumors successfully treated with limb preservation has been increasing. In addition to greatly improved survival rates, the quality of life for many survivors has become better.

It is assumed that at the time of diagnosis of an osteogenic sarcoma, patients already have microscopic foci of disease in their lungs. Although surgery can eliminate the primary tumor, chemotherapy is used to destroy these microscopic but undetectable areas of disease. In addition to being useful as an adjuvant modality for micrometastases in the treatment of primary bone tumors, chemotherapy can be employed preoperatively to shrink bulky primary and metastatic tumors rapidly.[34, 36, 40]

Many centers now give adjuvant chemotherapy to all patients with high-grade spindle cell sarcomas, which include osteogenic sarcomas, high-grade chondrosarcomas, high-grade fibrosarcomas, malignant fibrous histiocytomas, and malignant giant cell tumors (histologic grade III). Small cell sarcomas, which include Ewing's sarcoma, non-Hodgkin's lymphoma, angiosarcoma, rhabdomyosarcoma, and mesenchymal chondrosarcoma, are highly malignant and are very sensitive to modern multidrug chemotherapy.[35] In addition to employing surgery and chemotherapy, physicians use radiation

therapy as a means of obtaining local control of primary small cell sarcomas.

The current therapeutic approach to osteogenic sarcoma at Memorial Sloan–Kettering Cancer Center[34] is to treat all patients preoperatively with multicycle high-dose methotrexate with citrovorum factor rescue, bleomycin, cyclophosphamide, and dactinomycin (BCD) and adriamycin. This regimen is followed regardless of whether the patient is to have an amputation or a limb-sparing procedure. The effect of 4 to 12 weeks of preoperative chemotherapy is assessed by the histologic examination of the resected primary tumor. A grading system based on the extent of tumor destruction has been devised:[34] Grade I—little or no effect of chemotherapy noted; grade II—a partial response with up to 90% tumor necrosis noted and attributable to chemotherapy; grade III—greater than 90% tumor necrosis; grade IV—no viable-appearing tumor cells noted in any of the histologic specimens. In osteogenic sarcoma therapy, patients with grade III or IV response are continued on the same chemotherapy as used preoperatively. For those patients who have a grade I or II effect of preoperative chemotherapy on the primary tumor, the high-dose methotrexate is deleted from postoperative chemotherapy, and a regimen containing cis-platinum with mannitol diuresis combined with adriamycin is instituted. Thus, the patient's own tumor is evaluated in vivo for the efficacy of the chemotherapy protocol.

Combination chemotherapy also is used in the treatment of small cell sarcomas.[35] The patient is given early aggressive chemotherapy so that micrometastases are eliminated. Large, bulky tumors usually reduce significantly in size with this treatment. Local therapy is delayed for approximately 3 months, except in cases in which there is a poor response of the tumor as judged by frequent clinical examination, radionuclide imaging, x-rays, or any combination of these studies.

Although multidrug chemotherapy has provided a major advance in the treatment of cancer in general, it is associated with considerable toxicity. A regimen consisting of high-dose methotrexate with citrovorum rescue was associated with a mortality rate of approximarely 6% in the early days of its use.[17] Although mortality due to chemotherapy has declined with experience, significant temporary morbidity persists. Adriamycin may produce irreversible cardiomyopathy, and bleomycin can produce pulmonary fibrosis. *Cis*-platinum can cause permanent renal toxicity and ototoxicity. With chemotherapy, bone healing is delayed, so grafting procedures following resections require prolonged periods of immobilization. Because skin healing is protracted, chemotherapy should not be resumed until 2 weeks after surgery. Skin sutures are usually left in place for approximately 6 weeks.

Although the benefits of chemotherapy are not uniform and several groups do not use adjuvant chemotherapy, the consensus of orthopaedic oncologists is that adjuvant chemotherapy has a significant role in the treatment of high-grade malignant bone tumors, particularly osteosarcoma and Ewing's sarcoma.

Surgical Treatment

The choice of surgical procedures for malignant lesions depends on a number of factors. Accurate histologic diagnosis and surgical staging are paramount.[8] The size and extent of both osseous and soft-tissue involvement can be determined with biplane x-rays, arteriograms, bone and soft-tissue imaging procedures (see Figs. 21–2, 21–3, 21–5, and 21–6), and tomography.[18, 20] Perfusion CT scanning is a particularly sensitive method of determining whether or not the major neurovascular structures are involved and will help one decide whether resection or amputation is better. Preoperative chemotherapy may reduce the size of a tumor, rendering it resectable.[34, 36, 38] The age of the patient has a major role in determining the type of surgical procedure that should be employed. The projected limb length discrepancy in actively growing, very young children may make amputation the only realistic choice in proximal humeral lesions.

Despite advances in chemotherapy, amputation remains the most common surgical procedure performed for malignant tumors. The level of amputation is selected after x-rays and bone scans are carefully studied. The bone scan is particularly helpful in providing a good approximation of the proximal margin of the involved bone (Fig. 21–13).

Limb-sparing procedures involving en bloc resection are a valid alternative to amputation in carefully selected cases.[20, 25] Local resection of malignant lesions is still at the experimental stage and should be done

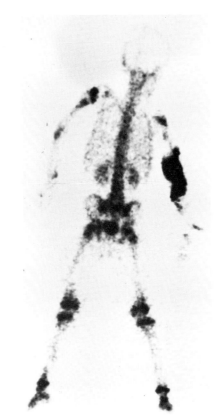

Figure 21–13. Bone scan of a 3-year-old female with an osteogenic sarcoma of the distal humerus.

only in centers with staff experienced with these techniques. In general, limb-sparing procedures involving en bloc excision may be considered in individuals with recurrent giant cell tumor, low-grade chondrosarcoma, parosteal osteogenic sarcoma, malignant fibrous histiocytoma, or a carefully selected localized high-grade malignancy. These patients must have a potential normal cuff of tissue around the tumor, no neurovascular involvement, and adequate skin coverage.

The first objective in tumor surgery in patients without evidence of skip areas or metastases is to obtain local control and avoid local recurrence. The second goal is to preserve as much function as possible without jeopardizing survival. Local recurrence after a high-grade sarcoma resection is associated with a poor survival rate. Limb-sparing surgery for malignant tumors should be performed with caution and only after careful evaluation of biplane x-rays, imaging studies, biplane arteriograms, and CT scans.

En bloc resection of malignant tumor entails the removal of the lesion with an intact cuff of normal tissue that completely surrounds the lesion. One must exercise careful judgment when deciding whether to implement such procedures. The patient and parents should appreciate the realistic functional goals of limb-sparing surgery. The patient will have definite impairment. In cases in which an alternative procedure such as amputation may become necessary, consent should always be obtained preoperatively.

The principles involved in en bloc resection of carefully selected malignant tumors are the same as those for all tumor surgery: The tumor must never be violated, and a surrounding margin of normal soft tissue and bone must be removed en bloc with the lesion.[8]

Malignant and aggressive benign neoplasms of the shoulder girdle can be surgically treated by forequarter amputation, scapulectomy, or shoulder disarticulation.[31] A limb-sparing procedure may be considered in cases in which the axillary artery and brachial plexus are free of tumor as evidenced by biplane arteriography and computed axial tomography. In addition, the lymph nodes should be clear. Invasion of the chest wall by tumor might even preclude a forequarter amputation as adequate therapy. The pro-

cedure of upper humeral interscapulothoracic resection was first reported in 1928 by Linberg, who credited Tikhoff with the initial description of the procedure in 1908.[22] Primary bone tumors as well as soft-tissue tumors adjacent to bone may be treated by this method. It may be performed for scapular and proximal humeral lesions (Fig. 21–14).[25] Lesser variations of en bloc procedures can include excision of part of the humerus, partial scapulectomy, or both. As in all other areas in which limb-sparing surgery is contemplated, consent for a forequarter amputation should be obtained preoperatively because the final decision about the resectability of the lesion can be made only during surgery.

The operative technique of the Tikhoff-Linberg resection for removal of malignant and locally aggressive tumors of the shoulder areas has been described.[22, 25] The site of the initial biopsy is chosen carefully so that any subsequent en bloc resection is not jeopardized. The initial incision is made so that the entire biopsy scar and tract are removed with the surgical specimen. The initial incision overlies the inner two thirds of the clavicle and is carried laterally to the acromioclavicular joint. It then continues anteriorly in the

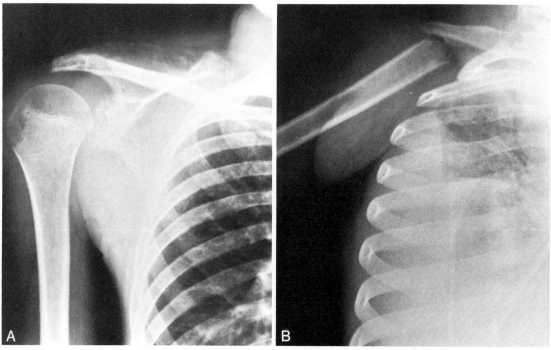

Figure 21–14. *A,* An 11-year-old male with a Ewing's sarcoma of the scapula who underwent a Tikhoff-Linberg resection of the proximal humerus and entire scapula. *B,* Postoperative x-rays show the humerus suspended from the clavicular remnant.

deltopectoral groove and distally along the anterolateral aspect of the arm. The posterior incision is carried over the midscapular region and distally to the angle of the scapula. The axillary artery and the brachial plexus are identified, and, if they are clear of tumor, the dissection is continued. Ligation of the anterior and posterior circumflex arteries is required for medial mobilization of the axillary artery. The musculocutaneous and radial nerves are identified and preserved if they are not involved in tumor. The muscles inserted into the proximal humerus are transected medially to the tumor mass. Posteriorly, mobilization of the scapula is started inferiorly and carried up the vertebral and lateral borders, with the surgeon taking care to control bleeding and to stay away from tumor. This part of the dissection is similar to that of a forequarter amputation. The level of scapula or humeral osteotomy varies with the location of the tumor and is judged on the basis of preoperative x-rays and bone scans. A subtotal scapulectomy is usually adequate for most humeral lesions. Similarly, for scapular lesions, osteotomy at the surgical neck of the humerus may give adequate margins. The clavicle is divided medially to its midpoint. Prior to proceeding with reconstructive procedures, the surgeon should confirm adequate margins by frozen sections. Frozen-section readings of the bone marrow from the remaining humerus are obtained so that it can be ascertained that no tumor remains.

Reconstruction following resection about the shoulder depends first on the age of the patient and second on the length of humerus resected. In small children and in patients in whom only a short segment of humerus has been resected, a soft-tissue reconstruction of the residual ends of muscles can add to the stability of the hanging humerus (Fig. 21–14B). The resected ends of the biceps and triceps may be sutured to the cut ends of the trapezius, pectoralis major, and latissimus dorsi. The patient sometimes obtains considerable arm function. When a large segment of humerus has been resected, the patient is left with considerable weakness and disability secondary to lack of shoulder function and loss of elbow function. Some stability is provided by insertion of a custom-made humeral prosthesis (Fig. 21–15) or a fibular graft (Fig. 21–16). The fibular graft may be either a nonvascularized autograft or a free vascularized autograft with microvascular anastomosis of its vascular pedicle to the

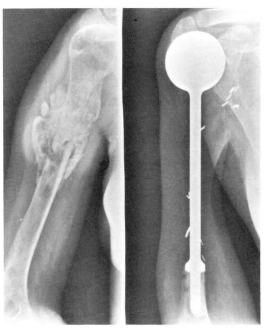

Figure 21–15. A 14-year-old female with osteogenic sarcoma of the proximal humerus (the patient shown in Figure 21–5) underwent a resection of the proximal three fourths of the humerus and reconstruction with a metallic implant. The large circumference of the prosthetic head rounds out the contour of the shoulder and also prevents migration of the metallic shaft through the skin.

brachial artery. In some cases, the peroneal artery may be anastomosed to the circumflex arteries. In the past, Küntscher nails inserted into the remains of the humeral stump were used to add stability to the arm (Fig. 21–17). Over the long term, they were associated with considerable morbidity, such as infection, protrusion of the rods through the skin, and on one occasion erosion of the subclavian artery. This method has been abandoned, and biologic, ceramic, and metal implants are available, with the choice depending on the treating surgeon's preference.

In limited resections that are confined to the humerus and only a short segment of scapula (e.g., the glenoid and coracoid), it is possible to reconstruct the arm with either an allograft (Fig. 21–18) or a custom modular design humeral prosthesis. Allografts, however, are suitable only in patients with low-grade lesions. Allografts inserted in patients undergoing adjuvant chemotherapy are associated with a high incidence of implant infection.[23] A fuller description of allografts is available in Chapter 23.

Diaphyseal lesions of the humerus are sometimes resectable, as shown in Figure

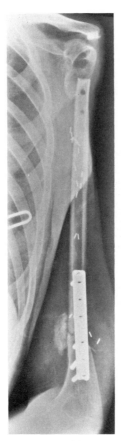

Figure 21–16. Reconstruction of the proximal humerus following a Tikhoff-Linberg resection using a free, vascularized fibular graft as a biologic strut.

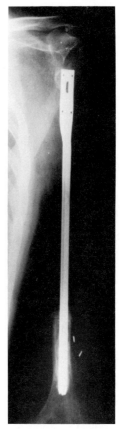

Figure 21–17. Reconstruction of a humeral shaft using a Küntscher rod. This patient's course was complicated by the rod's cutting through to the skin and a subsequent infection, which required removal of the rod.

21–19. The patient whose case is depicted in this illustration had a recurrent Ewing's sarcoma. The defect resected was filled with a vascularized fibular graft, which is a viable osseous unit that rapidly unites and hypertrophies, even with chemotherapy.[43]

Limb-sparing procedures have provided valid alternatives to amputations in selected tumors of the radius and ulna. After the distal femur and proximal tibia, the wrist is the next most common location for giant cell tumor of bone (Fig. 21–20). Curettage with or without bone grafting can result in a 40% to 50% recurrence rate. Recurrence often is associated with a more aggressive form of tumor. The best treatment for these lesions is wide resection of the distal radius.[33] En bloc procedures also may be performed in certain low-grade malignancies of the forearm and in carefully selected cases of high-grade tumors (Fig. 21–21A). As in all malignant tumors, accurate staging is critical in this decision. Principles for resection of the

tumor are the same as those for tumor surgery elsewhere. The lesion must be excised with a cuff of normal tissue without violation of the tumor itself. Any muscles, tendons, or fasciae adherent to the tumor are sacrificed. Tendon transfers may be performed primarily or at a later date as a secondary procedure.

Reconstruction of the forearm is necessary after resection of the tumor for preservation of function and normal alignment. Defects created by resection of the distal radius may be filled with corticocancellous autografts or a radial allograft. The proximal fibula can be transplanted to the forearm either as a free graft or as a vascularized graft (Fig. 21–21B). With the latter, the proximal radial artery or the anterior interosseous artery of the forearm is anastomosed to the distal end of the peroneal artery, and the proximal end of the peroneal artery is anastomosed to the distal stump of the radial artery at the wrist. This technique maintains two-vessel circulation to the hand, thus avoiding late cold intol-

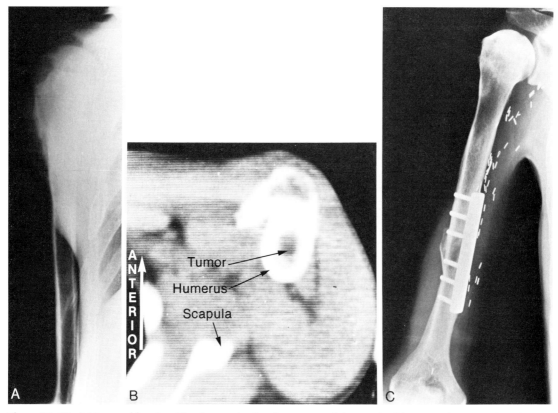

Figure 21–18. A 14-year-old male with a low-grade chondrosarcoma of the proximal humerus shown as a lytic lesion in the proximal humerus on a plain x-ray (A). A CT scan of the proximal humerus (B) revealing a lytic lesion surrounded by sclerotic new bone formation extending medially along the course of the subscapularis tendon. A postoperative X-ray of a proximal humeral reconstruction using cadaver allograft bone (C). This patient achieved an excellent functional result, with almost 80° of active forward flexion and abduction.

erance and maximizing vascular patency to the graft. For this procedure, extensive preoperative angiographic studies of vascular patterns of the forearm and the leg are required.

As an osseous transplant, the ipsilateral proximal fibula is the ideal replacement for the distal radius. The diameters of both diaphyses are approximately the same, and the fibular head conforms to the shape of the distal radius and provides reasonable congruity with the proximal row of carpal bones. Alternatively, a formal wrist arthrodesis may be performed. A more limited fusion of the fibular head with the scaphoid and lunate will retain some wrist function with motion at the intercarpal joints. Attempts at preserving even more wrist motion by ligamentous reconstruction for stabilization of the carpal bones on the fibula have not been successful in our hands or in the experience of others. The fibula is plated to the radius proximally.

The ipsilateral ulna also may be used to replace the resected radius. It is translocated into the gap created by the resection, and as a result the axis of forearm rotation is maintained and the hand remains centered on the forearm (Fig. 21–22). By preserving the soft-tissue attachments of the translocated portion of the ulna, this procedure provides a local vascularized bone graft without the need for microsurgical procedures. Another technique is to fuse the ulna to the proximal row of carpal bones. A plate is used proximally. Alternatively, the carpus may be centered on the distal ulna, resulting in a "one-bone forearm." The distal ulna is arthrodesed to the carpal bones, with the carpus fixed in the best functional alignment. Forearm rotation is eliminated, but the functional result is quite good. Prosthetic replacement of the distal end of the radius has been unsatisfactory.

Primary Malignant Tumors of the Hand. Primary malignant tumors of the hand are

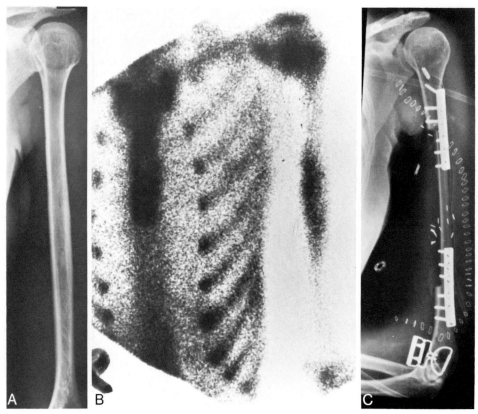

Figure 21–19. *A,* Preoperative x-ray of a 20-year-old female with recurrent Ewing's sarcoma, which presented as an irregularity in the middiaphysis of the humerus 5 years after initial treatment. *B,* A technetium-99m bone scan of a recurrent Ewing's sarcoma of the midshaft of the humerus. *C,* A postoperative x-ray following en bloc resection of the humeral diaphysis and reconstruction using a free vascularized fibular autograft.

extremely rare, accounting for fewer than 1% of reported large series.[8] Such tumors may be divided into lesions of soft-tissue or bony origin on the basis of their histology. However, because of the anatomy of the hand and proximity of all structures to one another, the methods of treating soft and bony lesions are apt to be the same.

The treatment of choice for such malignant tumors is adequate surgical excision followed by postoperative radiation or chemotherapy, depending on tumor type, stage, and grade.

The concept of adequate surgical excision has led to much debate, especially with respect to the hand. Because the hand is the most complex part of the musculoskeletal system, responsible for both afferent and efferent interactions with the environment, loss of hand function as a result of ablation is severe.

Enneking's concept of the hand as a single compartment would require amputation for

treatment of stage II or III lesions.[8] With the advent of improved adjuvant chemotherapy and with the desire to preserve more function, wide local (intracompartmental) resections are being performed.

Biplane x-rays and bone scans help one delineate the local extent of tumor. Unfortunately, the resolution of current CT scanners for evaluation of hand tumors has not been helpful because of the small size of the structures involved. The first generation NMR scanners likewise do not have sufficient resolving capabilities to be helpful in hand tumors. Thus, clinical means are relied on most heavily in the determination of margins for resection.

Malignant lesions of the fingers are best treated by ray resection/amputation (Fig. 21–23). Those tumors known to metastasize via lymph channels (e.g., melanoma, synoviosarcoma, and epithelioid sarcoma) also should undergo local/regional lymph node dissection for staging purposes.

Figure 21–20. *A,* An X-ray of a lytic lesion in the distal radius that was diagnosed on biopsy as giant cell tumor of the bone. *B,* The same patient 8 weeks following curettage, cryosurgery, and bone grafting, complicated by pathologic fracture through the distal radius. The complication of pathologic fracture following cryosurgery is common, and en bloc resection followed by reconstruction, with fibular graft and wrist arthrodesis or centralization of the carpus on the ulna, may be a better procedure.

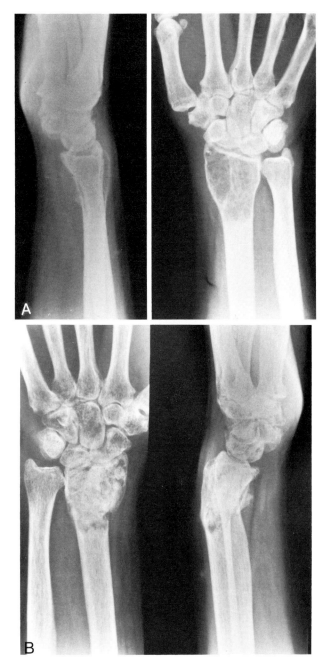

Amputations of the thumb ray can be reconstructed at a later date (e.g., after completion of chemotherapy) by pollicization of the index or toe-to-thumb microvascular free transfer.

Resection of the index ray gives an extremely functional result if preservation of the thumb and remaining middle, ring, and small fingers can be achieved.

The resected middle ray can be reconstructed by primary transfer of the index ray to the middle position, which widens the first web space and eliminates the "gap" in the palm (Fig. 21–24). Excellent cosmetic and functional results can be achieved. Lesions of the ulnar fingers and the ulnar border metacarpals can be treated by complete resection back to the carpal bones. Of course, one must take care to preserve the deep motor branch of the ulnar nerve. If the fixed unit of the hand (metacarpals 2 and 3) and the thumb can be preserved, the prehensile

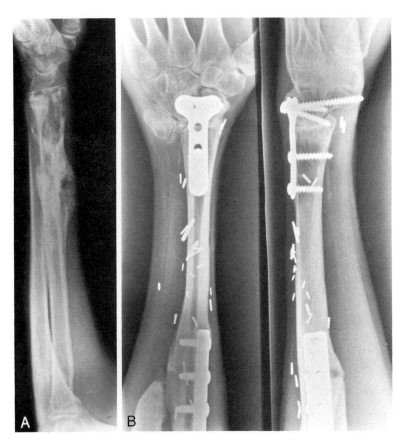

Figure 21–21. A, A fully malignant osteogenic sarcoma involving the distal radius in a 14-year-old boy who underwent preoperative chemotherapy followed by en bloc resection of the distal radius and ulna. B, Postoperative reconstruction using a vascularized fibular graft and an arthrodesis of the wrist (left). Note the hypertrophy of the vascularized graft two years after the surgery (right).

function of the hand will be spared. Even if the ulnar nerve must be sacrificed, median nerve innervation of the lumbricals to index and middle fingers will prevent claw deformities of the fingers. Thumb deformities and thumb flexion-adduction can be restored by a variety of tendon transfers.

Lesions of the central metacarpals (2 and 3) can be treated by deep resection back to the carpal bones. If the thumb and ulnar digits can be saved, an effective "pincer" hand remains despite the poor cosmetic result. Local rotation flaps, full-thickness skin graft, or microvascular free-flap transfer may be necessary for adequate soft-tissue coverage. If the median nerve must be sacrificed, sensation to the thumb may be restored by a neurovascular flap as a secondary reconstructive procedure.

Malignant tumors arising in, or extending to, the synovial flexor tendon sheath represent an additional problem with staging. Theoretically, a lesion of the flexor pollicis longus is continuous via the synovial sheath to the level of the wrist for which an above-wrist or midforearm amputation would be re-

quired. The rarity of malignant tumors of the hand makes it difficult for one to assess the efficacy of wide resection with chemotherapy compared with radical ablative amputation. There is no doubt that chemotherapy has enabled us to perform more limb-sparing surgery instead of amputation without any increase in the local recurrence rate. Treating the hand as a single compartment and performing complete amputations as suggested by Enneking probably give the best cure rate.[8]

Osteogenic Sarcoma. Osteosarcoma is the most common primary malignant sarcoma of the skeletal system.[13, 14, 15, 18, 20] The proximal humerus is the third most frequent site of involvement (15% of patients). The scapula and forearm bones are less often affected, and the hand is involved very rarely. The mean age of patients is 18 years for males and 17 years for females. Characteristically, the tumor is located in the metaphyseal area, causes trabecular destruction, breaks through the cortex, has little or no margination, elevates the periosteum (Codman's triangle) (see Fig. 21–2), and usually has evi-

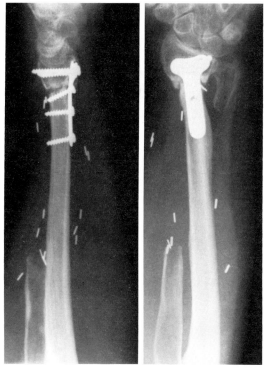

Figure 21–22. Postoperative x-rays of a reconstruction of a tumor in the distal radius similar to that in Figure 21–21, using a technique of transferring the distal radius to the proximal ulna, creating a one-bone forearm. Although this patient has no pronation and supination, the reconstruction was performed by placing the hand in the midprone position, which has left the patient with good function.

allows the surgeon to fabricate custom implants if limb preservation is anticipated (see earlier discussion). Recent data from Memorial Sloan–Kettering Cancer Center reports an 88% 4-year survival with no local recurrences in 32 consecutive limb preservation procedures for upper extremity osteosarcoma (stage IIB).

Chondrosarcoma. Chondrosarcomas, which occur in persons 20 to 60 years old, are the most common malignant lesions of the scapula and are frequently found in the proximal humerus.[2, 5, 10, 20, 27] Frequently, low-grade chondrosarcomas are incidental discoveries on chest x-rays or during arthritic evaluations of the shoulder. Chondrosarcomas are more likely than enchondromas when there is endosteal erosion, cortical breakthrough, areas of lysis, persistent pain at night, and changes on serial x-rays (see Fig. 21–18A). Although bone scans of chondrosarcomas are positive, scans of benign enchondromas in adolescents also can be positive.

High histologic grade III chondrosarcomas require very wide excisions or amputation. Histologic grades I and II tumors can be treated with curettage and cryosurgery or phenol or with limited resection, which results in a 90% to 95% five-year disease-free survival rate. Histologic grade II intermediate lesions require wide resections. This latter group does not respond to chemotherapy or radiotherapy, so adequate wide surgical margins are mandatory. This group of tumors has been frequently reconstructed with osteochondral allografts (see Fig. 21–18C) or custom implants (see Fig. 21–15). Cure rates for grade I tumors are excellent (65% to 85%); those for grade II lesions are adequate (40% to 65%); and those for high grade III tumors are poor (<20%).

Ewing's Sarcoma. Ewing's sarcoma may be found in any bone of the upper extremity but is most commonly encountered in the humerus and scapula (it is the second most common primary malignancy of the scapula).[3, 15, 35] Approximately 15% of Ewing's tumors occur in the shoulder girdle (see Fig. 21–14A), and they most frequently affect individuals between 5 and 25 years of age. The tumor arises in the marrow space and invades the cortex via the haversian system. It most commonly occurs in the diaphysis, but the metaphysis is involved in 25% of cases. Frequently, there is soft-tissue extension. Ewing's sarcoma is a permeative, destructive

dence of sarcomatous bone formation (except in telangiectatic osteosarcomas that are purely lytic). The majority of osteosarcomas present either as stage IIB or stage III (lung metastasis) lesions.

Prior to 1973, the 5-year survival rate among patients with osteogenic sarcoma was 10% to 25%, depending on the source of data.[26] Currently, cure rates approach 87%. Contributing to this optimistic turn of events has been the development of better preoperative staging techniques, including bone scanning and CT scanning, as well as the use of adjuvant chemotherapy. Systemic and arterial infusions of adriamycin, *cis*-platinum, and high-dose methotrexate, both prior to resection or ablation and after surgery, have led to improved survival rates.[6, 7, 19, 34] Preoperative chemotherapy permits the chemotherapist to judge the efficacy of the chosen agents at the time of definitive surgery and to adjust the agents if less than 90% necrosis is achieved. The preoperative program also

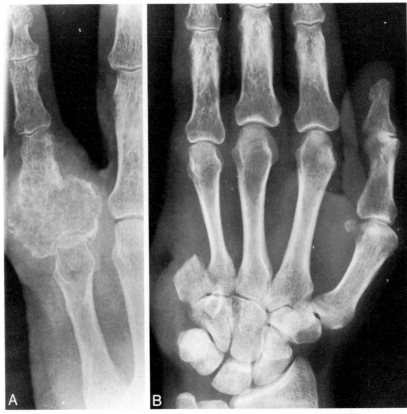

Figure 21–23. *A,* Preoperative x-ray of a grade II chondrosarcoma arising in the proximal phalanx of the fifth finger 3 years following currettage and bone grafting for an enchondroma. *B,* Postoperative x-ray following resection of the fifth ray.

lesion that can give rise to serial elevations of the periosteum and reactive bone formation (onion skinning) (Fig. 21–25). It can spread to the lungs and may affect the bone marrow (3%). Formerly, this tumor was associated with a very grim prognosis (15% 5-year survival), but with the advent of combination chemotherapy and radiation (in doses of 5000 rads), 5-year survivals of up to 75% have been reported. However, because of a continual fall-off even after 5 years and a local recurrence rate of 21% following radiation, wide surgical excision of the tumor mass has been combined with chemotherapy and low-dose radiation (3000 rads). The scapula is an expendable bone and can be closely resected partially or totally, depending on the location of tumor. Similarly, the humerus can be resected and an implant can be inserted, or radiation treatment can be used. Forearm bones can be resected and then reconstructed according to principles used for single bones.

Other Primary Bone Sarcomas. All sarcomas that primarily involve bone can involve the upper extremity. The combination of careful definition, wide excision, and adjuvant chemotherapy is utilized for all high-grade sarcomas (e.g., malignant fibrohistiocytomas). Cure rates are encouraging. Limb preservation can be achieved as long as adequate normal tissue coverage is available and the neurovascular bundle is spared.

SOFT-TISSUE TUMORS OF THE UPPER EXTREMITY

Tumors, benign and malignant, may arise from any tissue in the upper extremity.[9, 12, 13] Most are clinically characteristic (e.g., ganglions and warts) and can be diagnosed by physical examination. Others must be more carefully assessed, with extent of definitive treatment resting on pathological evaluation.

Benign Soft-Tissue Tumors

Benign lesions are quite common, and treatment consists of excision for relief of symptoms, which are usually due to pressure on

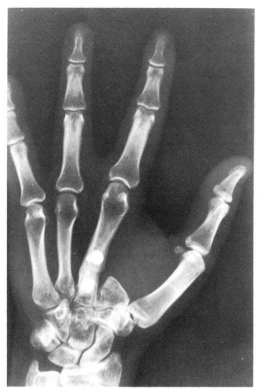

Figure 21–24. Postoperative x-ray of the hand of a 20-year-old female after resection of the middle ray for a malignant nerve sheath tumor. The index ray was transposed to the middle position, thus creating a functionally and cosmetically acceptable three-fingered hand.

adjacent structures. Excision will assure the patient and physician that malignancy is not present. Unsightly deformity is another indication for surgical removal of these lesions.

Ganglia. Ganglia, the most common tumors of the upper extremity, are located most frequently at the wrist (both volarly and dorsally at the radiocarpal joint area), at the flexor tendon sheath between the A1 and A2 pulleys (retinacular cyst), and at the base of the nail (mucous cyst) in association with degenerative changes in the DIP joint. Treatment consists of aspiration, aspiration with steroid installation, or careful resection that includes the degenerated portion of joint capsule or tendon sheath from which the lesions arise.

Epidermoid Inclusion Cyst. The epidermoid inclusion cyst is caused by trauma that drives the germinative epithelial cells deep into tissues, where a growth of skin and secretions of dermal appendages occur that cannot desquamate. Excision is the treatment of choice.

Keratoacanthoma. The keratoacanthoma is a skin lesion found on the dorsum of the arm and hand. It is frequently confused with squamous cell carcinoma. Simple excision is adequate treatment for these lesions.

Glomus Tumor. The glomus tumor is known for its paucity of signs but causes a tremendous amount of pain on exposure to trauma or changing temperature. Careful excision is the treatment of choice. Because these lesions commonly present in a subungual location, the surgeon may need to remove the nail plate and carefully elevate the nail bed to provide adequate exposure.

Arteriovenous Fistula. Arteriovenous fistula may be congenital or acquired as the result of trauma. The patient presents with a collection of dilated veins in the upper extremity. Blood flow, blood pressure, and skin temperature are higher in the affected arm. A pulsatile mass is the presentation of a pseudoaneurysm, which is most commonly found on the volar surface of the extremity secondary to repeated trauma to the hand or forearm.

Lipoma. Lipomas are soft, painless benign tumors of normal-appearing fat cells that may grow to enormous sizes and that can occasionally calcify.

Nodular Fasciitis. This lesion is most common in young adults and typically occurs in the forearm. The deep fascia appears somewhat like firm granulation tissue. Microscopically, the lesion is equivalent to Dupuytren's contracture. (It is discussed in greater detail elsewhere.)

Giant Cell Tumor of Tendon Sheath. Giant cell tumors of the tendon sheath are very common, are almost always benign, and are well defined, firm, and securely fixed to the deep structures (tendon sheath, ligament) but not to the skin. They usually arise from the tendon sheath and extend into the subcutaneous tissue of the digit. Full excision including all extensions usually results in cure. Recurrence of these tumors is probably related to incomplete excision.

Malignant Soft-Tissue Tumors

Fibrohistiocytoma. The most common malignant soft-tissue tumor of the upper extremity was originally thought to be fibrosarcoma. However, malignant fibrohistiocytoma is now believed to be the actual histologic diagnosis of the majority of those lesions formerly diagnosed as fibrosarcoma.

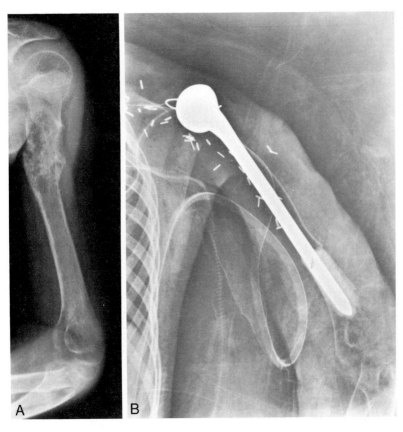

Figure 21–25. *A,* An 8-year-old female with Ewing's sarcoma of the proximal diaphysis of the humerus. Note the "onion skinning," a manifestation of successive elevations of the periosteum by tumor growth and periosteal new bone formation. *B,* Postoperative x-ray.

Rhabdomyosarcoma. Rhabdomyosarcoma arises from striated muscle and is the next most common malignant soft-tissue tumor. It occurs in children and young adults.

Epithelioid Sarcoma. Almost as common as rhabdomyosarcoma is epithelioid sarcoma, identified in 1970 by Enzinger.[9] Most of these tumors are located on the volar surfaces of the hand and attached to fascia or tendon sheaths. These tumors have a very high propensity to spread to noncontiguous areas, especially to regional lymph nodes.[9] Axillary node dissection is advised in the staging of these tumors.

Synovial Sarcoma. Synovial sarcomas arise adjacent to tenosynovial tissue of joints and tendons, most commonly in young adults. Calcified areas occur that may aid in radiographic diagnosis. Pain with a firm but cystic lesion is found, sometimes with multiple forearm metastasis.

Liposarcoma. Liposarcomas are malignant tumors of fat cell origin with a prospensity of local recurrence and distant metastatic spread. These tumors tend to be located in the deeper tissues of the extremity, in contrast to lipomas, which are superficial.

Melanoma. Melanoma arises from the skin and in children is a clinical oddity. The tumor most likely arises from a congenital melanotic lesion such as a giant hairy nevus. Depth of the lesion is a prime prognostic factor. Treatment includes excision and regional lymph node dissection if indicated.

Squamous Cell Carcinoma. Squamous cell carcinoma is extremely rare and when present in children usually occurs from predisposing conditions such as xeroderma pigmentosa and albinism. The lesion is most often found on the dorsum of the forearm and hand and frequently is associated with chronic exposure to sunlight, chemical irritants, or infection. It presents as a single, raised, crusted ulcer with a reddened base. Wide excision is the treatment of choice.

Treatment. Treatment of malignant soft-tissue lesions originally consisted of radical resection or amputation, resulting in a 70% cure and 10% local recurrence rate. Usually, forequarter amputation was performed after recurrence. Recently, the adjunctive use of preoperative, postoperative, or intraoperative radiation plus appropriate chemotherapy (Adriamycin) has provided 80% cure rates, with low recurrence rates in limb-preserving procedures.[13] However, in current protocols, amputation is still advised if there is neurovascular involvement.

PATHOLOGIC FRACTURES IN THE UPPER EXTREMITY

Pathologic fractures of the upper extremity may be divided into those resulting from benign lesions and those due to malignant lesions.[14, 21] The tendency for pathologic process and thus fracture is more common proximally in the appendicular skeleton and diminishes as one goes distally in the extremity. One exception to this rule is the high incidence of pathologic fracture of the phalanges with enchondroma, which is the most common presentation of this tumor.

A review of pathologic extremity fractures at Memorial Sloan–Kettering Cancer Center reveals that one of three were in the upper extremity. These were due to metastatic malignant disease and therefore did not include pathologic fracture secondary to benign processes such as simple bone cysts and aneurysmal bone cysts, which are more commonly seen in childhood.

The proximal humerus is the most common location of bony pathologic process in the upper extremity and it is not unusual for lesions to present as pathologic fractures in this location (see Fig. 21–2).

Fractures Secondary to Benign Processes

Unicameral and Aneurysmal Bone Cysts. Unicameral bone cyst often presents as a pathologic fracture in the proximal humerus (Fig. 21–26). The diagnosis can be made ra-

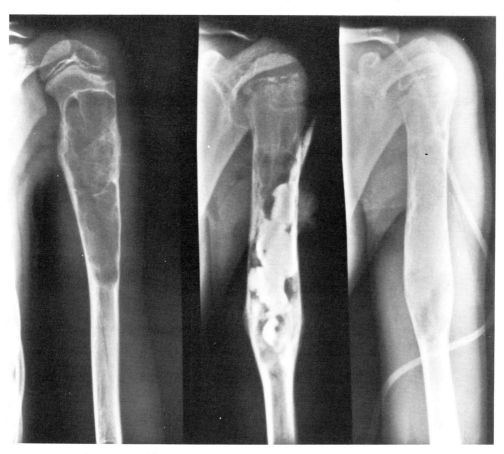

Figure 21–26. X-rays of a unicameral bone cyst of the proximal humerus in a 9-year-old boy complicated by a pathologic fracture extending into the humeral diaphysis. The middle picture shows intralesional contrast material used prior to the injection of methylprednisolone acetate. The third figure, 2 years after the initial injection, with healing of most of the cyst, reveals a persistent lytic lesion in the midshaft associated with a new pathologic fracture. This area was reinjected, and the patient went on to heal uneventfully.

diographically on the basis of the metadia-physeal location and the well-demarcated sclerotic rim of the lesion. The so-called fallen fragment sign is pathognomonic for unicameral cyst. A small percentage of cysts will heal spontaneously, especially following a fracture and immobilization in a sling and swathe or coaptation splints. Campanacci and colleagues have shown a 50% complete healing rate with multiple injections of methyl prednisolone acetate into the cystic cavity. Twenty-five percent of lesions resolve with small residual cysts, and another 25% fail to respond. The injections should be done in the operating room with the two-needle technique and radiographic control, and if the characteristic clear straw-colored fluid is not recovered, an open biopsy must be performed to confirm the diagnosis.

The injection technique has rare complications. The major criticism of the technique is that it fails to provide histologic diagnosis, and thus there is a risk of missing a malignant tumor. Therefore, we at Memorial suggest a Craig needle biopsy at the time of the first injection. For pathologic fractures resulting from benign processes, it is often helpful to wait 2 to 3 weeks for some early periosteal healing to take place before attempting treatment. Because the forces creating fracture through pathologic bone are usually small, the periosteum and overall alignment usually remain intact. During this period, the bone must be splinted externally for control of pain and maintenance of alignment. Attempts to inject fresh fractures occurring in unicameral cysts will not be effective because the methyl prednisolone acetate will leak out through the fracture site into the soft tissues. Similarly, pathologic fractures of the metacarpals and phalanges involved with enchondromas are more easily treated if some healing by periosteal new bone formation has been allowed to take place prior to curettage and bone grafting. This healing will obviate the need for internal fixation to control alignment and rotation in these potentially unstable fractures at the time of curettage and grafting.

For recurrent lesions of the distal radius, metacarpals, and phalanges with enchondroma or aneurysmal bone cyst, cryotherapy has been very helpful. The associated risks of skin and nerve complications prevent us from recommending its use for primary treatment except in giant cell tumor of bone. This technique is discussed elsewhere.

Fractures Secondary to Malignant Disease

The treatment of pathologic fracture of the long bones of the upper extremity due to malignant disease depends on whether or not the tumor is primary or metastatic and on its location.

Primary sarcomas of bone presenting with pathologic fracture in the upper extremity are associated with a poorer prognosis for en bloc resection than those without fracture because of contamination of soft-tissue planes by tumor-laden fracture hematoma. Therefore, special care must be taken in planning surgery for these cases, and amputation rather than en bloc resection may be required. The exception to this rule would be seen with Ewing's sarcoma, which can be controlled with radiation (prior to surgical excision).

Metastatic lesions of bone in the upper extremities (Fig. 21-27A) are less common than in the lower extremities, but they do occur, especially in patients with widespread metastatic disease.[14, 21] The philosophy of treating pathologic fractures advanced by Parrish and Murray is basically adhered to.[32] Although in their series Parrish and Murray aggressively treated pathologic fractures of the lower extremity with internal fixation and acrylic, humeral lesions were primarily treated nonoperatively. Of their total of 114 surgically treated pathologic fractures, only five humeral lesions were treated with intramedullary fixation.

One study of 137 surgically treated pathologic fractures of the humerus at Memorial Sloan-Kettering Cancer Center[44] revealed rapid and nearly complete pain relief in 86% of the patients, who had a median survival of 4.7 months. All patients in the series had metastatic tumors, and 25% survived over 1 year. Thus, pain relief and function were enhanced by operative intervention.

We have also treated with a functional humeral cast brace and radiation therapy 25 patients who were originally thought to be too ill for operative treatment or who had initially refused surgery. Most patients experienced dramatic pain relief within 48 hours of application of the brace and demonstrated gradual increase in function (Fig. 21-27B). Of this group, 50% went on to heal the fracture with abundant callus formation. Mean healing time was 8 weeks.

Thus, at this time we recommend humeral

Figure 21–27. *A*, An adult patient who has metastatic carcinoma of the breast presenting with a pathologic fracture of the humerus. She was treated with the humeral cast-brace technique outlined in the text. *B*, Posttreatment x-ray shows an abundant callus formation at the fracture site and clinical union 8 weeks following fracture.

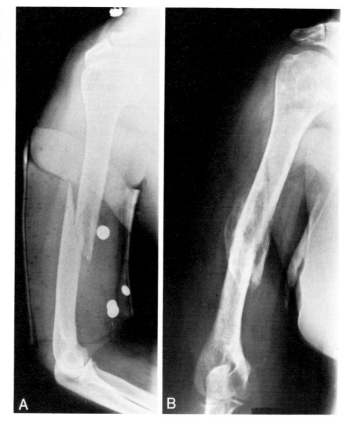

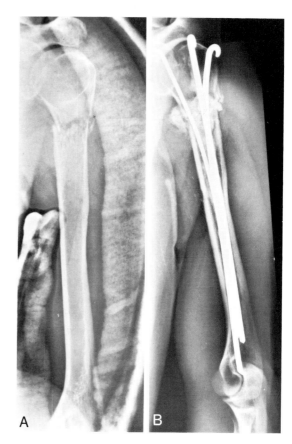

Figure 21–28. *A*, An x-ray of a female with metastatic epidermoid carcinoma of the cervix shows an impending pathologic fracture of the humerus. *B*, Because this patient needed her upper extremities for ambulation following fixation of pathologic fractures of the femur. it was elected to prophylactically fix the impending humeral fracture with an intramedullary nail and acrylic cement.

cast bracing of pathologic fractures with metastatic tumor in patients who are poor operative risks, who have less than 8 weeks' longevity, or who have a midshaft humeral fracture with a primary tumor that will respond well to radiation therapy (e.g., breast lesions, lymphomas). Those patients whose primary tumors are not very radiosensitive, whose fractures involve the surgical neck and head or the distal one third of the humerus (which are poorly controlled with bracing), or whose lower extremity involvement requires that they use the upper extremity for weight-bearing on crutches or a walker are more satisfactorily treated with internal fixation or endoprosthetic replacement and cement (Fig. 21–28).

SUMMARY

This chapter has described the staging and classification of benign and malignant tumors of the upper extremity. The principles of diagnostic work-up, including the critical biopsy and the current strategies of treatment, were outlined. Survival has improved for patients with high-grade malignant tumors, and techniques of limb preservation have become more successful. These advances have resulted from the combined use of defined surgery, adjuvant chemotherapy, and radiotherapy. Some guarded optimism is currently warranted.

References

1. Campanacci M, Di Sessa L, Trentani C. Scaglietti's method for conservative treatment of simple bone cysts with local injections of methylprednisolone acetate. Ital J Orthop Traumatol 3:27–36, 1977.
2. Campanacci M, Guernelli N, Leonessa D. Chondrosarcoma: a study of 133 cases, 80 with long-term follow-up. Ital J Orthop Traumatol 1:387–414, 1975.
3. Dahlin DC. Bone Tumors, General Aspects and Data on 6,221 Cases, 3rd ed. Springfield, IL, Charles C Thomas, 1978.
4. Dahlin DC, Coventry MB. Osteosarcoma: a study of 600 cases. J Bone Joint Surg 49A:101–110, 1967.
5. Dahlin DC, Salvador AH. Chondrosarcomas of bones of the hands and feet: a study of 30 cases. Cancer 34:755–760, 1974.
6. Eilber FR. Adjuvant treatment of osteosarcoma. Surg Clin North Am 61:1371–1378, 1982.
7. Eilber FR, Grant T, Eckhardt J. The Evolution of Limb Salvage at UCLA. 2nd International Workshop on Design and Application of Tumor Prostheses for Bone and Joint Reconstruction. Vienna, September 5, 1983.
8. Enneking WF, Spanier SS, Goodman M. Current concepts review: surgical staging of musculoskeletal sarcoma. J Bone Joint Surg 62A:1027–1030, 1980.
9. Enzinger FM. Soft Tissue Tumors. St. Louis, CV Mosby, 1983.
10. Gitelis S. Chondrosarcoma of bone. The experience at the Instituto Ortopedico Rizzoli. J Bone Joint Surg 63A:1248–1257, 1981.
11. Goldenberg RR, Campbell CJ, Bonfiglio M. Giant cell tumor of bone. An analysis of 218 cases. J Bone Joint Surg 52A:619–664, 1970.
12. Green DP. Operative Hand Surgery. New York, Churchill-Livingstone, 1982.
13. Hajdu SI. Pathology of Soft Tissue Tumors. Philadelphia, Lea & Febiger, 1979.
14. Harrington KD et al. Methylmethacrylate as an adjunct in internal fixation of pathological fractures. J Bone Joint Surg 58A:1047–1054, 1976.
15. Huvos AC. Bone Tumors—Diagnosis, Treatment and Prognosis. Philadelphia, WB Saunders, 1979.
16. Huvos AC, Marcove RC. Chondroblastoma of bone. A critical review. Clin Orthop 95:300–312, 1973.
17. Jaffee N, Frei E, Traggis D, Bishop Y. Adjuvant methotrexate and citrovorum-factor treatment of osteogenic sarcoma. N Engl J Med 294:994–997, 1974.
18. Lane JM. Malignant bone tumors, In Alfonson AE, Gardner E, eds. The Practice of Cancer Surgery. New York, Appleton-Century-Crofts, 1982:307–324.
19. Lane JM. Custom prosthetic segmental bone and joint replacement in malignant bone tumor patients. In Chao E, Ivins J, eds. Tumor Prosthesis—The Design and Application. New York, Thieme-Stratton, 1983.
20. Lane JM, Boland PJ. Tumors of bone and cartilage. In Goldsmith HS, ed. Practice of Surgery, vol. 1. New York, Harper & Row, 1983.
21. Lane JM, McCormack RR, Sundaresan N, et al. Treatment of pathological fractures. In Whitkoff H, ed. Current Concepts of Diagnosis and Treatment of Soft Tissue and Bone Tumors. New York, Springer-Verlag, 1984.
22. Linberg BE. Interscapulo-thoracic resection for malignant tumor of the shoulder joint region. J Bone Joint Surg 10:344–349, 1928.
23. Mankin HJ. Osteoarticular and intercalary allograft transplantation in the management of malignant tumors of bone. Cancer 50:613–630, 1982.
24. Mankin HJ, Lange TA, Spanier SS. The hazards of biopsy in patients with malignant primary bone and soft tissue tumors. J Bone Joint Surg 64A:1121–1127, 1982.
25. Marcove RC, Lewis MM, Huvos AC. En bloc upper humeral interscaplo-thoracic resection. The Tikhoff-Linberg procedure. Clin Orthop 124:219–228, 1977.
26. Marcove RC, Mike V, Hajek JV, et al. Osteogenic sarcoma under the age of 21. A review of 145 pre-operative cases. J Bone Joint Surg 52A:411–423, 1970.
27. Marcove RC, Mike V, Hutter RVP. Chondrosarcoma of the pelvis and upper end of the femur. An analysis of factors influencing survival time in 113 cases. J Bone Joint Surg 54A:561–572, 1972.
28. Marcove RC, Shaji H, Arlen M. Altered carbohydrate metabolism in cartilaginous tumors. Contemp Surg 5:53–54, 1974.
29. Marcove RC, Stoveli PB, Huvos AG. The use of cryosurgery in the treatment of low and medium grade chondrosarcoma. Clin Orthop 122:147–156, 1977.
30. Moore TM, Myers MH, Patzakis MJ, et al. Closed biopsy of musculoskeletal lesions. J Bone Joint Surg 61A:375–380, 1979.
31. Pack GT, McNeer G, Coley BL. Interscapulo-thoracic amputation for malignant tumors of the upper ex-

tremity. A report of 31 consecutive cases. Surg Gynecol Obstet 74:161–175, 1942.

32. Parrish FF, Murray JA. Surgical treatment for secondary neoplastic fractures. J Bone Joint Surg 52A:665–686, 1970.

33. Pho RW. Free vascularized fibular transplant for replacement of the lower radius. J Bone Joint Surg 61B:362–365, 1979.

34. Rosen G, Caparros B, Huvos AG, et al. Preoperative chemotherapy for osteogenic sarcoma. Selection of postoperative adjuvant chemotherapy based upon the response of the primary tumor to preoperative chemotherapy. Cancer 49:1221–1230, 1982.

35. Rosen G, Caparros B, Nirenberg N, et al. Ewing's sarcoma: ten-year experience with adjuvant chemotherapy. Cancer 47:2204–2213, 1981.

36. Rosen G, Marcove RC, Caparros R, et al. Primary osteogenic sarcoma. The rationale for preoperative chemotherapy and delayed surgery. Cancer 43:2163–2177, 1979.

37. Rosen G, Murphy ML, Huvos AG, et al. Chemo-

therapy, en bloc resection, and prosthetic bone replacement in the treatment of osteogenic sarcoma. Cancer 37:1–11, 1976.

38. Simon MA. Current concepts review, biopsy of musculoskeletal tumors. J Bone Joint Surg 64A:1253–1257, 1982.

39. Simon MA, Kirchner PT. Scintographic evaluation of primary bone tumors. J Bone Joint Surg 62A:758–764, 1980.

40. Souhami RL. What has adjuvant chemotherapy of osteosarcoma achieved? J R Soc Med 76:943–946, 1983.

41. Sweetnam R. Amputation in osteosarcoma. J Bone Joint Surg 55B:189–192, 1973.

42. Thompson HC, Garcia A. Myositis ossificans: aftermath of elbow injuries. Clin Orthop Rel Res 50:129–134, 1967.

43. Weiland A. Free vascularized bone grafts in surgery of the upper extremity. J Hand Surg 4:129–143, 1979.

44. Warren R. Unpublished data.

C H A P T E R ○ 2 2

Upper Limb Prostheses

MARTIN A. POSNER

Deficiencies of the upper limb in children are most often secondary to a congenital malformation. They can also follow trauma and can occasionally be the result of surgery. The objective of treatment in all cases is to enhance function of the affected limb. In many cases, this involves the fitting of a comfortable and, if possible, aesthetic prosthesis. An equally important objective of treatment is to instill within the child a positive self-image, which will enable him to pursue a satisfying and productive life. In order to accomplish these goals, one must initiate a multidisciplinary approach with the congenital amputee at birth and with other amputees at the time of limb loss.[14]

Emotional problems are common among these patients and their families and must be dealt with promptly and sympathetically. These problems are sometimes most difficult in parents whose child's limb deficiency is the result of a congenital defect. The joy and excitement experienced by the parents during pregnancy are replaced by shock, grief, and often guilt following the birth of a deformed child. The strains on the family increase as well-meaning relatives and friends make comments and offer advice that is often inaccurate and sometimes even callous. Professional psychiatric counseling may be helpful and, if needed, should be arranged for promptly.

ACQUIRED AMPUTATIONS (TRAUMATIC AND SURGICAL)

Limb deficiencies in the pediatric age group can be divided into two groups: acquired and congenital. Acquired limb deficiencies are most often secondary to trauma or to ablative surgery for malignant tumors, vascular malformations, or neurogenic disorders. In traumatic cases, the ratio of males to females is 12:1, and the injury usually involves the elbow area or the digits.[14] Accidents with power tools and machinery predominate in the traumatic group. Adverse sociologic and psychologic factors frequently exist in the homes of those children whose traumatic injury is the result of a train or motorcycle accident, or of a high-tension electrical burn.[9] Preventive measures, including educational programs, would help reduce the incidence of many traumatic amputations. Unfortunately, these programs have little impact when the problem is the child's home environment.

Surgical amputations in children, whether for disease or trauma, differ from those in adults because of future growth of the limb in the former group. Whenever possible, epiphyseal plates should be preserved. A disarticulation is therefore preferable to a metaphyseal or diaphyseal amputation in the growing child. In the elbow area, the prominent humeral condyles will atrophy as the child grows, and the initial bulbous appearance of the stump will lessen.[1, 3, 12]

The most frequent complication following amputations in children is terminal overgrowth of the bony stump. It is not due to overgrowth of the proximal epiphysis, so epiphyseodesis has no beneficial effect.[1, 46] The cause is probably related to mechanical stimulation of the periosteum at the amputation stump, which has a high osteogenic activity in children. Various techniques have been employed to control this problem, including the use of intramedullary implants of porous polyethylene or silicone rubber.[28, 42] Although these methods may become more effective in the future, the standard procedure at present is to resect the area of bony overgrowth. Recurrences are common, and stump revisions may be necessary until the child reaches maturity. Terminal overgrowth of the bone rarely occurs in congenital amputations.[1, 15]

Unlike congenital amputations, which are painless, surgical and traumatic amputations may result in a painful stump. This problem may be avoided by transection of the nerves proximal to the amputation level so that the cut end of the nerve will retract away from the stump end. Resection of a painful neuroma is sometimes necessary, particularly in traumatic cases, although adjustment of the prosthetic socket may suffice. Therapeutic programs for desensitization of the stump are rarely necessary in children. Phantom sensations of the absent part are frequent in all acquired amputations, but sensations disappear more rapidly in children, especially in those below the age of 10 years.[23]

Prior to prosthetic fitting, the stump should be wrapped with an elastic bandage so that edema is reduced. During this period, one should begin training the child in the activities of daily living, particularly if the dominant limb is the one that is lost. With respect to writing, the decision about

whether to retrain the dominant amputation side or to educate the child to use the nondominant hand should be deferred until the child has had the opportunity to practice with both extremities. If the interval between injury or surgery and definitive prosthetic fitting is expected to be long, a temporary prosthesis should be prescribed so that the training program can be started early. Amputees, particularly those with bilateral deficiencies, perspire more than normal children do owing to the loss of body surface area in the former group. Prostheses must therefore be light-weight and comfortable.

CONGENITAL AMPUTATIONS

There is scant information concerning the incidence of congenital upper limb amputation. A study in Scotland over a 5-year period showed an incidence of 1:3000.[33] Congenital malformations account for approximately 70% of upper limb deficiencies in children.[14] There is no known cause for many of these amputations, but 20% are due to established genetic factors, 5% result from chromosomal aberrations, and 5% are due to environmental cases such as teratogens. In those cases involving genetic factors, amputations are sporadic, and there is little risk of recurrence in future siblings.[22, 25] This is obviously comforting to the parents, who are naturally concerned about the outcome of subsequent pregnancies. In the unilateral amputee, the prosthesis serves as an assistive device of the normal limb, and it should not be expected to function as a normal limb, even under the best circumstances. In some situations, the prosthesis may compromise function because it reduces the remaining functional sensibility of the amputated limb. This situation is most likely to occur if the congenital amputation occurs at the terminal end of the limb.

Although each level of limb deficiency will be discussed separately, it should be noted here that there are several basic considerations in the use of prostheses. In congenital amputees, a prosthesis should be fitted when the extremity can be controlled by the child, usually at 6 months.[10] A primary objective of early prosthetic fitting is to integrate the brain and the extremity during early development. For this reason, many centers prescribe a passive terminal device in the form of a plastic- or plastisol-covered wafer capable of pushing objects or holding them with the aid of the opposite extremity. Other centers believe that the initial terminal device should be the small Dorrance plastisol-covered hook #12P. Advocates of this device consider it as effective as the mitten in facilitating pinch and believe that it helps the child pull himself up to a standing position. Another more practical advantage of the hook is that it can be activated when the child is older, which avoids the expense of purchasing a new terminal device. The Child Amputee Prosthetic Project (CAPP) at UCLA has developed its own terminal device that is unique in its appearance, control mechanism, and adaptability when compared with other commercially available terminal devices[38] (Figs. 22–1 and 22–2). In addition to having a closing spring that provides hold, the device is covered with a frictional, resilient covering that enhances control. Regardless of the device chosen, the child's attention is directed to the functional use of his extremity during his early development.[20]

By the time the child is 12 to 16 months of age, depending upon his development, one activates the terminal device by fitting with an appropriate cable and harnessing.[10] Initially, a child tends to open the terminal device accidentally, which makes him more aware of its functional capabilities. In time, the child will learn volitional control and

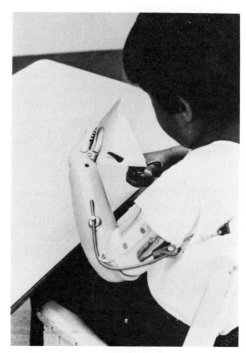

Figure 22–2. At a suitable age, the terminal device can be actively controlled with the addition of appropriate cable and harnessing.

how to open the device with the assistance of the opposite hand.

As the child grows, a prosthetic hand may be ordered to replace the hook. The hand is heavier than the hook and may be contraindicated for the child with a short forearm stump or for the child with an arm amputation and limited elbow flexion.[44] The prosthetic hand terminal devices are expensive, but the psychologic benefits to the child of having an aesthetic terminal device must be considered and may outweigh any economic and, in some cases, functional considerations.

Wrist units are usually manually controlled friction devices capable of providing pronation and supination. The degree of friction is adjusted by means of a ring around the base of the component (Fig. 22–3). In bilateral cases, a wrist flexion unit for at least one side is necessary to permit the amputee to reach the midline of the body for eating and personal hygiene activities (Figs. 22–4 and 22–5).

Flexible elbow hinges are used on most below-elbow prostheses because interference with stump pronation and supination is minimal with these devices. Regardless of the level of the below-elbow amputation, no

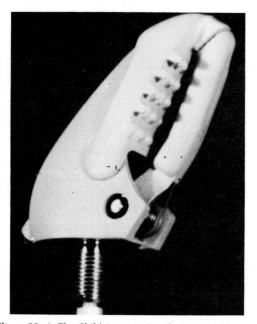

Figure 22–1. The Child Amputee Prosthetic Project (CAPP) terminal device.

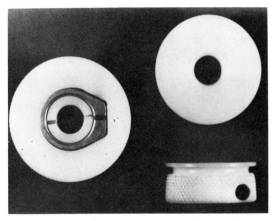

Figure 22–3. Nylon Hosmer-Dorrance frictional wrist.

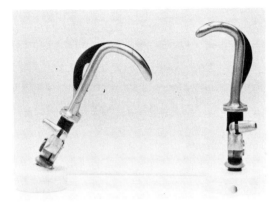

Figure 22–5. The preflexed wrist unit on the left with a Dorrance hook terminal device. The preflexed wrist unit has several advantages over a mobile wrist-flexion unit: lightness, which reduces weight at the terminal end of the prosthesis; simplified rotational positioning; and reduced energy expenditure, which is important in bilateral amputees.

more than 50% of pronation and supination can be transmitted with the prosthesis.[44] In children with very short forearm stumps and in those who use their prostheses for heavy lifting, rigid hinges are more suitable. Elbow components for above-elbow amputees are far more complex, and activation by muscular power is beyond the capabilities of the young child. Passive locking mechanisms or external power sources are often necessary. Understandably, the training program for the bilateral amputee is longer and more complex than that for the unilateral amputee, and it is essential that the goals for these children be realistic. Their ability to achieve independence depends on the level of the amputations, the agility of the rest of the body, and motivation. Motivation is a critical factor and can be enhanced by minimizing the level of the child's frustration. Adaptive aids for these severely handicapped children are essential and vary, depending on the amputation levels. One example is the use of a cuff splint on a forearm stump to permit holding a pen, pencil, or eating utensil. For the unilateral amputee, self-help devices are usually

not required, although a swivel spoon and fork for meals, a hook for buttoning clothing, and a nonskid pad for stabilizing paper when the child is writing may be helpful.

Although it is generally accepted that fitting a prosthesis at an early age increases the child's tolerance for wearing the device,[22] the discard rate of prostheses given to children before age 2 years is 25% by the time these children reach adolescence.[35] In those children fitted with a prosthesis after the age of 2 years, the discard rate approaches 50%. The appearance of the prosthesis, the realization that it does not satisfy their functional needs, and the discovery that they can manage as effectively without it are the major reasons that children discard a prosthesis. This is most likely to occur in the unilateral amputee whose limb deficiency is at, or more distal to, the wrist level.

Entire Limb Amputations

Absence of the entire limb, or amelia, is a rare condition. Usually, a portion of the shoulder girdle remains, such as the clavicle or acromion. These bony projections can be useful for manipulation of electrical switches in the socket of a prosthesis.[14] With unilateral involvement, the situation is similar to a shoulder disarticulation or a very short above-elbow amputation. Prosthetic fitting is recommended when the child is capable of sitting.

The child with bilateral amelia has the most severe functional impairment of all

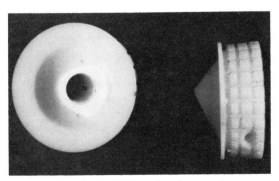

Figure 22–4. CAPP preflexed wrist unit.

upper limb deficiencies. The intelligent and well-motivated child will be able to substitute with foot function for such activities as personal hygiene and feeding. The use of feet for prehensile activities can be developed to an incredible degree provided that the spine and joints of the lower limbs, particularly the hip joints, are mobile. The children should always be encouraged in these activities, and adaptations in clothing such as the substitution of Velcro straps for laces are helpful for self-care. Although these children learn to do most of their daily activities with their feet, trunk, and mouth, prosthetic training for one of the absent limbs is recommended. The opposite limb can also be fitted with a light-weight prosthesis for cosmesis and for balance. These children may require another mode of prehension in later years because mobility of the spine and joints of the lower limbs tends to decrease with age.[22]

Prosthetic fitting in these children requires a combined effort of engineers, therapists, and physicians[36] (Figs. 22–6 and 22–7). The energy required to power a conventional prosthesis at the shoulder level is high and beyond the capabilities of small children. It is for this reason that externally powered prostheses using small cylinders of carbon dioxide gas have been developed.[27] Movements of the remaining portion of the shoulder girdle are used to manipulate the switches for this power supply. In spite of many advances in the design and fabrication of these devices, they remain cumbersome, and many children will eventually discard

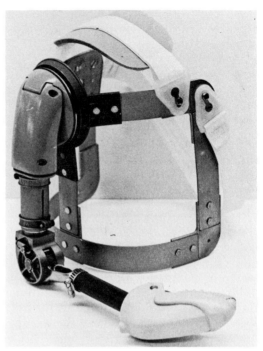

Figure 22–7. CAPP shoulder disarticulation prosthesis with a two-way shoulder component, a frame component, and a terminal device. The frame type of socket leaves most of the chest wall free, which reduces excessive perspiration, a frequent problem for children who wear this type of prosthesis. The design of the frame allows adjustments to be easily made.

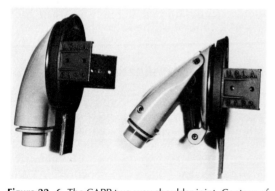

Figure 22–6. The CAPP two-way shoulder joint. Contour of this component closely parallels the natural shoulder profile and provides reliable friction in two places. Children with shoulder disarticulation prostheses require specific table-chair height relationship in order to function effectively. With this prosthesis, which allows shoulder abduction, the table-chair height relationship becomes less critical, increasing the functional work area for the child.

them. Myoelectric control prostheses are being researched and developed in many centers and may become the prosthesis of the future.

Phocomelia is considered with the category of a total limb deficiency. This term, derived from a combination of Greek and Latin words, refers to a "seal limb" in which the hand is attached to the trunk. In Frantz and O'Rahilly's classification,[13] it is an intercalary defect with shortening of the limb due to absence of all or a portion of the arm and forearm with a relatively normal hand.

This classification was based on two major categories, terminal and intercalary deficiencies. Since it used descriptive terms that were sometimes confusing and since all intercalary deficiencies have some terminal manifestations, however small, it was modified by the International Society of Prosthetics and Orthotics.[29] This international classification categorizes limb deficiencies into transverse and longitudinal groups.

In the transverse group, the limb deficiency is determined by the clinical appearance of the level at which the limb terminates. The longitudinal deficiencies are determined by the clinical and x-ray identification of the bones affected.

In cases of phocomelia that are the result of maternal ingestion of the teratogenic drug thalidomide, the developing somatic cells in the upper limb are affected between the thirty-ninth and forty-fourth days of gestation.[16] Almost all cases are bilateral, and none of the affected hands have a thumb. The little finger is the most well-developed of the digits, followed by the ring finger.[11] Although strength and function of these digits are rarely normal, there is usually enough intrinsic muscle power for manipulation of elbow- or shoulder-locking mechanisms or for operation of switches in powered units. It is for these reasons that surgical ablation of the digits is contraindicated. In those patients in whom the phocomelic limb is of sufficient length to reach the mouth, prosthetic fitting is probably unnecessary.[14]

Above-Elbow Amputations

Above-elbow amputations more frequently result from trauma or surgery than from a congenital defect. This amputation level has the highest incidence of bone overgrowth at its distal end for which surgery may be necessary.[14] A prosthesis is recommended at an early age. The mechanism for a prosthetic joint depends on the length of the humerus. For above-elbow amputations in children, unlike those in adults, a disarticulation through the elbow joint is preferred so that the distal humeral epiphysis can be preserved. If the amputation is through the elbow joint, a single-walled socket with an external locking joint is recommended. In children with shorter stumps, a double-walled socket and an elbow joint with internal control are best. The young child is unable to learn the complex movements necessary for active control of a prosthesis with an elbow joint and terminal device. Initial training is therefore directed toward control of the terminal device. Active control of the elbow joint is deferred until the age of 5 to 7 years, when the child has sufficient neuromuscular coordination to control a dual system. Prior to that age, elbow motions are carried out manually. A recent development is a prosthesis that combines both body power and myoelectric power. Body power is used to control the terminal device while

myoelectric signals from proximal muscles in the limb lock and unlock the elbow joint.[21]

Below-Elbow Amputations

Below-elbow amputations are the most common of congenital limb deficiencies,[14] and most are in the proximal third of the forearm. Although the epiphyses of the proximal radius and ulna are present, growth of the bones will be limited, and the length of the forearm will remain short. Prosthetic fitting is recommended at 6 months, and the appliance should be light, consisting of a plastic socket and a passive terminal device. The main difficulty in fitting is keeping the short forearm stump in the socket when elbow flexion exceeds 90°. The standard method of fitting is use of a preflexed socket, which permits positioning of the terminal device near the midline of the body. This prosthesis prevents forearm slippage, but its curved appearance, commonly referred to as a"banana arm," is considered by some to be objectionable.[44] Another technique, used primarily in bilateral cases, is a split socket with stepped-up hinges, which provide 10° of forearm flexion for each 5° of stump flexion. Although this device improves stability, the durability of the hinges and lifting power of the prosthesis are poor. The Münster prosthesis (named for the German city in which it was developed) is probably the most popular choice for the elbow amputation with a short forearm stump in the unilateral amputee. This prosthesis has a socket shaped in 35° of flexion and permits further active flexion up to 90°. This limitation in flexion precludes its use in bilateral amputees. The prosthesis provides normal arm contour, lifting power, and excellent stability because the socket conforms to the biceps tendon, the humeral epicondyles, and the stump itself.[10] If properly fitted, harnessing is provided with a single axillary loop that obviates the need for the more cumbersome figure-of-eight harness.

The Münster socket has also been used successfully for the control of myoelectric terminal devices, a paradox because in these cases the socket is least necessary.[10, 22, 41] The recognition that electrical impulses are present in the musculature of amputees has stimulated experiments in this country and in Europe to manufacture electromyographically controlled hands, wrist rotation units, and, in some cases, elbow mechanisms. With proper fitting and training, patients are able to demonstrate excellent function in research settings, but use of these devices in clinical settings has not been as satisfactory. Difficulties include the high cost of these devices (four times greater than body-powered devices) as well as the increased cost of maintenance. Although the prosthesis is capable of mechanically substituting for joint motion, it has yet to replace satisfactorily the sensory and proprioceptive abilities of a normal limb. The body-powered arm and hand have the advantage of a voluntary muscle feedback system that is an extension of our physiologic proprioception pathway.[24] In contrast, the feedback loop of a myoelectric device is incomplete. Efferent control occurs by sequential action of motor nerves, muscles, and electrodes that are amplified to the actuators, but the prosthesis fails to provide any afferent information. The patient compensates with visual monitoring, with cues he receives from motor vibrations and sound, and with recall of opening-closing time of the terminal device. Research is in progress to provide for a feedback system. Tendons in the amputation stump may be capable of supplying information on forced proprioception, and transcutaneous electrical stimulation may provide useful sensory feedback.[6]

Any discussion of forearm amputations must include mention of the Krukenberg procedure (see Chapter 3 for description). Devised by Krukenberg in 1917, it converts the forearm into an active pincer covered by skin with good sensibility. Traditionally, it has been considered the procedure of choice for at least one limb in the blind patient with bilateral hand loss. It is also useful for patients of normal sight, particularly in regions of the world where prosthetic fitting is unavailable. However, because the appearance of the forearm after surgery is unattractive, the procedure has been rarely performed in Western countries.[45] Despite the aesthetic problems, the functional results can be excellent: a strong pinch with good sensibility. In children, surgery has been recommended as early as age 2 years, and if digits remain at least one should be preserved at the tip of each pincer to assist in pinch. It has been suggested that the criticism of the aesthetic problems with this procedure is exaggerated. If desired later by the patient, a prosthesis can still be fitted without difficulty.[43] The patient then has the advantage of a Krukenberg stump for functional activities and a prosthesis for social occasions.

Wrist and Hand Amputations

Amputation through the wrist with complete absence of the hand (acheiria) is rare. Far more common is a transverse loss occurring at the midcarpal area with motion remaining at the radiocarpal joint. Amputations limited to absence of digits only are called adactylia. In cases of amputation with a large mobile carpal remnant, wrist flexion and extension provide excellent bilateral holding activities and may permit some unilateral prehension. Prosthetic fitting for patients with these deformities is not only unnecessary but also contraindicated because it interferes with the normal sensory appreciation between the stump and other objects. When flexion and extension of the stump are limited, a prosthetic post anchored around the distal forearm enables the child to hold objects between his palm and the opposing surface of the post. The CAPP program has developed a post that is multipositional so that the child can alter the position of the post with respect to his hand to accommodate objects of varying sizes. When not in use, the post can be folded back against the forearm. The prosthesis enables the child to hold various objects, such as eating utensils, and it helps older children tie shoelaces and participate in sports activities, including bicycle riding, golf, archery, and skiing. This type of post or plate prosthesis is fitted after age 2 years (Fig. 22–8).

Digit Amputations

Partial or complete amputations of a digit are usually the result of trauma. Most of these injuries are confined to the digit tip, which is the anatomic area distal to the base of the nail. The injury may involve a loss of skin or skin and pulp tissue and include a portion of the distal phalanx and nail bed. Many articles have been written on the acute treatment of these injuries, including reports on the use of partial- or full-thickness skin grafts, local flaps, or distant flaps. The specific procedure employed depends on the nature of the injury, the digit involved, the patient's age, and the expertise of the treating physician. Frequently, careful cleaning and good hygiene are the best treatment for fingertip injuries in children, and in such cases healing will occur within 3 to 4 weeks. Even if the underlying phalanx is partially amputated, re-epithelialization will occur, pro-

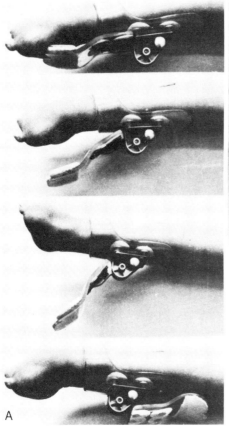

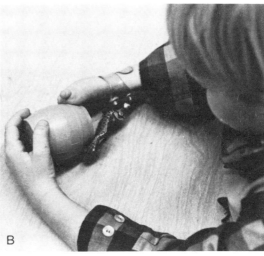

Figure 22–8. The CAPP multipositional post (*A*) and its use (*B*). This device permits prehension between the post, which can be set at different positions, and the mobile carpal remnant. When not in use, the post can be folded back against the forearm (*A*, bottom picture). (Figures 1 through 8*A* were generously provided by the Child Amputee Prosthetics Project at University of California Rehabilitation Center, 1000 Veteran Avenue, Los Angeles, California 90024.)

vided that the remaining bone is not protruding distal to the level of soft tissue loss.

When the amputation is through the more proximal portion of the digit, replantation should be considered, particularly for injuries involving the thumb. Revascularization of a partially amputated part is a reasonable option in children, and the return of sensibility following repair of the digital nerves is superior to that obtained in older patients. Epiphyseal growth of the replanted bone has been shown to continue, and in some cases overgrowth occurs. It is unclear whether this epiphyseal overgrowth is secondary to transient hypoxia or to the increased vascularity that accompanies the healing process.[19]

The treatment of single digit amputations, whether they are the result of trauma or a congenital deformity, depends on the digit involved and the impact that its loss has on overall hand function. With amputation of the thumb, there is a marked impairment in prehension involving key and tip pinch. Surgery is necessary in most cases, and the procedure of choice depends on the level of amputation. Congenital amputations generally involve the entire ray, and pollicization of

the index finger is the preferred operation. Surgery is also advised for amputations of one of the central digits, the middle or ring finger. Loss of one of these fingers produces a deformity that is unattractive because of the loss of symmetry, which is most apparent when the fingers are extended. Objects may fall from grasp, and, when the amputation is near the metacarpophalangeal joint, the adjacent fingers will eventually scissor. Ulnar transposition of the index finger with loss or absence of the middle finger or radial transposition of the little finger with loss or absence of the ring finger is usually indicated (Figs. 22–9 and 22–10).

Prosthetic replacements for an entire finger or a portion of a finger are commercially available, but these devices interfere with the sensibility of the stump and are easily soiled, damaged, and dislodged in the active child. The single digit prosthesis may be used for social occasions, but it impedes hand function and is therefore rarely used by the child when engaged in activities.[30]

In the child with an amputation of all fingers, a partial prosthesis will provide a post for pinch if there is a thumb. A similar device

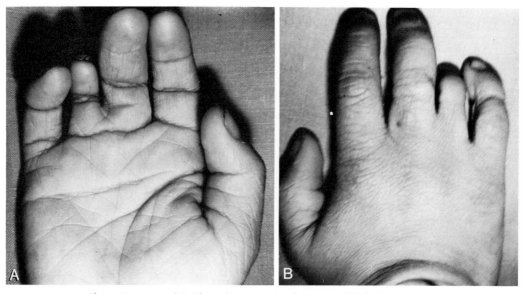

Figure 22–9. *A* and *B*, The rudimentary ring finger was of little functional use.

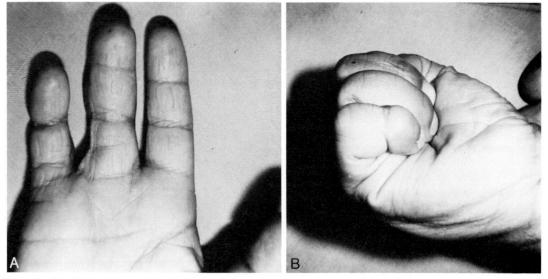

Figure 22–10. *A*, After ray resection of the ring finger and ulnar transposition of the little finger. *B*, By osteotomizing the fourth metacarpal at a more distal level than the fifth metacarpal, the little finger is lengthened when transposed, improving the symmetry of the hand.

can also be used for pinch if there is only one finger present.

SUMMARY

Acquired and congenital amputations of the upper limb are complex problems requiring a multidisciplinary approach involving physicians, therapists, and prosthetists. The emotional impact of the limb loss for the child—particularly during adolescence—and for the parents is often difficult. Prompt recognition and effective management of any emotional problem are the first essential steps in a successful rehabilitation program. It is also important to establish realistic functional goals for the congenital amputee at birth and for other amputees at the time of their limb loss. Only then can prosthetic fitting be planned, which should be aimed at enhancing the child's functional capabilities both immediately and throughout his life into adulthood.

References

1. Aitken GT. Amputation or a treatment for certain lower extremity congenital abnormalities. J Bone Joint Surg 41A:1267–1285, 1959.
2. Aitken GT. Management of the child amputee. AAOS Instructional Course Lectures 17:246–198, 1960.
3. Aitken GT. Surgical amputation in children. J Bone Joint Surg 45A:1735–1741, 1963.
4. Baumgartner RF. Surgery of arm and forearm amputations. Orthop Clin North Am 12(4):805–817, 1981.
5. Beasley RW. Surgery of hand and finger amputations. Orthop Clin North Am 12(4):763–803, 1981.
6. Beeker TW, During J, Den Hertog A. Artificial touch in a hand prosthesis. Med Biol Eng 5:47–49, 1967.
7. Brooks B, Beal L, Ogg L, Blakeslee B. The child with deformed or missing limbs: his problems and prosthesis. Am J Nurs 62:89, 1962.
8. Clarke SD, Patton JG. Occupational therapy for the limb-deficient. Clin Orthop 148:47–54, 1980.
9. Cummings V, Molnar G. Traumatic amputation in children resulting from "train/electrical burn" injuries: a social-environmental syndrome? Arch Phys Med Rehab 55:72, 1974.
10. Downie GR. Limb deficiencies and prosthetic devices. Orthop Clin North Am 7(2):465–473, 1976.
11. Fletcher I. Review of the treatment of thalidomide children with limb deficiencies in Great Britain. Clin Orthop 148:18–25, 1980.
12. Frantz, CH, Aitken GT. Management of the juvenile amputee. Clin Orthop 9:30–47, 1959.
13. Frantz CH, O'Rahilly R. Congenital skeletal limb deficiencies. J Bone Joint Surg 43A:1202–1224, 1961.
14. Gillespie R. Congenital limb deformities amputation surgery in children. In Kostuia JP, Gillespie R, eds. Amputation Surgery and Rehabilitation: The Toronto Experience. New York, Churchill-Livingstone, 1981:105–136.
15. Glassner JR. Spontaneous intra-uterine amputation. J Bone Joint Surg 45A:351–355, 1963.
16. Harris JM, Pashayan HM. Teratogenesis. Orthop Clin North Am 7(2):281–289, 1976.
17. Harrison SH, Mayou B. Bilateral Krukenberg operations in a young child. Br J Plast Surg 30:171–173, 1977.
18. Hubbard S. In Kostuia JP, Gillespie R, eds. Amputation Surgery and Rehabilitation: The Toronto Experience. New York, Churchill-Livingstone, 1981.
19. Jaeger SH, Tsai TM, Kleinert HE. Upper extremity replantation in children. Orthop Clin North Am 12(4):897–907, 1981.
20. Klopsteg PE, Wilson PD. Human Limbs and Their Substitutes. New York, McGraw-Hill, 1954.
21. Lamb DW. Prosthetics in the upper extremity. J Hand Surg 8(5):774–777, 1983.
22. Lamb DW, Scott H. Management of congenital and acquired amputations in children. Orthop Clin North Am 12(4):973–993, 1981.
23. Lambert CN. Amputation surgery in the child. Surg Clin North Am 3:473–482, 1972.
24. Law HT. Engineering of upper limb prostheses. Orthop Clin North Am 12(4):929–951, 1981.
25. Lenz W. Genetics and limb deficiencies. Clin Orthop 148:9–17, 1980.
26. Marquardt EG. A holistic approach to rehabilitation for the limb-deficient child. Arch Phys Med Rehab 64:237–240, 1983.
27. Marshall M. The upper extremity in children. In Kostuia JP, Gillespie R, eds. Amputation Surgery and Rehabilitation: The Toronto Experience. New York, Churchill-Livingstone, 1981:347–366.
28. Meyer LC, Saver BW. The use of porous high-density polyethylene caps in the prevention of appositional bone growth in the juvenile amputee. A preliminary report. Inter-Clinic Information Bulletin 14:1–4, 1975.
29. Mital MA. Classification and treatment. Orthop Clin North Am 7(2):457–464, 1976.
30. Pillet J. Esthetic hand prostheses. J Hand Surg 8(9):778–781, 1973.
31. Posner MA. Ray transposition for central digital loss. J Hand Surg 4(3):242–257, 1979.
32. Robinson KP, Andrews BG, Vitali M. Immediate operative fitting of upper limb prostheses at the time of amputation. Br J Surg 62:634–637, 1975.
33. Rogala ET, Wynne-Davies R, Little-John A. Congenital limb anomalies: frequency and aetiological factors. J Med Genet 11:221, 1974.
34. Rosenfelder R. Infant amputees: early growth and care. Clin Orthop 148:41–46, 1980.
35. Scotland TR, Galway HR. A long-term review of children with congenital and acquired upper limb deficiency. J Bone Joint Surg 65B(3):346–349, 1983.
36. Setoguchi Y, Sumida C, Shaperman J. Child Amputee Prosthetic Project-Research. Los Angeles, University of California Rehabilitation Center, 1982.
37. Shaperman J. Learning patterns of young children with above elbow prostheses. Am J Occup Ther 33(5):299–305, 1979.
38. Shaperman J, Sumida CT. Recent advances in research in prostheses for children. Clin Orthop 148:26–33, 1980.
39. Simpson DC, Lamp DW. A system of powered prostheses for severe upper limb deficiencies. J Bone Joint Surg 47B:442–447, 1965.
40. Smith RJ, Lipke RW. Treatment of congenital deformities of the hand and forearm. New Engl J Med 300(8):344–348, 1978.
41. Sorbye R. Myoelectric prosthetic fitting in young children. Clin Orthop 148:34–40, 1980.
42. Swanson AB. Bone overgrowth in the juvenile amputee and its control by the use of silicone rubber implants. Inter-Clinic Information Bulletin 8:9–16, 1969.
43. Swanson AB, Swanson GD. The Krukenberg procedure in the juvenile amputee. Clin Orthop 148:55–61, 1980.
44. Tooms RE. The amputee. In Lovell WW, Winter RB, eds. Pediatric Orthopaedics, 2nd ed. Philadelphia, JB Lippincott, 1978.
45. Tubiana R. Krukenberg's operation. Orthop Clin North Am 12(4):819–826, 1981.
46. VanSoal G. Epiphyseodesis combined with amputation. J Bone Joint Surg 21:442–443, 1939.
47. Zhong-Wei C, Meyer VE, Kleinert HE, Beasley R. Present indications and contraindications for replantation as reflected by long-term functional results. Orthop Clin North Am 12(4):849–870, 1981.

CHAPTER ○ 2 3

Allografts in the Upper Extremity

GARY E. FRIEDLAENDER

During the course of musculoskeletal disease or following reconstructive surgery, circumstances may arise in which the integrity of the skeleton is compromised, threatened, or deficient, and the use of a bone graft represents a reasonable therapeutic alternative. Inadequacies of bone for which grafting procedures may be considered include failure of anticipated biologic function, such as a nonunion of a fracture, and loss of biomechanical attributes, exemplified by segmental bone loss following trauma or tumor resection. The types of bone graft available for reconstructive purposes vary widely with respect to tissue architecture (cortical versus cancellous), vascular status, immunogenetics, and mechanical properties (e.g., different shapes and sizes and preservation-induced changes); the surgical approaches by which these tissues are implanted are equally heterogeneous. The selection and proper application of these various transplantable osseous tissues are based on an understanding of their biology, particularly the sequence of physiologic events that occur between the times of implantation, incorporation, and remodeling. Furthermore, influence of these biologic events on mechanical properties of bone as a material also must be considered in the course of developing and implementing clinical applications and methods of long-term storage.

GENERAL CONSIDERATIONS

The vast majority of bone grafts accomplished at the present time are autogenous; that is, tissue is removed from one portion of the skeleton and transferred to another location in the same individual. By definition, autografts are biologically compatible and represent maximal obtainable physiologic properties, but they require sacrifice of normal structures at one site in favor of their availability at a second location. The most frequent donor site is the pelvis, particularly the iliac crest, and there is generally little morbidity associated with acquisition. Wound infection, prolongation of the operative procedure with additional blood loss, weakening of the donor bone or herniation of soft tissues through an osseous defect, and increased post-operative discomfort must be considered, but these *potential* complications rarely seem sufficient justification for avoiding the use of bone autografts when the material is required clinically. Limitations in the size, shape, and quantity of transplantable tissue available from the ilium or from alternative locations that also may serve as donor sites (e.g., the proximal tibia, proximal humerus, or distal radius) represent more practical obstacles to reliance on autogenous bone. For these reasons, other sources of graft material have been sought, and these have generally been allogeneic.

Allografts are tissues transferred from one member of a species to a second member of the *same* species (e.g., rabbit to rabbit, rat to rat, or human to human). This transfer, by definition, involves an incompatibility of tissue types between donor and recipient, except for the special circumstance presented by inbred animals or identical twins. In addition to causing concern for immunologic responses and their potentially adverse consequences, the use of allografts raises the possibility of transferring disease between donor and recipient, and there remains an important question as to whether the biologic capacity of these grafts is comparable with that of autogenous tissues or, at least, satisfactory for their intended application. There is sufficient evidence to suggest that all these concerns can be minimized and that bone allografts do, indeed, represent an acceptable alternative to fresh autogenous bone in properly selected cases.[34]

Bone xenografts, formerly termed heterografts, are characterized by transfer of tissue between species, but there has been no practical enthusiasm in the United States for this approach since the demonstrated clinical failure of Boplant.

BIOLOGIC CONSIDERATIONS

Autografts

Incorporation of bone grafts, regardless of anatomic type (cortical versus cancellous) or genetic considerations, depends on a predictable but poorly understood sequence of events.[9, 14, 18, 41, 44, 54] In general, revascularization of the transferred tissue must occur first and is then followed by appropriate, relative amounts of resorption and formation activity.

The primary, or initial, phase of incorporation begins with hematoma formation, graft cell necrosis (if cell viability was actually present at the time of transplantation), and an inflammatory response. The magnitude and character of the cellular infiltrate reflect both local cell death and histocompatibility differences. These events are a prelude to vascular invasion and the recruitment of osteoprogenitor cells that appear in the fibrovascular response replacing the organizing hematoma. Up to this point, the incorporation process is similar for cortical and cancellous grafts, but subsequent events differ for these two types of bony tissue.

The second phase of events associated with fresh autogenous cancellous graft material is a rapid revascularization in which invading blood vessels are accompanied by differentiated cell populations capable of osteoblastic and osteoclastic activity. Cancellous grafts first undergo deposition of new bone on the surface of dead or dying trabecula and subsequently experience osteoclastic activity with resorption of pre-existing donor mineral and matrix. Eventually, the ongoing process of formation and resorption leads to nearly complete remodeling of the original graft material and replacement by host-derived bone.

Fresh autogenous cortical tissues also revascularize, but at a slower rate than cancellous tissues do. In general, the pattern of blood vessel ingrowth follows pre-existing haversian canals and begins in the more peripheral locations directly in contact with the host bed. Resorption activity predominates initially, causing loss of dead bone, widening of the haversian canals, and a general increase in porosity. The subsequent stage of "creeping substitution" involves deposition of new bone and reconstitution of bone mass, although the remodeling process rarely affects more than half of the original graft. Nonetheless, the incorporation process is sufficient to ensure the structural integrity of the graft and its ability to withstand physiologic stresses over indefinite periods of time. Compared with incorporation of cancellous bone, cortical bone incorporation is slower, is characterized by resorption activity prior to new bone deposition, and is less complete in terms of the extent of bone eventually remodeled.[7]

It should be kept in mind that virtually all the resources required for graft incorporation emanate from the host bed; consequently, factors that adversely influence the recipient site will also interfere with the normal sequence of bone graft repair. Radiation therapy, for example, results in soft-tissue scarring that is incompatible with the normal revascularization required for optimal graft incorporation. Many chemotherapeutic agents negatively influence cell metabolism, cell division, or both, and this systemic effect includes osteoprogenitor cells as well as differentiated osteoblastic and osteoclastic populations in addition to neoplastic cells.[37] Infection in its more aggressive form is accompanied by tissue necrosis, and this circumstance also interferes with normal revascularization and recruitment of appropriate cell populations required for bone graft repair.

The exception to dependence on host-bed characteristics for graft incorporation is the revascularized free tissue transplant in which bone remains biologically viable at its site of implantation and needs only to repair at its osteosynthesis sites.[67] This is, in theory, accomplished by a process analogous to fracture repair rather than graft incorporation, and the approach has been addressed more fully in a previous chapter.

Allografts

Histologic aspects of allograft incorporation vary with the magnitude of genetic disparity between donor and recipient and with the preservation techniques applied.[14, 20, 41, 42] In general, allografts evoke a more intense inflammatory response, undergo more resorption activity, and repair more slowly than autografts. Nonetheless, grafts between closely matched donor-recipient pairs or bones subjected to a preservation technique such as deep-freezing or freeze-drying may proceed to very satisfactory incorporation, albeit at a slower rate.[44]

Initial events following allograft implantation are similar to those observed with autografts. The bone is surrounded by a hematoma and evokes an inflammatory cellular infiltrate. Marked genetic disparity in the absence of graft preservation results in an intense cellular reaction that may lead to a chronic inflammatory response characterized by mononuclear cells and fibrosis with little or no new bone formation and eventual resorption of the implant. Although it is difficult to monitor bone allograft "rejection" precisely, this type of histologic response must approximate the biologic consequences of an immunologically mediated rejection

phenomenon in bone. The other end of the spectrum in allograft incorporation is virtually indistinguishable from normal autograft repair—that is, an orderly sequence of revascularization, new-bone accretion, and resorption occur at appropriate rates, and the allograft functions biologically and biochemically as autogenous tissue.[7]

Burchardt and his colleagues have classified the histologic patterns of graft repair into three groups, and these in turn reflect three distinct types of repair observed clinically.[7, 67] Type 1 repair exemplifies the events seen with more fresh autografts; type 2 repair includes a greater incidence of nonunion or delayed union and is characterized by predomination of resorption over new-bone formation; and type 3 repair is characterized by high rates of non-union, fatigue fractures, and intense resorption activity. It is tempting to classify all observed deviations from type 1 activity as reflections of immunologic differences, especially when genetic disparities exist between donor and recipient. Indeed, the role of histocompatibility-related responses is inescapable. In Burchardt's studies of the canine fibula, however, autografts demonstrated type 2 repair approximately 15% of the time, and the behavior of 20% of freeze-dried allografts was indistinguishable from that of autografts in terms of histology and clinical course. Fresh allografts, however, nearly always demonstrated a type 3 repair in these studies.

BIOMECHANICAL CONSIDERATIONS

Biomechanical correlates of the histologic pattern clearly exist. Grafts begin with mechanical properties identical with those of normal bone, except as altered by preservation techniques such as freeze-drying; however, ensuing resorption activity leads to increased porosity that in turn results in decreased structural integrity. As new bone formation builds, the resorption becomes compensated for, and the mechanical strength of the graft returns toward normal. In the canine fibula model, this biomechanical sequence takes 1 to 2 years, and in the human the process appears to take approximately twice as long.[7, 8] It is important to recognize the normal physiologic loss of strength and subsequent repair pattern so that the nature of the surgical procedure and its goals are compatible with stresses on the bone that can be tolerated. The choice of preservation method also must be consistent with mechanical goals, as will be explained further on in more detail.

IMMUNOLOGIC CONSIDERATIONS

The nature and significance of immune responses associated with osteochondral allografts have been pursued experimentally for over 30 years by methods reflecting the current state of transplantation immunology in general.[14, 22, 24] Consequently, attempts at evaluating allograft immunogenicity were initially based on histologic descriptions of the evoked cellular response[2, 15, 17, 44] and later progressed through the application of techniques based on skin graft rejection patterns[6, 13] and lymph node responses.[16, 17] More recently, in vitro and in vivo assays of humoral and cell-mediated responses have been applied.[4, 22, 24, 35, 45]

Evaluation of immune responses evoked by osteochondral allografts requires attention to variables in the animal models, assay techniques, and antigens chosen as targets. There are clearly species-related idiosyncrasies in immune responsiveness as well as differences observed by various routes of sensitization, timing, dosage, and graft preparation. The potential sources of bone graft immunogenicity can include matrix components and collagen,[31, 63, 68] but cell-surface antigens are assumed to predominate. The cell types present in bone are heterogeneous, but, for the most part, all cell populations represented carry consistent surface markers related to the major histocompatibility complex. Assays for evoked responses are numerous and are influenced by the nature and concentration of antigen, effector cell representation, timing, and numerous other method-related variables.

Despite this heterogeneity, there is surprising uniformity in the conclusions regarding immunogenicity of fresh and preserved bone allografts; that is, fresh allografts are highly sensitizing, deep-freezing considerably reduces observed responses, and freeze-drying decreases responses to lower and often immeasurable levels (Fig. 23–1). The significance of these observed responses, however, remains uncertain despite considerable data from a variety of animal

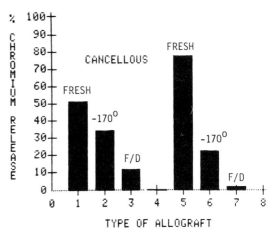

Figure 23–1. Immune responses to fresh, frozen (−170°C), and freeze-dried (F/D) cancellous bone in a rabbit model using a chromium-release microcytotoxicity assay for cell-mediated lymphocytotoxicity (columns 1–3) and humoral antibody (columns 5–7).

models and even preliminary observations in humans.[36, 46, 56]

BONE BANK CONSIDERATIONS

Clinical application of bone allografts requires that a safe and effective banking approach be implemented. Safety refers to avoidance of disease transfer from donor to recipient and efficacy reflects predictable maintenance of biologic and biomechanical properties compatible with intended use of the graft. The current state of knowledge pertaining to bone graft biology and to the effects of various preservation techniques is insufficient to allow rigorous definition of approaches to banking; however, sufficient direction can be gleaned from available information to establish flexible, yet meaningful, guidelines. The American Association of Tissue Banks has provided a forum for most of the peer-group discussions leading to these recommendations, which are summarized here in terms of approaches to donor selection, tissue recovery, preservation, and long-term storage.[32] These issues have been addressed in more detail elsewhere.[21, 33, 61]

Donor Selection

In the United States, a person 18 years of age or older may, by an antemortem statement, provide authorization of postmortem donation of tissues and organs for either research or transplantation. Following death, and in the absence of an antemortem statement by the individual, the responsible next-of-kin may provide permission for tissue and organ donation. The laws that facilitate this process are known collectively as the Uniform Anatomic Gift Act and have been adopted by all 50 states since being drafted by the Commissioners on Uniform State Laws in 1968. The Gift Act underscores the need for appropriate authorization for removal of tissues and organs following death and at the same time establishes a simple, rapid vehicle for documenting permission while protecting individuals acting in good faith from any subsequent liability.[19]

Donor selection requires criteria by which potentially harmful transmittable diseases can be excluded. This is accomplished for both living and deceased donors through review of the medical history and by appropriate laboratory tests. When cadavers are used as donors, autopsies also may provide valuable information. Disorders in the potential bone donor to be avoided include infections, malignancies, venereal diseases, diffuse collagen disorders, the presence of toxic substances in toxic amounts, and significant diseases of unknown etiology. The rationale for these contraindications has been provided elsewhere, but the intent is to prevent transmission of potentially harmful illness to the recipient. It must be remembered that some of these concerns can be minimized by the method of tissue recovery and the manner in which grafts are subsequently processed. For example, one may apply methods of secondary sterilization to contaminated tissues to eliminate bacterial pathogens.

Tissue Recovery

Tissue recovery may be accomplished in an aseptic fashion consistent with routine operating room technique or in a clean but not sterile environment in which a method of secondary sterilization is required. In the case of sterile tissue recovery, one must rely on the donor-screening process and subsequent bacteriologic cultures to confirm the clinical impression of sterility and the fact that it was present at the time tissues were placed in storage containers. The author personally favors this approach, but it is clear

that several other acceptable methods of sterilization also can be applied. These include high doses of ionizing radiation (in the 1.5- to 5-megarad range),[5] the use of ethylene oxide,[55] and the chemosterilization approach recommended by Urist.[64] In such cases, the methods must be demonstrated effective by appropriate laboratory tests, the absence of any lingering toxic substances must be confirmed, and any changes in the biologic or biochemical function of the graft caused by the sterilization technique must be recognized and taken into account when the material is used clinically.

Regardless of sterile or nonsterile tissue recovery, virtually any bone or joint can be removed from a cadaver donor in anticipation of its intended clinical applications. This is generally accomplished through longitudinal incisions down extremities leading to subperiosteal dissection and followed by either disarticulation or transection of the bone at any desired level. Sufficient capsule and ligament are retained at articular locations to aid in reconstruction at the time of implantation. Bones may be saved as intact specimens for replacement of segmental defects or cut and shaped to reflect potential applications, including filling for cystic defects, onlay plates, wafers, blocks, and numerous other configurations. Each graft should be cultured, and the defects in the cadaver should be reconstructed (e.g., with wooden dowels) so that deformity is minimized.

Preservation Techniques

Long-term preservation of bone can be achieved by several means, especially because cell viability is not required for biologic functions such as osteoconduction and osteoinduction. The most popular approaches to storage include deep-freezing,[21, 33, 61] freeze-drying,[5] and the AAA technique of chemical extraction, sterilization, and demineralization developed by Urist.[64] Each method has advantages and disadvantages that must be recognized so that appropriate clinical application is ensured (Fig. 23–2). For example, freezing alone is simple and does not interfere with the biochemical integrity of bone. It is also compatible with cryopreservation of articular cartilage. Disadvantages of freezing include the need to maintain specimens in a frozen state until

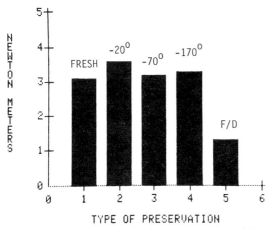

Figure 23–2. The maximum load in compression to failure of rat tail vertebrae was not influenced by freezing ($-20°$C, $-70°$C or $-170°$C) but was significantly less in fresh specimens following freeze-drying.

used, preferably around $-80°$ C, and this makes shipment between transplant centers more problematic than with other methods of preservation. In contrast, freeze-drying permits storage in vacuum-sealed containers at room temperature for indefinite periods of time so that shipping is easy. Structural changes, however, are created in the material, making its application in segmental defects more dependent on internal fixation than frozen grafts,[53] and preservation of cartilage is not possible. Changes in the biomechanical parameters do not interfere with use of fragments in filling cystic defects. AAA-prepared bone is thought to present optimal osteogenic stimulation to the host bed, and this freeze-dried preparation is easy to store, although it is also devoid of strength and incompatible with articular cartilage preservation.

Cartilage Preservation

Cartilage preservation requires attention to chondrocyte viability so that the specialized articular matrix is maintained. To accomplish this, one must expose cartilage to a cryoprotectant agent, such as dimethyl sulfoxide (DMSO), prior to freezing. At present, immersion of articular cartilage in 10% DMSO followed by an uncontrolled freeze probably results in 30% to 40% chondrocyte viability.[62] Under more controlled circumstances in the laboratory, cell viability can be greatly enhanced. However, it is not clear what percentage of cells is required to main-

tain the matrix or what tests of cell viability are most appropriate for predicting retention of "functional" properties.

Other Issues

The issues of storage, distribution, and record keeping are discussed elsewhere,[5, 33] but their importance is not meant to be minimized by lack of attention in this discussion.

CLINICAL CONSIDERATIONS

Clinical applications of osseous and osteochondral allografts have been described in relation to traumatic, degenerative, congenital, and neoplastic disorders.[34] In general, success rates have been comparable with those achieved with fresh autografts when alternative choices were feasible (e.g., filling cystic defects) and have been considered satisfactory in cases in which acceptable results could not be obtained with autogenous tissues because of size, shape, or quantity constraints (e.g., massive segmental loss). Indeed, it must be remembered that the efficacy of allografts is properly compared with that of autografts or with results consistent with the particular host or bed characteristics, and that these control circumstances do not necessarily represent completely favorable or unqualified successes.

Applications

One of the most common and well-documented clinical applications of allogeneic bone is the filling of benign cystic defects (Fig. 23–3), especially unicameral bone cysts. Spence and coworkers reviewed 177 cases treated by curettage and freeze-dried cancellous allografts and 144 cases treated by freeze-dried cortical allografts.[59, 60] No significant differences were observed between these cases and cases in which similar treatment with fresh autogenous bone was used. Healing of these lesions was most dependent on thoroughness of curettage and the activity status of the cyst. Latent cysts completely curetted and packed with freeze-dried cortical bone healed in approximately 90% of cases. Similarly, anterior cervical fusions accomplished with either autograft or preserved allograft developed radiographic ar-

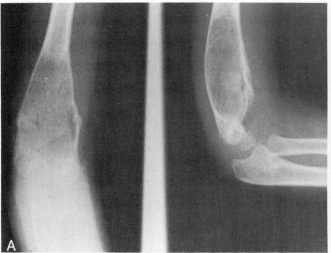

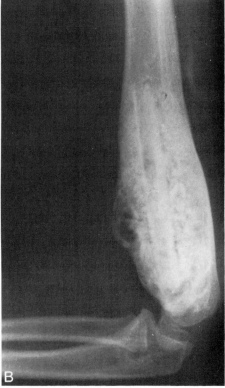

Figure 23–3. A benign cystic defect in the distal humerus of a 7-year-old boy caused by fibrous dysplasia; preoperatively (*A*) and 23 months following curettage and grafting with F/D cortical bone chips and a fibular strut (*B*).

throdesis in 90% of cases reviewed by Schneider and colleagues, regardless of the type of graft material inserted.[57] Allografts used as onlays for fracture repair (Fig. 23–4),[39] for small wedges and blocks used with midface advancements,[23] for repair of periodontal defects,[58] and for mandibular reconstructions[43] have provided predictable success rates, comparable with those obtained with autogenous alternatives.

Massive Allografts

Perhaps the most exciting and certainly the most challenging applications of massive segmental allografts have been in the reconstruction of large traumatic skeletal deficits, especially those encountered during the course of limb-sparing tumor resections (Fig. 23–5). The pioneering efforts of Parrish[52] have been most notably expanded by Mankin at the Massachusetts General Hospital,[48–50] by Gross at the University of Toronto,[40] and by Murray[51] in an on-going series at the M.D. Anderson Hospital and Tumor Institute.

Mankin has accomplished and reviewed his experience with over 200 massive frozen bone and cartilage allografts performed since

1971.[48–50] Most cases in his series involved reconstruction following tumor resection, but traumatic deficits can be treated by a similar approach with comparable results, provided there is an appropriate soft-tissue bed. From both an anatomic and technical point of view, two types of grafts were implanted: (1) osteoarticular, including a segment of bone with a cartilage surface, and (2) intercalary, in which no articular tissue was involved. Osteoarticular grafts required attention to cryopreservation of the cartilage as well as reconstruction of periarticular ligaments and capsule. Most osteoarticular segments were used to reconstruct the distal femur, proximal tibia, and proximal humerus, but virtually any anatomic location could be similarly approached. A major limiting factor with this technique is the need to mate joint surfaces congruently. These considerations do not exist for intercalary replacements.

Several trends have been supported by Mankin's experience and by that of others using a similar approach with massive allografts. First, the basic concept is feasible if careful attention is paid to banking principles and if patient selection is appropriate.

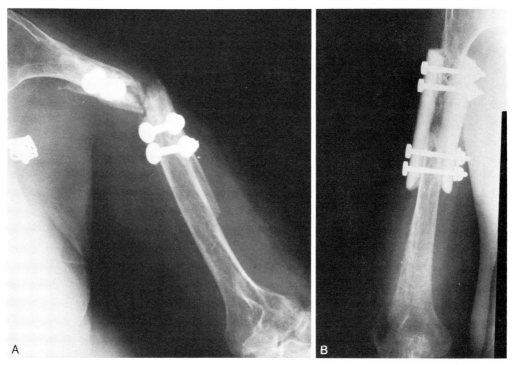

Figure 23–4. A fractured humerus in a 63-year-old woman was unsuccessfully treated by open reduction and fixation, first with a plate and screws and subsequently by autogenous cortical plates (*A*). Two years after the application of freeze-dried cortical allografts the bone is united (*B*).

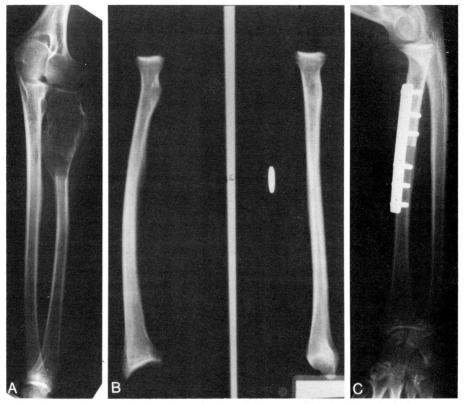

Figure 23–5. A unicameral bone cyst in the proximal radius of a 15-year-old male after multiple fractures (*A*). A frozen allograft (*B*), shown with a nickel as a reference marker, was used to replace the postresection deficit (*C*).

This latter point emphasizes the need for satisfactory vascularity and an uncontaminated soft-tissue bed. Both radiation therapy and systemic chemotherapy have adverse effects on the clinical course of allograft incorporation. Satisfactory results, either good or excellent by Mankin's criteria, occurred in 70% to 80% of cases, and the quality of results stabilized by 2 years following implantation and held up during 8 to 10 years of observation.[49] Three graft-related complications were identified, all of which became apparent within the first 2 years of follow-up: nonunion at the osteosynthesis site, fracture of the graft, and deep-wound infection.[47] The incidence of each of these complications was between 10% and 15%. Most non-unions could be salvaged by replacement of internal fixation or supplementation with autograft or both, and none of these techniques ever had a poor result. Fractures through the allograft could similarly be retrieved as satisfactory in over half of the cases in which this problem arose. In contrast, deep-wound infection usually meant failure. The apparently high incidence of infection may, in part, have represented a manifestation of "immunologic rejection" but was also correlated with compromised soft tissue and the magnitude of surgery required to first resect the neoplasm and to then reconstruct the deficit.

Additional long-term compromise of recipient function is likely to arise with further observation, especially with respect to articular surfaces. Further improvement in cryopreservation of cartilage is required. Nonetheless, results already achieved are sufficient to commend this approach. One must also keep in mind the reconstructive goals for which preserved osteochondral allografts are not well suited. They cannot, for example, include a predictably functional physis, a potential problem if longitudinal growth is required. Preserved allografts are also unsatisfactory when the soft-tissue bed is compromised by trauma, treatment (chemotherapy, radiation therapy), or infection, in which cases the use of vascularized bone grafts should be considered.

ADJUVANT THERAPY CONSIDERATIONS

In predicting clinical applications of bone allografts, various authors have considered and partially addressed three special influences on the reparative processes of bone: systemic chemotherapy, immunosuppression, and local irradiation. Each of these modalities has been evaluated with respect to physiologic turnover of intact bone, and the data derived permit speculation concerning the fate of bone grafts under similar therapeutic circumstances. Only limited information is available for direct assessment of the biologic consequences of these treatment approaches on bone allografts, all in animal models.

Chemotherapy

Most chemotherapeutic agents are antimetabolites, affecting normal biologic processes to the point at which either cell proliferation or homeostasis is disrupted. This impact is apparent on neoplastic cells but also influences active but normal cells, including those responsible for bone formation and resorption. The susceptibility of specific cell populations (osteoblasts versus osteoclasts) varies according to the type of drug used, and thus the measurable changes in bone also differ with respect to scope and magnitude. Normally, bone formation and resorption are coupled such that the net activity results in maintenance of bone mass. If both activities are increased or decreased similarly, there is no net change in mass (bone volume). If, however, this activity is uncoupled (normal resorption but suppressed formation, decreased resorption but an even greater reduction of formation activity, etc.) the net result will change bone mass in a predictable direction.[27, 28]

Both methotrexate and doxorubicin (Adriamycin) decrease bone formation rates by as much as 40% to 50%.[26, 30, 37] Osteoclastic activity also is diminished by methotrexate, but even more intensely by Adriamycin. This results in a substantial decrease in net bone volume during methotrexate treatment (markedly decreased formation with a lesser effect on resorption), but a less profound net change subsequent to Adriamycin chemotherapy (despite a greater influence on cellular metabolism). It would be reasonable to predict that bone allograft incorporation is adversely affected by systemic chemotherapy; indeed, this is supported by studies in a dog model by Burchardt and coworkers[11] and by limited experience in clinical situations.[38, 47]

Immunosuppression

Immunosuppression would be of theoretic value for bone allografts if histocompatibility differences caused immune responses with direct detrimental impact on biologic aspects of bony repair. As was discussed, there are clearly immune responses generated against antigens associated with bone allografts, but the biologic significance of these reactions remains unresolved.[3, 4, 10] Furthermore, the clinical application of traditional immuno-suppression for viable organ transplantation, with use of steroids and azathioprine, has not been justified in view of the morbidity and mortality associated with these drugs and because of the degree of success likely without this approach.

The introduction of cyclosporin-A, an immunosuppressant believed to cause selective inhibition of helper–T cell populations required to generate an effective allogeneic immune response, has been associated with less morbidity and enhanced efficacy. It will not be long before researchers evaluate this drug in appropriate animal models to assess its influence on vascularized bone allografts and on traditional nonvascularized bone. Although it has demonstrated only subtle biomechanical effects on the late remodeling normally associated with fracture repair in a rat model and has produced no detectable influence on early callus formation,[66] cyclosporin-A has extremely profound suppressive effects on both osteoblastic and osteoclastic activity.[25] These rates were slowed by up to 80% (synchronously), suggesting either that the drug affects both cell populations equally and profoundly or, more likely, that it produces an inhibition of the signal that activates bone turnover. If the latter is true, one could reasonably predict that bone allograft incorporation would not be enhanced, and would probably be inhibited, by cyclosporin-A. In children, there might also be a negative influence on normal skeletal growth. None of these hypotheses has been confirmed in humans; in fact, none has even been the subject of a reported investigation.

Irradiation

Radiation also is known to interfere with cellular metabolism, especially replication. Histomorphometric evaluation of intact bone suggests that both formation and resorption are impaired, in a coupled fashion, but that osteoclastic activity is re-established more quickly than formation of new bone.[28, 29] This causes a transient loss of bone mass. Because the repair of bone grafts depends on local host site–derived responses, both vascular radiation and cellular radiation are detrimental to graft incorporation. This has been observed in humans and in animal models with respect to both hard- and soft-tissue healing.[1, 47]

Thus, a variety of therapeutic modalities, both systemic and local in nature, may have adverse consequences on bone allograft biology. Preliminary studies in animal models and available clinical observations suggest that bone allografts will fare less well in patients receiving systemic chemotherapy and in cases in which bone is placed in an irradiated host bed. The influence of immunosuppression provides some theoretic advantages, but with cyclosporin-A these may be outweighed by direct suppression of normal homeostatic and reparative mechanisms.

SUMMARY

Bone and cartilage allografts represent satisfactory therapeutic alternatives in properly selected cases. Their appropriate application reflects a basic understanding of biologic, biomechanical, and, perhaps, immunologic considerations and a rational banking approach. Consequently, there is every reason to suspect that continued attention to these principles and improved understanding will increase the efficacy, indications, and frequency of osteochondral allografts in the future.

References

1. Ariyan S, Krizek TJ. Radiation effects, biological and surgical considerations, In Converse JM, ed. Reconstructive Plastic Surgery, 2nd ed, vol 1. Philadelphia, WB Saunders, 1977:531.
2. Bonfiglio M, Jeter WS, Smith CL. The immune concept: its relation to bone transplantation, Ann NY Acad Sci 59:417, 1955.
3. Bos GD, Goldberg VM, Powell AE, et al. The effects of histocompatibility matching on canine frozen bone allografts. J Bone Joint Surg 65A:89, 1983.
4. Bos GD, Goldberg VM, Zika JM, et al. Immune responses of rats to frozen bone allografts. J Bone Joint Surg 65A:239, 1983.
5. Bright RW, Friedlaender GE, Sell KW. Current concepts: tissue banking: the United States Navy Tissue Bank. Milit Med 142:503, 1977.

6. Brooks DB, Heiple KG, Herndon CH, Powell AE. Immunological factors in homogenous bone transplantation. IV. The effect of various methods of preparation and irradiation on antigenicity. J Bone Joint Surg 45A:1617, 1963.

7. Burchardt H. The biology of bone graft repair. Clin Orthop 174:28, 1983.

8. Burchardt H. Biology of cortical bone graft incorporation. In Friedlaender GE, Mankin HJ, Sell KW, eds. Osteochondral Allografts: Biology, Banking and Clinical Applications. Boston, Little, Brown, 1983:51.

9. Burchardt H, Enneking WF. Transplantation of bone. Surg Clin North Am 58:403, 1978.

10. Burchardt H, Glowczewskie FP, Enneking WF. Allogeneic segmental fibular transplants in azathioprine immunosuppressed dogs. J Bone Joint Surg 59A:881, 1977.

11. Burchardt H, Glowczewskie FP Jr, Enneking WF. The effect of adriamycin and methotrexate on the repair of segmental cortical autografts in dogs. J Bone Joint Surg 65A:103, 1983.

12. Burchardt H, Jones H, Glowczewskie FP, et al. Freeze-dried allogeneic segmental cortical-bone grafts in dogs. J Bone Joint Surg 60A:1082, 1978.

13. Burwell RG. Studies in the transplantation of bone. V. The capacity of fresh and treated homografts of bone to evoke transplantation immunity. J Bone Joint Surg 45B:386, 1983.

14. Burwell RG. The fate of bone grafts. In Apley AG, ed. Recent Advances in Orthopaedics. Baltimore, Williams & Wilkins, 1969:115.

15. Burwell, RG, Gowland G. Studies in the transplantation of bone. III. The immune responses to lymph nodes draining components of fresh homologous cancellous bone and homologous bone treated by different methods. J Bone Joint Surg 44B:131, 1962.

16. Burwell RG, Gowland G, Dexter F. Studies in the transplantation of bone. VI. Further observations concerning the antigenicity of homologous cortical and cancellous bone. J Bone Joint Surg 45B:597, 1963.

17. Chalmers J. Transplantation immunity in bone grafting. J Bone Joint Surg 41B:160, 1959.

18. Chase SW, Herndon CH. The fate of autogenous and homogenous bone grafts. J Bone Joint Surg 37A:809, 1955.

19. Curran WJ. The Uniform Anatomical Gift Act. N Engl J Med 280:36, 1969.

20. Curtiss PJ Jr, Chase SW, Herndon CH. Immunological factors in homogeneous bone transplantation: II. Histological studies. J Bone Joint Surg 38A:324, 1956.

21. Doppelt SH, Tomford WW, Lucas AD, Mankin HJ. Operational and financial aspects of a hospital bone bank. J Bone Joint Surg 63A:244, 1981.

22. Elves MW. Newer knowledge of the immunology of bone and cartilage. Clin Orthop 129:232, 1976.

23. Epker BN, Friedlaender GE, Wolford LM, West RA. The use of freeze-dried bone in mid third face advancement. Oral Surg 42:278, 1976.

24. Friedlaender GE. Immune responses to osteochondral allografts. Current knowledge and future directions. Clin Orthop 174:58, 1983.

25. Friedlaender GE. Unpublished observations.

26. Friedlaender GE, Baron R, Doganis AC, et al. Chronic effects of Adriamycin on bone volume in rats. Trans Orthop Res Soc 8:297, 1983.

27. Friedlaender GE, Baron R, Pelker RR. Effects of chemotherapy on bone. In Friedlaender GE, Mankin HJ,

Sell KW, eds. Osteochondral Allografts: Biology, Banking and Clinical Applications. Boston, Little, Brown, 1983:319.

28. Friedlaender GE, Baron R, Pelker RR, Doganis AC. The effects of chemotherapy and radiation therapy on physiologic bone turnover and fracture repair. In Hunt TK, Heppenstall RB, Pines E, Reeve DT, eds. Soft and Hard Tissue Repair: Biologic and Clinical Aspects. New York, Praeger, 1984.

29. Friedlaender GE, Doganis AC, Baron R, Kapp D. Histomorphometric changes in cancellous bone following palliative doses of radiation. Trans Orthop Res Soc 6:310, 1981.

30. Friedlaender GE, Doganis AC, Baron R, Kirkwood J. Histomorphometric changes in rat bones following chronic methotrexate chemotherapy. Trans Orthop Res Soc 7:98, 1982.

31. Friedlaender GE, Ladenbauer-Bellis I, Chrisman OD. Cartilage matrix components as antigenic agents in an osteoarthritis model. Transact Orthop Res Soc 5:170, 1980.

32. Friedlaender GE, Mankin HJ. Guidelines for the banking of musculoskeletal tissues. Am Assoc Tissue Banks Newsletter 4(suppl.):30, 1980.

33. Friedlaender GE, Mankin, HJ. Bone banking: current methods and suggested guidelines. AAOS Instruct Course Lect 30:36, 1981.

34. Friedlaender GE, Mankin HJ, Sell KW. Osteochondral Allografts: Biology, Banking and Clinical Applications. Boston, Little, Brown, 1983.

35. Friedlaender GE, Strong DM, Sell KW. Studies on the antigenicity of bone. I. Freeze-dried and deep-frozen bone allografts in rabbits. J Bone Joint Surg 58A:854, 1976.

36. Friedlaender GE, Strong DM, Sell KW. Studies on the antigenicity of bone. II. Donor specific anti-HLA antibodies in human recipients of freeze-dried bone allografts. J Bone Joint Surg 66A:107, 1984.

37. Friedlaender GE, Tross RB, Doganis AC, et al. Effects of chemotherapy on bone. I. Short-term methotrexate and doxorubicin (Adriamycin) treatment in a rat model. J Bone Joint Surg 66A:602, 1984.

38. Grant TT, Eilber FR, Johnson EE. Limb salvaging in osteosarcoma. Orthop Trans 5:427, 1981.

39. Gresham RB. The freeze-dried cortical bone homograft: a roentgenographic and histologic evaluation. Clin Orthop 37:194, 1964.

40. Gross AE, McKee NH, Pritzker KPH, Langer F. Reconstruction of skeletal deficits at the knee: a comprehensive osteochondral transplant program. Clin Orthop 174:96, 1983.

41. Heiple KG, Chase SW, Herndon CH. A comparative study of the healing process following different types of bone transplantation. J Bone Joint Surg 45A:1593, 1963.

42. Herndon CH, Chase SW. Experimental studies in the transplantation of whole joints. J Bone Joint Surg 43A:564, 1952.

43. Kelly JF, Friedlaender GE. Preprosthetic bone graft augmentation with allogeneic bone: a preliminary approach. J Oral Surg 35:268, 1977.

44. Kruez FP, Hyatt GW, Turner TC, Bassett AL. The preservation and clinical use of freeze-dried bone. J Bone Joint Surg 33A:863, 1951.

45. Langer F, Czitrom A, Pritzker KP, Gross AE. The immunogenicity of fresh and frozen allogeneic bone. J Bone Joint Surg 57A:216, 1975.

46. Lee EH, Langer F, Halloran P, et al. The immunology of osteochondral and massive allografts. Transact Orthop Res Soc 4:61, 1979.

47. Mankin HJ. Complications of allograft surgery. *In* Friedlaender GE, Mankin HJ, Sell KW, eds. Osteochondral Allografts: Biology, Banking and Clinical Applications. Boston, Little, Brown, 1983:259.
48. Mankin HJ, Doppelt SH, Sullivan TR, Tomford WW. Osteoarticular and intercalary allograft transplantation in the management of malignant tumors of bone. Cancer 50:613, 1982.
49. Mankin HJ, Doppelt SH, Tomford WW. Clinical experience with allograft implantation. Clin Orthop 174:69, 1983.
50. Mankin HJ, Fogelson FS, Trasher AZ, Jaffer F. Massive resection and allograft transplantation in the treatment of malignant bone tumors. N Engl J Med 294:1247, 1976.
51. Murray JA. Techniques of osteochondral allograft reconstruction following resection of skeletal neoplasms. *In* Friedlaender GE, Mankin HJ, Sell KW, eds. Osteochondral Allografts: Biology, Banking and Clinical Applications. Boston, Little, Brown, 1983:275.
52. Parrish FF. Allograft replacement of all or part of the end of a long bone following excision of a tumor: report of twenty-one cases. J Bone Joint Surg 55A:1, 1973.
53. Pelker RR, Friedlaender GE, Markham T. Biomechanical properties of preserved allografts. Clin Orthop 174:54, 1983.
54. Phemister DB. The fate of transplanted bone and regenerative power of its various constituents. Surg Gynecol Obstet 19:303, 1914.
55. Prolo DJ, Oklund SA. Sterilization of bone by chemicals. *In* Friedlaender GE, Mankin HJ, Sell KW, eds. Osteochondral Allografts: Biology, Banking and Clinical Applications. Boston, Little, Brown, 1983:233.
56. Rodrigo JJ, Fuller TC, Mankin HJ. Cytotoxic HL-A antibodies in patient with bone and cartilage allografts. Transact Orthop Res Soc 1:131, 1976.
57. Schneider JR, Bright RW. Anterior cervical fusion using preserved bone allografts. Transplant Proc 8(suppl. 1):73, 1976.
58. Sepe WW, Bowers GM, Lawrence JJ, et al. A clinical evaluation of freeze-dried bone allografts in periodontal osseous defects. Part II. J Periodontol 49:9, 1978.
59. Spence KF Jr, Bright RW, Fitzgerald SP, Sell KW. Solitary unicameral bone cyst: treated with freeze-dried crushed cortical bone allograft: a review of one hundred forty-four cases. J Bone Joint Surg 58A:636, 1976.
60. Spence KF, Sell KW, Brown RH. Solitary bone cyst: treatment with freeze-dried cancellous bone allograft. J Bone Joint Surg 51A:87, 1969.
61. Tomford WW, Friedlaender GE. 1983 bone banking procedures. Clin Orthop 174:15, 1983.
62. Tomford WW, Mankin HJ. Investigational approaches to articular cartilage preservation. Clin Orthop 174:22, 1983.
63. Trentham DE, Townes AS, Kang AH, David JR. Humoral and cellular sensitivity to collagen in type II collagen induced arthritis in rats. J Clin Invest 61:89, 1978.
64. Urist MR. Practical applications of basic research on bone graft physiology. AAOS Instruct Course Lect 25:1, 1976.
65. Urist MR, Silverman BG, Buring K, et al. The bone induction principle. Clin Orthop 53:243, 1967.
66. Warren SB, Friedlaender GE, Pelker RR, et al. The effects of cyslosporin-A on intact and fractured bone. Trans Orthop Res Soc 9:302, 1984.
67. Weiland AJ, Moore RJ, Daniel RK. Vascularized bone autografts: experience with 41 cases. Clin Orthop 174:87, 1983.
68. Yablon IG, Brandt KD, DeLellis RA. The antigenic determinants of articular cartilage: their role in the homograft rejection. Trans Orthop Res Soc 2:90, 1977.

Index

Note: Page numbers in *italics* refer to illustrations; page numbers followed by t refer to tables.